HANDBOOK

NOTICE

Medicine is an ever-changing science. As new research and clinical experience broaden our knowledge, changes in treatment and drug therapy are required. The authors and the publisher of this work have checked with sources believed to be reliable in their efforts to provide information that is complete and generally in accord with the standards accepted at the time of publication. However, in view of the possibility of human error or changes in medical sciences, neither the authors nor the publisher nor any other party who has been involved in the preparation or publication of this work warrants that the information contained herein is in every respect accurate or complete, and they disclaim all responsibility for any errors or omissions or for the results obtained from use of the information contained in this work. Readers are encouraged to confirm the information contained herein with other sources. For example and in particular, readers are advised to check the product information sheet included in the package of each drug they plan to administer to be certain that the information contained in this work is accurate and that changes have not been made in the recommended dose or in the contraindications for administration. This recommendation is of particular importance in connection with new or infrequently used drugs.

PEDIATRIC ANESTHESIA HANDBOOK

Editor:

Terrance A. Yemen, MD
Associate Professor of Anesthesia and Pediatrics
University of Virginia
Director of Pediatric Anesthesia
University of Virginia Health Sciences Center
Charlottesville, Virginia

McGraw-Hill
Medical Publishing Division

New York Chicago San Francisco Lisbon London Madrid Mexico City
Milan New Delhi San Juan Seoul Singapore Sydney Toronto

McGraw-Hill

*A Division of The **McGraw·Hill** Companies*

Pediatric Anesthesia Handbook

Copyright © 2002 by **The McGraw-Hill Companies, Inc.** All rights reserved. Printed in the United States of America. Except as permitted under the United States Copyright Act of 1976, no part of this publication may be reproduced or distributed in any form or by any means, or stored in a data base or retrieval system, without the prior written permission of the publisher.

1 2 3 4 5 6 7 8 9 0 DOCDOC 0 9 8 7 6 5 4 3 2

ISBN 0-07-158687-3

This book was set in Times Roman at Pine Tree Composition, Inc.
The editors were Martin Wonsiewicz, Kitty McCullough, and Nicky Panton.
The production supervisor was Lisa Mendez.
The cover designer was Eve Siegel.
The index was prepared by Coughlin Indexing Services, Inc.

R. R. Donnelley & Sons Company was the printer and binder.

This book is printed on acid-free paper.

Cataloging-in-Publication Data is on file for this book at the Library of Congress.

To my loving wife, Gerry, and our three sons, Cory, Ryan, and Sean, for the meaning they give my life.

To my parents for providing me the opportunities to grow.

To my Departmental Chairmen, past and present, for providing the time and support to succeed.

CONTENTS

Contributors — xi
Foreword — xvii
Preface — xix
Acknowledgments — xxi

CHAPTER 1 — 1
Risk and Outcome in Pediatric Anesthesia
Robert S. Holzman

CHAPTER 2 — 13
Ethical and Legal Issues in Pediatric Care
David B. Waisel

CHAPTER 3 — 26
Selecting the Suitable Pediatric Outpatient
Ramesh I. Patel / Raafat S. Hannallah

CHAPTER 4 — 35
Appropriate Laboratory and Radiologic Testing in Children
Ramesh I. Patel / Raafat S. Hannallah

CHAPTER 5 — 41
Preanesthetic Sedation for Pediatric Patients Lacking Intravenous Access
George D. Politis

CHAPTER 6 — 56
Providing for the Child, Parent, and Family in Difficult Situations
Barbara A. Castro / Frederic A. Berry

CHAPTER 7 — 80
The Child With Respiratory Problems
Jennifer E. O'Flaherty / Terrance A. Yemen

CHAPTER 8
The Child With Stridor
Andrew M. Woods / Terrance A. Yemen
107

CHAPTER 9
Perioperative Management of the Former Preterm Infant
Leila G. Welborn
130

CHAPTER 10
Management of the Child With a Difficult Airway
Barbara A. Castro / Frederic A. Berry
143

CHAPTER 11
The Child With Congenital Heart Disease
Victor C. Baum
167

CHAPTER 12
Dysrhythmias in the Pediatric Patient
Denise Joffe
179

CHAPTER 13
Anesthetic Considerations for the Child With Multiple Trauma
Aisling Conran / Madelyn Kahana
196

CHAPTER 14
Management of the Child With Thermal Injury
Tracy Koogler
206

CHAPTER 15
The Child With Cancer
Joseph Rossi
219

CHAPTER 16
The Child With Neurosurgical Problems
Frank Mazzeo / Bruno Bissonnette
261

CHAPTER 17
Systemic Disorders Commonly Seen in Pediatric Anesthesia
Terrance A. Yemen / James Michael Jaegar
275

CHAPTER 18　300
The Child With Allergies
Robert S. Holzman

CHAPTER 19　312
The Four Hs: Hypertension, Hypotension, Hypoxia, and Hypercarbia
Josée Lavoie

CHAPTER 20　322
Blood Salvage and Conservation Techniques in Children
Josée Lavoie

CHAPTER 21　338
Malignant Hyperthermia in Pediatric Anesthesia
Barbara Brandom

CHAPTER 22　358
Monitoring and Discharge Criteria From the Recovery Room
Denise Joffe

CHAPTER 23　374
Problems With Pediatric Postoperative Pain Control
Joëlle F. Desparmet / Terrance A. Yemen

CHAPTER 24　389
The Anesthesiologist and Sedation: Who, What, When, Where, and Why?
Myron Yaster / Lynne G. Maxwell / Richard F. Kaplan

Index　*401*

CONTRIBUTORS

Victor C. Baum, MD
Associate Professor of Anesthesia and Pediatrics
Director of Cardiac Anesthesia
University of Virginia
Department of Anesthesiology
University of Virginia Medical Center
Charlottesville, Virginia
(CHAPTER 11)

Frederic A. Berry, MD
Department of Anesthesia and Pediatrics
University of Virginia Medical Center
Charlottesville, Virginia
(CHAPTERS 6 & 10)

Bruno Bissonnette, MD
Professor of Anesthesia
University of Toronto
Staff Anesthetist
Director of Neurological Anesthesia
Department of Anesthesia
The Hospital for Sick Children
Toronto, Ontario
Canada
(CHAPTER 16)

Barbara Brandom, MD
Professor of Anesthesiology
University of Pittsburgh School of Medicine
Attending Anesthesiologist
Department of Anesthesiology
Children's Hospital of Pittsburgh
Pittsburgh, Pennsylvania
(CHAPTER 21)

Barbara A. Castro, MD
Assistant Professor of Anesthesia and Pediatrics
Department of Anesthesia and Pediatrics
University of Virginia Medical Center
Charlottesville, Virginia
(CHAPTERS 6 & 10)

Aisling Conran, MD
Assistant Professor of Clinical Anesthesia
University of Chicago
Department of Anesthesia and Critical Care
University of Chicago Hospitals
Chicago, Illinois
(CHAPTER 13)

Joëlle F. Desparmet, MD
Associate Professor
McGill University
Staff Anesthesiologist
Department of Anesthesia
Director, Pain Management Center
Montreal Children's Hospital
Montreal, Quebec
Canada
(CHAPTER 23)

Raafat S. Hannallah, MD
Chairman of Anesthesiology
Professor of Anesthesiology and Pediatrics
Children's National Medical Center and
George Washington University Medical Center
Washington, DC
(CHAPTERS 3 & 4)

Robert S. Holzman, MD, FAAP
Senior Associate in Anesthesia
Chairman, Risk Management Committee
Department of Anesthesia
Children's Hospital
Associate Professor of Anesthesia
Harvard Medical School
Boston, Massachusetts
(CHAPTERS 1 & 18)

James Michael Jaegar, MD, Ph.D.
Associate Professor of Anesthesia and Neurological Surgery
University of Virginia
Department of Anesthesia and Pediatrics
University of Virginia Medical Center
Charlottesville, Virginia
(CHAPTER 17)

Denise Joffe, MD
Assistant Professor of Anesthesiology
Division of Anesthesiology
Children's National Medical Center and
George Washington University Medical Center
Washington, DC
(CHAPTERS 12 & 22)

Madelyn Kahana, MD
Professor of Clinical Anesthesia and Pediatrics
Director of the Pediatric Intensive Care Unit
Department of Anesthesia and Critical Care
University of Chicago Hospitals
Chicago, Illinois
(CHAPTER 13)

Richard F. Kaplan, MD
Associate Professor of Anesthesiology and Pediatrics
Children's National Medical Center and
George Washington University Medical Center
Washington, DC
(CHAPTER 24)

Tracy Koogler, MD
Assistant Professor
Department of Anesthesia and Critical Care
University of Chicago Hospitals
Chicago, Illinois
(CHAPTER 14)

Josée Lavoie, MD, FRCPC
Director, Cardiac Anesthesia
Assistant Professor in Anesthesia
McGill University Health Centre
Montreal Children's Hospital
Montreal, Quebec
Canada
(CHAPTERS 19 & 20)

Lynne G. Maxwell, MD
Associate Professor of Anesthesiology, Critical Care Medince, and
Pediatrics
Johns Hopkins Medical Institutions
Baltimore, Maryland
(CHAPTER 24)

Frank Mazzeo, MD
Clinical Fellow
Department of Anesthesia
The Hospital for Sick Children
University of Toronto
Toronto, Ontario
Canada
(CHAPTER 16)

Carol Brown Michael
Freelance Writer
Brookline, Massachusetts
(CHAPTER 6)

Jennifer E. O'Flaherty, MD, MPH
Assistant Professor of Anesthesia and Pediatrics
Department of Anesthesia and Pediatrics
University of Virginia Health Sciences Center
Charlottesville, Virginia
(CHAPTER 7)

Ramesh I. Patel, MD
Professor of Anesthesiology and Pediatrics
George Washington University
Attending Anesthesiologist
Department of Anesthesiology
Children's National Medical Center
Washington, DC
(CHAPTERS 3 & 4)

George D. Politis, MD
Assistant Professor of Anesthesiology
Department of Anesthesiology
Wake Forest University School of Medicine
Winston-Salem, North Carolina
(CHAPTER 5)

Joseph Rossi, MD
Attending Anesthesiologist
Columbia Children's Hospital
Columbia, Ohio
(CHAPTER 15)

David B. Waisel, MD
Assistant in Anesthesia
Children's Hospital
Instructor in Anesthesia
Harvard Medical School
Boston, Massachusetts
(CHAPTER 2)

Leila G. Welborn, MD
Professor of Anesthesiology and Pediatrics
George Washington University
Department of Anesthesiology
Children's National Medical Center
Washington, DC
(CHAPTER 9)

Andrew M. Woods, MD
Associate Professor of Anesthesia and Pediatrics
University of Virginia
Department of Anesthesia
University of Virginia Health Sciences Center
Charlottesville, Virginia
(CHAPTER 8)

Myron Yaster, MD
Associate Professor of Anesthesiology, Critical Care Medicine, and Pediatrics
Johns Hopkins Medical Institutions
Baltimore, Maryland
(CHAPTER 24)

Terrance A. Yemen, MD
Associate Professor of Anesthesia and Pediatrics
University of Virginia
Director of Pediatric Anesthesia
University of Virginia Health Sciences Center
Charlottesville, Virginia
(CHAPTERS 7, 8, 17 & 23)

FOREWORD

The frequent complaint about medical practice at any university is that it bears little relation to what goes on in the real world. Subspecialists practice in a rarified atmosphere in which they do not have to deal with the everyday problems of patients or the health care delivery system. But for the specialty of anesthesiology, and particularly at this time in North American health care delivery, the situation is far from "special." Frequently, as anesthesiologists, we do not enjoy such protection and we end up being the front-line troops in a variety of settings. Patients and their families, even if they are not more thoroughly informed by the media and the Internet, are more demanding of explanations that require thoughtful responses. Parents may well ask more questions about their child's anesthetic and surgery than they would about their own, so we end up providing education at a variety of levels and face a complex anesthetic challenge.

At various children's hospitals, anesthesia care is limited strictly to pediatrics. At the University of Virginia, our Children's Medical Center is integrated into the overall hospital and health care system per se. Despite a busy service that includes complex pediatric cardiac repairs and sophisticated craniofacial and spinal surgeries, our pediatric anesthesiologists take care of adults. We nonpediatric anesthesiologists take care of a number of healthy children with a variety of problems in addition to their sometimes confused or worried parents and grandparents. This nonsegregated practice means that no one is cloistered from the real world and we all come to understand its variety of problems. It is in this atmosphere of continuous interaction between all types of anesthesiologists that the contrasts and parallels between pediatric and adult anesthetic practice are more clearly defined. It is such an interactive milieu that gives rise to books such as *Anesthetic Management of the Difficult and Routine Pediatric Patient* by Fritz Berry (now out of print) and *Anesthesia for Genetic, Metabolic, & Dysmorphic Syndromes of Childhood* by Vic Baum and Jenny O'Flaherty. This book by Terry Yemen continues in that vein—trying to bring the lessons from the sophisticated practice of the Children's Medical Center to the anesthesiologist with a broader spectrum of practice. The important point to be made is that this is a task at which Terry is an expert because he does it every day with his colleagues and the residents at every level of experience. Many of the contributors have had to practice not only in the cloisters of the pediatric hospital but also in the more cosmopolitan world of the "general hospital." As a consequence, this book provides ways of dealing with the practical problems of pediatric anesthesia that confront all of us from time to time.

This book is for all of us who occasionally have to face the 2-year-old patient with the inspired peanut at 9:30 P.M. (with her parents) or the 6-year-old patient with an unknown dystrophy needing a pinning of a fractured elbow. I commend your attention to the insights, principles, and pearls in this book.

Carl Lynch III, MD, PhD
Robert M. Epstein Professor and Chair
University of Virginia
Department of Anesthesia
Charlottesville, Virginia

PREFACE

The practice of pediatric anesthesia requires sound knowledge of pediatric medicine and surgery and a solid base of anesthesia. I have practiced, and taught, pediatric anesthesia for more years than I want to admit—at least to my children. I have come to the conclusion that the everyday practice of this specialty is not unlike many others. The day-to-day problems in pediatric anesthesia are, in general, finite but with an infinite variety of presentations. It is not unlike the expression, "It's not that it's always something everyday, but rather it's the same thing everyday." The purpose of this *Pediatric Anesthesia Handbook* is to identify those pediatric anesthesia problems that occur day to day, week to week. These are the challenges that all pediatric anesthesiologists must master to practice successfully, regardless of their practice setting. These are the problems that my residents have repeatedly presented to me throughout my teaching years.

Most of these complications are addressed in standard pediatric textbooks, so why another book? My co-authors and I believe our approach will expand the breadth of discussion related to common pediatric problems. All of the contributors are practicing pediatric anesthesiologists. They have presented information in a practical and sound way, with each offering sage advice about a particular aspect. Their work is not only based on peer-reviewed literature but also tempered by their own interpretation and experience. Each has attempted to tell the reader, "This is not only what I have read, this is how I practice."

The field of pediatric anesthesia is diverse. There are many pediatric illnesses and problems that are not addressed in this text. Unfortunately, practicality requires that I select those issues that I believe are most important to the current practice of pediatric anesthesia. I certainly acknowledge that many other aspects could have been included but those would have distracted from the original intent. In addition, the contributors have addressed their topics primarily from a pediatric anesthesia as opposed to a surgical perspective. It is my belief that the anesthetic implications of a given surgery are important, but the problems addressed in this book occur without deference to the type of surgery. I have attempted to provide a handbook that residents and practitioners alike can carry in their coat pockets. It is not intended to be an encyclopedia of pediatric care. There are many excellent expansive textbooks on the market that can act as reference textbooks. In this instance, I hope the reader will find a useful handbook to carry throughout the day, with corners worn with use and the pages marked and highlighted from everyday reference.

Like all multiauthor works, the contributors have their own writing styles and teaching methods. Although considerable effort has been made to provide consistency in reaching the goals for this book, no apologizes are offered for the diversity in approach or the thoughts provided. I hope that one of the valued aspects of this handbook will be the variety and overlap of opinions offered on a select group of problems. This is truly representative of pediatric anesthesia; each aspect is unique but not separable from the whole.

Terrance A. Yemen, MD
May, 2002

ACKNOWLEDGMENTS

As editor, I acknowledge the expertise and support of my secretarial staff, especially Joanne Zabihaylo for all her hard work in organizing the original text and communication with my co-authors, and Patty Jenkins for putting all the pieces together, more than once, and making my deadlines her deadlines. I am extremely grateful to both.

PEDIATRIC ANESTHESIA
HANDBOOK

1 | Risk and Outcome in Pediatric Anesthesia

Robert S. Holzman, MD, FAAP

Reports of anesthetic risk are fraught with conceptual and methodologic inconsistencies: definitions of mortality (intraoperative? perioperative? within 24 h? 48 h? 1 month?) and morbidity, changing practices of anesthesia (e.g., routine endotracheal intubation rather than mask anesthesia), study design (prospective vs. retrospective, case review vs. preestablished and rigorously defined criteria), and method of acquisition of information (voluntary vs. compulsory). Studies have been published that are single versus multiinstitutional and based on claims data and outcome. Some investigators have limited themselves to deaths thought to have been the result of anesthesia, whereas others have included all cardiac arrests in the operating room and postanesthesia care unit (PACU). In one study, two deaths were included as "associated with anesthesia" wherein *no anesthetic had been given*; it was considered by the investigators that, *had* the anesthetist become involved and given an anesthetic after adequate resuscitation, a more favorable outcome would have ensued!

MORTALITY STUDIES OF ANESTHETIC RISK (Figure 1–1)

In the middle of the 20th century, deaths due to anesthesia were more numerous in the first decade of life than at any other time, with an incidence of cardiac arrest as high as 1:719 in infants younger than 1 year. One-fifth of the pediatric deaths occurred within the first week of life. Leaders in pediatric anesthesia at that time felt that most of those accidents were preventable.

Chopra et al. found a cardiac arrest incidence attributable to anesthesia of 1.3:10,000 (*n* = 113,074), with a mortality of 0.62:10,000.[1] Aubas et al. found a mortality rate due to cardiac arrest of 1.1:10,000.[2] The main causes were overdose with or without hypovolemia, hypoxemia, and multifactorial sudden cardiac arrest. At Vrije University Hospital, Amsterdam, perioperative death was related in part to anesthetic administration in 16 patients (2.5:10,000), exclusively to anesthetic administration in 2 patients (0.3:10,000), and to anesthesia and surgical factors in 14 patients (2.2:10,000).[3] In Western Australia, deaths due mainly to anesthetic factors are estimated to occur once in every 40,000 operations.[4] In Italy an overall mortality rate of 7.54:10,000 was reported, with a distribution of mortality inversely related to age.[5,6] Infants younger than 1 month (3.6% of the total) had twice the mortality of infants 2 to 6 months of age. Respiratory complications occurred with three times the frequency of cardiocirculatory complications (180:10,000 vs. 62:10,000). Typical respiratory complications included laryngospasm (65:10,000), bronchospasm (47:10,000), respiratory depression (44:10,000), and difficult or impossible intubation (20:10,000).

Recently, the Pediatric Perioperative Cardiac Arrest (POCA) Registry reported an anesthesia-related cardiac arrest incidence of 1.4:10,000, with a mortality rate of 26% (0.35:10,000). Medication-related (37%) and cardiovascular (32%) causes were most common, with halothane-related cardiovascular depression causing two-thirds of the medication-related cardiac arrests. Infants younger than 1 year accounted for 55% of all anesthesia-related car-

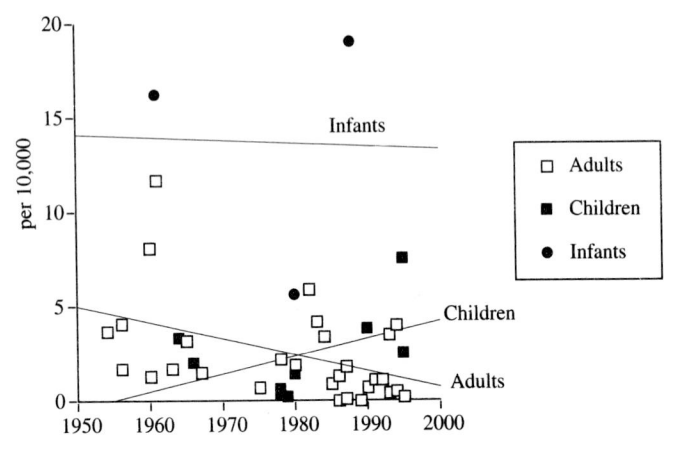

FIG. 1-1 Composite of studies in mortality related to anesthesia. Whereas adult data show a decrease in anesthetic-related mortality over the past 50 years, anesthetic mortality in infants has not changed, although there are few studies. For children, the data are even more disturbing because of the increase in mortality rate. Even if the 1995 study with a child mortality rate of 7.5:10,000 were eliminated as an outlier, the line of best fit for this group is parallel to that of infants.

diac arrests. Although severe underlying disease (Physical Status [PS] Categories 3–5) and emergency surgery were the factors most strongly associated with mortality after cardiac arrest, it is noteworthy that PS 1–2 patients accounted for one-third of the anesthesia-related cardiac arrests. Medication-related arrests were more common and cardiovascular etiologies were less common in PS 1–2 patients than in PS 3–5 patients.

Closed Claim and Single Institution Studies

The Committee on Professional Liability of the American Society of Anesthesiologists (ASA) found that 10% of 2400 closed claims reviewed since 1985 were for children 15 years or younger (Table 1-1).[7] Differences between children and adults were found in claims for inadequacy of ventilation (20% of pediatric closed claims vs. 9% of adult closed claims) and unexplained cardiovascular events (6% of pediatric closed claims vs. 1% of adult closed claims). Although not achieving statistical significance, trend differences also were seen in airway obstruction, inadvertent or premature extubation, and equipment problems. Cohen et al. in a large ($n = 29,220$) single-institution survey found that infants younger than 1 month had the highest rate of adverse events intraoperatively and in the recovery room, with the main problem related to the respiratory and cardiovascular systems.[8] In children older than 5 years, postoperative nausea and vomiting were very frequent, with about one-third of the children experiencing this problem. When all events were considered (major and minor), there was a risk of an adverse event in 35% of the pediatric cases versus 17% for adults. The Australian Incident Monitoring Study showed a similar pattern.[9] Of the first 2000 incidents reported, 90% involved adults, 7% involved children, and 3% involved infants. Healthy children accounted for a greater proportion of adverse events in the pediatric group than did healthy adults in the

TABLE 1–1 Risks of Pediatric Anesthesia

Damaging events	Pediatric (n)	%	Adults(n)	%	p
Total no. of patients	238		1953		
Inadequate ventilation	47	20	179	9	<0.01
Esophageal intubation	13	5	110	6	NS
Airway obstruction	11	5*	40	2*	NS
Difficult intubation	9	4	125	6	NS
Inadvertent extubation	8	3*	16	1*	NS
Premature extubation	8	3*	24	1*	NS
Aspiration	5	2	33	2	NS
Endobronchial intubtion	2	1	13	1	NS
Bronchospasm	0	0	40	2	NS
Inadequate F_{IO_2}	0	0	7	0	NS
Unexplained cardiovascular	14	6	27	1	< 0.01
Inadequate/inappropriate fluid therapy	9	4*	26	1*	NS
Excessive blood loss	2	1	18	1	NS
Air embolism	2	1	11	1	NS
Electrolyte imbalance	2	1	5	0	NS
Inadvertent intravascular injection	1	0	1	0	NS
Wrong blood	0	0	13	1	NS
Other cardiovascular event	0	0	1	0	NS
Equipment problem	30	13*	189	10*	NS
Wrong drug/dose	7	3	68	3	NS
Convulsion	5	2	35	2	NS

F_{IO_2}, fraction of inspired oxygen; NS, not significant.
*Trend difference, but not statistically significant.
Source: Morray JP, Geiduschek JM, Caplan RA, et al: A comparison of Pediatric and Adult Anesthesia Closed Malpractice Claims. *Anesthesiology* 78:461, 1993.

adult group. Children comprised 10% of the total claims in the Australian and ASA Closed Claims studies. In both studies, incidents involving the respiratory and breathing circuit systems accounted for nearly half of the problems. The mortality rate was greater in pediatric claims, and anesthetic care was judged inadequate more often in comparison with adult claims. Bradycardia frequently was a sentinel sign of inadequate ventilation. Claims involving children 6 months or younger accounted for more claims than any other age group. There were also more ASA PS 1 patients but fewer PS 2 and 3 patients than in adult claims.

COMPLICATIONS DURING ANESTHESIA

Bronchospasm, laryngospasm, and aspiration are said to occur twice as much in children as in adults and in even greater proportion in relation to certain preoperative conditions, type of surgery, and use of endotracheal intubation. Milross et al. found the incidence of gastroesophageal reflux in children to be 2.5%, without progression to an adverse respiratory event.[10] Bradycardia, traditionally a heralding sign of catastrophe, has, in the first year of life, been found to be twice that of children in the third year and almost 10-fold higher than in 4 year olds.[11] Preoperative disease or specific type of surgery, dose of inhalation agent, and hypoxemia were the most common etiologies of bradycardia, and significant morbidity included hypotension, asystole or ventricular fibrillation, with death in 8%.

DOES IT MATTER WHO ADMINISTERS THE ANESTHETIC?

Keenan et al. retrospectively compared anesthetics and cardiac arrests in patients 1 year or younger during a 7-year period in a large university hospital.[12] In each case, it was determined whether a pediatric anesthesiologist (those with pediatric fellowship training or the equivalent) was in attendance and whether a cardiac arrest due to anesthesia occurred. No anesthesia-related cardiac arrests occurred in the pediatric anesthesiologist group; four anesthetic cardiac arrests occurred in the nonpediatric anesthesiologist group (19.7 per 10,000 anesthetics, $p = 0.048$). The inhalation anesthetic drug was judged to be the immediate cause of arrest in each case; hypoxemia was not judged to be a factor in the four cases. Bradycardia was less than half as likely when the supervising anesthesiologist was a member of the Pediatric Anesthesia Service.[11] In an accompanying editorial, Morray underscored the controversial implication of the article by introducing the notion of a pediatric anesthesia subspecialty care of children.[13] It has been suggested more bluntly that those who don't care for children regularly shouldn't care for them at all.[14] Although the validity of this suggestion remains uncertain, as performance-based practice evolves, outcome-based scrutiny with practitioner profiles may be a logical result.

Clearly a delicate area because of the implications of exclusivity, the studies cited above suggest that there are distinctly greater risks for pediatric patients younger than a certain age, although that age is not well defined. Our anesthesia colleagues in the United Kingdom have taken steps to develop guidelines for defining pediatric cases appropriate for the "district hospital" as distinct from the "specialist hospital" including experience-based criteria for pediatric anesthetists.[15] These criteria have been met with guarded enthusiasm on both sides of the debate in the United Kingdom.[16–18]

Does experience, aside from training, lower the complication rate of pediatric anesthesia? Auroy et al. asked this question in France, and in a self-report survey found a significantly higher incidence of complications in groups that performed 1–100 ($7.0 \pm 24.8:1,000$ anesthetics) and 100–200 pediatric anesthetics ($2.8 \pm 10.1:1,000$ anesthetics) than in the group that administered more than 200 pediatric anesthetics per year ($1.3 \pm 4.3:1,000$ anesthetics).[19] Guidelines suggesting competency by a minimum number of pediatric anesthetics in various age categories annually have been proposed in the United Kingdom.[15] In the meantime, guidelines for the pediatric perioperative anesthesia *environment* (excluding specific training or experience recommendations for members of the anesthesia care team) have been published by the Section on Anesthesiology of the American Academy of Pediatrics.[20]

ARE THERE SAFER ANESTHETIC AGENTS AND TECHNIQUES?

Although halothane remains the historical standard against which all other inhalation agents are judged in pediatric anesthesia, sevoflurane has been embraced enthusiastically in the pediatric anesthesia community because of its rapidity of induction, ease of acceptance by patients, and the continued advantages of the ether anesthetics.[21-25] There are some suggestions that, as a nonirritating inhalation agent accepted with at least the same rate as halothane,[26] vital signs may be more stable during induction with sevoflurane[27] and its use during induction may preserve myocardial function better than halothane.[28]

Regional anesthesia is incorporated more than ever before in pediatric anesthesia. A rare choice as the sole anesthetic for surgery, regional techniques are most often combined with a general anesthetic and primarily serve to provide excellent perioperative analgesia.[29] Although recovery of pulmonary function may not differ between patients treated with neuraxially delivered versus parentally delivered opioids, the quality of analgesia has been found to be better.[30] It appears to offer an excellent alternative to general anesthesia for preterm or former preterm babies with histories of apnea and bradycardia and immaturity of ventilatory drive.[31-33] Because intravenous injection of local anesthetic occurred in 9% of medication-related cardiac arrests in the POCA study, local anesthetics with less myocardial toxicity such as ropivacaine or an altered ratio of enantiomeric to bupivacaine may enhance patient safety in the future.

PEDIATRIC ANESTHETIC RISK AND COEXISTING CONDITIONS

Upper Respiratory Tract Infections

Most anesthesiologists are wary of upper respiratory infections (URIs) in surgical candidates. Patients with symptoms of URI have a greater incidence of decreased SpO2 (<95%) after anesthetic induction. Even with uncomplicated URI symptoms, symptomatic patients had increased risks for the development of mild hypoxemia during anesthesia.[34] Although there was no increase in *major* desaturation events (SpO2 ≤ 85% for ≥30 s), *minor* desaturation events (SpO2 ≤ 95% for ≥60 s) were increased in patients with URI.

The incidence of hypoxemia (SpO2 < 93%) is greater during the transfer from the operating room to the PACU in children with acute and recent URI and during recovery in the acute group compared with asymptomatic children.[35] In addition, children with URI are two to seven times more likely to experience respiratory-related adverse events during the intraoperative, PACU, and postoperative phases.[36] If a child had a URI and endotracheal anesthesia, the risk of a respiratory complication increased 11-fold (95% confidence intervals 6.8–18.1).

Congenital Heart Disease and Noncardiac Surgery

Special considerations for children with uncorrected, palliated, or corrected congenital heart disease include a propensity to cerebrovascular accidents, altered ventilatory control and mechanics, neurobehavioral consequences of the underlying disease, chronic elevation of endogenous catecholamine levels, and possible electrophysiologic abnormalities as a result of progression of the disease or previous surgical intervention. The post–cardiac transplant patient requires a sound understanding of the management of the denervated heart.[37] It is particularly important to remember that children will not always respond in an identical fashion as adults given the same presenting signs and it is risky to treat them the same way without specific knowledge about pediatric cardiac disease. Children demonstrate remarkable adaptability after surgical correction, however, and may recover significantly from an earlier, poorly functional cardiac status.

The child with complex congenital heart disease should have a summary referral letter from a cardiologist, including past corrective surgery, results of recent investigations, and specific recommendations for perioperative subacute bacterial endocarditis (SBE) prophylaxis and arrhythmia control. Even children with uncomplicated heart murmurs may be candidates for SBE prophylaxis. The latest guidelines from the American Heart Association clarify many previously nebulous areas such as tympanostomy, gastrointestinal or pulmonary endoscopy, transesophageal echocardiography, cardiac catheterization, and circumcision, all of which no longer require routine SBE prophylaxis.[38]

Masseter Muscle Spasm and Malignant Hyperthermia

Isolated masseter muscle spasm (MMS) after the administration of intravenous succinylcholine during volatile agent anesthetic induction in children may occur as frequently as 1 per 100 cases. In the past, clinicians had assumed that these patients were at imminent risk for developing malignant hyperthermia (MH) and therefore discontinued the anesthetic. However, failure of the masseter muscles to relax after succinylcholine is not uncommon in children.[39] Even if MMS is part of the clinical spectrum of MH, it has been suggested[40] that anesthesia can be continued in cases of isolated MMS when careful monitoring accompanies diagnostic evaluation for hypercarbia, metabolic acidosis, elevation of serum creatine kinase, and myoglobinuria. Moreover, it has been recognized that incomplete jaw relaxation is different from masseter muscle rigidity (MMR), and trismus is not uncommon in children after a halothane–succinylcholine sequence and should be considered a normal response. In contrast, MMR and trismus should continue, for the present, to be *possible* sentinel signs of malignant hyperthermia susceptibility until proven otherwise. Such proof might consist of further evaluation by in vitro contracture testing, which has a diagnostic sensitivity of 99% and a specificity of 94%.[41]

Preterm and Former Preterm Infants and Apnea

Former preterm infants are at risk for postoperative apnea after general anesthesia, leading some to advocate the putatively safer alternative of spinal anesthesia.[32,42] However, the use of spinal anesthesia may reduce, but not eliminate, the perioperative risk: supplementary anesthesia or airway control may become necessary to provide optimal operating conditions[43] or postoperative care.[44] That caution is required in administering adjuncts with spinal anesthesia was shown by Welborn when eight of nine infants (89%) who received spinal anesthesia and intraoperative sedation with ketamine developed prolonged apnea with bradycardia.[31] Two of the eight infants had no prior history of apnea.

Coté et al. combined the original data from eight prospective studies of former preterm infants undergoing inguinal herniorrhaphy under general anesthesia and concluded that no fewer than 5% of former preterms are at risk for apnea if their postconceptual age is 48 weeks with a gestational age of 35 weeks and no fewer than 1% for that same subset until postconceptual age is 56 weeks with gestational age of 32 weeks or postconceptual age is 54 weeks with gestational age of 35 weeks.[33] One significant cofactor for perioperative apnea is anemia; the use of intravenous caffeine base (10 mg/kg) appears to decrease the risk of apnea.

Neuromuscular Disease

Progressive muscle weakness due to myopathy, muscular dystrophy, or myotonia typically results in respiratory system dysfunction, scoliosis and cervical spinal changes, dysphagia, reflux, cardiomyopathy and cardiac conduction defects. In addition, some confusion has arisen over signs and symptoms during or after anesthesia that are similar to MH. Increases in body temperature, abdominal pain with dark urine after surgery, and perioperative courses resembling malignant hyperthermia have been seen in patients with Duchenne's muscular dystrophy (DMD), occasionally occurring years before the neuromuscular disease was diagnosed. Larach et al. reviewed pediatric (age < 18 years) cardiac arrests occurring within 24 h of anesthesia and found that 25 patients (92% male, median age 45 months) had arrested. *Before receiving a potent inhalational anesthetic (92%) and/or succinylcholine (72%), those patients were evaluated by the anesthesiologist as being healthy, with no personal or family history of myopathy.* Previously unrecognized DMD ($n = 8$) or unspecified myopathy ($n = 4$) was diagnosed in 12 (48%) patients.[45] Thus, an unusual course of anesthesia in male children or unexpected cardiac arrest after succinylcholine administration calls for further investigation.

DOES PATIENT PREPARATION HAVE A ROLE IN DECREASING RISK?

Ironically, in these times of "safer anesthesia," it has been questioned whether a preoperative clinic evaluation is even necessary for PS 1 or 2 patients.[46] Great reliance continues to be placed on the pediatrician for optimal preoperative preparation. Rather than viewing the pediatric anesthesiologist as inaccessible,[47] pediatricians must feel that their surgery and anesthesiology colleagues are readily accessible; likewise, anesthesiologists, through telephone consultations, preoperative clinics, and education programs, must be at the forefront of educating their medical colleagues about the special issues in pediatric anesthesia, including newer techniques and agents,[48] lest they be treated as mere technicians to whom medical clearance is being granted.[47] Various booklets are available from commercial vendors in addition to the ASA booklet *When Your Child Needs Anesthesia*.[49] An excellent guideline for pediatricians describing the evaluation and preparation of pediatric patients undergoing anesthesia has been published by the Section on Anesthesiology of the American Academy of Pediatrics. It details typical considerations for preoperative preparation that may be asked of the pediatrician or other primary health care provider.[50]

POSTANESTHESIA CARE

Anesthesia problems were found in 18% of more than 12,000 patients in the operating room and the PACU in one institution. After the introduction of pulse oximetry, rates of recovery room impact events (RRIEs; "an unanticipated, undesirable, possibly anesthesia-related effect that required intervention, was pertinent to PACU care, and did or could cause mortality or at least moderate morbidity") decreased, although a clear cause-and-effect relationship was not demonstrated. Indeed, when feedback was given to anesthesiologists during the study about the rate and type of complications encountered, there was no change in the rate of RRIEs. In an adult PACU study, an overall PACU complication rate of 23.7% was found, with an overall intraoperative complication rate of 5.1%. Nausea and vomiting (9.8%), the need for upper airway support (6.9%), and hypotension requiring treatment (2.7%) were the most frequently encountered PACU complications.[51] Cohen et al. noted that the profile of adverse events experienced by children in the PACU differed from that of adults, with children less likely to experience problems with arrhythmias or hypotension but much more likely to have problems related to the respiratory system. Overall, the rate of PACU complications was 13:10,000 for children and 5.9:10,000 for adults.

Because the "major" risks appear to have been reduced over the past decade principally through diligence in safety monitoring, the "minor" risks of anesthesia are an emerging area of interest. Selby et al. found a higher incidence of the minor sequelae of anesthesia in children than had previously been reported, with the three most common sequelae being nausea (48.1%), vomiting (35.0%), and sore throat (31.4%).[52] Perioperative nausea and vomiting are distressing and may make perioperative pain management more difficult and contribute to surgical morbidity because of the increasing tendency toward bleeding, particularly for head and neck procedures, or disruption of the surgical repair. It is a common perioperative problem, although perhaps less common at younger ages,[53] and it may be possible to anticipate perioperative difficulties based on female sex, previous history of postoperative sickness, longer duration of surgery, nonsmoking, and history of motion sickness.[54] Strategies for management include the administration of antiemetics, promotility drugs, avoidance of nitrous oxide, use of propofol, and avoidance of narcotics, or various combinations of the foregoing.[55-60]

The rapidity of recovery, which we not only favor as clinicians but also are pressured into because of the demand for rapid turnover and efficient operating room use, has some drawbacks. Surveys done after their children underwent ambulatory surgery showed that rapid recovery from anesthesia and quick discharge from the hospital were not key parental expectations.[61] For example, parents associated a rapid recovery with more pain, and they were justifiably concerned. In at least one report, 29% of children experienced severe or unbearable pain or experienced pain for all of the 24 h after surgery.[62] Although parents should be more fully informed of the advantages of rapid recovery and reassured that children can recover quickly and completely, we have yet to provide a longer-term option for perioperative patient comfort.

As the recovery phase is shifted more toward outpatient management, we can expect to see a redistribution of problem focus to the outpatient setting, with the parents as primary managers. For example, after adenoidectomy, Kokki et al. found that 83% of children had pain at home and 17% of them had moderate or severe pain on a four-point verbal rating scale; 80% of children used pain medication at home.[63] In another study, problematic behavioral changes postoperatively had an incidence of 47%. These behavior problems, not surprisingly, were most common in the 1.0 to 2.9 year olds and the incidence decreased from 46% on the day of the operation to 9% 4 weeks later. Predictors were age, mild pain at home after surgery, severe pain, and a prior bad experience, which adversely affected the attitude of the child toward doctors or nurses. Pain on the day of the operation predicted the occurrence of behavioral problems up to the fourth week, 2 to 4 weeks longer than the duration of pain itself.[64] In another study, 23% of children undergoing ambulatory tonsillectomy did not have adequate pain control at home, but only 7% of parents contacted a physician. The majority of the children experienced restless sleep (62%), behavior changes (75%), and difficulty taking oral fluids because of complaints of pain (56%).[65] Postoperative nausea and vomiting occurred in 13% of children in the former study and in 26% in the latter study. Predictors were emetic symptoms in the hospital, pain at home, age older than 5 years, and administration of postoperative opioid. Opioid given during anesthesia (fentanyl or alfentanil) did not increase the incidence. Emetic symptoms were most common after tonsillectomy (31%), with emetic symptoms in the hospital being the most significant predictor of nausea and vomiting at home.[66]

THE COST OF ANESTHETIC ACCIDENTS IN PEDIATRIC ANESTHESIA

In a provocative paper, Dexter and Tinker speculated whether it would be cost effective to eliminate adverse anesthetic outcomes from high-risk but not from low- or moderate-risk surgical operations.[67] Looking simply at the hospital costs, they concluded that, for low- and moderate-risk procedures (laparoscopic cholecystectomy, cesarean section, total hip replacement), improvements in the quality of anesthetic care would not significantly reduce costs and that improving the quality of perioperative care may be cost efficient for high-risk operations such as lung lobectomy, coronary artery bypass, and kidney transplant. This strategy may beg the issue in pediatric anesthesia, however, because of the relatively high rate of medication-related adverse events in healthy children undergoing routine procedures.[7,68,69] With the mortality rate greater in pediatric claims than in adult claims and anesthetic care judged less than appropriate more frequently, the distribution of payments to the plaintiff was different (median payment of $111,234 in pediatric claims vs. $90,000 in adult claims; Table 1-2).

RISK DISCLOSURE AND INFORMED CONSENT

Having reviewed the current landscape of morbidity and mortality in pediatric anesthesia, the generally verified increased risks, and the favorably changing profile, clinicians are left with the question: What do I tell the patient and parents? The answer is not at all clear. Litman et al. determined that 87% of parents wanted to know the chances of death as a result of anesthesia.[70] Mothers were more likely to want to hear all possible risks, whereas fathers were more likely to want to know only about those that were likely to occur. After discussions with an anesthesiologist, including the possibility of death as a result of anesthesia, 88% of parents stated that they wanted that information. Waisel and Truog pointed out that the explanation of the risks of anesthesia appear to be rooted in satisfying parental responsibility and understanding, and not necessarily in providing information for decision making or anxiety relief.[71] Anesthesiologists, therefore, should seek to satisfy individual parental needs as an integral part of the consent process.

TABLE 1–2 Payment in ASA Closed Claim Study: Pediatric Versus Adult Payment Data

	Pediatric	Adult	p
Median payment	$111,234.00	$90,000.00	< 0.05
Median payment by severity of injury			
Temporary	$9000.00	$11,000.00	NS
Permanent	$554,000.00	$120,000.00	< 0.01
Death	$88,000.00	$200,000.00	< 0.01

ASA, American Society of Anesthesiologists; NS, not significant.
Source: Morray JP, Geiduschek JM, Caplan RA, et al: A Comparison of Pediatric and Adult Anesthesia Closed Malpractice claims. *Anesthesiology* 78:461, 1993.

REFERENCES

1. Chopra V, Bovill JG, Spierdijk J: Accidents, near accidents and complications during anaesthesia. A retrospective analysis of a 10-year period in a teaching hospital. *Anaesthesia* 45:3, 1990.
2. Aubas S, Biboulet P, Daures JP, et al: [Incidence and etiology of cardiac arrest occurring during the peroperative period and in the recovery room. Apropos of 102,468 anesthesia cases]. *Ann Fr Anesth Reanim* 10:436, 1991.
3. de Lange JJ, Scheffer GJ, Zuurmond WW, et al: [Perioperative mortality and the role of anesthesiologic activity at the Vrije University Hospital in Amsterdam]. *Ned Tijdschr Geneeskd* 142:701, 1998.
4. Eagle CC, Davis NJ: Report of the Anaesthetic Mortality Committee of Western Australia 1990–1995. *Anaesth Int Care* 25:51, 1997.
5. Bonoli P, Grillone G, Fossa S, et al: [Complications of pediatric anesthesia. Survey carried out by the Study Group SIAARTI for anesthesia and intensive therapy in children]. *Minerva Anestesiol* 61:115, 1995.
6. Leykin Y, Franceschelli N, Grillone G, et al: [A prospective study of pediatric anesthesia and complications observed in Italy over a period of 18 months (January 1990–June 1992)]. *Cah Anesth* 41:543, 1993.
7. Morray JP, Geiduschek JM, Caplan RA, et al: A comparison of pediatric and adult anesthesia closed malpractice claims. *Anesthesiology* 78:461, 1993.
8. Cohen MM, Cameron CB, Duncan PG: Pediatric anesthesia morbidity and mortality in the perioperative period. *Anesth Analg* 70:160, 1990.
9. Van der Walt JH, Webb RK, Osborne GA, et al: The Australian Incident Monitoring Study. Recovery room incidents in the first 2000 incident reports. *Anaesth Int Care* 21:650, 1993.
10. Milross J, Negus B, Street N, et al: Gastro-oesophageal reflux and adverse respiratory events in children under anaesthesia. *Anaesth Int Care* 23:587, 1995.
11. Keenan RL, Shapiro JH, Kane FR, et al: Bradycardia during anesthesia in infants. An epidemiologic study. *Anesthesiology* 80:976, 1994.
12. Keenan RL, Shapiro JH, Dawson K: Frequency of anesthetic cardiac arrests in infants: effect of pediatric anesthesiologists. *J Clin Anesth* 3:433, 1991.
13. Morray J: Implications for subspecialty care of anesthetized children. *Anesthesiology* 80:969, 1994.
14. Gough M: Perioperative deaths among children. *Br M J* 300:1606, 1990.
15. Lunn J: Implications of the national confidential enquiry into perioperative deaths for paediatric anaesthesia. *Paediatr Anaesthiol* 2, 1992.
16. McNicol R: Paediatric anaesthesia—who should do it? The view from the specialist hospital. *Anaesthesia* 52:513, 1997.
17. Rollin A: Paediatric anaesthesia—who should do it? The view from the district general hospital. *Anaesthesia* 52:515, 1997.
18. Arul G, Spicer R, McDonald P, et al: Where should paediatric surgery be performed? *Arch Dis Child* 79:65, 1998.
19. Auroy Y, Ecoffey C, Messiah A, et al: Relationship between complications of pediatric anesthesia and volume of pediatric anesthetics. *Anesth Analg* 84:234, 1997.
20. Hackel A, Badgwell J, Binding R, et al: Guidelines for the pediatric perioperative anesthesia environment. *Pediatrics* 103:512, 1999.
21. Sarner JB, Levine M, Davis PJ, et al: Clinical characteristics of sevoflurane in children. A comparison with halothane. *Anesthesiology* 82:38, 1995.
22. Welborn L, Hannallah R, Norden J, et al: Comparison of emergence and recovery characteristics of sevoflurane, desflurane, and halothane in pediatric ambulatory patients. *Anesth Analg* 83:917, 1996.
23. Lerman J, Davis P, Welborn L, et al: Induction, recovery, and safety characteristics of sevoflurane in children undergoing ambulatory surgery. A comparison with halothane. *Anesthesiology* 84:1332, 1996.
24. Kataria B, Epstein R, Bailey A, et al: A comparison of sevoflurane to halothane in paediatric surgical patients: results of a multicentre international study. *Paediatr Anaesthiol* 6:283, 1996.

25. Taivainen T, Tiainen P, Meretoja OA, et al: Comparison of the effects of sevoflurane and halothane on the quality of anaesthesia and serum glutathione transferase alpha and fluoride in paediatric patients. *Br J Anaesth* 73:590, 1994.
26. Doi M, Ikeda K: Airway irritation produced by volatile anaesthetics during brief inhalation: comparison of halothane, enflurane, isoflurane and sevoflurane. *Can J Anaesth* 40:122, 1993.
27. Epstein R, Mendel H, Guarnieri K, et al: Sevoflurane versus halothane for general anesthesia in pediatric patients: a comparative study of vital signs, induction, and emergence. *J Clin Anesth* 7:237, 1995.
28. Holzman R, van der Velde M, Kaus S, et al: Sevoflurane depresses myocardial contractility less than halothane during induction of anesthesia in children. *Anesthesiology* 85:1260, 1996.
29. Pietropaoli JA, Jr., Keller MS, Smail DF, et al: Regional anesthesia in pediatric surgery: complications and postoperative comfort level in 174 children. *J Pediatr Surg* 28:560, 1993.
30. Chabas E, Gomar C, Villalonga A, et al: Postoperative respiratory function in children after abdominal surgery. A comparison of epidural and intramuscular morphine analgesia. *Anaesthesia* 53:393, 1998.
31. Welborn LG, Rice LJ, Hannallah RS, et al: Postoperative apnea in former preterm infants: prospective comparison of spinal and general anesthesia. *Anesthesiology* 72:838, 1990.
32. Sartorelli KH, Abajian JC, Kreutz JM, et al: Improved outcome utilizing spinal anesthesia in high-risk infants. *J Pediatr Surg* 27:1022, 1992.
33. Coté C, Zaslavsky A, Downes J, et al: Postoperative apnea in former preterm infants after inguinal herniorrhaphy. A combined analysis. *Anesthesiology* 82:809, 1995.
34. Taguchi N, Matsumiya N, Ishizawa Y, et al: [The relation between upper respiratory tract infection and mild hypoxemia during general anesthesia in children]. *Masui* 41:251, 1992.
35. Levy L, Pandit UA, Randel GI, et al: Upper respiratory tract infections and general anaesthesia in children. Peri-operative complications and oxygen saturation. *Anaesthesia* 47:678, 1992.
36. Cohen MM, Cameron CB: Should you cancel the operation when a child has an upper respiratory tract infection? *Anesth Analg* 72:282, 1991.
37. Lyons J, Chambers F, MacSullivan R, et al: Anaesthesia for non-cardiac surgery in the post-cardiac transplant patient. *Irish J Med Sci* 164:132, 1995.
38. Dajani A, Taubert K, Wilson W, et al: Prevention of bacterial endocarditis. *JAMA* 277:1794, 1997.
39. van der Spek A, Reynolds P, Fang W, et al: Changes in resistance to mouth opening induced by depolarizing and non-depolarizing neuromuscular relaxants. *Br J Anaesthesiol* 64:21, 1990.
40. Littleford JA, Patel LR, Bose D, et al: Masseter muscle spasm in children: implications of continuing the triggering anesthetic. *Anesth Analg* 72:151, 1991.
41. Ording H, Brancadoro V, Cozzolino S, et al: In vitro contracture test for diagnosis of malignant hyperthermia following the protocol of the European MH Group: results of testing patients surviving fulminant MH and unrelated low-risk subjects. The European Malignant Hyperthermia Group [see comments]. *Acta Anaesthesiol Scand* 41:955, 1997.
42. Krane E, Haberkern C, Jacobson L: Postoperative apnea, bradycardia, and oxygen desaturation in formerly premature infants: prospective comparison of spinal and general anesthesia. *Anesth Analg* 80:7, 1995.
43. Webster A, McKishnie J, Kenyon C, et al: Spinal anaesthesia for inguinal hernia repair in high-risk neonates. *Can J Anaesthesiol* 38:281, 1991.
44. Cox R, Goresky G: Life-threatening apnea following spinal anesthesia in former premature infants. *Anesthesiology* 73:345, 1990.
45. Larach MG, Rosenberg H, Gronert GA, et al: Hyperkalemic cardiac arrest during anesthesia in infants and children with occult myopathies. *Clin Pediatr* 36:9, 1997.
46. O'Connor M, Drasner K: Preoperative laboratory testing of children undergoing elective surgery. *Anesth Analg* 70:176, 1990.

47. Fisher Q: "Clear for surgery": current attitudes and practices of pediatricians. *Clin Pediatr* 30:35, 1991.
48. Browning R, Triebwasser A, Weissburg A: What every pediatrician should know about pediatric anesthesia. *R I Med* 75:81, 1992.
49. Anonymous: *When Your Child Needs Anesthesia.* Park Ridge, IL, American Society of Anesthesiologists, 1993.
50. Anonymous: Evaluation and preparation of pediatric patients undergoing anesthesia. American Academy of Pediatrics. Section on Anesthesiology. *Pediatrics* 98:502, 1996.
51. Hines R, Barash PG, Watrous G, et al: Complications occurring in the postanesthesia care unit: a survey. *Anesth Analg* 74:503, 1992.
52. Selby IR, Rigg JD, Faragher B, et al: The incidence of minor sequelae following anaesthesia in children. *Paediatr Anaesthesiol* 6:293, 1996.
53. Karlsson E, Larsson LE, Nilsson K: Postanaesthetic nausea in children. *Acta Anaesthesiol Scand* 34:515, 1990.
54. Koivuranta M, Laara E, Snare L, et al: A survey of postoperative nausea and vomiting. *Anaesthesia* 52:443, 1997.
55. Ferrari LR, Donlon JV: Metoclopramide reduces the incidence of vomiting after tonsillectomy in children. *Anesth Analg* 75:351, 1992.
56. Lin DM, Furst SR, Rodarte A: A double-blinded comparison of metoclopramide and droperidol for prevention of emesis following strabismus surgery. *Anesthesiology* 76:357, 1992.
57. Martin TM, Nicolson SC, Bargas MS: Propofol anesthesia reduces emesis and airway obstruction in pediatric outpatients. *Anesth Analg* 76:144, 1993.
58. Mendel HG, Guarnieri KM, Sundt LM, et al: The effects of ketorolac and fentanyl on postoperative vomiting and analgesic requirements in children undergoing strabismus surgery. *Anesth Analg* 80:1129, 1995.
59. Morton NS, Camu F, Dorman T, et al: Ondansetron reduces nausea and vomiting after paediatric adenotonsillectomy. *Paediatr Anaesthesiol* 7:37, 1997.
60. Watcha MF, Simeon RM, White PF, et al: Effect of propofol on the incidence of postoperative vomiting after strabismus surgery in pediatric outpatients. *Anesthesiology* 75:204, 1991.
61. Sikich N, Carr A, Lerman J: Parental perceptions, expectations and preferences for the postanaesthetic recovery of children. *Paediatr Anaesthesiol* 7:139, 1997.
62. Romsing J, Walther-Larsen S: [Parents' expectations and evaluation of their children's postoperative pain treatment]. *Ugeskr Laeger* 159:419, 1997.
63. Kokki H, Ahonen R: Pain and activity disturbance after paediatric day case adenoidectomy. *Paediatr Anaesthesiol* 7:227, 1997.
64. Kotiniemi L, Ryhanen P, Moilanen I: Behavioural changes in children following day-case surgery: a 4-week follow-up of 551 children. *Anaesthesia* 52:970, 1997.
65. Sutters K, Miaskowski C: Inadequate pain management and associated morbidity in children at home after tonsillectomy. *J Pediatr Nurs* 12:178, 1997.
66. Kotiniemi L, Ryhanen P, Valanne J, et al: Postoperative symptoms at home following day-case surgery in children: a multicentre survey of 551 children. *Anaesthesia* 52:963, 1997.
67. Dexter F, Tinker J: The cost efficacy of hypothetically eliminating adverse anesthetic outcomes from high-risk, but neither low- nor moderate-risk surgical operations. *Anesth Analg* 81:939, 1995.
68. Holzman RS: Morbidity and mortality in pediatric anesthesia. *Pediatr Clin North Am* 41:239, 1994.
69. Morray JP, Geiduschek J, Ramamoorthy C, et al: Anesthesia-related cardiac arrest in children: initial findings of the Pediatric Perioperative Cardiac Arrest (POCA) Registry. *Anesthesiology* 93:6, 2000.
70. Litman RS, Perkins FM, Dawson SC: Parental knowledge and attitudes toward discussing the risk of death from anesthesia. *Anesth Analg* 77:256, 1993.
71. Waisel DB, Truog RD: The benefits of the explanation of the risks of anesthesia in the day surgery patient. *J Clin Anesthesiol* 7:200, 1995.

2 | Ethical and Legal Issues in Pediatric Care

David B. Waisel, MD

Inherent in the care of children is an understanding of those ethics that shape and influence the manner in which we approach, discuss, and perform the medical services we provide to patients on a daily basis. The objective of this chapter is to provide the reader with a sound knowledge of a broad assortment of problems that pediatric anesthesiologists need to understand and address to provide appropriate care. Many of these issues are similar to those regarding adult medical practice; many are not. This chapter addresses the commonality and differences of that care.

INFORMED CONSENT*

The Informed Consent Process for Pediatric Patients

The core of medicine lies at the interaction between patient and physician and the basis of this interaction is informed consent. The doctrine of informed consent centers on the belief that patients have a right to self-determination. Anesthesiologists facilitate this right by explaining to the patient the risks, benefits, and alternatives to the procedure and obtaining from the patient an active, voluntary, informed authorization to perform a specific plan[1] (Table 2-1).

Informed Permission

Applying this template to pediatric patients may be confusing. Pediatric patients range from the newborn to the teenager and different standards describe the various techniques for informed consent. Depending on the age and maturity of the patient, tenets of pediatric informed consent may include obtaining informed permission from parents, using the best-interests standards for children who cannot offer an informed opinion, and obtaining informed assent from children with decision-making capacity[2] (Table 2-2).

Parents traditionally make medical decisions and give consent for their children. To acknowledge that this practice does not fulfill the spirit of consent, which requires obtaining an autonomous decision from the person receiving treatment, it may be more proper to think in terms of parents giving *informed permission*. Informed permission has the same requirements as informed consent, but it acknowledges that one person is giving permission for another. The practical difference to this distinction is that, whereas society will permit individuals to make any choice (such as a Jehovah's Witness's decision to refuse potentially life-saving blood products), society has determined that there are certain decisions that fall outside the boundary of parental decision-making. Thus, the decision-making process for pediatric patients may involve patients, parents, caregivers, and, at times, the courts.

---

*Throughout this discussion, the terms *parent* and *parents* describe the individual who provides the legal informed permission for the child. It should be understood, however, that in some situations, parents might not always be the legal surrogate decision-makers, as when a child is in the custody of the state.

TABLE 2-1 Elements of Consent and Assent as Defined by the American Academy of Pediatrics Committee on Bioethics

Consent
  Adequate provision of information including the nature of the ailment or condition, the nature of the proposed diagnostic steps or treatment, and the probability of their success; the existence and nature of the risks involved; and the existence, potential benefits, and risks of recommended alternative treatments (including the choice of no treatment)
  Assessment of the patient's understanding of the above information
  Assessment, if only tacit, of the capacity of the patient or surrogate to make the necessary decisions
  Assurance, insofar as it is possible, that the patient has the freedom to choose among the medial alternatives without coercion or manipulation

Assent
  Helping the patient achieve a developmentally appropriate awareness of the nature of his or her condition
  Telling the patient what he or she can expect with tests and treatment
  Making a clinical assessment of the paitent's understanding of the situation and the factors influencing how he or she is responding (including whether there is appropriate pressure to accept testing or therapy)
  Soliciting an expression of the patient's willingness to accept the proposed care

Source: Committee on Bioethics, American Academy of Pediatrics. *Pediatrics* 95:315, 1997.

Best-Interests Standard

When children cannot express an informed preference, parents, physicians, and other caregivers use the *best-interests standard* to guide their decision-making. The best-interests standard requires the parent to weigh the benefits and the burdens of clinical options and determine what is in the best interests of the child. The difficulties lie in assuming there is one best choice. The determination of the best option is affected by medical judgment, the

TABLE 2-2 Approaches to Pediatric Consent

Age	Decision-making capacity	Techniques
Young children	None	Best-interests standard
Children unable to participate in the decision-making process	Not accessible	Best-interests standard
7–12 years	Developing	Informed permission, informed assent
12–18 years	Mostly developed	Informed assent, informed permission
Mature minor	Developed, as legally determined by a judge	Informed consent
Emancipated minor	Developed, as legally determined by a situation	Informed consent

Note: When children are in the upper range of an age bracket, limited or full inclusion of a higher technique, such as the use of assent for a 6 year old, may be appropriate. This table provides a broad outline. Specific circumstances should be taken into consideration.
Source: Committee on Bioethics, American Academy of Pediatrics. *Pediatrics* 95:315, 1997.

specific situation, and the decision-maker's preferences. In most cases, it is natural for the parents to make decisions for their children, and in a society that respects the family unit and multiculturalism there is considerable latitude in what is considered acceptable decision-making. There is rarely one right decision. More often, there is a continuum of acceptable decisions. For this reason, a common approach is to define the parameters of acceptable decision-making and rely on parents to choose within those parameters.

The criteria used to determine the parameters of acceptable decision-making include the amount of harm to the child by the intervention or its absence, the likelihood of success, and the overall risk-to-benefit ratio.[3] For example, on the one hand, it is nearly always considered unacceptable under treatment for Jehovah's Witnesses to refuse a life-sustaining blood transfusion for their children. On the other hand, parents may decline to have an epidural placed in their child for postoperative pain management, thus depriving the child of an optimal source of pain control. This is not considered unacceptable undertreatment, in part because the harm is limited by other adequate methods of pain control. It may be difficult to resolve these dilemmas.

However, there are times when caregivers believe that the parents are making a choice that falls *outside* the range of acceptable decision-making. Some parents, intentionally or unintentionally, do not do what is in the best interests of their children. The anesthesiologist who believes that parents are choosing an unacceptable treatment should find out why they have made such a decision, address those specific concerns, and involve other caregivers to offer an assessment of the appropriateness of care and engage the parent in discussion. If clinicians believe that parents are incapable of making decisions that fall within the continuum of acceptability, they should consider contacting the proper child protective services to determine whether a different surrogate decision-maker would be more appropriate.

Informed Assent

Informed assent becomes relevant when children approach age 7 years and begin to develop decision-making ability, which is the capacity to make a specific decision at a specific time. The participation of children increases as they grow older and depends on the patient's age, maturity, decision-making ability, and the consequences involved in the decision (e.g., an 8 year old may decide whether to have an inhalation or intravenous induction of anesthesia, a choice of lower risk, but may not decide whether to have the surgical procedure, a choice of higher risk). A patient gives evidence of decision-making capacity by being able to appreciate one's situation, to understand the proposed procedure and the alternatives, and to communicate a decision based on internally coherent reasoning. Anesthesiologists should tailor the assent process to the patient's needs and abilities.

Some adolescents older than 14 years will have developed extensive decision-making capacity and anesthesiologists should try to fulfill the ethical requirements of consent while obtaining assent. However, although adolescents have sufficient ability to weigh and compare the benefits and burdens of a choice, they may have insufficient life experiences to place the decision in proper perspective and thus may make impulsive decisions. Anesthesiologists should make adolescents full participants in decision-making but should not acquiesce to questionable decision-making without critically evaluating the patient's position and obtaining appropriate consultative help.

Anesthesiologists should respect the right of adolescents to refuse elective care and should avoid coercing or forcing patients into proceeding. For example, if a 15 year old scheduled for an elective knee arthroscopy comes to the preoperative holding area and starts refusing care, it is wrong to forcibly proceed by intramuscularly injecting ketamine, even if that is the parents' wishes. The patient should be treated with respect, and the reason for the refusal should be determined and addressed. Techniques for diffusing the situation center on giving the patient control, often by removing the patient from the situation and allowing the patient to get dressed. The next step is to clarify the patient's concerns and pay particular attention to likely sources of problems such as misinformation, misunderstanding, desire for control, or fear. Although it is inappropriate to chemically force an adolescent into surgery and anesthesia (e.g., by intramuscular ketamine or midazolam), it is not inappropriate to make an agreement with the patient to receive sedation before arriving in the holding area to better enable that individual to undergo the experiences. There is a sharp and critical distinction between the use of involuntary chemical force and the use of voluntary and chosen chemical sedation to ease anxiety before surgery.

This situation becomes more complicated when the patient expresses significant decision-making capacity and refuses an urgent or emergent procedure. Anesthesiologists should use caution when adolescents make questionable decisions and seek help from ethics consultation services and hospital general counsel. Most importantly, because obviating an adolescent's decision-making is not benign, anesthesiologists should be wary that the urgency of the situation is rooted solely in patient care and not in the convenience of the anesthesiologist, surgeon, or operating room.

Disclosure

It is often difficult to know what information to disclose to a patient. The reasonable-person standard requires disclosure to be to the level that would be desired by the hypothetically reasonable person. It does not, however, define what should be told, and it is often unclear who the "reasonable" person is and what the "reasonable person" would want to know. Some suggest that using the subjective-person standard may be more successful at fulfilling the spirit of informed consent.[4] This standard holds that informed consent should be matched to the wants and needs of the individual person giving consent. Although this may be considered the ideal form of disclosure, it requires greater effort and is more difficult to use (Table 2-3).

A tiered approach may be prudent. Anesthesiologists should discuss common events relevant to anesthesia practice, such as complications of airway management, invasive monitoring, and the risks and benefits of the possible anesthetic plans.[5] They should avoid the rote listing of less relevant risks that clutter the informed consent process. After a standard presentation relevant to the patient, anesthetic, and surgical procedure, the anesthesiologist should ask the patient whether hearing the less likely, more dangerous risks (e.g., death in the healthy patient having a low-risk procedure) is preferable. The goal is to focus on information that patient wants to know.

Parents may use the informed consent process not to make decisions but to know more about the procedure or because they feel they are obligated to participate in the patients' care.[6,7] These issues can be addressed by frankly discussing parents' desires to the point of asking (particularly in the face of an unusual question), Why do you want to know that? In this vein, some advocate discussing the low risk of death from anesthesia in a healthy child as a way of reassuring parents. By knowing what the goals are for the informed consent discussion, anesthesiologists are more capable of satisfying the patients and parents.

TABLE 2–3 The Concept of Negligence

Four elements necessary to sustain a cause of action for negligence	Routine clinical care	Informed consent
Presence of a duty A duty to meet a standard was owed	To provide a certain level of care such as to use standard monitors for routine anesthetic management	To provide information and circumstances sufficient to satisfy the "reasonable person"*
Breach of duty The standard was not met	Standard monitors were not used when they should have been used	Information given or the circumstances in which information was given in were insufficient[†]
Causation The failure to meet the standard was the proximate cause of an injury and the injury was a foreseeable result of failing to meet the standard	The failure to use standard monitors resulted in late diagnosis of cardiac dysrhythmia	If the patient had known the information or if circumstances were different (i.e., if the standards were met), the patient would have chosen differently (not given informed consent) for a specific procedure
Proof of damage An actual damage or injury occured	The cardiac dysrhythmia led to harm to the patient's heart and brain	Harm occurred as result of the decision (it does not matter whether the harm occurred as a result of other clinical malpractice)

Note: Obtaining informed consent does not, nor is it intended to, protect a clinician from being successfully sued for malpractice. Obtaining informed consent is relevant only to informed consent malpractice. Most medical malpractice suits are based on negligence, which is defined as the unintentional failure of one party to fulfill a legal standard owed to a second party. To sustain a cause of action for negligence, four elements must be met. The table compares the elements of negligence in routine clinical care and informed consent.

*Assuming this occurs in a jurisdiction that uses the reasonable-patient standard.

[†]Circumstances are important, too. For example, negligence can occur if the patient is not given time or opportunity to ask questions about the information.

Source: Flamm MB: Health care provider as a defendant. *Legal Medicine,* 3rd ed. In Sanbar SS, Gibofsky A, Firestone MH, Leblang TR (eds). St. Louis, Mosby-Yearbook, 1995, p 118.

Using Pediatric Informed Consent

Anesthesiologists should attempt to achieve informed permission from the parent and assent as appropriate from the pediatric patient (Table 2-2). Because infants and young children have no decision-making capacity, assent is not a viable option, and anesthesiologists should obtain informed permission from the parent. When obtaining informed consent, anesthesiologists should realize that informed consent does not have to be fully and perfectly achieved for it to be valid. It is more than sufficient for the patient to achieve a *substantial* level of informed consent. Anesthesiologists should also use their experience and superior knowledge to offer opinions. At the same time, they should explain the rationale behind those opinions so the patient and parents can independently evaluate the reasons and values behind the recommendation.

Situations in Pediatric Informed Consent

Mature Minors and Emancipated Minor Status

Certain adolescents have legal health care decision-making authority for themselves. Under the mature minor doctrine, a court may award to the patient the legal right to make a specific health care decision if the court believes the patient is capable of fulfilling the requirement of giving informed consent. As the patient nears the age of majority, decisions of greater weight and risk tend to be permitted. Evidence in determining mature minor status is whether the patient is of sufficient age (usually 14 years or older) and whether the patient appreciates and understands the proposed procedure and the benefits and burdens of proceeding and not proceeding.

Emancipated minor status is automatically awarded to minors who have undergone certain events and gives the minor all the rights of adulthood with regard to health care decision-making. Precise definitions differ by state. Events that may confer emancipated minor status include marriage, being in the military, being economically self-supporting, and possibly pregnancy. Mature minors and patients who are emancipated have a right to complete confidentiality.

Jehovah's Witnesses

Jehovah's Witnesses value life and the medical treatments that optimize or maintain life. At the same time, Jehovah's Witnesses interpret biblical scripture as prohibiting blood transfusions.[8] Acting in ways inconsistent with their interpretation of scripture jeopardizes believers' ability to earn eternal salvation. Thus, the decision to refuse transfusion therapy is not based on a disrespect of life but on the greater value placed on eternal salvation. The concept of respect for autonomy allows competent patients to refuse any treatment and for the most part the courts have faithfully upheld the rights of nonpregnant adults to refuse blood transfusions.

Children, however, are different. In the United States, governments have an obligation to protect the interests of those who are unable to protect themselves. The courts have generally granted physicians the right to transfuse minors over the objections of their parents. The key to obtaining informed assent and informed permission for the care of a Jehovah's Witness's child is preparation and documentation. Addressing transfusion therapy preoperatively helps avoid a crisis situation later; although the discussion may be adjusted depending on the likelihood of transfusion, it cannot be ignored. Anesthesiologists should determine with great specificity what type of care is acceptable to the patients and parents and should try to give care consistent with their preferences. Commonly accepted therapy includes deliberate hypotension, deliberate hypothermia, and hemodilution. Synthetic colloid solutions, dextran, erythropoietin, desmopressin, and preoperative iron therapy are usually acceptable, and blood removed and returned in a continuous loop, such as with a cell saver, may be acceptable. The patient and family should be informed that, although attempts will be made to comply with their specified wishes, the physicians would seek a court order to authorize a transfusion if faced with a life-threatening situation. When there is a high likelihood of transfusion and parents will not consent to potentially life-sustaining transfusion therapy, anesthesiologists may want to consult with the hospital general counsel about establishing appropriate legal arrangements. Precise documentation forces the issue to be clearly defined and helps bring forth misunderstandings before they cause harm.

Adolescents nearing the age of majority may be able to consent to refusal of blood products under the mature minor doctrine, and anesthesiologists faced with that decision should consult ethics services and hospital general counsel for guidance about local procedures. Anesthesiologists should ensure that the surgeon, other operating room caregivers, and postoperative ward or intensive care unit caregivers are willing to abide by the patient's decisions if that individual has the right to refuse transfusion therapy. In these cases, anesthesiologists should not proceed without a good faith belief that they and the system can support the patient's preferences. When providing emergency care, nearly all commentators believe that anesthesiologists should proceed with potentially life-sustaining transfusions in minors and in patients who have not made their preferences clear, based on the ethical belief that the patient has not made an informed decision to forgo transfusion therapy.

Confidentiality, Pregnancy Testing, and Abortion

Confidentiality requires physicians to protect patient information from unauthorized and unnecessary disclosure. Adolescents are prone to inadequate treatment when they believe their interactions will not be confidential, particularly when it concerns sensitive medical problems such as sexually transmitted diseases and contraceptive services. Confidentiality strengthens an adolescent's trust in a physician, which allows for greater honesty and better care. Possible exceptions to the principle of confidentiality include those required by law; reporting statutes, parental notification requirements, and when the patient makes a credible threat to another person.

Confidentiality is relevant when considering preoperative pregnancy testing. To determine the potential for pregnancy in the adolescent woman, anesthesiologists may (1) ask if she could be pregnant with her parents present, (2) ask if she could be pregnant without her parents present, or (3) do routine pregnancy testing on adolescents. Although opinions differ, the consensus is that pediatric patients of childbearing age should be routinely tested before anesthesia and surgery. It is unrealistic to assume that an anesthesiologist can determine whether an adolescent is telling the truth about sexual activity, particularly with her parents present. If she says she cannot be pregnant, the anesthesiologists must (1) believe her, (2) send her to surgery with doubts, (3) imply she is not to be believed by overtly ordering the pregnancy test, or (4) deceive her by covertly ordering the test. Because it is impossible to make a determination of sexual activity or truthfulness in a short preoperative visit, the safest route is a policy of routine testing.

Pragmatically, anesthesiologists should inform the patient and family that a pregnancy test will be performed. Patients have a right to know when they are being tested, particularly if they would want to know that the test is occurring. If the parents object to obtaining the pregnancy test, explain to them the concerns of anesthetizing a pregnant patient. Emphasize there is no way to determine who needs a pregnancy test and the decision to order the test is not an appraisal of the patient or her family.

If the test is positive, it is ethically appropriate to inform the patient of the positive test in private and encourage her to tell her parents. In some states, laws relating to reproductive services make it a legal breach of confidentiality if the anesthesiologist tells the parents. Notwithstanding the legal requirements, if the patient chooses not to tell her parents, it is my opinion that that is her right. However, the anesthesiologists should encourage the patient to tell her parents and provide her with professional resources such as names of obstetricians, adolescent specialists, and social workers who are experienced in dealing with these matters.

For elective abortions, most states require some form of parental involvement such as parental consent or parental notification.[9] If a state requires parental involvement, the ability of the minor to circumvent parental involvement through judicial intervention must be available. Requirements and enforcement of statutes differ from state to state and some statutes are enjoined or not enforced. Depending on the jurisdiction, abortion may be a restricted procedure for the emancipated or mature minor. To prevent problems, anesthesiologists should know the law in their jurisdiction, know how to obtain ethical and legal advice, and consider beforehand whether they are willing to provide anesthesia services for abortion.

FORGOING LIFE-SUSTAINING CARE

The decision to forgo potentially life-sustaining care is often based on the perceived benefits and burdens of proceeding with therapy. For example, some may value an extra few weeks of life at the expense of pain and suffering, whereas others may value a reduction in suffering at the expense of extending life. Perceived benefits may include reduction in pain or suffering, improved quality of life, or an increased enjoyment of life.[10] Perceived burdens may include intractable pain and suffering, disability, events that cause a decrement in the quality of life.

Relevant factors when considering whether a therapy may be futile focus on the specific therapy, the desired outcome, the perceived magnitude of the benefits and burdens, and the likelihood of the outcomes, benefits, and burdens occurring. For example, consider an adolescent with a life expectancy of less than 1 year who presents with a bowel obstruction. He is currently active and fully enjoys his life. The primary benefit of relieving the obstruction is the high likelihood of eliminating the disease, with the burden of a relatively small risk of morbidity, even in the face of a terminal illness. Most people would weigh the value of being alive with minimal risk and discomfort to be significantly more valuable (and therefore "worth it") than the high likelihood of the severe morbidity and discomfort associated with dying of bowel obstruction. However, if he were unable to be extubated in the postoperative period, than the balance of benefits and burdens in favor of continued therapy may change. The longer he remains intubated in the intensive care unit, the greater the burdens associated with the therapy. At some point, he or his surrogate decision-makers may decide that the benefits of continued therapy may not be worth the increasing suffering and the decreasing likelihood that the patient will be discharged or returned to a "desirable" status. At this point, further therapy may become "futile" in that it will not achieve benefits within acceptable burdens. Contrast this with the decision made to have the surgery, in which it appeared that the goals of a limited surgery to decrease pain and improve function for his remaining life would be "worth it" or the decision to continue therapy in an otherwise similar patient who does not have cancer and therefore may have more to gain to counterbalance the increased burden.

Anesthesiologists may have questions about futile care when a patient is brought to the operating room for what may be a "futile" operation.[11] Anesthesiologists should test their assumptions. Why do they think the procedure is futile? What can be gained by the procedure? How does the patient value that gain? If the answers to these questions are not satisfactory, anesthesiologists should voice their concerns to their surgical colleagues. If anesthesiologists still consider the answers unsatisfactory, they are free not to provide elective care.

Perioperative Do-Not-Resuscitate (DNR) Orders

The American Society of Anesthesiology and the American College of Surgeons endorse the right of patients to have DNR orders reevaluated for the perioperative period. Automatic revocation of the DNR order is inappropriate.[12] To tailor the perioperative DNR order to the patient, anesthesiologists must be able to offer multiple options. The following options are appropriate for all patients, including all ages of pediatric patients.

Options for Obtaining and Documenting Perioperative DNR Orders

Option 1: Full resuscitation The patient desires that full resuscitative measures be employed during anesthesia and surgery and in the postanesthesia care unit, regardless of the clinical situation.

There are a number of reasons patients and parents may prefer this option. By establishing a clear reference, such as revocation, the difficult question of determining "what is resuscitation" can be avoided. Patients, parents, and physicians then do not have to worry if a certain intervention is considered to be resuscitative, and they do not have to worry about limiting anesthetic or surgical interventions. Perhaps more importantly, physicians do not need to worry about having their hands tied if an easily reversible event occurs. In addition, outcomes from witnessed arrests are much better than outcomes from those that are unwitnessed, especially when the cause of the arrest is iatrogenic. As such, the chance of quality survival after an arrest in the operating room is higher than after an arrest elsewhere.

Option 2: Goal-directed order *The patient desires resuscitative efforts during surgery and in the pediatric anesthesia care unit only if the adverse events are believed to be both temporary and reversible, in the clinical judgment of the attending anesthesiologists and surgeons.*

Although this statement suffices for the great majority of patients, the goals and values of patients and parents also can be detailed by using a statement like the following: *The patient desires resuscitative efforts during surgery and in the postanesthesia care unit only if, in the clinical judgments of the attending anesthesiologists and surgeons, such resuscitative procedures will support the following goals and values of the patient (a statement of values).*

The goal-directed approach arose from the idea that it is often more effective to talk about goals and outcomes than about procedures.[13] By taking advantage of the operating room environment, in which specific physicians take care of a patient for a defined period, patients may guide therapy by prioritizing outcomes rather than procedures.[14,15] After defining desirable outcomes in individual discussions with the physicians who will be in the operating room, patients and parents authorize those physicians to use their clinical judgments to determine how specific interventions will affect achieving these goals.

The strength of the goal-directed approach is that physicians should feel that they could truly honor the declared values without having to worry about getting "caught" in a technicality requiring them to act inconsistently with those values. Even better, predictions about the success of interventions that are made by the anesthesiologist at the time of the resuscitation are likely to be more accurate than predictions made preoperatively, when the quality and nature of the problems are not known. The problem, of course, is that the goal-directed approach is not as explicit as a procedure-directed approach.

Option 3: Procedure-directed *During anesthesia and surgery, the patient refuses the following specific resuscitative interventions: (a list of interventions may be written here).*

Some patients and parents may prefer the security of being able to define precisely what interventions would be permitted. The procedure-directed approach imitates the well-recognized techniques used for ward DNR orders. Patients and parents choose, often from a checklist, which specific interventions may be used. Anesthesiologists advise them based on the benefit and burden of the intervention as well as the likelihood of that intervention allowing them to achieve their desired goals. Interventions frequently on such lists include tracheal intubation or other airway management, postoperative ventilation, chest compressions, defibrillation, vasoactive drugs, and invasive monitoring. When certain procedures are considered mandatory for the anesthetic and surgery to occur, such as tracheal intubation, patients and parents should be informed about which procedures are "essential to the success of anesthesia" and thus cannot be refused.[12]

Procedure-directed orders are unambiguous and clearly define which procedures are desired. Procedure-directed orders, however, do not allow for clinical subtleties that may be difficult to precisely document and define.

Postoperative Planning: Using the Opportunity to Withdraw Care to the Patient's Advantage

Regardless of how the DNR order is managed during the perioperative period, preoperative discussion should include preferences for continuing with and withdrawing from postoperative care. The ability to give the patient a trial of therapy, such as mechanical ventilation, is one of the better ways to fulfill end-of-life requests to the recipient of resuscitative efforts without the possibility of "getting stuck on the ventilator." After an unsuccessful intervention, patients and patents then know with as much certainty as possible that continued therapy would be inconsistent with their goals. Choosing that option, for example, is a way of declaring that the burden of a few days of ventilatory support may be worth the potential benefit of extubation of the trachea, but that the burden of long-term ventilation is not worth it, especially if there is a decreasing likelihood of success. If the time-limited trial is deemed unsuccessful in light of the declared goals, then mechanical ventilation may be withdrawn.

Most ethicists consider withholding treatment, i.e., the act of not starting it, to be ethically and morally equivalent to withdrawing it, or removing if it is found not to be successful.[4] Nonetheless, physicians find withdrawing care more difficult than withholding care. Withdrawing such treatment may make them feel they are breaching expectations or that they have personally failed in their duties to the patient. Or, perhaps they view any death as a failure and thus are reluctant to even tacitly sanction their "failure" by withdrawing care. They may inappropriately believe they are more legally culpable when they stop unsuccessful therapy than when they do not start therapy. In reality, these feelings and beliefs are misplaced. The act of withholding therapy requires greater certainty in the likelihood that a therapy will fail than does withdrawing a therapy after it has been shown to be unsuccessful.

Response to Iatrogenic Arrest and Emergencies

Physicians may feel that, although it is acceptable for patients to refuse care for their diseases, it may be somewhat less acceptable for that wish to be honored when the causal event is iatrogenic.[16] This is untrue. Patients choose based on the lives they want to lead, not how they got to that point. Thus, to patients and their decision-making processes, it is wholly irrelevant whether the cardiac arrest was iatrogenic; what is relevant is the physical and mental status after the arrest.

In an emergency situation, the traditional bias of providing treatment in the absence of a clear communication not to resuscitate should hold. After stabilization, patients' wishes may be clarified and followed. Although this may lead to a brief period of going against patients' wishes, this is a worthwhile trade to be able to be more certain of patients' desires.

OTHER COMMONLY ENCOUNTERED PROBLEMS

Suspicion of Child Abuse

Anesthesiologists are legally required to report the suspicion of child abuse or neglect to appropriate authorities. Signs of physical child abuse include mouth or dental injuries, injuries in the shape of objects, injuries to upper arms or legs, and fractures in infants. Children with physical and mental handicaps and hospitalized children with histories of being abused are at greater risk for receiving further abuse.

Pediatric Pain Management

Anesthesiologists are obligated to manage pain, fear, and apprehension in individual children with acute or chronic pain and to implement hospitalwide pain management systems.[17] Pediatric patients are prone to undertreatment. Neonates may still be harmed by the fallacious belief that they are not affected by or do not have a response to pain. Older children may have difficulty in articulating the source or quantity of the pain and are unable to demand adequate treatment.

Risk factors for deficient pediatric pain management include inexperienced and undereducated caregivers, inadequate postoperative care facilities, and no designated pain service. Anesthesiologists should assume that the behaviors consistent with pain, fear, and apprehension indicate pain, fear, and apprehension, and we should do everything possible to manage the patient's condition. Although individual effort may overcome these inadequacies and achieve good pain management for a specific patient, anesthesiologists should seek to minimize the reliance of patients on the motivated caregiver by working toward systemwide improvements in pain management.

Personal Integrity Issues: Refusing Cases and Production Pressure

Acceptable reasons to refuse to provide care center on issues that violate the physician's personal convictions. The classic example is abortion. Sincere, caring, thoughtful people disagree strongly about if and how abortion services should be provided. The motivation for an individual not to provide anesthesia for abortions may come from fundamental beliefs and deserves to be respected. It is controversial whether an alternate caregiver needs to be found. Some argue that requiring a physician to find a replacement caregiver is inappropriate because the physician then becomes obligated to facilitate therapy that he or she morally opposes; this is especially true in the case of providing anesthesia for abortion. The emergent situation is more complex. In an emergent situation, the requirements to permit an anesthesiologist not to provide care in an emergency are less clear-cut and more rigorous. In general, anesthesiologists should make every effort to comply with the patient's wishes in an emergency.

Production pressure is the pressure anesthesiologists feel to keep the operating room running efficiently.[18] Production pressures arise from internal pressures, such as financial (e.g., loss of case load), concern for professional reputation (e.g., does not want to be difficult to work with), and familial obligations. Production pressure may be from colleagues concerned about decreased group revenue or loss of time off. Surgical, medical, or administrative colleagues may be concerned that delaying or canceling cases might be inconvenient or not cost effective. Nursing and ancillary services may be concerned about increased overtime. Patients and families also may pressure to proceed, perhaps out of limited concern about the anesthetic risk or greater concern of delay or cancellation.

Effects of production pressure may include rushing through preoperative interviews, hastily performing procedures, and making questionable management choices. Production pressure also may push anesthesiologists to anesthetize patients they do not feel qualified to anesthetize. This may occur, for example, when a child with complicated or severe coexisting diseases is scheduled for a routine procedure such as a herniorrhaphy in a community hospital. Anesthesiologists are not required to provide elective care they believe is inappropriate or dangerous.[19]

Facing production pressure is stressful. Internal stress arises from deviating from internal convictions or from not deviating and having to face the ramifications. Techniques to mange production pressure include (1) acknowledging its presence, (2) designing systems that reduce production pressure, (3) remembering primary obligations, and (4) being cognizant of decision-making practices to see if they are being affected by production pressure. In the long run, providing good care and not bowing to inappropriate production pressure will more likely secure professional and financial success.

Seeking Help

Managing conflicting obligations can be difficult. Anesthesiologists prepare for ethical conflicts by developing a practiced way of thinking about these issues, by anticipating and preparing for potential problems, and by reviewing policies to help prevent untenable situations. Resources for help with ethical dilemmas include the ethics consultation service and medical law (also known as hospital general counsel). Both services can clarify statutes and policies, define options, and assist in resolution, and both services often "take call" and are available through paging systems.

REFERENCES

1. Waisel DB, Truog RD: Informed consent. *Anesthesiology* 87:968, 1997.
2. Committee on Bioethics, American Academy of Pediatrics: Informed consent, parental permission, and assent in pediatric practice. *Pediatrics* 95:314, 1995.
3. McMenamin JP, Bigley GL: Children as patients. In *Legal Medicine*, 3rd ed. Sanbar SS, Gibofsky A, Firestone MH, LeBlang TR, eds. St. Louis, Mosby-Year Book, 1995, p 456.
4. Beauchamp TL, Childress JF: *Principles of Biomedical Ethics*, 4th ed. New York, Oxford University Press, 1994.
5. Hirsh HL: A visitation with informed consent and refusal. In *Legal Medicine 1995.* Wecht CH, ed. Charlottesville, VA, Michie, 1995, p 147.
6. Kain ZN, Wang SM, Caramico LA, Hofstadter M, Mayes LC: Parental desire for perioperative information and informed consent a two-phase study. *Anesth Analg* 84:299, 1997.
7. Litman RS, Perkins FM, Dawson SC: Parental knowledge and attitudes toward discussing the risk of death from anesthesia. *Anesth Analg* 77:256, 1993.
8. Rothenberg DM: The approach to the Jehovah's Witness patient. *Anesthesiol Clin North Am* 8:589, 1990.
9. Committee on Adolescence, American Academy of Pediatrics: The adolescent's right to confidential care when considering abortion. *Pediatrics* 97:746, 1996.
10. Committee on Bioethics, American Academy of Pediatrics: Guidelines on forgoing life-sustaining medical treatment. *Pediatrics* 93:532, 1994.
11. Tomlinson T, Czlonka D: Futility and hospital policy. *Hastings Cent Rep* 25(3):28, 1995.
12. American Society of Anesthesiologists: *Ethical Guidelines for the Anesthesia Care of Patients with Do-Not-Resuscitate Orders or Other Directives That Limit Care, 1999 Directory of Members.* Park Ridge, IL, American Society of Anesthesiologists, 1999.
13. Clemency MV, Thompson NJ: Do not resuscitate orders in the perioperative period: patient perspectives. *Anesth Analg* 84:859, 1997.
14. Truog RD, Waisel DB, Burns JP: DNR in the OR: a goal-directed approach. *Anesthesiology* 90:289, 1999.
15. Bastron RD: Ethical concerns in anesthetic care for patients with do-not-resuscitate orders. *Anesthesiology* 85:1190, 1996.
16. Casarett DJ, Stocking CB, Siegler M: Would physicians override a do-not-resuscitate order when a cardiac arrest is iatrogenic? *J Gen Intern Med* 35:8, 1999.
17. Schecter NL, Berde CB, Yaster M: Pain in infants, children and adolescents: an overview. In *Pain in Infants, Children and Adolescents.* Schecter NL, Berde CB, Yaster M, eds. Baltimore, Williams and Wilkins, 1993, p 3.
18. Gaba DM, Howard SK, Jump B: Production pressure in the work environment: California anesthesiologists' attitudes and experiences. *Anesthesiology* 81:488, 1994.
19. Flamm MB: Health care provider as a defendant. In *Legal Medicine*, 3rd ed. Sanbar SS, Gibofsky A, Firestone MH, Leblang TR, eds. St. Louis, Mosby-Year Book, 1995, p 118.

3 | Selecting the Suitable Pediatric Outpatient

Ramesh I. Patel, MD
Raafat S. Hannallah, MD

More than 70% of all pediatric surgical procedures are currently performed on an outpatient basis. Therefore, preoperative evaluation and selection of suitable patients for outpatient surgery is an important part of the practice of anesthesiology. The psychological, medical, and financial benefits of minimizing the time spent in the hospital have been cited as reasons to allow many more children including those with significant underlying medical problems to undergo outpatient surgery. Many children with chronic diseases benefit substantially from outpatient treatment. For example, immunocompromised patients benefit from limited contact with a hospital environment. Physically handicapped, psychologically disturbed, and mentally retarded children also benefit from not being separated from the continued support of a parent or guardian, which is usually fostered in outpatient facilities.[1]

The criteria for selecting patients for pediatric outpatient surgery are especially important because outpatient surgical procedures are performed not only on patients classified as Physical Status (PS) 1 or 2 according to the American Society of Anesthesiologists (ASA) but also many ASA PS 3 and even PS 4 patients. Therefore, it is important to use an effective screening method that determines the child's fitness to undergo the proposed outpatient surgery. Failure to determine the appropriateness of outpatient surgery in advance and to prepare the child for surgery [i.e., nil per os (NPO) guidelines, consultations, laboratory tests, and radiologic studies] result in delays and cancellations on the day of surgery. Such delays and cancellations lead to anger and frustration among surgeons, patients, and their families. It also causes disruption of the operating room schedule, resulting in loss of time and money.

A presurgical evaluation is vital for the efficient functioning of an outpatient surgical center. The primary care physician, the surgeon, and the anesthesiologist share this responsibility. The anesthesiologist is responsible for coordinating preoperative evaluation and acting as a gatekeeper to ensure that undue risks are minimized. After an evaluation, all patients are assigned to one of three groups : (1) suitable and ready for outpatient surgery, (2) suitable but not ready for surgery, or (3) not suitable for outpatient surgery.

Patients in group 1 are ready for surgery. Children in group 2 are suitable for ambulatory surgery but may need additional laboratory or radiologic tests or optimization of a medical condition such as control of asthma or seizures. Children in group 3 are not suitable for outpatient surgery and their surgeries should be performed as an inpatient. Examples of such patients are those with severe cardiac disease or infants younger than 46 weeks in conceptual age.

Guidelines for outpatient surgery differ across institutions and are usually influenced by the views of the local community, patient population mix, ease with which hospital admission is possible, and staff expertise.[2] Individual selections of patients depend on the condition of the patient, the attitude of the parents, the type of surgical procedure, and special considerations concerning the anesthetic management and required postoperative care.[1]

The surgical site also has to be considered. Certain limitations affect patient or procedure selection in a free-standing center or office-based location. Lack of a critical care unit, inpatient beds, an extensive laboratory, or a blood bank as an immediate backup may alter selection criteria. Whereas a hospital-based ambulatory center can offer outpatient surgery to higher risk patients, the free-standing or office-based location is less likely to accept higher risk patients and procedures. As the number of day surgery patients rise and their surgical care becomes more complex, it becomes increasingly important to have clear guidelines on common problems such as NPO times, patient selection, prophylaxis for subacute bacterial endocarditis, and discharge criteria.

SCREENING METHODS

The child should be in good physical health (ASA PS 1 and 2). When patients with moderately severe illness are accepted (ASA PS 3), their medical conditions must be well controlled. There are many methods to screen patients scheduled for outpatient surgery.

1. Some centers require a preoperative visit by the parents and the child to the anesthesiologists' office.
2. At our institution, we depend on the careful evaluation by the surgical staff and telephone screening.[3] A nurse or an associate screens patients with a preprinted form 3 to 5 days before the scheduled date of surgery. An anesthesiologist is consulted if a medical problem is detected from the telephone screening. The anesthesiologist then reviews the medical records of that child and interviews the parents by telephone. A visit to the anesthesiologist's office may be required for physical examination. Consultation from other services may also be requested.

    The needs of specific groups of patients are detected and individual strategies developed to minimize difficulties. The oncologist, for example, provides a special summary sheet for patients with cancer. The summary includes the names and dosages of chemotherapeutic agents, including steroids and adriamycin, and results of cardiac evaluation, including echocardiographic findings and ejection fraction. This summary is incorporated into the preoperative evaluation. Another telephone call is made on the evening before surgery to confirm NPO guidelines and time of arrival and to detect symptoms of acute illness. A final preoperative evaluation is done by the anesthesiologist before the induction of anesthesia.
3. Another approach gaining popularity is the use of computerized information-gathering systems. For example, the Tele-Pad (a pen-based mobile computer) is used as the platform for a paperless perioperative screening record for use in the outpatient setting.[4]

    The HealthQuiz is a computerized device that displays a series of screening questions on a small liquid crystal display screen, and the patient responds by using three buttons labeled *yes*, *no*, or *don't know*. A summary report is produced at the end of the screening session with suggestions for laboratory tests.[4]

AGE

Adult patients over a certain age (e.g., >85 years) often are considered not suitable for outpatient surgery despite a stable medical condition because of concerns regarding adequate postoperative care at home. What about the other extreme? Is a 3-day-old, full-term, otherwise healthy newborn of a

16-year-old mother an suitable candidate for outpatient surgery? The first month of life is marked by rapid and profound physiologic changes such as closure of the patent ductus arteriosus, decreased pulmonary vascular resistance, increased functional residual capacity, increased glomerular filtration rate, and physiologic jaundice. The literature does not provide any conclusive data on how to formulate guidelines concerning the minimum acceptable age for outpatient surgery. Individual evaluation and counseling are necessary in such cases. At the Children's National Medical Center, we have arbitrarily set the minimum age limit for outpatient surgery for full-term infants at 2 weeks. By 2 weeks of age, any physiologic jaundice would have abated, pulmonary vascular resistance would have decreased, and the ductus arteriosus would have closed. We believe that outpatient surgery is safer when these conditions have been resolved. However each center, in consultation with their neonatologists and surgeons, should set their own guidelines.

Sudden Infant Death Syndrome (SIDS)

Full-term infants have a risk of developing SIDS during their first years of life. There is no evidence that anesthesia or surgery increases the risk of SIDS.[5] Isolated case reports[6] of full-term infants developing apneic spells in the postoperative period should increase our awareness with regard to SIDS in infants. Moreover, a fatal apneic episode could occur coincidentally in an infant during the postoperative period, with no cause-and-effect relationship between anesthesia and mortality. The cause of SIDS is not known and there is no diagnostic test available to identify SIDS-prone infants. Certain risk factors, however, are well established. If the patient has a sibling with a history of SIDS or if the mother has abused drugs during her pregnancy, the risk of SIDS increases many fold. Infants whose histories suggest a high risk for SIDS should be monitored closely for a longer postoperative period and the parents must be counseled. It is not unreasonable to send such infants home with an apnea monitor.

SPECIAL PROBLEMS

The Child With a Runny Nose

A child who presents for surgery with a runny nose usually has a benign, noninfectious seasonal or vasomotor rhinitis, in which case elective surgery can be safely performed. The runny nose, however, may signal an infectious process or a lower respiratory infection, in which case elective surgery should be postponed.[7] Because 20% to 30% of all children have runny noses for a significant part of the year, every child with a runny nose must be evaluated on an individual basis.

The preanaesthetic assessment of these patients consists of a complete history, a physical examination, and appropriate laboratory tests. Early in the clinical course of infection, the child's history is the single most important factor in the differential diagnosis. Information on allergies should be actively sought. Parents usually can tell whether their child's runny nose is a chronic condition or something different. A finding of fever, rales, or ronchi on physical examination or an elevated white blood cell count indicates a more serious condition and surgery should be postponed. If surgery is postponed because of simple nasopharyngitis, it can be usually rescheduled in 1 to 2 weeks. If symptoms of lower respiratory tract infection are present, surgery should be postponed until at least 1 month after resolution of symptoms.[1]

A situation that often poses a dilemma is that of a child with a severe runny nose who presents for insertion of ventilation tubes for chronic serous otitis media. We usually do not postpone surgery in such children.[7–9] There is no increase in perioperative complications associated with uncomplicated upper respiratory infections.[8,9] Because children with upper respiratory infections are at increased risk of transient postoperative hypoxemia, they should be given supplemental oxygen or have their oxygen saturation monitored during transport after surgery and in the postanesthesia care unit.[10]

The Ex-Premature Infants

The ex-premature infant may not be a suitable candidate for outpatient surgery because of potential immaturity of its respiratory center, temperature control, and gag reflexes. In a retrospective chart review of healthy infants undergoing herniorrhaphy, Steward[11] reported that 12% of preterm infants had prolonged apnea up to 12 h after anesthesia. Subsequently, prospective studies have shown that postoperative apnea after anesthesia occurs in infants 46 to 55 weeks of conceptual age undergoing inguinal herniorapy.[12–14] The infants at greatest risk are those younger than 46 weeks postconceptual age who have histories of apnea. Between 25% to 70% of formerly premature infants younger than 46 weeks develop postoperative apnea.[12–14] Infants at 55 weeks' gestational age or younger scheduled for more invasive procedures, such as abdominal or neurosurgical procedures, are at risk for developing postoperative apnea.[15] In general, the younger the infant's gestational and postconceptual ages, the more frequent the incidence of periodic breathing.[16] However, the clinical significance of apneic episodes that result in bradycardia and arterial oxygen desaturation but eventually self-correct before cardiorespiratory arrest develops is not known. The risk of postoperative apnea is present at least 12 to 18 h postoperatively, so such patients are not suitable for outpatient surgery.[17]

In brief, the anesthesiologist must be aware that a history of prematurity is a "red flag"; such infants must be observed carefully for episodes of postoperative apnea. Until more extensive, meticulous, prospective studies are carried out, it seems prudent to admit to the hospital all ex-premature infants younger than 46 weeks' postconceptual age who are scheduled for surgery and then monitor them for postoperative apnea, bradycardia, and oxygen desaturation. If the infant has bronchopulmonary dysplasia (BPD), this period should be extended for as long as the infant is symptomatic. It is also appropriate to individualize all decisions and, when in doubt, to err on the side of caution. Should any questions arise, inpatient care is recommended.

A single intravenous dose of 10 mg/kg of caffeine at the beginning of surgery may control postanesthetic apnea in former premature infants.[18] However, until more extensive studies with this approach are available, all infants at risk should be monitored for apnea or bradycardia after anesthesia.

The age at which the premature infant attains physiologic maturity and no longer presents an increased risk must be determined individually. As the child matures, the tendency toward apnea greatly diminishes, but no one knows the age when all infants can be anesthetized safely on an outpatient basis. Factors that govern decision-making include the infant's growth and development, problems during feeding, frequency of upper respiratory infections, and a history of apnea or metabolic, endocrine, neurologic, or cardiac disorders.

Bronchopulmonary Dysplasia

The infant with BPD presents several problems, including decreased pulmonary function with airway hyperreactivity, residual lung disease that may cause hypoxia and hypercarbia, and an abnormal response to hypoxia, which can lead to apnea, further hypoxia, bradycardia, and sometimes death.[16] Decisions regarding a patient's suitability for outpatient surgery must be made on an individual basis. Patients with persistent wheezing, hypercarbia, and oxygen dependency are generally unsuitable for outpatient surgery. They should be admitted to the hospital for preoperative treatment that will optimize their physical condition. Cardiorespiratory monitoring often is required after surgery.

THE CHILD WITH A HEART MURMUR

More than 50% of children will have a heart murmur some time before adolescence. Many such murmurs are first heard during the preanesthetic examination. Even if the child is asymptomatic, the cause of the murmur should be diagnosed before anesthesia and surgery. Newburger et al. concluded that a pediatric cardiologist can reliably confirm an innocent murmur by physical examination alone.[19] Whether other physicians including general pediatricians can consistently diagnose an organic murmur is debatable. At the Children's National Medical Center, the form shown in Table 3-1 serves as a guide to determine the need for a cardiology consultation. It is generally safe to proceed with surgery if the child has normal growth and activity patterns and the murmur is characterized as low intensity, nonradiating, and early systolic. When in doubt, it is best to consult a cardiologist.

A child with a murmur may not require specific preoperative cardiac therapy or even a modification in the selection of anesthetic agents and technique. However, such a child usually does need antibiotic prophylaxis to prevent subacute bacterial endocarditis. Children who have innocent heart murmurs do not require subacute bacterial endocarditis prophylaxis. Prophylaxis also is not required for orotracheal intubation and myringotomy.

The most recent guidelines from the American Heart Association do not recommend a second dose of antibiotics, thereby eliminating the need for medication at home[20] (Table 3-2). For quick reference, every anesthesiology department should have available the most recent guidelines from the American Heart Association for the prevention of bacterial endocarditis[20] (Table 3-3).

CONGENITAL OR ACQUIRED HEART DISEASE

Congenital heart disease occurs in 0.08% of newborn infants. The decision to schedule a child with heart disease for outpatient surgery must be made only after communication with the cardiologist and surgeon. If the cardiac status

TABLE 3–1 The Child With a Heart Murmur

Clinical Diagnosis by	No heart disease	Possible heart disease		Definite heart disease
Anesthesiologist	Yes	Yes	No	Yes
Pediatrician	Yes	No	Yes	Yes
Cardiology consult?	No	Yes	Yes	Yes

TABLE 3–2 Prophylactic Regimens for Dental, Oral, Respiratory Tract, or Esophageal Procedures

Situation	Agent	Regimen
Standard general prophylaxis	Amoxicillin	Audlts: 2.0 g; children: 50 mg/kg orally 1 h before procedure
Unable to take oral medications	Ampicillin	Adults: 2.0 g IM or IV; children: 50 mg/kg IM or IV within 30 min before procedure
Allergic to penicillin	Clindamycin* or	Adults: 600 mg; children: 20 mg/kg orally 1 h before procedure
	Cephalexin[†] or cefadroxil[†] or	Adults: 2.0 g; children; 50 mg/kg orally 1 h before procedure
	Azithromycin or clarithromycin	Adults: 500 mg; children: 15 mg/kg orally 1 h before procedure
Allergic to penicillin and unable to take oral medications	Clindamycin or	Adults: 600 mg; children: 20 mg/kg IV within 30 min before procedure
	Cefazolin[†]	Adults: 1.0 g; children: 25 mg/kg IM or IV within 30 min before procedure

IM, intramuscular; IV, intravenous.
*Total children's dose should not exceed adult dose.
[†]Cephalosporins should not be used in individuals with immediate-type hypersensitivity reaction (urticaria, angioedema, or anaphylaxis) to penicillins.
Source: American Heart Association. *Prevention of Bacterial Endocarditis: AHA Medical/Scientific Statement,* 1998.

TABLE 3–3 Prevention of Bacterial Endocarditis

Endocarditis prophylaxis recommended
  High-risk category
    Prosthetic cardiac valves, including bioprosthetic and homograft values
    Previous bacterial endocarditis
    Complex cyanotic congenital heart disease (e.g., single ventricle states, transposition of great arteries, tetralogy of Fallot)
    Surgically constructed systemic pulmonary shunts or conduits
  Moderate-risk category
    Most other congenital cardiac malformations (other than those above and below)
    Acquired valvar dysfunction (e.g., rheumatic heart disease)
    Hypertrophic cardiomyopathy
    Mitral valve prolapse with valvar regurgitation and/or thickened leaflets
Endocarditis prophylaxis not recommended
  Negligible-risk category (risk not greater than in the general population)
    Isolated secundum atrial septal defect
    Surgical repair of atrial septal defect, ventricular septal defect, or patent ductus arteriosus (without residua beyond 6 mo)
    Previous coronary artery bypass graft surgery
    Mitral valve prolapse without valvar regurgitation
    Physiologic, functional, or innocent heart murmurs
    Previous Kawasaki disease without valvar dysfunction
    Previous rheumatic fever without valvar dysfunction
    Cardiac pacemakers (intravascular and epicardial) and implanted defibrillators

Source: American Heart Association. *Prevention of Bacterial Endocarditis: AHA Medical/Scientific Statement,* 1998.

is stable and a cardiologist has been following the child, outpatient surgery may be appropriate. The responses to four questions should determine the anesthetic plan[21]: (1) Is there a cardiac shunt? (e.g., ventricular septal defect); (2) Is there obstruction to blood flow? (e.g., valvular stenosis, coarctation); (3) What are the consequences of the defect? (e.g., congestive heart failure, cyanosis); and (4) What is the relation of pulmonary vascular resistance to systemic vascular resistance?

If there is a cardiac shunt, meticulous attention should be paid to eliminating air bubbles from the intravenous lines and to maintain a left-to-right shunt flow. Patients with congestive heart failure must continue to receive all medications until the morning of surgery. If the child is cyanotic due to decreased blood flow to the lungs secondary to increased pulmonary vascular resistance, hyperventilation and a high fraction of inspired oxygen will improve blood flow to the lungs. If pulmonary flow is excessive due to the cardiac defect, then ventilation with positive end-expiratory pressure and reducing inspired oxygen concentration will decrease pulmonary blood flow.

Patients with the following risk factors have increased rates of complications after ambulatory surgery and, hence, may not be suitable for outpatient surgery.[22]

1. Cyanotic heart disease
2. Pulmonary hypertension
3. Congestive heart failure
4. Younger than 2 years
5. Poor general health

If there is any question about the stability of the cardiac lesion, hospital admission should be advised. Patients requiring routine supplemental oxygen should be hospitalized.

ASTHMA

The prevalence of asthma among children in the United States is 7.6%. It is the most common major disease among children. Most children have their first attack before their third birthday.[23] The prevalence of asthma is rising, as are hospitalization and mortality rates associated with this condition. Asthma is one of the four most common problems identified during preoperative telephone screening for pediatric outpatient surgery.[1] Patients with asthma may be subgrouped into one of the following three categories.

1. Patients who have infrequent attacks, often associated with a cold, exercise, or allergies. They require minimal medication, and inhalers easily controls their wheezing. Such patients are suitable candidates for outpatient surgery.
2. These patients have moderately severe asthma that requires continuous therapy. It is important to know their baseline status and communicate directly with their primary physicians before scheduling them for outpatient surgery. Should outpatient surgery be scheduled, these children must receive their medications until the morning of surgery. A β-agonist should be administered in the operating room holding area. If the patient has persistent cough, wheezing, or tachypnea on the day of surgery, it is best to reschedule surgery.
3. Children with severe asthma who are never completely free of wheezing. If surgery is needed, they usually require admission to the hospital.

MALIGNANT HYPERTHERMIA

Many children are presumed to be malignant hyperthermia susceptible (MHS) because of a family history suggestive of MH or a previously suspected MH reaction. Few patients actually have biopsy-proven MHS. Children otherwise suitable for outpatient surgery often are hospitalized overnight solely because of known or suspected to be MHS. Yentis et al.[24] concluded from their retrospective analysis that postoperative admission to the hospital solely on the basis of MHS labels is not warranted. Intraoperative use of nontriggering agents and 4 h of postoperative observation are recommended.

CONCLUSION

The experiences of the past decade have proved that outpatient surgery is safe and cost effective. The number of patients undergoing outpatient surgery has climbed to more than 70%. Although the future growth rate is not likely to be as exponential as in the 1980s, payors will continue to exert pressure to perform more procedures on an outpatient basis. Performing more complex procedures on sicker patients will be a continuing challenge for outpatient surgery centers. The keys to success are careful patient selection and meticulous intraoperative and postoperative care.

REFERENCES

1. Hannallah RS, Epstein BS. Management of the pediatric patient. In *Anesthesia for Outpatient Surgery*, 2nd ed. Wetchler BV, ed. Philadelphia, JB Lippincott, 1991, p 131.
2. Everett LL, Kallar SK: Presurgical evaluation and laboratory testing. In *The Ambulatory Anesthesia Handbook*. Twersky RD, ed. St. Louis, Mosby, 1995, p 1.
3. Patel RI, Hannallah RS: Preoperative screening for pediatric outpatient surgery: evaluation of a telephone questionnaire method. *Anesth Analg* 75:258, 1992.
4. White PF: Ambulatory anesthesia and surgery: past, present and future. In *Ambulatory Anesthesia and Surgery*. White PF, ed. London, Saunders, 1997, p 9.
5. Steward DJ: Is there risk of general anesthesia triggering SIDS? Possibly not! *Anesthesiology* 63:326, 1985.
6. Tetzlaff JE, Anand DW, Pudimat MA, Nicodemus HF: Postoperative apnea in a full term infant. *Anesthesiology* 69:426, 1989.
7. Berry FA: The child with the runny nose. In *Anesthetic Management of Difficult and Routine Pediatric Patients*, Berry FA, ed. New York, Churchill-Livingstone, 1986, p 349.
8. Tait AR, Knight PR: Intraoperative respiratory complications in patients with upper respiratory tract infections. *Can J Anaesth* 34:300, 1987.
9. Tait AR, Knight PR: The effect of general anesthesia on upper respiratory tract infections in children. *Anesthesiology* 67:930, 1987.
10. DeSoto H, Patel RI, Soliman IE, Hannallah RS: Changes in oxygen saturation following general anesthesia in children with upper respiratory infection signs and symptoms undergoing otolaryngological procedures. *Anesthesiology* 68:276, 1988.
11. Steward DJ: Pre-term infants are more prone to complications following minor surgery than are term infants. *Anesthesiology* 56:304, 1982.
12. Liu LMP, Cote CJ, Goudsouzian NG, et al: Life-threatening apnea in infants recovering from anesthesia. *Anesthesiology* 59:506, 1983.
13. Welborn LG, Ramirez N, Oh TH, et al: Postanesthetic apnea and periodic breathing in infants. *Anesthesiology* 65:658, 1986.
14. Welborn LG, DeSoto H, Hannallah RS, et al: The use of caffeine in the control of post-anesthetic apnea in former premature infants. *Anesthesiology* 68:796, 1988.

15. Kurth CD, Spitzer AR, Broennle AM, et al: Postoperative apnea in preterm infants. *Anesthesiology* 66:483, 1987.
16. Coté CJ, Zaslavsky A, Downes JJ, et al: Postoperative apnea in former preterm infants after inguinal herniorrhaphy. *Anesthesiology* 82:809, 1995.
17. Berry FA. Preoperative assessment of pediatric patient. In *Outpatient Anesthesia.* White PF, ed. New York: Churchill-Livingstone 1990, p 147.
18. Welborn LG, Hannallah RS, Fink R, et al: High-dose caffeine suppresses postoperative apnea in former preterm infants. *Anesthesiology* 71:347, 1989.
19. Newburger JW, Rosenthal A, Williams RG, et al: Noninvasive tests in the initial evaluation of heart murmurs in children. *N Engl J Med* 308:61, 1983.
20. American Heart Association: *Prevention of Bacterial Endocarditis: AHA Medical/Scientific Statement,* 1998.
21. Campbell FW, Schwartz AJ: Anesthesia for non-cardiac surgery in the pediatric patient with congenital heart disease. *Refresher Course Lectures Anesthesiol* 14:75, 1986.
22. Warner MA: The ex-premie, the congenital heart disease patient or the pediatric patient with asthma for outpatient surgery. Paper presented at the 14th Annual Meeting of the Society for Ambulatory Anesthesia, 1999.
23. Gerge PJ, Mullally DI, Evans R III: National survey of prevalence of asthma among children in the United States, 1976 to 1980. *Pediatrics* 81:1, 1988.
24. Yentis SM, Levine MF, Hartley EJ: Should all children with suspected or confirmed malignant hyperthermia susceptibility be admitted after surgery? A 10-year review. *Anesth Analg* 75:345, 1992.

4 | Appropriate Laboratory and Radiologic Testing in Children

Ramesh I. Patel, MD
Raafat S. Hannallah, MD

Preoperative evaluation of pediatric patients consists of a history, physical examination, and appropriate laboratory and radiological tests. Such testing should be based on the patient's history and physical findings in addition to objective criteria for laboratory tests. Data from the Mayo Clinic indicated that patients undergoing minimally invasive surgery have little to benefit from additional laboratory testing, if a careful medical history has been obtained and a physician has decided that no preoperative tests are required.[1] In general, a patient's medical history and physical examination are far more important than a battery of tests to make a diagnosis. About 85% of diagnoses depend on the history provided by the patient or parents, another 6% of diagnoses are made by physical examination, and tests add another 8% of the diagnosis in medical outpatients.[2] The practice of ordering batteries of tests unnecessarily has many disadvantages: it is not cost effective, it decreases health care funds for others, it may lead to inadequate or inappropriate care as a result of the time-consuming follow-up of test results, it increases risk to the patient, and it increases medicolegal risk to the health care provider.[3] Asymptomatic patients are more likely to be harmed by unwarranted tests and the physician's actions in response to the abnormal results of those tests. Despite lack of evidence that routine preoperative testing of healthy children before elective surgery is warranted, this practice continues in many health care facilities. State- or institution-mandated testing is far less prevalent than previously reported, but physician-recommended testing still comprises a large part of routine tests.

INDICATIONS FOR TESTING

Assuming that a medical history has been obtained and the physical examination performed, the possible medical reasons for preoperative investigations are:

1. to detect unsuspected conditions. A finding of a new condition may alter the risk of surgery. The previously unidentified condition may be correctable or not correctable. If the condition is corrected preoperatively, it leads to a lower risk of surgery. If the condition is not modifiable, it is simply noted for the sake of completing medicolegal records[4];
2. to obtain baseline results that may be helpful in decision-making during and after surgery (e.g., preoperative hemoglobin value to determine allowable blood loss during surgery)[4];
3. to screen for conditions unrelated to the planned surgery;
4. to satisfy institutional or legislative criteria;
5. habit.[5]

However, healthy children who are scheduled to undergo surgical procedures that are not associated with the possibility of extensive blood loss require only minimal preoperative laboratory testing. In some instances, such testing is governed by hospital or state policy.

HEMOGLOBIN AND HEMATOCRIT

Until recently, the routine measurement of blood hemoglobin (Hb) concentration or hematocrit (Hct) before elective surgery had been a widely accepted practice. It was assumed that routine preoperative Hb/Hct testing would detect a significant number of anemic children and that the risk of general anesthesia increased with even mild anemia. It has been since noted that the incidence of anemia in otherwise healthy children is extremely low in most parts of the North America and Europe and mild degrees of anemia do not require therapeutic intervention or modification of the anesthetic technique.[6] Most anesthesiologists now accept Hct levels of 25 mg/dL or so for elective surgical procedures, provided there are no other systemic problems. Our current practice is not to order routine Hb/Hct tests in any patient but to obtain tests after evaluation of the medical history and any proposed surgical procedure. The most common reason to obtain a preoperative Hb/Hct is to assess allowable blood loss during surgery.

The usefulness of routine preoperative Hb/Hct determinations has been evaluated and the value of this test has been questioned.[7-10] Baron et al. in a retrospective review found that only 1.1% of the 1863 children studied had Hct values of less than 30% or greater than 50%.[11] Roy et al. studied 2000 patients with ages from 1 month to 18 years scheduled for minor surgery.[7] Eleven patients (three younger than 1 year and eight 1 to 5 years old) had a Hb less than 10 g/%. Of these, three patients had their surgeries postponed and rescheduled after oral iron therapy; the remaining eight underwent anesthesia and surgery without complications. Those investigators concluded that healthy pediatric patients 5 years and older who are scheduled for minor surgery do not require routine Hb determinations. Further, the low incidence of anemia and low rate of deferral for surgery in anemic children 1 to 5 years of age led them to question the value of routine preoperative Hb testing in this age group.[7] Hackmann et al. found anemia in 0.5% of the 2648 pediatric day-surgery patients studied.[9] Only two of the anemic patients had their surgeries postponed (one also had a respiratory infection). They reported three observations from their study:

1. The incidence of anemia is rare but is more likely to occur in those younger than 1 year.
2. A mild degree of anemia does not alter the decision to proceed with day surgery.
3. Physicians cannot reliably detect anemia clinically.[9]

The present view is that a thorough medical history and physical examination are more important than routine laboratory tests in determining a child's fitness for surgery.

There are three groups of patients who are at increased risk of having anemia:

1. infants younger than 1 year;
2. adolescent menstruating females;
3. children with chronic disease.[12,13]

One of the common causes of anemia in adolescent females is heavy menstrual periods. The precise incidence of anemia in presurgical patients in this group is not known. Preoperative Hb/Hct testing may be indicated in such patients and those undergoing surgical procedures associated with considerable blood loss. A recent survey of pediatric anesthesiologists in the United States found that only 50% order routine Hb/Hct tests in infants younger than 1 year and only 33% require routine Hb/Hct tests in adolescents.[14]

COMPLETE BLOOD COUNT

We rarely order a complete blood count before ambulatory surgery. The possible benefits of performing a complete blood count routinely would be the detection of leukopenia or leukocytosis reflecting hematologic malignancies or infection.[4] O'Connor and Drasner found abnormal white blood cell counts in 13 of 486 (2.7%) patients.[8] None of the children in that study had their surgeries canceled. One instance of elevated white blood cell count was thought to be secondary to chronic otitis media. The remaining 12 elevated counts were unexplained, with no documented follow-up.

URINE ANALYSIS

Urinanalysis (UA) is rarely ordered preoperatively. The rationale for performing routine US before surgery is detecting and then treating children with unsuspected renal disease and urinary tract infections. However, O'Connor and Drasner found clinically abnormal UA results in 36 of 453 (8%) patients.[8] Of those abnormal results, 12 were related to known conditions, and repeat studies in another 12 patients showed normal UA. The remaining 12 patients had no documented follow-up. Surgeries were canceled in two children. One infant returned a week later for emergency surgery and another infant was operated on after treatment of a urinary tract infection. The researchers concluded that routine UA adds little to the preoperative evaluation of a healthy child and should be omitted. Our survey indicated that the practices of most institutions reflect this recommendation in that routine UA is ordered by only 15% of physicians.[14]

COAGULATION TESTING

Because of the conflicting results of the studies and individual clinical experiences, the hemostatic evaluation of patients undergoing surgery, especially tonsillectomy, has not been uniform despite recommendations by the American Academy of Otolaryngology–Head and Neck Surgery that coagulation studies should be performed only in patients with positive histories and physical examinations.[15] Despite those recommendations, approximately 40% to 50% of respondents to a questionnaire on hemostatic laboratory tests before tonsillectomy stated that they continue to obtain prothrombin time (PT) and partial thromboplastin time (PTT) before tonsillectomy.[14] We order hemostatic tests before tonsillectomy only when the child'd medical history suggests a bleeding problem.

The incidence of posttonsillectomy bleeding ranges from 0.28% to 2.15%.[16,17] It is arguable whether routine preoperative hemostatic (PT/PTT) tests should be performed in all children scheduled for tonsillectomy. Even if the hemostatic tests are performed for all such children, there is evidence that those tests will not predict all cases of posttonsillectomy bleeding. Excessive bleeding associated with tonsillectomy usually is not a result of an identifiable coagulation disorder.[16] Close et al. suggested that routine measurements of the activated PTT (APTT) and PT in asymptomatic patients undergoing tonsillectomy are not useful for predicting postoperative bleeding.[15] Houry et al. prospectively compared the results of four standard preoperative hemostatic screening tests (PT, APTT, platelet count, and bleeding time) with medical history and clinical data in a multicenter study of 3242 patients.[18] Their results suggested that preoperative hemostatic screening tests should not be performed routinely, but only in patients with abnormal clinical data. In contrast, Bolger et al. found that 21% of patients undergoing tonsillectomy had an abnormal APTT, PT, or bleeding time and suggested that these tests be performed in all patients to detect possible coagulation disorders.[19] Most pediatric anesthesiologists do not order hemostatic profiles for healthy children undergoing tonsillectomy.

PREGNANCY TEST

Even though the overall pregnancy rate in the presurgical patient may be low, there are many social, ethical, and medicolegal concerns when an adolescent scheduled for outpatient surgery tests positive for pregnancy just before surgery. For this reason, it is not surprising that pregnancy tests are routinely required by about 45% of anesthesiologists.[14]

At our institution, we do not perform routine pregnancy testing in adolescent patients. Instead, we rely on the medical history provided by the patient. On the morning of surgery, the nursing staff of the outpatient surgical admissions unit escort the adolescent away from the parents and confidentially elicit her history of sexual activity and the possibility of pregnancy. The patient is informed of the risks of anesthesia and surgery for a pregnant patient. The anesthesiologist or the operating room nursing staff again try to confirm the history just before induction of anesthesia. Whenever the history is suggestive of pregnancy or if the medical history is inconclusive, a urine pregnancy test is obtained. If this test is negative, no further action is necessary and the surgery proceeds without further delay. However, if the urine pregnancy test is positive, then a blood pregnancy test is ordered with parental approval to verify the results of the urine test. If the blood test is positive, then the adolescent and her parents are informed and the plan for elective surgery is modified.

The rate of teenage pregnancies in the United States is high, not only in urban populations but also in non-urban areas. Teenage pregnancy represents 13% to 23% of total pregnancies in the United States.[20] Because of the potential concerns over teratogenicity and miscarriages, elective surgery under general anesthesia is not advised. An accurate medical history often is not obtained because adolescents may not believe that they could be pregnant and are reluctant to disclose their sexual behavior or pregnancy.

Azzam et al. retrospectively examined the results of 2 years of mandatory pregnancy testing in 412 adolescent surgical patients.[21] Pregnancy testing was performed without patients' or their parents' specific consent, as it was deemed a component of the preoperative evaluation and the practice had been approved by the medical staff bylaws. The overall incidence of positive tests was 1.2%. Five of 207 patients who were older than 15 years tested positive for pregnancy, an incidence of 2.4% in that group. None of the 205 patients younger than 15 years had a positive pregnancy test. The surgical procedure was postponed in three patients, performed under local anesthesia in one patient, and general anesthesia without nitrous oxide was administered to another patient. The investigators concluded that mandatory pregnancy testing is advisable in adolescent surgical patients 15 years and older.[21] In an editorial comment in response to that study, Duncam and Pope questioned the ethical, financial, and legal grounds of performing pregnancy tests without consent from each patient or her parents.[22]

In contrast, Malviya et al. prospectively evaluated the reliability of the preoperative history obtained from adolescent patients in ruling out pregnancy.[23] Four hundred fourty-four adolescent patients who underwent 525 procedures were questioned preoperatively regarding the possibility of pregnancy. Regardless of the history, urine pregnancy tests were ordered. In 514 cases, patients or their parents denied the possibility of pregnancy. Eight patients stated that they might be pregnant. Seventeen patients were not tested due to patient or parental refusal. All pregnancy tests were negative. There was not a single patient who was pregnant. They concluded that adolescents educated about the potential risks of anesthetics may provide a reliable history with regard to the possibility of pregnancy.[23]

SICKLE CELL DISEASE

Routine preoperative sickle cell testing is not performed, but we order Hb/Hct testing and electropheresis for Hb-SS for children known to have sickle cell disease. The incidence of sickle cell disease is estimated to be 0.2% to 0.5% among the African American population. The incidence of sickle cell trait is about 8% in the same population. Routine testing for sickle cell disease often is done by the neonatologist or pediatrician. The diagnosis usually is made in the first year of life and it is rare for an undiagnosed child to be scheduled for routine surgery. African American children with low Hb/Hct levels, however, should be tested. Frequently, the diagnosis of sickle cell disease is known before surgery but the child has not had any preoperative preparation. It is crucial that the severity of the sickle cell disease is known and that the hematologist has adequately prepared the child for general anesthesia and surgery.

CHEST RADIOGRAPH

Of all the preoperative tests, the chest radiograph has been most objectively studied in adults. This was never a routine test in children before surgery. The American Academy of Pediatrics recommended eliminating this test as part of a routine preoperative assessment as long ago as 1983. However, the increasing incidence of infections such as human immunodeficiency virus and tuberculosis raises concerns for the protection of other patients who share the same playroom or holding area and health care workers.

LEGISLATIVE MANDATE

The Joint Commission on Accreditation of Healthcare Organizations, which is responsible for the accreditation of health care facilities in the United States, only requires that any indicated laboratory or x-ray examination be completed preoperatively.[24] There are no specifically mandated tests before surgery. Similarly, the American Society of Anesthesiologists, the American College of Surgeons, and the American Academy of Pediatrics have no guidelines recommending specific routine preoperative laboratory tests.[4] Individual states and local requirements may differ.

In conclusion, routine laboratory and radiologic tests are not necessary. Test results are obtained on the basis of the patient's medical history and physical examination.

REFERENCES

1. Warner MA, Shields SE, Chute CG: Major morbidity and mortality within 1 month of ambulatory surgery and anesthesia. *JAMA* 270:1437, 1993.
2. Mamton JR, Harrison MJB, Mitchell JRA, et al: Relative contributions of history taking, physical examination and laboratory investigation to diagnosis and management of medical outpatients. *BMJ* 31:486, 1975.
3. Roizen MF, Fischer SP: Preoperative evaluation: adults and children. In *Ambulatory Anesthesia and Surgery*. White PF, ed. London, WB Saunders, 1997, p 155.
4. Hannallah RS: Preoperative investigations: clinical review. *Paediatr Anaesth* 5:325, 1995.
5. Macpherson DS: Preoperative laboratory testing: should any tests be "routine" before surgery? *Med Clin North Am* 77:289, 1993.
6. Steward DJ: Screening tests before surgery in children. *Can J Anesth* 38:693, 1991.
7. Roy WL, Lerman J, McIntyre BG: Is preoperative hemoglobin testing justified in children undergoing minor elective surgery? *Can J Anaesth* 38:700, 1991.
8. O'Connor ME, Drasner K: Preoperative laboratory testing of children undergoing elective surgery. *Anesth Analg* 70:176, 1990.
9. Hackmann T, Steward DJ, Sheps SB: Anemia in pediatric day-surgery patients: prevalence and detection. *Anesthesiology* 75:27, 1991.
10. Livesey JR: Are hematological tests warranted prior to tonsillectomy? *J Laryngol Otol* 107:205, 1993.
11. Baron MJ, Gunter J, White P: Is the pediatric preoperative hematocrit determination necessary? *South Med J* 85:1187, 1992.
12. Welborn LG, Hannallah RS, Luban NLC, et al: Anemia and postoperative apnea in former preterm infants. *Anesthesiology* 74:1003, 1991.
13. Patel RI, Hannallah RS: Patient selection criteria for pediatric ambulatory surgery. *Ambulat Surg* 1:183, 1993.
14. Patel RI, DeWitt L, Hannallah RS: Preoperative laboratory testing in children undergoing elective surgery: analysis of current practice. *J Clin Anesth* 9:569, 1997.
15. Close HL, Kryzer TC, Nowlin JH, et al: Hemostatic assessment of patients before tonsillectomy: a prospective study. *Otolaryngol Head Neck Surg* 111:733, 1994.
16. Crysdale WS, Russell D: Complications of tonsillectomy and adenoidectomy in 9409 children observed overnight. *Can Med Assoc J* 35:1139, 1986.
17. Maniglia AJ, Kushner M, Cozzi L: Adenotonsillectomy—a safe outpatient procedure. *Arch Otolaryngol Head Neck Surg* 15:92, 1989.
18. Houry S, Georgeac C, Hay JM, et al: A prospective multicenter evaluation of preoperative hemostatic screening tests. *Am J Surg* 170:19, 1995.
19. Bolger WE, Parsons DS, Potempa L: Preoperative hemostatic assessment of the adenotonsillectomy patients. *Otolaryngol Head Neck Surg* 3:396, 1990.
20. Stevens-Simon C, White MM: Adolescent pregnancy. *Pediatr Ann* 20:322, 1991.
21. Azzam FJ, Padda GS, DeBoard JW, et al: Preoperative pregnancy testing in adolescents. *Anesth Analg* 82:4, 1996.
22. Duncan PG, Pope WDB: Medical ethics and legal standards. *Anesth Analg* 82:1, 1996.
23. Malviya S, D'Errico C, Reynolds P, et al: Should pregnancy testing be routine in adolescent patients prior to surgery? *Anesth Analg* 83:854, 1996.

5 | Preanesthetic Sedation for Pediatric Patients Lacking Intravenous Access

George D. Politis, MD

Preanesthetic sedative administration is commonly practiced in all age groups but is arguably most important in the pediatric population. More than 90% of healthy infants and children in the United States who come for anesthesia with no intravenous line in place receive an inhalation induction.[1] They rarely comprehend our good intentions when we separate them from their families and force them to inhale harsh anesthetic gases. Frightening induction experiences are not only unpleasant for pediatric patients and operating room personnel, they also appear to cause negative behavioral manifestations that persist for weeks or months after surgery. Preanesthetic sedatives can quell separation fears, facilitate acceptance of inhalation agents, and decrease the incidence of postoperative behavioral and sleep disturbances.[2] Also, laryngospasm may occur less frequently when a preoperative sedative has been administered.[3] As with all good things, the benefits of preanesthetic sedation may come at a price. Depending on the sedative and the route chosen, administration of preanesthetic sedation may affect the respiratory and cardiovascular systems, leading to a need for heightened vigilance or even monitoring in the preoperative area. Surgery may be delayed while waiting for adequate sedative effect, and anesthetic emergence and recovery can be delayed. As outlined in this chapter, the potential negative effects of preanesthetic sedation can be nearly eliminated when certain sedatives and routes are chosen, and when the time courses of sedative effects are understood.

Despite the many good reasons noted above for administration of preoperative sedation to pediatric patients, children are less likely than adults to receive it.[4] In fact, in the United States only 40% to 50% of children between 6 months and 7 years of age receive a preanesthetic sedative.[5] Various factors may contribute to this deficiency, including the mistaken beliefs that presence of a parent at induction may substitute for preanesthetic sedation and that children who are calm in the presence of their parents will remain calm with separation and anesthetic induction. Another contributing factor may be cost and efficiency requirements of the managed care environment, as shown by less use of premedication in geographic regions where penetration of managed care is greatest.[5] Lack of knowledge regarding the benefits of preanesthetic sedation and the means to minimize its potential negative effects also may limit its usage.

The presence of a parent during induction may improve cooperation in some children who have not received preanesthetic sedation, but it does not provide the same degree of cooperation and anxiolysis achieved with sedation. A comparison of parental presence without sedation versus midazolam preanesthetic sedation without a parent present found anxiety levels to be greater in patients and parents in the parent-present group.[6] In addition, patient cooperation at induction was greater in the midazolam group. When no preanesthetic sedative has been given, the presence of a parent may increase or decrease patient anxiety levels depending on whether the parent is anxious or calm, respectively.[7,8] Because some parents strongly desire to be present at induction and satisfaction of families is an important goal, parental participation should be considered when requested by a family. Usually, parents no longer feel the need to be present at induction after witnessing the calming effects of a good preanesthetic sedative. Evidence clearly suggests that the decision regarding whether to administer a preanesthetic sedative should not be based on whether a parent will be present.

Deciding which children will cooperate without sedation is difficult, if not impossible. Busy schedules of surgical suites rarely allow time for premedication when the need is first recognized at the time of separation. Therefore, a practical approach is to administer preanesthetic sedation to all children between the ages of 9 months and 8 years who have no medical contraindication. Whether to administer a sedative to infants in the 7- to 9-month age range can be based on their degree of stranger anxiety, which can be accessed by holding the infant. Infants younger than 7 months generally tolerate induction without sedation. Children 8 years and older often cooperate even without having received a sedative, so the decision on whether to sedate can be individualized according to the child's maturity and anxiety levels. Because preanesthetic sedatives administered in the doses discussed below rarely cause unconsciousness, establishing rapport and maintaining verbal contact with patients throughout the preinduction and induction periods is crucial for alleviating fears and achieving satisfactory patient cooperation.

Whether to coadminister muscarinic blockers such as atropine or glycopyrulate with preanesthetic sedatives has been controversial. The ability of atropine to decrease secretions during induction is suspect because peak decrease in salivation occurs at 2 h,[9] as does time-to-peak serum concentration.[10] Recent evidence has demonstrated that 40 mg/kg of oral atropine decreases laryngospasm during halothane induction,[11] but dosing was 1 h before induction, which would be impractical for coadministration with sedatives such as oral midazolam, which lose effectiveness by that time. Whether or not atropine can prevent laryngospasm during sevoflurane induction is unknown. Oral atropine may attenuate cardiovascular depression associated with halothane anesthesia in infants when given at 20 or 40 µg/kg and administered 30 to 90 min before induction.[12] Oral glycopyrulate appears to be less effective than oral atropine at attenuating the bradycardia associated with halothane induction, even when glycopyrulate is administered at 50 µg/kg as opposed to 20 µg/kg of atropine.[13] Rectally administered atropine has a more rapid onset than orally administered atropine, with the peak level occurring at approximately 30 min.[14] The favorable time course of rectal atropine may be advantageous in patients who are suitable for rectal dosing, but the dose required to achieve desired effects is not known. Intramuscular dosing of atropine also has a peak level near 30 min, requires approximately half the oral dose,[9] but is infrequently considered because of the unpleasant aspect of the injection. Reasons to consider avoiding antimuscarinic premedication are the unpleasant side effects of dry mouth, pyrexia, flushing, and tachycardia. Drug-induced rapid heart rate may decrease the anesthesia practitioner's ability to assess the patient's depth of anesthesia and volume status.

A perfect pediatric preanesthetic sedative would be readily accepted by all children, have an instantaneous onset of action, and a duration brief enough to avoid delay of anesthetic emergence and post-anesthetic recovery, even for short procedures. Anxiolysis, amnesia, and cooperation would be certain, and side effects such as nausea and vomiting would be nonexistent. Of course, the sedative would work without causing respiratory or cardiovascular depression, thereby obviating heightened vigilance or monitoring after its administration. Unfortunately, such a perfect agent does not exist, and we must select from medications and routes of administration that have specific strengths and shortcomings. To assist in that choice, this chapter examines the most commonly used preanesthetic sedatives and routes. Material is organized according to routes of administration. Strengths and weaknesses of each sedative and route will be considered, with emphasis on the drugs and routes most frequently used. Dosage ranges, timing of dosages, degree of effectiveness, potential for delaying emergence and recovery, and need for monitoring will be considered. Recommendations in this chapter pertain to children who do not manifest medical conditions that make preanesthetic sedation dangerous. Those situations require exercising clinical judgment based on knowledge of the disease process and the effects of the sedative.

ORAL AND SUBLINGUAL TRANSMUCOSAL ROUTES

The oral route comprises approximately 80% of all pediatric preanesthetic sedation in the United States, and midazolam is overwhelmingly the most commonly used oral premedication.[4] Other commonly administered sedatives include ketamine and fentanyl. The popularity of oral administration is largely due to the nonthreatening and nonpainful nature of this route. However, most sedatives are unsavory, and a lack of patient cooperation can make oral administration impossible. Gradual absorption after oral administration reduces the likelihood of serious respiratory or cardiovascular side effects. In fact, preoperative monitoring does not appear to be necessary when appropriate doses of oral midazolam or ketamine are administered to healthy patients. Oral fentanyl nonetheless may produce such side effects and requires heightened vigilance and use of pulse oximetry. Observation by parents and nurses and restriction of activity are always warranted regardless of the sedative used.

Oral Midazolam

Oral midazolam's popularity is a result of its rapid onset, short duration of action, high efficacy, and wide therapeutic index. An oral formulation is available, but the parenteral solution also may be administered, and the bitterness masked with fruit-flavored syrup or flavored acetaminophen elixir. The recommended dose range for preanesthetic sedation is 0.4 to 0.75 mg/kg. Children heavier than 20 kg seem to require a dose at the lower end of the range, with 15 mg serving as a prudent maximum. Sedative effect is present after 10 min, with maximal effect occurring at 30 min.[15] In one study, 0.5 mg/kg achieved satisfactory sedation for separation from parents in 85% and 96% of patients at 15 and 30 min, respectively, with clinical effect waning by 45 min[15] (Figure 5-1). In addition to sedation, midazolam provides anterograde amnesia[16,17] and anxiolysis.[18] Across a dose range of 0.5 to 1.0 mg/kg, similar sedation and anxiolysis result[18]; however, doses at the higher end of the range may be slightly more efficacious[17] (Figure 5-2). Even at 1.0 mg/kg no adverse hemodynamic or respiratory effects occur, but doses of 0.75 mg/kg or greater may produce more dysphoria, blurred vision, and loss of balance and head control.[18] Oral midazolam in doses as high as 1.0 mg/kg does not appear to delay emergence or recovery after ambulatory

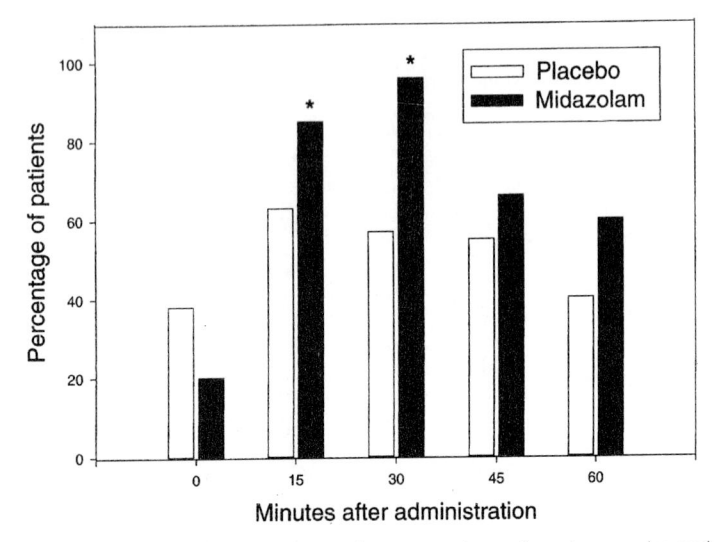

FIG. 5-1 Percentage of patients who were calm and awake or calm and asleep versus time after receiving 0.5 mg/kg of oral midazolam. *Midazolam group greater than placebo group, $p < 0.05$. *(Adapted with permission from Weldon BC, Watcha MF, White PF: Oral midazolam in children: Effect of time and adjunctive therapy.* Anesth Analg *75:51, 1992.)*

anesthesia with halothane plus nitrous oxide,[15,18] but 0.5 mg/kg may delay emergence by 10 min after sevoflurane plus nitrous oxide.[19] Also, preanesthetic sedation with oral midazolam 0.5 mg/kg may delay emergence by 6 to 19 min and recovery by 26 to 60 min if propofol or thiopental is used for induction.[20–22] No information is available regarding the effect of midazolam preanesthetic sedation on the quality of the emergence. However, during the first week after surgery, children who receive a midazolam premedication appear to have less of the negative behavioral effects that are seen in as many as 54% of all children during that period.[2] The behaviors most affected appear to be separation anxiety and eating disturbances.

Optimal timing of oral midazolam administration is 30 min before separation to produce maximal drug effect when most needed and to allow waning of effects by the end of surgery. Due to midazolam's bitter taste, patients frequently spit out part or all of the dose. Redosing once, after most of a dose has been expelled, is safe considering the wide therapeutic index, but consideration should be given to alternative administration routes that require less patient cooperation.

Oral Ketamine

Ketamine is often administered as an oral premedication, although it is considerably less popular than midazolam. As with midazolam, intravenous solutions can be mixed with flavored syrups, but tend to be better accepted than midazolam. Poor bioavailability of oral ketamine requires administration of 3 to 6 mg/kg, which produces adequate sedation for separation in 80% of patients and for induction in 65% to 80%.[23,24] The higher end of this dose range is more efficacious than the lower end, but is still 10% to 15% less effective

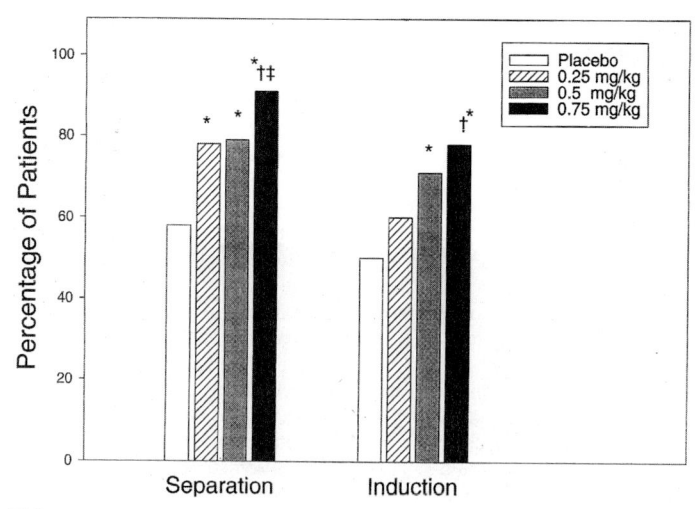

FIG. 5-2 Effectiveness of various doses of oral midazolam given as a preanesthetic sedative to children ages 1 to 10 years. The figure shows the percentage of patients who were calm or easily calmed at the time of separation from parents and during inhalational induction of anesthesia. *Percentage greater than for placebo group, $p < 0.05$. †Percentage greater than for 0.25 mg/kg midazolam group, $p < 0.05$. ‡Percentage greater than for 0.5 mg/kg midazolam group, $p < 0.05$. *(Adapted from Feld LH, Negus JB, White PF: Oral midazolam preanesthetic medication in pediatric patients. Anesthesiology 73:831, 1990.)*

at producing satisfactory sedation than standard doses of oral midazolam.[23] Time to onset of sedation with oral ketamine is approximately 10 min, with maximal sedative effect occurring at 16 to 20 min.[25,26] Oral ketamine at 6 mg/kg reliably achieves amnesia and provides adequate analgesia to allow minimal or no resistance to venous cannulation in two-thirds of patients.[24,26] Common undesirable side effects include nystagmus and tongue fasciculations, and families should be warned to expect these innocuous occurrences. In addition, ketamine causes increased oral secretions. Coadministration of oral atropine does not provide effective antisialagogue activity due to its slow absorption.[26] Emergence delirium has occurred after oral ketamine, albeit rarely. Delayed patient recovery may occur, with delays of 10 to 20 min after approximately 1 h of anesthesia with halothane and nitrous oxide.[23] Oral ketamine 6 mg/kg administered to healthy patients appears to produce no adverse hemodynamic or respiratory effects.[24,26] The recommendations for readministration of an expelled oral ketamine dose is therefore the same as for midazolam.

Oral Transmucosal Fentanyl Citrate (OTFC)

Oral narcotics have been used as pediatric preanesthetic sedatives for more than 50 years but have lost popularity with the introduction of midazolam. Oral transmucosal fentanyl citrate is the narcotic that has gained interest most recently. It is available in 200-, 300-, and 400-µg lollipop formulations, which has created considerable controversy regarding the social implications of a narcotic lollipop despite reasonable efficacy as a sedative premedication[27,28] (see Table 5-1). Oral transmucosal fentanyl citrate has not gained popularity because of its narrow therapeutic range and numerous troublesome side effects. The optimal dose of OTFC appears to be 15 to 20 µg/kg, with a maximum of 400 µg, because this dose provides a balance between efficacy and limited side effects. At that dose, onset and peak sedative effects occur at 18 and 34 min, respectively.[28] However, even 15 to 20 µg/kg increases postoperative nausea and vomiting[28,29] and may precipitate preoperative emesis.[30] Prophylactic antiemetics may partly counter the emetogenic effects of OTFC, although firm evidence remains lacking.[27] Preoperative pruritus occurs in nearly all patients receiving OFTC, and postoperative pruritus occurs in approximately half.[28] Oral transmucosal fentanyl citrate 15 to 20 µg/kg decreases respiratory rate, may lead to oxygen desaturation,[27] has caused chest rigidity,[30] and may delay emergence. Although patient compliance with ingestion is good, approximately 15 min is required for consumption of an oralet. Because OTFC has numerous shortcomings compared with the oral sedatives discussed above, careful consideration should be given before its administration. Oral transmucosal fentanyl citrate should be avoided in patients younger than 2 years or with less than 15 kg of body weight.

Oral Combinations

Combinations of premedications have been used in an effort to enhance effectiveness. For several decades, oral meperidine combined with phenergan and thorazine had been used as a sedative and analgesic cocktail, although it was originally developed as a preanesthetic sedative. It has fallen out of usage due to a high incidence of life-threatening events and because of its excessive duration of action.[31] Oral meperidine 1.5 mg/kg has been combined with 0.5 mg/kg of oral midazolam and does not appear to enhance sedation when compared with midazolam alone, but may slow anesthetic recovery.[15] Oral ketamine (4 mg/kg) combined with oral midazolam (0.4 mg/kg) may be a good choice for patients with previous oral midazolam failure because this combination offers more effective sedation than standard doses of either drug alone.[32] Although these more recently used sedative combinations have not produced serious respiratory or cardiovascular side effects when used in the above doses, studies contain small patient enrollments, so I recommend close observation after their administration.

NASAL TRANSMUCOSAL ROUTE

Nasal administration is the second most common method of pediatric preanesthetic sedative administration in the United States, but comprises only 8% of all those given.[4] The sedative most commonly administered by the nasal route is midazolam, but intranasal sufentanil and ketamine have also been used. Nasal administration has the advantage of a rapid onset and the limited ability of the child to expel the drug. Therefore, it is useful as a primary technique and after other techniques have failed. However, concern has been expressed regarding nasal administration of drugs not approved for that route. That concern is based on a theoretical potential of causing neurotoxicity by direct passage of drugs or preservatives through the cribriform plate and into the spinal fluid.[31] Further, nasal dosing can cause burning and epistaxis. Rapid absorption of nasally administered sedatives leads to greater

TABLE 5–1 Dosages, Time to Onset and Peak Effect, Efficacy, and Monitoring Recommendations for Preanesthetic Sedatives and Routes Most Often Used

Agent	Route	Dosage	Onset (min)	Peak effect (min)	% Efficacy at separation	% Efficacy at induction	Monitoring/observation recommendations[§]
Midazolam	PO	0.4–0.75 mg/kg	10	30	70–89	83	Minimal
	IN	0.2–0.3 mg/kg	5	10	97	81	Close observation
	PR	0.5–1 mg/kg	5–7	12[*]	100	89	Close observation
	IM	0.08–0.15 mg/kg	2–3	22[*]	78	79–90	Close observation
Ketamine	PO	3–6 mg/kg	10–12	16–20	65–90	65–80	Minimal
	IN	5–6 mg/kg	NDA	11	NDA	86	Close observation
	IM	2–3 mg/kg	1–2	2.7[†]	100	100	Close observation
Fentanyl	PO	15–20 μg/kg	18[‡]	34	92	70	Close observation + monitoring
Methohexital	PR	15–30 mg/kg	6	8[†]	> 95	> 95	Close observation + monitoring

IM, intramuscular; IN, intranasal; NDA, no data available; PO, per oral; PR, per rectal.
[*]Time to peak serum level; no data available on time to peak effect.
[†]Time to induction of anesthesia.
[‡]Onset related to dose; larger dose leads to more rapid onset.
[§]Minimal, parental observation required; close observation, constant nurse or physician observation required; close observation + monitoring, close observation plus monitoring with minimum of pulse oximetry.

Intranasal Midazolam

Intranasal midazolam is administered in a dose of 0.2 to 0.3 mg/kg when using the 5 mg/mL intravenous preparation. A 1- or 3-mL syringe containing the midazolam should be placed at the entrance to the nostril, preferably with the head tilted back, and then sprayed rapidly intranasally without the syringe entering the nostril. Crying follows instillation of intranasal midazolam in 71% of recipients and lasts for an average of 45 sec.[33] Peak midazolam levels are achieved at 10 to 13 min after administration,[34,35] but satisfactory sedation generally occurs 5 min sooner.[36] Ten minutes after nasal administration, serum midazolam concentration is 57% of that of an equal dose of intravenous midazolam[34] (Figure 5-3). After intranasal midazolam, 0.2 to 0.3 mg/kg, successful separation from parents occurs in 97% of patients, and 81% are adequately sedated for induction.[33] Amnesia and anxiolysis are presumed to occur at this dose because serum levels achieved generally exceed the levels obtained with doses of oral midazolam known to produce those effects.[36] Adverse respiratory effects are rare, but respiratory depression and even apnea may occur.[36] Nasal midazolam 0.2 to 0.3 mg/kg does not appear to delay emergence or recovery times after brief halothane and nitrous oxide anesthetics.[37]

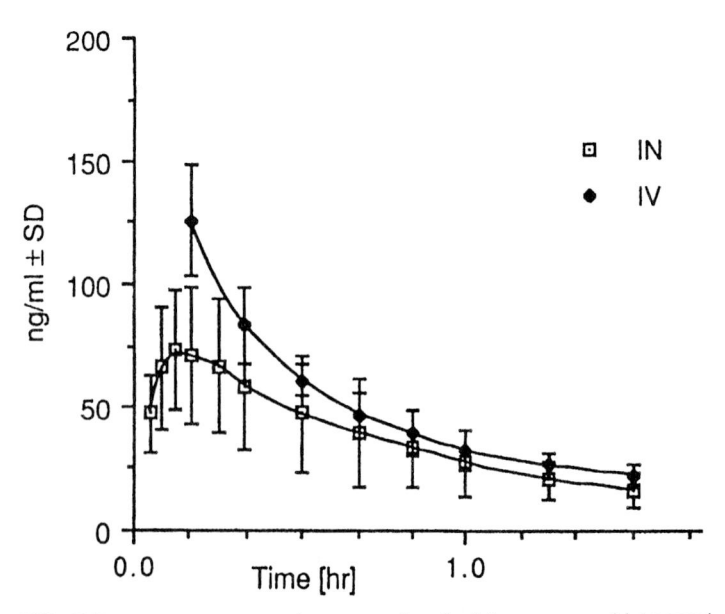

FIG. 5-3 Plasma concentration versus time for intravenous and intranasal midazolam. *(Reprinted with permission from Walbergh EJ, Wills RJ, Eckhert J: Plasma concentrations of midazolam in children following intranasal administration.* Anesthesiology *74:233, 1991.)*

Intranasal Sufentanil

Sufentanil has been administered intranasally with a dose range of 1.5 to 3.0 µg/kg and has a time course similar to that for nasal midazolam. Compared with nasal midazolam, sufentanil causes less nasal irritation. Sufentanil also lessens the reaction to tracheal intubation in patients intubated without muscle relaxants, is associated with decreased maintenance requirements for inhalation anesthetics, and decreases requirements for postoperative analgesics.[38] Nasal sufentanil has not gained popularity because it can decrease chest wall compliance, cause arterial oxygen desaturation, and not infrequently results in postoperative respiratory depression requiring naloxone administration.[38] Intranasal sufentanil is less reliable than nasal midazolam for achievement of adequate sedation,[38,39] may increase the incidence of postoperative nausea and vomiting, and is reported to prolong recovery times.[40] For those reasons, there appears to be little reason to use intranasal sufentanil.

Intranasal Ketamine

Ketamine also has been administered intranasally, but data regarding that route are limited. A dose of 5 to 6 mg/kg is recommended because 3 mg/kg did not produce better patient cooperation for separation and induction when compared with placebo.[41] Either the 5% or 10% solution can be diluted with saline to make a total of 1 to 2 mL for nasal instillation. Maximal sedation occurs at 10 min after administration.[25] Concentration versus time curves have been generated for intranasal and other routes of ketamine administration[42] (Figure 5-4). Intranasal ketamine at 5 to 6 mg/kg allowed minimal or no resistance during induction in 86% of patients. In addition, patients did not experience excessive sedation or emergence reactions, but nasal burning was problematic.[43] No ad-

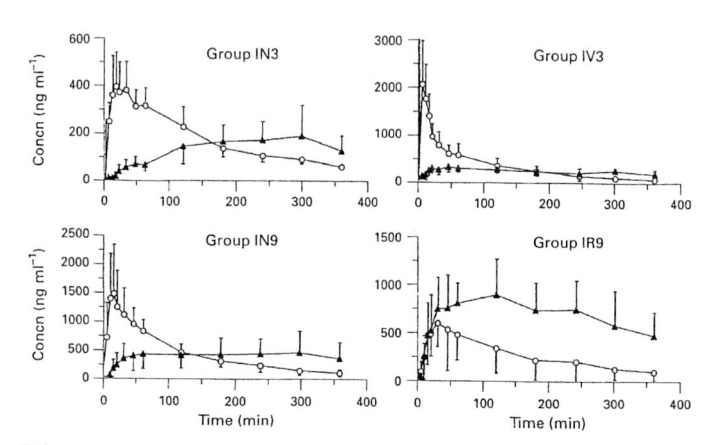

FIG. 5-4 Plasma concentration versus time for intravenous, rectal, and two doses of intranasal ketamine. IN3, intranasal ketamine at 3 mg/kg; IN9, intranasal ketamine at 9 mg/kg; IV3, intravenous ketamine at 3 mg/kg; IR9, intrarectal ketamine at 9 mg/kg; o, ketamine; ∆, norketamine. *(Reprinted with permission from Malinovsky JM, Servin F, Cozian A, Lepage JY, et al: Ketamine and norketamine plasma concentrations after i.v., nasal and rectal administration in children.* Br J Anaesth *77:203, 1996.)*

verse cardiovascular or respiratory events occurred in the few studies performed. However, no data exist regarding the effects of 5 to 6 mg/kg of intranasal ketamine on respiratory and cardiovascular parameters or on the rapidity of anesthetic emergence and postanesthetic recovery.

RECTAL TRANSMUCOSAL ROUTE

The rectal route of administration of preanesthetic sedatives is used less commonly than those discussed above but is often chosen for children younger than 4 years. Children of that age are accustomed to rectal thermometers and in general have not developed a sense of modesty that eventually precludes this route. Rectal administration remains a possibility for older patients if they are developmentally delayed. A lubricated pediatric feeding tube can be inserted 5 to 10 cm past the rectal opening to administer sedative. Advantages of the rectal route include the relative lack of patient discomfort, the inability of the child to spit the medication out, and a faster onset of action than with oral ingestion. Disadvantages include inconsistent absorption, potential premature evacuation of the drug due to defecation, and slower onset than with other transmucosal routes. Premature evacuation occurs frequently in patients with patulous anal sphincters and leads to a high incidence of failed sedation. Premature evacuation can be attenuated by manually squeezing the buttocks together for several minutes after administration or by administration into the upper rectum.[44] However, higher administration may result in greater first-pass hepatic metabolism. Because rectal methohexital can cause apnea, heightened vigilance, monitoring with a minimum of pulse oximetry, and availability of equipment for airway management are recommended. Close observation appears to be adequate after rectal midazolam or ketamine.

Rectal Methohexital

Rectal methohexital has been used as a preanesthetic sedative and an induction agent in children for more than three decades. The dose range is between 15 and 30 mg/kg with solutions anywhere from 1% to 10%. Larger volumes of more dilute solutions may reduce dose requirements,[45] but a 5% or 10% solution is generally easier to administer. A dose of 30 mg/kg of a 10% solution produces sleep in 85% of recipients, with an onset that averages 6 min and ranges from 2 to 12 min.[46] In those patients who do not fall asleep, moderate or heavy sedation is achieved in two-thirds. Unsuccessful sedation is uncommon but does occur in nearly half of all patients who have been maintained on anticonvulsant drugs. Cardiovascular effects are generally benign, with heart rate increasing by 20 to 30 beats per minute and arterial blood pressure unchanged; however, bradycardia can occur.[45,47] Untoward respiratory effects are uncommon, but airway compromise occurs in as many as 4% of patients, occasionally requiring positive pressure ventilation.[47] Apnea has been reported in patients with myelomeningocele[48] but also can occur in patients without preexisting illness.[45] Methohexital has epileptogenic effects that are thought to be limited to individuals with psychomotor seizures. Seizures have occurred in such individuals after receiving rectal methohexital,[49] so another sedative should be used for patients with that history. Hiccups occur frequently but appear to be of no particular consequence. Emergence and recovery after short cases may be delayed because full recovery from the sedative effects requires 60 to 90 min.

Rectal Midazolam

Midazolam can be administered rectally as a preanesthetic sedative at a dose of 0.5 to 1 mg/kg when using the 5 mg/mL intravenous solution diluted with saline to make a total of 10 mL. Onset of sedation occurs at 5 to 7 min after dosing, with patients uniformly calm for separation after 10 min. With the use of 1 mg/kg, the success rate for achieving calm induction approaches 90%, and only at higher doses is recovery delayed after halothane, nitrous oxide, and fentanyl anesthesia[50] (Figure 5-5). As with oral midazolam, delayed recovery may result when rectal midazolam premedication is combined with intravenous induction agents.[51] No clinically significant cardiovascular or respiratory effects seem to occur even when 5.0 mg/kg is used.

Rectal Ketamine

Rectal ketamine has been used as a preanesthetic sedative, but data are limited. At a dose of 3 mg/kg rectal ketamine appears to be no better than placebo.[51] Although one series of patients documented that 8 to 10 mg/kg of the 1% and 5% ketamine solutions was safe, previous administration of di-

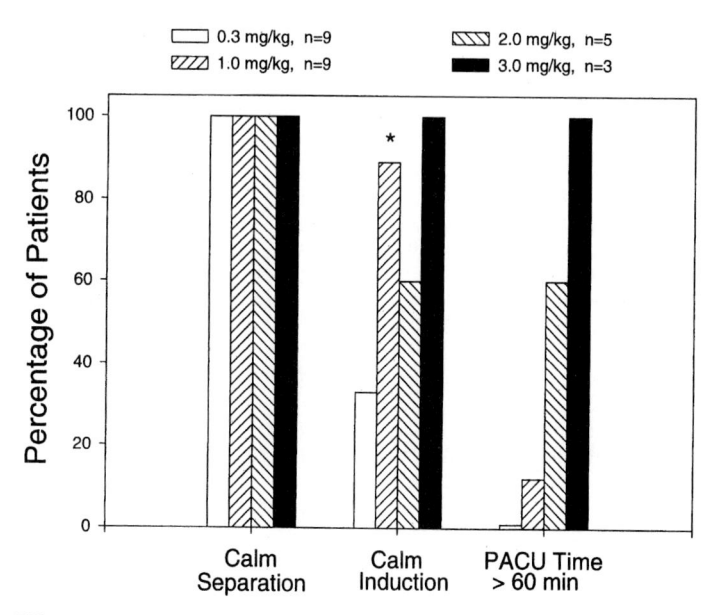

FIG. 5-5 Effectiveness of various doses of rectal midazolam given as a preanesthetic sedative to children aged 8 months to 5 years. The figure shows the percentage of patients who were calm at the time of separation from their parents and during inhalational induction of anesthesia. Also shown is the percentage of patients with recovery room stays longer than 60 min after an average of 163 min of halothane/nitrous oxide anesthesia. *Percentage greater for midazolam 1.0 mg/kg group versus 0.3 mg/kg group, $p < 0.05$. *(Adapted with permission from Spear RM, Yaster M, Berkowitz MB, et al: Preinduction of anesthesia in children with rectally administered midazolam. Anesthesiology 74:670, 1991.)*

azepam obscured their data on clinical efficacy, and no data exist regarding the potential to delay awakening and recovery.[52] Delay may be more likely when ketamine is administered by this route because first-pass hepatic metabolism leads to high concentrations of norketamine, an active metabolite with a longer course of action than ketamine[42] (Figure 5-4). When a rectal preanesthetic sedative is desired, use of methohexital or midazolam, when available, may be more predictable than ketamine.

INTRAMUSCULAR ROUTE

Intramuscular injection is the third most popular route of administration of preanesthetic sedation in the United States, after the oral and nasal routes. Advantages include its rapid onset and the ability to administer it to uncooperative patients. Historically, morphine, demerol, ketamine, pentobarbital, and the combination of demerol with phenergan and thorazine have been popular intramuscular preanesthetic sedatives. However, discomfort and fear caused by injections and availability of equally effective alternative routes[25,53,54] have led to decreased popularity. In general, intramuscular administration of preanesthetic sedation should be reserved for patients who are unable to cooperate with other routes or for those who struggle due to a failed premedication. Intramuscular ketamine and midazolam will be discussed briefly because they appear to be superior to narcotic counterparts.[55,56] Because of the small potential for respiratory embarrassment after most intramuscular sedative injections, close patient observation and the availability of airway management equipment are essential.

Intramuscular Ketamine

Ketamine can be administered intramuscularly in a dose of 2 to 3 mg/kg of the 50 or 100 mg/kg solution. Higher doses may result in lengthy recovery times and appear unnecessary because acceptable sedation can consistently be achieved with 2 to 3 mg/kg.[57] That dose, even when administered at induction, does not delay emergence and only slightly prolongs discharge time after halothane and nitrous oxide anesthesia for myringotomy tube placement.[57] Higher doses also appear to increase the likelihood of unpleasant emergence phenomena and excessive salivation, which rarely occur at the above dose. As with other routes of administration, nystagmus and tongue fasciculations often occur. Sedative effects are easily appreciated in just under 3 min, although peak plasma concentration occurs at 22 min.[58] Although data are lacking with regard to hemodynamic and respiratory variables after intramuscular injection of ketamine, experience indicates that instability is rare when ketamine is used as a single agent. Nonetheless, close patient observation should be maintained after administration.

Intramuscular Midazolam

Midazolam has been administered intramuscularly by needle or Biojector Jet Injector,[59] with the effective dose being between 0.08 and 0.15 mg/kg. Onset is rapid, with approximately 78% of children calm for separation from parents at 10 min after injection[59] and 70% to 90% offering complete cooperation during inhalation induction.[55] Jet injection results in less crying, with only one-third of patients crying after injection, and may also increase the efficiency and rate of drug absorption. Even at doses as high as 0.3 mg/kg, intramuscular midazolam has an excellent safety profile and does not prolong discharge time after halothane and nitrous oxide anesthesia for myringotomy tube placement.[59] However, doses above 0.15 mg/kg do not significantly improve efficacy of sedation, but may increase pain of injection when administered by the Biojector.

In summary, a variety of sedatives and numerous effective routes are available for pediatric preanesthetic sedation. Because there are many reasons for administration of preanesthetic sedation and because of the excellent safety profiles of the agents most frequently used, preanesthetic sedation should always be considered for pediatric patients. Choice of sedative and route should be dictated by patient and situational factors. The need for close observation and monitoring must be tailored according to the sedative and the route of administration chosen.

REFERENCES

1. Politis GD, Tobin JR, Morell RC, et al: Tracheal intubation of healthy pediatric patients without muscle relaxant: a survey of technique utilization and perceptions of safety. *Anesth Analg* 88:737, 1999.
2. Kain ZN, Mayes LC, Wang SM, et al: Postoperative behavioral outcomes in children: effects of sedative premedication. *Anesthesiology* 90:758, 1999.
3. Schreiner MS, O'Hara I, Markakis DA, et al: Do children who experience laryngospasm have an increased risk of upper respiratory tract infection? *Anesthesiology* 85:475, 1996.
4. Kain ZN, Mayes LC, Bell C, et al: Premedication in the United States: a status report. *Anesth Analg* 84:427, 1997.
5. Kain ZN, Bell C, Rimar S, et al: Use of premedication in the United States: status report on pediatric patients. *Anesthesiology* 85:A1070, 1996.
6. Kain ZN, Mayes LC, Wang SM, et al: Parental presence during induction of anesthesia versus sedative premedication: which intervention is more effective? *Anesthesiology* 89:1147, 1998.
7. Bevan JC, Johnston C, Haig MJ, et al: Preoperative parental anxiety predicts behavioural and emotional responses to induction of anaesthesia in children. *Can J Anaesth* 37:177, 1990.
8. Kain ZN, Mayes LC, Caramico LA, et al: Parental presence during induction of anesthesia. A randomized controlled trial. *Anesthesiology* 84:1060, 1996.
9. Mirakhur RK: Comparative study of the effects of oral and i.m. atropine and hyoscine in volunteers. *Br J Anaesth* 50:591, 1978.
10. Saarnivaara L, Kautto UM, Iisalo E, et al: Comparison of pharmacokinetic and pharmacodynamic parameters following oral or intramuscular atropine in children. Atropine overdose in two small children. *Acta Anaesthesiol Scand* 29:529, 1985.
11. Shaw CA, Kelleher AA, Gill CP, Murdoch LJ, et al: Comparison of the incidence of complications at induction and emergence in infants receiving oral atropine *vs* no premedication. *Br J Anaesth* 84:174, 2000.
12. Miller BR, Friesen RH: Oral atropine premedication in infants attenuates cardiovascular depression during halothane anesthesia. *Anesth Analg* 67:180, 1988.
13. Cartabuke RS, Davidson PJ, Warner LO: Is premedication with oral glycopyrrolate as effective as oral atropine in attenuating cardiovascular depression in infants receiving halothane for induction of anesthesia? *Anesth Analg* 73:271, 1991.
14. Bejersten A, Olsson GL, Palmer L: The influence of body weight on plasma concentration of atropine after rectal administration in children. *Acta Anaesthesiol Scand* 29:782, 1985.
15. Weldon BC, Watcha MF, White PF: Oral midazolam in children: effect of time and adjunctive therapy. *Anesth Analg* 75:51, 1992.
16. Twersky RS, Hartung J, Berger BJ, et al: Midazolam enhances anterograde but not retrograde amnesia in pediatric patients. *Anesthesiology* 78:51, 1993.
17. Feld LH, Negus JB, White PF: Oral midazolam preanesthetic medication in prediatric outpatients. *Anesthesiology* 73:831, 1990.

18. McMillan CO, Spahr-Schopfer IA, Sikich N, et al: Premedication of children with oral midazolam. *Can J Anaesth* 39:545, 1992.
19. Viitanen H, Annila P, Viitanen M, et al: Premedication with midazolam delays recovery after ambulatory sevoflurane anesthesia in children. *Anesth Analg* 89:75, 1999.
20. Bevan JC, Veall GR, Macnab AJ, et al: Midazolam premedication delays recovery after propofol without modifying involuntary movements. *Anesth Analg* 85:50, 1997.
21. McCluskey A, Meakin GH: Oral administration of midazolam as a premedicant for paediatric day-case anaesthesia. *Anaesthesia* 49:782, 1994.
22. Cray SH, Dixon JL, Heard CM, et al: Oral midazolam premedication for paediatric day case patients. *Paediatr Anaesth* 6:265, 1996.
23. Alderson PJ, Lerman J: Oral premedication for paediatric ambulatory anaesthesia: a comparison of midazolam and ketamine. *Can J Anaesth* 41:221, 1994.
24. Sekerci C, Donmez A, Ates Y, et al: Oral ketamine premedication in children. *Eur J Anaesth* 13:606, 1996.
25. Cioaca R, Canavea I: Oral transmucosal ketamine: an effective premedication in children. *Paediatr Anaesth* 6:361, 1996.
26. Gutstein HB, Johnson KL, Heard MB, et al: Oral ketamine preanesthetic medication in children. *Anesthesiology* 76:28, 1992.
27. Friesen RH, Lockhart CH: Oral transmucosal fentanyl citrate for preanesthetic medication of pediatric day surgery patients with and without droperidol as a prophylactic anti-emetic. *Anesthesiology* 76:46, 1992.
28. Streisand JB, Stanley TH, Hague B, et al: Oral transmucosal fentanyl citrate premedication in children. *Anesth Analg* 69:28, 1989.
29. Stanley TH, Leiman BC, Rawal N: The effects of oral transmucosal fentanyl citrate premedication on preoperative behavioral responses and gastric volume and acidity in children. *Anesth Analg* 69:328, 1989.
30. Epstein RH, Mendel HG, Witkowski TA, et al: The safety and efficacy of oral transmucosal fentanyl citrate for preoperative sedation in young children. *Anesth Analg* 83:1200, 1996.
31. American Academy of Pediatrics Committee on Drugs: Alternative routes of drug administration—advantages and disadvantages. *Pediatrics* 100:143, 1997.
32. Warner DL, Cabaret J, Velling D: Ketamine plus midazolam, a most effective paediatric oral premedicant. *Paediatr Anaesth* 5:293, 1995.
33. Karl HW, Rosenberger JL, Larach MG, et al: Transmucosal administration of midazolam for premedication of pediatric patients. Comparison of the nasal and sublingual routes. *Anesthesiology* 78:885, 1993.
34. Walbergh EJ, Wills RJ, Eckhert J: Plasma concentrations of midazolam in children following intranasal administration. *Anesthesiology* 74:233, 1991.
35. Malinovsky JM, Lejus C, Servin F, et al: Plasma concentrations of midazolam after i.v., nasal or rectal administration in children. *Br J Anaesth* 70:617, 1993.
36. Malinovsky JM, Populaire C, Cozian A, et al: Premedication with midazolam in children. Effect of intranasal, rectal, and oral routes on plasma midazolam concentrations. *Anaesthesia* 50:351, 1995.
37. Davis PJ, Tome JA, McGowan FX Jr, et al: Preanesthetic medication with intranasal midazolam for brief pediatric surgical procedures. Effect on recovery and hospital discharge times. *Anesthesiology* 82:2, 1995.
38. Karl HW, Keifer AT, Rosenberger JL, et al: Comparison of the safety and efficacy of intranasal midazolam or sufentanil for preinduction of anesthesia in pediatric patients. *Anesthesiology* 76:209, 1992.
39. Henderson JM, Brodsky DA, Fisher DM, et al: Pre-induction of anesthesia in pediatric patients with nasally administered sufentanil. *Anesthesiology* 68:671, 1988.
40. Zedie N, Amory DW, Wagner BK, et al: Comparison of intranasal midazolam and sufentanil premedication in pediatric outpatients. *Clin Pharmacol Ther* 59:341, 1996.
41. Diaz JH: Intranasal ketamine preinduction of paediatric outpatients. *Paediatr Anaesth* 7:273, 1997.

42. Malinovsky JM, Servin F, Cozian A, et al: Ketamine and norketamine plasma concentrations after i.v., nasal and rectal administration in children. *Br J Anaesth* 77:203, 1996.
43. Weksler N, Ovadia L, Muati G, et al: Nasal ketamine for paediatric premedication. *Can J Anaesth* 40:119, 1993.
44. Khalil SN, Florence FB, Van den Nieuwenhuyzen MC, et al: Rectal methohexital: concentration and length of the rectal catheters. *Anesth Analg* 70:645, 1990.
45. Laishley RS, O'Callaghan AC, Lerman J: Effects of dose and concentration of rectal methohexitone for induction of anaesthesia in children. *Can Anaesth Soc J* 33:427, 1986.
46. Audenaert SM, Montgomery CL, Thompson DE, et al: A prospective study of rectal methohexital: efficacy and side effects in 648 cases. *Anesth Analg* 81:957, 1995.
47. Audenaert SM, Wagner Y, Montgomery CL, et al: Cardiorespiratory effects of premedication for children. *Anesth Analg* 80:506, 1995.
48. Yemen TA, Pullerits J, Stillman R, et al: Rectal methohexital causing apnea in two patients with meningomyeloceles. *Anesthesiology* 74:1139, 1991.
49. Rockoff MA, Goudsouzian NG: Seizures induced by methohexital. *Anesthesiology* 54:333, 1981.
50. Spear RM, Yaster M, Berkowitz ID, et al: Preinduction of anesthesia in children with rectally administered midazolam. *Anesthesiology* 74:670, 1991.
51. Beebe DS, Belani KG, Chang PN, et al: Effectiveness of preoperative sedation with rectal midazolam, ketamine, or their combination in young children. *Anesth Analg* 75:880, 1992.
52. Saint-Maurice C, Laguenie G, Couturier C, et al: Rectal ketamine in paediatric anaesthesia. *Br J Anaesth* 51:573, 1979.
53. Guldbrand P, Mellstrom A: Rectal versus intramuscular morphine-scopolamine a premedication in children. *Acta Anaesthesiol Scand* 39:224, 1995.
54. De Jong PC, Verburg MP: Comparison of rectal to intramuscular administration of midazolam and atropine for premedication of children. *Acta Anaesthesiol Scand* 32:485, 1988.
55. Rita L, Seleny FL, Mazurek A, et al: Intramuscular midazolam for pediatric preanesthetic sedation: a double-blind controlled study with morphine. *Anesthesiology* 63:528, 1985.
56. Ryhanen P, Kangas T, Rantakyla S: Premedication for outpatient adenoidectomy: comparison between ketamine and pethidine. *Laryngoscope* 90:494, 1980.
57. Hannallah RS, Patel RI: Low-dose intramuscular ketamine for anesthesia preinduction in young children undergoing brief outpatient procedures. *Anesthesiology* 70:598, 1989.
58. Grant IS, Nimmo WS, Clements JA: Pharmacokinetics and analgesic effects of i.m. and oral ketamine. *Br J Anaesth* 53:805, 1981.
59. Greenberg RS, Maxwell LG, Zahurak M, et al: Preanesthetic medication of children with midazolam using the Biojector jet injector. *Anesthesiology* 83:264, 1995.

6 | Providing Care for the Child, Parent, and Family in Difficult Situations

Barbara A. Castro, MD
Frederic A. Berry, MD

All anesthesiologists are cognizant of the psychological stress endured by children and their families during the perioperative period. As a matter of fact, it is not unusual for them to express a greater concern about the anesthesia than the surgery itself. The ability of a particular child and family to cope with the stress of surgery and anesthesia depends on many factors including the child's developmental and behavioral status and the family dynamics and cultural biases. Because of the multiple factors involved, it is safe to say that every case is unique. Numerous preoperative educational programs, for children and adults, have evolved with the intention of alleviating some of these fears and anxiety. The programs offered differ from one hospital to the next and include preoperative tours of operating rooms, educational videos, play therapy, puppet shows, and anesthesia consultations.

Eventually all anesthesiologists are confronted with the particularly difficult child or parent. This can be very challenging. First of all, there is no set definition for difficult child or parent. Previous experience, gut reaction, or one's own personal beliefs may influence what one may consider outside the realm of normal behavior and therefore a difficult situation. Second, identifying a difficult child or parent in advance is not always easy. Occasionally, the anesthesiologist may receive a warning from the surgeon or nursing staff based on their previous encounters with the family. However, more often than not, the anesthesiologist first meets the child or family just before surgery and has limited time to assess the situation. With experience, some anesthesiologists will be able to identify those difficult children and parents during that short preoperative assessment and plan accordingly. However, the child or parent likely will not be recognized as difficult until "the moment of truth": induction of anesthesia. Third, how does one deal with these situations so as to avoid psychological distress in the child, family, and health care team?

The objectives of this chapter are to help the anesthesiologist define and identify which are the difficult or potentially difficult child and parent and how to assist them and the entire health care team through the enormous stress of the perioperative period. Suggestions are offered on how to manage these situations to avoid long-standing psychological impairment.

IDENTIFYING THE DIFFICULT CHILD OR PARENT

Child Development and Behavior

Understanding normal child development and behavior provides a framework for working with children of different ages. *Child development* refers to the unfolding of broadly defined human capabilities and unique characteristics over time. *Psychological development* can be defined as the progressive organization of cognitive, emotional, and social aspects of behavior.[1] Many factors influence development and the debate surrounding the significance of nature versus nurture continues. Nature emphasizes the genetically preprogrammed capabilities of an individual, whereas nurture emphasizes learning and environment. Also controversial is whether development occurs as a gradual, continuous process or in a stepwise fashion.

Initially, the field of developmental psychology was merely descriptive. In 1787 Dietrich Tiedemann produced the very first diary recording the growth and development of his own child. In the 18th and 19th centuries, many parent scientists, including Charles Darwin (1877), collected data on the development of their own children. Arnold Gesell was particularly instrumental in documenting normal physical and mental development as a process of maturation.[2] By the mid-19th century a transformation occurred in the field and the focus shifted from descriptive to explanatory. As a result, numerous theories and models have been proposed to explain child development and behavior.[1] Three of the most influential models and their proponents are outlined in Table 6-1. Behavioral development by age is concisely outlined in Table 6-2,[3] with some of the expected behavioral responses, positive and negative.

Understanding normal child development and behavior may help the anesthesiologist anticipate how a child of a given age might cope or respond to the stress of surgery. For example, at the age of 6 to 9 months infants start to have anxiety when separating from their parents. Toddlers are prone to have temper tantrums if they do not get their way. Preschool children may enjoy imaginative play and story-telling, whereas the older school age children might want detailed explanations of the facts surrounding surgery and tend to interpret everything literally. Adolescents are very independent yet have issues regarding self-esteem and bodily image.

Developmental and Behavioral Disorders

Unfortunately all children do not follow the path of "normal" development and behavior. For various reasons, genetic and environmental, many children are prone to have delays in their development or behavioral problems. Identifying and interacting with these children and their families, in the acute care setting, can be very challenging. A brief review of three of the more common disorders follows: attention-deficit hyperactivity disorder (ADHD), learning disabilities, and pervasive developmental disorders, commonly referred to as autism.

Attention-Deficit/Hyperactivity Disorder

In 1902, George Still identified a group of children with "incapacity for sustained attention" and "defects in moral control."[4] Since that time, the symptoms of inattention, overactivity/hyperactivity, and impulsivity have been defined as "minimal brain damage," "minimal brain dysfunction," "hyperkinetic reaction of childhood," "attention deficit disorder," and "attention-deficit/hyperactivity disorder." This reflects the fact that the emphasis has shifted away from the relationship of these symptoms to brain insult or injury toward the role of information processing and response generation. The current belief is that the central deficit may be in the processing between incoming information and the response that is generated or in the failure to inhibit appropriately responding until all information is considered. Neurobiologic studies suggest that the circuitry involving frontal cortical and basal ganglia connections may be structurally or functionally different in ADHD.[5]

TABLE 6–1 Developmental Models

	Organismic	Psychoanalytic	Mechanistic
Focus of development	Cognitive	Emotional/personality	Cognitive/social
Basis of development	Maturation	Conflict resolution	Learning
Nature of change	Qualitative	Qualitative	Quantitative
	Unidirectional	Bidirectional	Continuous
	Irreversible	Reversible	Stimulus driven
	Universal		
Role of individual versus environment	Active versus passive	Interactive	Passive versus active
Proponents	**Jean Piaget**	**Sigmund Freud**	**Ivan Pavlov and B. F. Skinner**
	Develpmental progression through discrete periods in which the rate may vary but the sequence is invariant	Orderly, cummulative progression of development based on tension resolution in each stage	Development dependent on level of stimulation, type of stimulation, and history of organism
	Developmental periods	Progression of the mind	*Classical conditioning*
	Sensorimotor (birth–2 years) exploration of the world	*Id (infancy)*	Normally neutral stimulus evokes a specific responce
	Concrete (2–11 years)	Primitive drives and instincts, pleasure principle	*Operant conditioning*
	Preoperational (2–6 years)	*Ego (childhood)*	Consequences of behavior affect learning
	Egocentric	Self	Behavior influenced by the events that follow them rather than those that precede them
	Formation of mental representations of objects and actions	Discover acceptable ways to express the basic drives of the id	**Reinforcement** follows a behavior and <u>increases</u> the likelihood of the behavior occuring again
	Concrete operational (7–11 years)	*Superego (adolescence)*	**Punishment** follows a behavior and <u>decreases</u> the likelihood of the behavior occuring again
	Development of logical thinking	Conscience	
	Ability to perform logical operations concrete objects	Internal representation of familial and societal rules	
	Formal operations		
	Abstract thinking		

TABLE 6-2 Examples of Behavioral Development and Responses

	Behavior development	Behavior responses
Infant (birth to 1 year)	Bonding Security Trust Awareness of environment	Thumb-sucking Pacifier use Cuddling	Dependence on caretakers Eating/sleep problems Colic Differences in temperament
Toddler 1–4 years	Learns control of bodily functions (e.g., toilet training), impulses (e.g., waiting), and behavior (e.g., frustration) Develops language Increased mobility	Negativity (says no) Short attention span, indecisive, active (explores environment, gets into things), play, not sharing, taking turns Releases tension by thumb-sucking Sleep problems Toilet training Tantrums/aggression	Increased self-care (wants to do more on their own) Cognitive development and increased language Magical thinking Problems: contrary/stubborn, tantrums, bedtime fears
Preschool (4–6 years)	Learning social rules, learns to express anger and emotions more appropriately Thinking more organized/conceptual	Bossy/boastful Tells stories, imaginative Asks "how" and "why" Takes things	Argues, demands attention, disobedient, jealous, fears, shows off, shy, whines
School age (6–11 years)	Learns to read, write, etc. Adjusts to out-of-home situation (school, neighborhood), cooperative play Increased importance of peer group	Bedwetting Noncompliant, asks "why," resists rules Shyness or aggressiveness	Inattention/nonconforming to school rules Problems: achievement, school phobia/refusal
Adolescent (11–late teen years)	Develops some independence from family Sexual maturation Abstract thought Development of life skills, commitment to vocation	Dealing with body and self-image	Talks back noncompliant/rebellious Responsibilities/irresponsible Sexual activity

Source: Cruikshank BM, Cooper LJ, Greydanus DE, Wolraich ML: Common behavioral problems. In *Behavioral Pediatrics*, Greydanus DE, Wolraich ML (eds). New York, Springer Verlag, 1992.

The reported prevalence of ADHD varies, from a low of 2% to 3% to a high of 15% to 17%. The most commonly quoted rate in the United States, based on criteria in the *Diagnostic and Statistical Manual of Mental Disorders,* 4th ed. (DSM-IV), is 5% of school-age children. Attention-deficit/hyperactivity disorder is four to nine times more common in males than in females. There is a hereditary component to ADHD, although it is most likely multifactorial as opposed to a single genetic defect. The incidence of comorbid disorders in children with ADHD is reported to be anywhere from 50% to 90%. These include antisocial disorders, anxiety disorders, mood disturbances, and learning disorderss. The diagnosis of a comorbid condition influences prognosis and treatment.[5–7]

Attention-deficit/hyperactivity disorder is purely a behavioral diagnosis; there are no clear biologic markers or diagnostic tests. The three key elements are inattention, hyperactivity, and impulsivity. The DSM-IV diagnostic criteria are outlined in Table 6-3.[8] It is imperative that the symptoms be pervasive, present before the age of 7 years, persistent for longer than 6 months, outside the range of normal development, and represent a significant impairment to social and academic functioning. The diagnosis is usually made clinically based on history, examination, observation, and reports from parents and teachers including behavior-rating scales.

There is ongoing controversy regarding the treatment of children with ADHD, particularly with regard to the use of stimulant medications. The use of stimulants for the treatment of ADHD dates back to the 1930s, when a serendipitous observation revealed that stimulant therapy reduced the disruptive symptoms of ADHD. Stimulants affect the central norepinephrine and dopamine (DA) pathways by occupying and blocking the DA transporter, which leads to an increase in the intrasynaptic concentration of DA. The increased concentration of DA enhances functioning of the executive control processes, which helps overcome the deficits in inhibitory control and working memory present in children with ADHD.[9] Many subsequent studies have proven the short-term beneficial effects of stimulants on behavior and school performance in children with ADHD. Unfortunately, the long-term benefits of stimulant therapy in terms of academic achievement and social skills are not as promising. By 1995, an estimated 2.8% of U.S. children between the ages of 5 and 18 years were prescribed stimulant medication.[9] Table 6-4 lists the four most commonly used stimulants. Side effects of stimulant therapy include anorexia, weight loss, headaches, insomnia, and tics. Some children with ADHD do not respond to stimulant therapy or have a contraindication to stimulant use. Other drugs, which have been used with some success, are clonidine and tricyclic antidepressants.[10] Children with ADHD and comorbid conditions may be on additional antipsychotic medications.

Behavioral approaches, including positive reinforcement, reprimands and redirection, family training, cognitive behavior training, environmental stimulation, and biofeedback, have been studied in children with ADHD. The evidence suggests short-term benefit when behavioral modification is used in association with stimulant therapy.[11] However, behavioral therapy alone does not seem to be as effective.

Over the years many alternative therapies have been suggested, including dietary restrictions (the Feingold diet), megavitamins, oculovestibular treatment, auditory stimulation, and homeopathy. There is no scientific evidence to support such treatment; however, it may be worth questioning families about the use of these treatments.

TABLE 6–3 Diagnostic Criteria for Attention-Deficit/Hyperactivity Disorder

A. 1 or 2 (or both):
  1. Six or more of the following symptoms of inattention have persisted for at least 6 months to a degree that is maladaptive and inconsistent with development level:
      a. Often fails to pay close attention to details or makes careless mistakes in schoolwork, work, or other activities
      b. Often has difficulty sustaining attention in tasks or play activities
      c. Often does not seem to listen when spoken to directly
      d. Often does not follow through on instructions and fails to finish school work, chores, or duties in the workplace (not due to oppositional behavior or failure to understand instructions)
      e. Often has difficulty organizing tasks and activities
      f. Often avoids, dislikes, or is reluctant to engage in tasks that require sustained mental effort (such as schoolwork or homework)
      g. Often loses things necessary for tasks or activities (e.g., toys, school assignment, pencils, books, or tools)
      h. Is often easily distracted by extraneous stimuli
      i. Is often forgetful in daily activities
  2. Six or more of the following symptoms of hyperactivitiy or impulsivity have persisted for at least 6 months to a degree that is maladaptive and inconsistnet with developmental level:
      Hyperactivity
      a. Often fidgets with hands or feet or squirms in seat
      b. Often leaves seat in classroom or in other situations in which remaining seated is expected
      c. Often runs about or climbs excessively in situations in which it is inappropriate (in adolescents or adults, may be limited to subjective feelings of restlessness)
      d. Often has difficulty playing or engaging in leisure activities quietly
      e. Is often on the go or often acts as if driven by a motor
      f. Often talks excessively, impulsivity
      g. Often blurts out answers before the question has been completed
      h. Often has difficulty awaiting turn
      i. Often interrupts or intrudes on others (e.g., butts into conversations or games)
Additional criteria:
B. Some hyperactive-impulsive or inattentive symptoms that caused impairment were present before age 7 years
C. Some impairment from symptoms is present in two or more settings (e.g., school or work and at home)
D. There must be clear evidence of clinically significant impairment in social, academic, or occupational functioning
E. The symptoms do not occur exclusively during the course of pervasive developmental disorder, schizophrenia, or other psychotic disorder and are not better accounted for by another mental disorder (e.g., mood disorder, anxiety disorder, dissociative disorder, or personality disorder)

Source: Reproduced with permission from American Psychiatric Association: *The Diagnostic and Statistical Manual of Mental Health Disorders,* 4th ed. Washington, DC, American Psychiatric Association, 1994.

There is no doubt that every anesthesiologist who provides care for children will need to be familiar with ADHD. The complex medical environment presents quite a challenge for these children. The anesthesiologist's approach to these children may depend on the situation. One of the major issues is whether or not the child should take his/her usual medication before elective

TABLE 6-4 Commonly Used Stimulants in Children and Adolescents

	Dextroamphetamine (Dexedrine)	Methylphenidate (Ritalin)	Amphetamine/Dextroamphetamine (Adderall)	Pemoline (Cylert)
How supplied (mg)	5; Spansule 5, 10, 15	5, 10, 20; 20 SR	5, 10, 20, 30	18.75, 37.5, 75
Single-dose range (mg/kg)	0.15–0.5	0.3–0.7	0.15–0.5	0.5–2.5
Daily dose range (mg/d)	5–40	10–40	40	18.75–112.5
Initial dose	2.5–5 mg, 1–2 times/day Spansule 5 mg every morning	5 mg, 2 times/day	2.5–5 mg, 1–2 times/day	18.75 mg every morning
Peak plasma level	2–3 h	1.5–2.5 h	2–3 h	2–4 h
Plasma half-life	4–6 h	2–3 h	4–6 h	7–8 h (children)
Peak clinical effect	1–2 h	1–3 h	1–2 h	Variable
Onset of behavioral effect	30–60 min	30–60 min	30–60 min	Variable
Duration of behavioral effect	4–6 h	3–5 h	4–6 h	6–8 h

Source: Morgan AM: Attention deficit/hyperactivity disorder. *Pediatr Clin North Am* 46 (5), 1995.

surgery. For instance, if the child is scheduled as a first case, the anesthesiologist may choose to withhold the usual medication and give a sedative premedication, if necessary. Conversely, if surgery is scheduled later in the day, one may choose to have the child take his/her usual medication to have a more cooperative, attentive patient in the waiting area. In this case, the anesthesiologist must be familiar with the medication, usually a stimulant or clonidine, and understand potential side effects and drug interactions.

Learning Disabilities

The term *learning disabilities* refers to a heterogeneous group of disorders characterized by difficulties in the acquisition and use of listening, speaking, reading, writing, reasoning, or mathematical abilities. A 1991 estimate by the U.S. Department of Education identified 4% to 5% of school-age children as learning-disabled. Learning disabilities are commonly classified into one of two categories. Language-based disabilities, primarily associated with problems in reading and spelling, are the most common. Nonverbal learning disabilities, characterized by problems in arithmetic and deficits in neurocognitive and adaptive functions attributed to the right hemisphere, represent fewer than 10% of all learning disabilities.[12]

Recent studies have challenged the commonly held view that learning disabilities are more prevalent in boys than in girls. However, genetic factors definitely play a significant role in the acquisition of learning disabilities. Studies have shown that as many as 35% to 40% of first-degree relatives of reading-disabled children also have reading disabilities. Comorbid conditions are not uncommon in children with learning disabilities, the most common being ADHD. Recent evidence actually supports a common underlying genetic origin for ADHD and reading disabilities. In addition, externalizing disorders, such as conduct disorders and delinquency, and internalizing disorders, such as anxiety disorders and depression, have been observed in children with learning disabilities.[12]

The fundamental deficit in learning-disabled children is a deficit in processing rapidly changing information in several sensory channels. The complex environment of the hospital may be particularly challenging for these children. It is also important to realize that learning disabilities persist into adolescence and adulthood.

Although some of these children have obvious comorbid conditions, such as ADHD or behavioral disorders, many have isolated learning disabilities, which are not apparent. Unfortunately, many of these children are mistakenly labeled as uncooperative, although they may simply have difficulty understanding the usual preoperative explanations, especially when they are rushed. These children are likely to benefit from preoperative educational programs that allow time for questions and present the information in alternative ways. A preoperative questionnaire may help to identify these children and refer them to the appropriate services, i.e., child life programs or anesthesia preoperative clinics, when available. Otherwise, just taking the time preoperatively to provide explanations in a manner the child can understand will avoid frustration for the child and anesthesiologist.

Pervasive Developmental Disorders

The pervasive developmental disorders (PDDs) are a heterogeneic group of developmental disabilities characterized by impairments in reciprocal social interactions, communication, and imaginative activity and by a markedly restricted repertoire of activities and interests. The term *autism*, first introduced in 1943, describes the most severe form. These children are usually mentally retarded, nonverbal, and engage in stereotypy or self-injurious behavior. At the opposite end of the spectrum are those children with Asperger's syndrome. These children have normal intelligence and good verbal skills but pedantic speech and idiosyncratic interests. They also exhibit subtle deficits in interpersonal interactions. The term *pervasive developmental disorder* not otherwise specified is reserved for those children with qualitative impairment in the three major areas (social interactions, communication skills, and behavioral flexibility) but do no meet the DSM-IV diagnostic criteria for autistic disorder as outlined in Table 6-5.[13]

The prevalence of autism is 5 per 10,000. Pervasive developmental disorder *not otherwise specified* (PDD-NOS) is believed to be twice as common. The

TABLE 6–5 Diagnostic Criteria for Autistic Disorder

A. Six (or more) items from (1), (2), and (3), with at least two from (1), one each from (2) and (3):
  1. Qualitative impairment in social interaction, as manifested by at least two of the following:
     a. Marked impairment in the use of multiple nonverbal behaviors such as eye-to-eye gaze, facial expression, body postures, and gestures to regulate social interaction
     b. Failure to develop peer relationships appropriate to developmental level
     c. A lack of spontaneous seeking to share enjoyment, interests, or achievements with other people (e.g., by a lack of showing, bringing, or pointing out objects of interest)
     d. Lack of social or emotional reciprocity
  2. Qualitative impairments in communication as manifested by at least one of the following:
     a. Delay in, or total lack of, the development of spoken language (not accompanied by an attempt to compensate through alternative modes of communication such as gesture or mime)
     b. In individuals with adequate speech, marked impairment in the ability to initiate or sustain a conversation with others
     c. Stereotyped and repetitive use of language or idiosyncratic language
     d. Lack of varied, spontaneous make-believe play or social imitative play appropriate to developmental level
  3. Restricted repetitive and stereotyped patterns of behavior, interests, and activities, as manifested by at least one of the following:
     a. Encompassing preoccupation with one or more stereotyped and restricted patterns of interests that is abnormal either in intensity or focus
     b. Apparently inflexible adherence to specific, nonfunctional routines or rituals
     c. Steroptyped and repetitive motor mannerisms (e.g., hand or finger flapping or twisting, or complex whole-body movements)
     d. Persistent preoccupation with parts of objects
B. Delays or abnormal functioning in at least one of the following areas, with onset before age 3 years: (1) social interaction, (2) language as used in social communication, or (3) symbolic or imaginative play
C. The disturbance is not better accounted for by Rett's disorder or childhood disintegrative disorder

Source: American Psychiatric Association: *Diagnostic and Statistical Manual of Mental Disorders,* 4th ed. Washington, DC, American Psychiatric Association, 1994.

prevalence of Asperger's syndrome may be as high as 28.5 per 10,000.[14] Autism appears to be more common in boys than in girls by a ratio of 3 to 4:1.[13] Evidence supports a genetic predisposition for PDD. The risk of PDD in siblings of individuals with PDD is 2% to 8.6%, or 50 to 215 times the risk in the general population.[15] Several genetic syndromes are associated with PDD including Fragile X, Williams, Rett, Cornelia de Lange, Moebius, and Noonan.[13,15] Seizure disorders occur in approximately one-fourth of children with autism, usually presenting in adolescence.[14–16] The precise etiology of PDD remains unknown. Neurochemical studies have found elevated serum serotonin levels and reduced central serotonergic responsiveness in children with autism. Other studies have found elevated DA turnover in addition to brain and plasma opioid abnormalities. Neuropathologic studies point to abnormalities in the limbic system and cerebellum. Some studies have suggested an autoimmune process.[13,15,16] Whether or not prenatal factors play a role in the etiology remains questionable. Clearly the etiology is complex and multifactorial.

The diagnosis of autism/PDD is made clinically. The children may present in infancy or childhood. Infants usually avoid eye contact and are stiff, irritable, and indifferent to caregivers. Children may display normal development until ages 12 to 18 months, at which time they may present with delays in attaining language milestones or loss of previous language skills; stereotypes such as toe walking, arm flapping, and rocking; ritualistic behaviors; social isolation; and unusual response to sensory information such as lack of response to pain. Older children may exhibit self-injurious or aggressive behaviors.[13,15] The treatment of PDD is primarily behavioral and cognitive training. However, pharmacologic treatment is sometimes necessary. Serotonin uptake inhibitors, risperidone and fluoxetine, have been used to suppress aggression and repetitive behaviors.[14,16,18] Naltrexone has been used to treat autism based on the theory that certain patients may be hypersecreting brain opioids, specifically B endorphins.[17,18] Sedatives or hypnotics such as clonazepam may be necessary to control hyperactivity and aggression.[15,18] Central nervous system stimulants have been studied to improve attention.[15,16,18] Neuroleptic agents may be used in the most severe forms.[15,18] In addition, many of these children are on anti-epileptic medications to control seizures.

The anesthesiologist's approach to the autistic child will depend on the severity of the disorder. The noncommunicative, severely retarded child who displays self-injurious behaviors is best served by a sedative premedication. Occasionally, it may even be necessary to medicate these children before they leave their homes because the unfamiliar hospital environment may trigger behaviors that jeopardize the safety of the child and health care workers. Conversely, the child with Asperger's syndrome may do well during the perioperative period as long as they have a parent or familiar caregiver with them. Needless to say, the child with a PDD is complex and challenging at the very least. Parents and caregivers are often the anesthesiologist's best allies in predicting the child's behavior and reactions. However, even they can be fooled at times, making pharmacologic backup a necessity.

Chronic Illness

The advances in medical and surgical technology over the past two decades have led to an increasing number of children with severe medical problems surviving to young adulthood. Studies indicate that approximately 12% of children, or 7.5 million children younger than 18 years, have a chronic illness. Approximately 10% of those children have functional limitations that affect their daily lives.[19]

Chronic illness usually is defined by (1) the duration of the illness, usually at least 3 to 12 months, and (2) the severity of the illness as indicated by the need for long or frequent hospitalizations or extensive nursing care.[19,20] A chronic illness may be congenital (cystic fibrosis or inborn errors of metabolism) or acquired (sequelae of prematurity or trauma). A chronic illness may present at birth (trisomy 21, myelomeningocele) or later in childhood (asthma, diabetes, or leukemia). A child with a chronic illness may appear well (symptom-free infant with human immunodeficiency virus or a child with well-controlled epilepsy) or disabled (ventilator-dependent child with muscular dystrophy or wheelchair-dependent child with cerebral palsy). Although the disease processes may be substantially different, the fact that the child with a chronic illness must learn to cope and adapt to this situation while also trying to negotiate the normal process of development remains constant. Table 6-6 outlines some of the factors that influence child development and behavior in the face of chronic illness.

The child's age is important for two reasons. First, it will affect how they understand or perceive their illness. Second, the presence of a chronic illness may affect normal child development. Hospitalization during infancy may interfere with the development of a trusting relationship between caregiver

TABLE 6–6 Factors That Influence Development and Behavior Among Children With Chronic Health Conditions

Illness or condition characteristics (other than specific diagnosis)
  Severity (physiologic or sensory impact)
  Duration
  Age of onset
  Interference with age-appropriate activities
  Expected survival
  Course (stable vs. progressive)
  Certainty (predictable vs. uncertain)
  Impact on morbidity
  Impact on cognition and communication
  Pain
Child factors
  Gender
  Intelligence and communication skills
  Temperament
  Coping skills and patterns
Family factors
  Family functioning
  Parental mental health
  Household structure (number of adults and children)
  Socioeconomic status
Social factors
  Cultural attitudes
  Access to health care
  Community resources
  Geography
  School and day care systems

Source: Perrin JM, Thyen U: Chronic illness. In *Behavioral Pediatrics.* Levine MB, Carey WB, Crocker AC (eds). Philadelphia, W.B. Saunders, 1999.

and infant. The toddler (18 to 36 months old) with a chronic illness may have restrictions not imposed on other children of the same age and as a result may fail to develop any independence, be very clingy, and fail to interact with peers of the same age. Preschool children (3 to 6 years old) tend to think illness is caused by something they did or did not do or think. Due to physical limitations they may not master certain skills and end up being passive and fearful. The major focus of the school-age child (6 to 12 years old) is peer acceptance and approval. A child with a chronic illness may be perceived as different and therefore teased or avoided. Children at this age perceive illness as an external contamination (germ theory). They also begin to understand the meaning and irreversibility of death. The focus of adolescence (13 to 18 years old) is the establishment of personal identity and independence. This can be troublesome because adolescents with chronic illness may still need to rely on parents. They also begin to understand the physiologic and psychologic bases of disease.[19–21]

Temperament, or how one behaves spontaneously and in reaction to various situations, also influences development and behavior in children with chronic illness. Three constellations of temperament have been described. The *easy child* is characterized by regularity, positive approach and response to new stimuli, good adaptability, and a predominantly good mood. The *difficult child* is characterized by irregularity of biologic functions, negative withdrawal responses to new stimuli or people, poor adaptability, and primarily negative mood. The *slow-to-warm up* child is characterized by negative responses of mild intensity to new stimuli, slow but eventual adaptability, and a tendency toward irregularity of biologic function. Temperament characteristics are genetically determined and relatively stable but not entirely fixed. In the presence of a chronic illness, temperament may be helpful in predicting how a child may cope and adapt. Even so, environment and physical condition may actually influence temperament over time.[22]

Over all, children with chronic illness are two to three times more likely than their healthy peers to have some behavioral or psychiatric disturbance.[19] It is important to note that this holds true for all children with chronic illness regardless of the specific diagnosis.[20] However, there are a few disease-specific concerns worth mentioning. First, any child with a chronic condition involving the central nervous system, such as epilepsy, hydrocephalus, or head trauma, has an even greater risk for behavioral and psychiatric problems.[19,20] Second, the advances in neonatal medicine have led to increased survival of very premature infants with very low birthweight (VLBW; <1500 g) and extremely low birthweight (ELBW; <1000 g). Psychological outcomes for these children remain unclear. One recent report has estimated approximately one-fourth of VLBW children have severe or multiple psychological problems and another fourth have moderate to mild problems. Lowered intelligence quotient and attention deficit and schooling problems are the most prevalent psychological problems. In addition, it is unlikely that a favorable postdischarge environment will allow for catch-up or compensation in the VLBW children.[23] Children with congenital heart disease represent a third group known to have neurologic sequelae. Although improvements in anesthetic and surgical techniques have led to earlier corrective surgery and improved survival, neurologic abnormalities are still found. In a recent study comparing children with corrected dextro-transposition of the great vessels to normal siblings, the children with dextro-transposition of the great vessels were more likely to have abnormal neurologic examination findings, learning disabilities, and behavioral disorders.[24] Fourth, previously normal children may develop psychologic or behavioral difficulties as a result of specific treatment. For example, the treatment of leukemia has been associated with a decline in cognitive function and the use of steroids in childhood asthma has been associated with attention deficit and aggressive behavior.[20] Fifth, adolescents with chronic illnesses have an increase in depression, suicidal ideation, and suicides.[19]

Overall, the manner in which children cope and adapt to chronic illness depends on multiple factors. The nature and severity of the disease itself; the child's stage of cognitive development, temperament, and coping styles; and the reaction of the family and society play a crucial role.

Family Dynamics

Every child must be considered in the context of the "family." In today's society, family compositions vary tremendously; however individual children are very familiar and comfortable with their own families and the role of each member. Although the current medical environment does not allow much time for interaction with the family, it is extremely important for health care providers to observe the family dynamics to better understand the child. One often can get a feel for parenting styles, parental relationships, grandparent involvement, and sibling interactions by simple observation. At the very least, one can usually decide who is in control, the parent or the child.

As anesthesiologists we are often confronted with families in the midst of a large deal of stress. They may be angry, guilt-ridden, or simply exhausted. Whether the family is confronted with a sudden catastrophic event, such as an accident or premature birth, or dealing with a chronic illness, the emotional reactions follow a similar pattern: (1) shock, (2) disbelief, (3) grieving and anger, (4) stabilization, and (5) maturation and acceptance. It is important to realize that these stages are not mutually exclusive; there may be setbacks and at any given time different family members may be at different stages.[19,20,25] How any individual ultimately copes will depend on previous experience, temperament, and coping styles. Obviously, dealing with the different temperaments and attitudes of multiple family members can be quite challenging. Nurses and other care providers who already have developed a relationship with the family may be able to provide some insight into the best ways to communicate with any particular family member.

External factors also can influence a family's ability to cope with an acute or chronically ill child. The family with a single parent may rely on community resources for support. School systems may need to be flexible so that children with illnesses are not left behind. The health care community may be able to provide information on support groups for parents and siblings of sick children. Religious beliefs may influence how a family makes decisions on certain health care issues, for example, Jehovah's Witnesses' reluctance to use blood products.

The care of a chronically ill child can be particularly burdensome for a family. The actual physical care of the child can lead to feelings of fatigue, isolation, and depression. Healthy siblings may be deprived of quality parental time. Marital relations may be strained. Financial constraints may be significant secondary to increased expenses or loss of income. All of these issues are superimposed on the primary illness and can lead to dissolution or dysfunction.

Ultimately, the manner in which a family copes with an illness or hospitalization largely determines how a child will cope.[26] Children identify with certain family members and learn by example. The well-organized, open, and communicative family tends to be supportive and resourceful, whereas the disorganized, noncommunicative, and dysfunctional family tends to be angry and frustrated. Clearly, dealing with a family and a child from the latter situation will be quite challenging.

MANAGEMENT OF THE DIFFICULT CHILD OR PARENT
Preanesthetic Evaluation

There is no question but that same-day surgery has been a boon in many ways to the psychological and physical well-being of parents, family, patients, etc. Nevertheless, this often delays the preanesthetic evaluation to a time immediately before the surgery, a time that is clearly a very stressful one for the child and family. In some practice situations, the entire patient population lives in the local community near the hospital. Therefore, preanesthetic visits with the anesthesiologist or tours organized by child-life specialists may be possible. However, for many medical centers, particularly for teaching institutions, patients often come from far away. This makes a visit to the hospital for anesthetic consultation and preparation often impossible. With the time constraints of today's practice, it is helpful to always have one's goals in mind. The three goals of the preanesthetic evaluation are as follows: (1) review of illness, previous experiences, and current state of health; (2) assessment of child's behavior and interactions; and (3) bonding with the parents or caregivers.

The first goal, review of illness, previous experiences, and current state of health, is largely achieved by chart review, history and physical examination, and consultation with other care providers. Many of these issues are discussed in detail in other chapters of this book.

The second goal, assessment of child's behavior and interactions, can be achieved through observation and a brief, age-appropriate conversation with the child. By simple observation one can usually tell whether or not the child's behavior is age appropriate. For example, 12-month-old infants are usually upset if they are separated from their parents, whereas preschool children can be engaged in some form of imaginative play. One also should be able to determine whether or not a child has behavioral or developmental disorders, e.g., the school-age child with ADHD who did not take Ritalin on the morning of surgery and cannot sit still in the waiting area, or the child with cerebral palsy and learning disabilities who has difficulty with self-expression. The way a child interacts with you (whether or not they will warm up to you with time) and his/her parents (whether or not the parents can set limits and follow through) are key in establishing an anesthetic plan. In older children and teenagers, independence is very important, so it is crucial to involve them in the decision-making process.

At this point it is worth mentioning one particularly difficult subset of patients, the veterans of anesthesia. These are the children who have played the "anesthesia and surgical game" before and are not interested in participating again. Their previous experiences usually have been negative. Often, they are upset from the minute they walk in the door or may not even get out of the car upon arrival to the hospital. These are the children who benefit most from pharmacologic intervention and may require a sedative before leaving home.

The third goal, bonding with parents or caregivers, is the most challenging and time-consuming. The biggest concern for parents often involves the anesthesia, not the surgery. This is especially true when you consider that, at this point, the parents and child have met with the surgeon before, under calmer circumstances, and have had a chance to consider and digest the information that was provided. This same family is meeting with the anesthesia team for the first time, often with little or no understanding of the anesthesia events that are shortly to occur. Whether it is an elective surgery or an unanticipated surgery, this is a very stressful time for parents. Therefore, it is very important to take the time to address parental concerns and establish a trusting relationship with the family. Most parents know and understand their children well and are upset when they are not allowed to participate in medical decisions for their children. The senior author remembers one experience poignantly. It involved a child who had had two kidney transplants, chronic dialysis, and more. One of the routine preoperative questions that we ask of parents is: Is there anything special that we should know about your child, or that you can think of, that can help us to help you, and your child, to get through this period any better? The parent was rather amazed; her child was a new patient in our medical center, and she turned to her sister and said, "this is the first time anybody has ever asked me, was there anything that would help me or my child get through these difficult times."

Parents do have knowledge about what can make their and their child's lives easier in these difficult times. Of course, we all know that there is the occasional parent who is particularly difficult. Some parents are just overbearing and demand total control of the situation. These parents usually have had previous bad experiences or are just frustrated with "the system." In these situations, it is important to be empathetic and understanding and to set limits and clearly define the parent's role. For example, some parents not only ask to be present for the induction of anesthesia but also want to know why they cannot stay for the entire procedure. It is very important, early on, to clearly set the boundaries of parental involvement to avoid confrontations at crucial periods such as immediately after the anesthetic induction.

One potentially difficult situation involves the children whose parents are practicing Jehovah's Witnesses. A full discussion with the family regarding the use of blood products and fluid replacement will be required if the surgery is of such a nature that a blood transfusion may be needed. Many state laws at the present time will not allow a family to let their child die because of the lack of blood transfusion. These states have laws whereby the child is made a ward of the court for the time of the surgery and blood transfusions can be given, as determined by the attending physicians, without the parent's permission. This is done with a court order. It must be obtained preoperatively, or, in the case of an emergency, it can be obtained as the operation is proceeding. There are several philosophies in dealing with parents of a Jehovah's Witness and the issue of transfusion. Our approach is that there is no question but that the parents would like their child to survive, but their religion is an extraordinarily important point of their lives, if not their whole lives. Those who follow the teaching of Jehovah's Witness believe that blood transfusion(s) cause the recipient to effectively lose their soul. These parents are extraordinarily committed to their religion and to their child. Rather than challenging their religious beliefs and convictions, it is our practice to explain to the parents that we are not as strong as they are and would be unable to allow their child to die from a lack of blood transfusion. We explain that we will do everything possible not to transfuse their child, that we understand they do not want their child transfused, but that, if it becomes a question of life and survival, by the authority of an appropriate court order we will administer blood products as needed. This is done in a nonconfrontational, empathetic manner that avoids hostility and anger and encourages understanding and acceptance. It also allows parents the opportunity to reconsider their choices. Some families, having been given a forthright discussion of the anesthetic plan, may opt to seek care in those institutes where anesthesiologists and surgeons are willing to provide all care, no matter what the risk, without giving blood products.

Options in Premedication

The decision to administer a premedication to a child should be made on an individual basis. Some institutions routinely premedicate all of their pediatric patients, whereas others rarely use premedication. These arbitrary policies do not take into consideration the uniqueness of each case. The decision to administer a premedication to a child should be made by the anesthesiologist in consultation with the parents and the child, when appropriate. Many factors should be considered, including the age of the patient, the type of surgery, the length of surgery, the child's previous experience with hospitalization or surgery, and the family's expectations.

The overly anxious, very uncooperative child presents a somewhat different issue with premedication. Often these children will refuse to take an oral premedication. Thus, the very child who would benefit from premedication, to achieve some degree of sedation, anxiolysis, and amnesia, simple won't take it. One is then left with combining techniques of premedication and induction, such as the use of intramuscular ketamine. If the child will not take premedication and if it is evident that there is a good chance that, even with the parents there for induction, the child may become totally disruptive, then the use of intramuscular ketamine for induction should be discussed. In our practice, we knew parents who, because of the recurrent nature of the need for surgery, often would inform us, up-front, that they thought intramuscularly administered ketamine was the easiest way to manage their child.

There are several important aspects to the administration of the ketamine. The first is that it would be important to give it in the upper extremity because the uptake from the upper extremity is more rapid than the uptake from lower extremity. The second is that it will take at least two people to hold the child while the intramuscular injection is given. The operator secures the upper arm with the left hand and holds the syringe with the ketamine in the right hand. We use a 3-mL luer lock syringe with a 21-gauge needle. The skin is not wiped with alcohol because doing so warns the child that trouble is coming. The thumb is held on the plunger and, with one quick motion, the injection is made. There is no need for aspiration of blood; the medication is injected directly; it takes 2 to 4 min for the ketamine to become effective. The description of what is going to occur should be given to the parents before the drug is administered. They should be told that their child will develop a far-off gaze, may or may not close the eyes completely, and will just relax and become very cooperative, although the child may still be mumbling a few words while being wheeled into the operating room. It should be remembered that it takes approximately 2 h for the effects of this ketamine to completely dissipate. To decrease secretions, it is helpful to administer an antisialagogue with the ketamine. To the uninitiated, intramuscular ketamine can seem aggressive, insensitive, and even barbaric, but used appropriately it is, at worst, the least of evils. At one time or another each of us will be challenged by an uncooperative child in whom a single small needle injection is the least painful and frightening method of induction.

Options for Induction

One of the more controversial topics in pediatric anesthesia is parental presence during induction of anesthesia. Some anesthesiologists are strong proponents and encourage all parents to be present, whereas others are uncomfortable with the concept and will not allow any parents to be present for the induction of anesthesia. Similar to the issue of premedication, each child and family must be looked at individually. What is good for one child and family may not be ideal for the next.

The early proponents of parental presence during induction believed that it would reduce preoperative anxiety, in particular separation anxiety, and decrease the use of sedative premedication, which would be advantageous in the ambulatory setting. However, as this practice became more popular, several questions were raised and eventually studied. Three of the most commonly asked questions are: (1) Is parental presence during induction really beneficial to the child? (2) Is this a positive experience for the parents? (3) How do anesthesiologists and other health care professionals feel about parental presence for induction?

Early studies supported the beliefs that parental presence reduced anxiety and decreased the use of heavy premedication.[27,28] However, subsequent studies have challenged whether parental presence truly makes a difference[29] and even suggested that parents with a high level of anxiety preoperatively may actually cause their child to be more upset at induction.[30] Recent studies by Kain et al. concluded that parental presence benefited children older than 4 years, children whose parent had low trait anxiety, and children with a low baseline level of activity or temperament.[31] In subsequent studies they concluded that oral midazolam was more effective than parental presence in reducing a child's anxiety preoperatively[32] and that parental presence combined with oral midazolam was no more beneficial in reducing a child's anxiety than oral midazolam alone.[33] Interestingly, there are still no data to support that parental presence has a positive impact on postoperative behavioral outcomes in the short or long term. Obviously, the benefit to the child of having a parent present during induction is not as simple as originally believed. Many factors come into play and must be considered, including the age of the child, the temperament of the child, the anxiety level of the parents, and the experience of the anesthesiologist.

All anesthesiologists who allow parents to be present for induction probably have experienced parents getting upset during induction. This prompts one to ask: Is this practice beneficial to the parents? When surveyed, most parents who were present for an anesthetic induction admitted to being upset at some point even if they did not appear so. Most reported being upset by leaving the child after induction, watching the child get very limp, or watching their child get upset during induction. However, these same parents strongly believed that they helped their child and the anesthesiologist during the induction and, if need be, they would do it again.[34,35] In addition, although Kain et al. reported that parental presence in addition to sedative premedication does not provide added benefit to the children, the parents who were present for induction were less anxious and more satisfied with the care than those who did not accompany their children.[33] In today's competitive health care environment, parental satisfaction cannot be ignored.

The final issue to consider is the attitude of the staff, anesthesiologists and operating room personnel, toward parental presence for induction. Most institutions do not have written policies regarding parental presence and the decision is left to the individual anesthesiologist. Overall, parental presence in more widely accepted and practiced in Great Britain than in the United States.[36] The concerns expressed by anesthesiologists include the stress placed on the anesthesiologist when being watched and potentially criticized by parents, the effects of parental presence on resident education, and the legal implications of having parents present for induction. Some anesthesiologists are uncomfortable with the idea of parents watching a critical procedure, such as the induction of anesthesia, and feel that, if something goes wrong, they will be distracted by having the parents present or even be criticized by the parents.[37,38] More experienced anesthesiologists, anesthesiologists who practice pediatric anesthesia exclusively, and anesthesiologists who practice in pediatric hospitals are more likely to favor parental presence during induction.[36] Interestingly, one survey of residents showed that the overwhelming majority favors parental presence and does not feel that it has a negative impact on their education. It is important to note that the residents surveyed belonged to a program in which most anesthetic inductions were performed with parents present.[39] With regard to legal implications, an Illinois Supreme Court ruling in response to a mother who fainted in a treatment room and suffered a head injury, stated that a hospital that *allows* a nonpatient to accompany a patient during treatment does not have a duty to protect the nonpatient. However, if medical personnel *invite* the nonpatient to participate in the treatment, the hospital then has a legal responsibility toward the nonpatient.[40] Does this mean that, if we invite parents to be present for induction of anesthesia, we are legally responsible for their well-being during the induction?

It is worthwhile to review a few logistical concerns regarding parental presence for induction. First, the decision on whether or not to have parents present for induction must be made by the anesthesiologist in consultation with the parents. During the preanesthetic evaluation, the anesthesiologist may invite the parents to be present or the parents may ask to be present. Either way, the anesthesiologist and other members of the team must be comfortable with the concept. If this is not the way they usually practice, they should communicate this to the family and inform the family that they would prefer to stay with their usual practice. In contrast, no parent should ever be forced to be present for induction. If a parent is uncomfortable with the idea, other options are discussed including the use of sedation. The parents should be supported in their decision and assured that someone will be there to hold and talk to their child during the induction. Second, once the decision to have parents present for induction is made, the team must decide where to induce and whether to allow more than one parent, grandparent, etc. Some institutions have induction rooms where more than one family member may be present. However, many institutions must take the parent to the operating room for induction, so it may only be feasible to allow one parent. This must be clearly communicated to the family. Third, the parents must be instructed on what to expect as their child is induced. This includes noisy breathing, eye rolling, and excitatory movements. They also must be told that, once their child is asleep, they must leave the room so that the team can perform the remaining tasks in caring for their child. It is helpful to appoint one person in the room the job of escorting the parents to the waiting area.

To summarize, parental presence during anesthetic induction is controversial and complex. As discussed, the benefits of parental presence for the child and the parents are a topic of debate. Although the short-term benefits to the child are questionable, the benefits for the parents appear to be real, at least as perceived by the parents themselves. The effect of parental presence on the relationship between parent and child in the long run has not been adequately studied. For example: Is there anything wrong with children getting upset with the idea that they are about to undergo surgery that they don't want? It would seem that this negative reaction is normal. Nonetheless, overcoming this challenge with the help of one's parents may actually strengthen the relationship between parent and child.

Despite one's best efforts to alleviate a child's anxiety, including premedication, parental presence, or preoperative tours, every now and then an anticipated smooth induction goes sour. Even though the child may hold the mask preoperatively and seem completely cooperative, when the moment of truth comes, the child decides differently. This makes for a very difficult situation, particularly if parents are present. Realistically, there are three options at this point. First, one can renegotiate with the child. The key to the induction of a difficult child is to give the child the options whenever possible. By talking with the child, one can offer to hold the mask slightly farther from the face or offer an intravenous induction if the mask is too annoying. One can also consider sedation, if it hasn't already been used, and let the child choose the administration technique, oral or intramuscular. Frequently, when all the options are proposed to the child, including a shot or intravenous induction, the child decides to cooperate with the mask induction. At times, however, the situation is completely out of hand and the child will not listen or cooperate. Now there are only two options left. If the surgery is elective, you can postpone the procedure and attempt to reschedule for another day when the child is better prepared. This is obviously not a popular choice because schedules are usually tight and families have planned time off work and school. If the surgery were emergent or the parents would prefer to proceed, one would have to resort to intramuscular ketamine, as described previously.

Parents in the Postanesthetic Care Unit

At the beginning of the previous decade, very few postanesthesia care units (PACUs) allowed parents to be present for the period shortly after their children were extubated and thought to be stable. Now, at the beginning of the new millennium, many PACUs allow parents to be present for the recovery of their children. There is no question that some PACUs were doing the right thing but for the wrong reason; there was a shortage of nurses so parents would help during the shortage. Many, however, did the right thing for the right reason: to let parents be present to help in the recovery of their child because this is a particularly vulnerable period for the child who may or may not be awakening in pain but certainly is awakening in strange surroundings with people that the child does not know. The problem with the emergence of an uncooperative child is even of a greater magnitude and often compounded by previously negative experiences. The appropriate use of parents in the PACU can certainly make the transition of this child, from surgery to recovery, much smoother. One of the issues in many PACUs therefore is when to allow the parents to be reunited with their children.

Most PACUs will not allow parents to be present if the child is still intubated or has an artificial airway of any kind. This seems a reasonable approach because there may be an urgency or emergency that arises which would be inappropriate for a parent to be observing. However, shortly after all the artificial airways are removed and the child is beginning to arouse, the presence of a parent is appropriate because they can help the child return to orientation with a familiar person. Some PACUs require that the child be almost fully recovered before allowing parents to the child's bedside. This philosophy is somewhat puzzling and seems rather arbitrary. If the object of the parents' presence is to help the child to reorient, then it seems reasonable that parents should be present while the child is reorienting. Clearly each case should be examined individually so that parents who are present during the recovery of their child are of help and not emotionally distraught, which hinders the child's recovery. In addition, the parent can be of assistance in helping to determine whether the child's upset is secondary to pain or due to another factor. Parents often can make the distinction between "normal distress" and that which is more serious or distressing.

Postoperative Discussion

It is very useful to debrief with parents in the recovery room so that the members of the anesthesia care team can have an unhurried, meaningful discussion with the parents about the perioperative care of their child. What do the parents think might make the preoperative preparation easier? Was there anything about the premedication that might be improved? Are there any suggestions for improving the type of induction? It is very important to ask parents for their input about how things might have been better for themselves and the child, especially for those with difficult emotional and physical issues.

In summary, the management of the difficult child or difficult parent challenges the ingenuity of the anesthesiologist. The important issues for the anesthesiologist are: (1) being a very attentive listener to the spoken and unspoken messages of the parents and the child and (2) empathy and support because this might be an extraordinarily difficult time for the entire family. Many parents think they know, and often they do know, what is best for their child. Many health care givers are, unfortunately, offended when parents tell them how they think their child should be managed. Unless the parent is suggesting an approach that is harmful to the child, every effort should be made to accommodate, in some way, the wishes of the parent. It is also very important to find out why parents are angry, whether the message comes from the nurse or from your own perception. Often the air can be cleared quite easily with empathy for the situation and by directly addressing the problem. Sometimes the parent simply desires an apology regarding the fact that they were asked to come 3 h early and had to sit and wait for what seemed to them to be forever to receive their medical care. If we were to find ourselves in the same position, we might have the same emotions.

The well-trained and experienced anesthesiologist often has a number of options for accomplishing various steps in the perioperative period: premedication versus no premedication, the type of premedication, and the choice of induction agents. By using all possible skills and options, the clever and innovative anesthesiologist often can manage the difficult child or difficult parent in a way that is satisfying to all and often results in a more cooperative and less frightened child at the next occasion. In addition, there is a certain satisfaction to meeting a formidable challenge and managing it in a very thoughtful and effective way to the satisfaction of the entire health care team, as well as the child and the parents.

APPENDIX: A PARENT'S PERSPECTIVE

Carol Brown Michael, Freelance Writer

> All happy families resemble one another, but all unhappy families are unhappy in their own way.
>
> (Leo Tolstoy, *Anna Karenina*)

It's 6:00 A.M. and my husband and I are in an examining room waiting for our son Josh to be sedated for spinal fusion surgery. Josh, severely affected by tuberous sclerosis, is tired and hungry and scared, and so are we. With a complex chronic disease, Josh is a frequent patient at this hospital and has a thick chart. This morning we gave Josh's history to a nurse, a surgical resident, and a medical student, but the anesthesiologist doesn't seem to know anything about Josh when he arrives to sedate him. The doctor is not focused on communicating with him, which takes concentration in far less stressful situations, or with us, or on how he can best approach Josh for the needle prick. He has difficulty finding a vein and Josh becomes agitated.

> "Don't worry, it will just feel like a bee sting, and then it will be over," the doctor says lightly.
> "No bees, no bees, no bees!!!" Josh cries.

In a panic, he flails his arms as if there were a swarm in the room. Although I have no doubt that the doctor intended to minimize his fear, with Josh it only serves to inflame his anxiety. It takes a long time to calm Josh and then sedate him. We are all miserable, the anesthesiologist included, by the time he is wheeled away to the operating room.

Two days later, that same anesthesiologist came to Josh's room to speak to us. He wanted to know how to do it differently the next time. How do you approach a child with limited language? What do you say to the family? In addition to medical skill and technical competence, what do patients need from their physicians? What do parents look for? How much can doctors give? There is no one correct answer to these tough questions, no one way for doctors to act, no one way that works best for all families. But we must take an approach that looks beyond the illness and diagnosis to see the whole child and family rather than an isolated health problem.

> The things we cannot measure may be the things that ultimately sustain our lives.[41]

In our professional lives, in medicine, in law, in education, we use case studies to illustrate important points. In our personal lives, we use stories—bedtime stories, folk tales, Bible stories, war stories, legends. Telling stories is how we teach our children about their family history, our moral values, and spiritual and religious beliefs. They listen to our stories and make personal connections through them to understand the world. Sometimes parents tell the stories to make loss meaningful.

Taking a medical history is like hearing a story. Good doctors listen carefully. They know that not everything a doctor needs to know is contained in the answers to specific questions. Good doctors understand that the stories parents tell often contain the details they need to approach a child successfully, make them comfortable, and help a procedure go more smoothly.

Parents want to make their children well. In general, they are excellent observers and reporters of their children's behavior. They know them better than anyone else, spend more time with them, and have a vested interest in their health. Parents know and deal with the side effects of the medication their children take. They see and report the seizures their children have. They deal with their children's behavior and know the interventions that do and don't work. They know what comforts their children, what frightens them, and what infuriates them. In the medical world, this information is called *anecdotal evidence*. But calling it *anecdotal evidence* minimizes it, as if it's not as important because it's not hard data. It should never replace data, but sometimes vital information is missed because it serves a different purpose than the one the doctor has in mind.

Parents look to the experts for the information they do not have and to the doctors to heal what they cannot. Experts and doctors need to listen carefully to the information parents have. Crucial details often are not captured on a questionnaire or a form. Doctors must make the time to hear the story, to watch how it is told. That relationship between the doctor and the patient and family is a partnership with great power. Making the child's life easier often makes the doctor's life easier.

Of course, life is often more complicated than this. Even with the best of intentions and interventions, it may not be possible to calm a child. Often children will misunderstand what a doctor has said and be unable or too afraid to voice their fears. After hearing a devastating diagnosis or a bad outcome, a family may be unable to remember anything directly after that statement or may remember only one particularly painful comment. Physicians need to choose their words carefully. They must have patience for the time it takes to understand complicated medical procedures and integrate information that may change a family's life dramatically. Anesthesiologists must understand that they are the front line in many procedures so their ability to communicate is particularly important. Enabling a patient or family to ask more questions, to plan the next steps, is not simply thoughtful or an extra dose of kindness but rather good medicine that in the end can save time.

Good communication is challenging in the best of circumstances, with normally developing children, but is much more difficult with a child who may not understand what is being said or a family with a different cultural or value system than your own. That said, sometimes the simplest questions provide the most information. When my typical child was 16 years old and in preop for knee surgery due to a sports injury, the anesthesiology fellow introduced herself to us, turned directly to my daughter, and asked, "What are you most scared of right now?" Without a moment's hesitation, Rachel replied, "the pain after my surgery," something she hadn't said to us. The doctor could then talk about pain management, answer Rachel's unasked questions, and allay her anxiety. It was exactly the right question for her, and for us, at that moment.

To listen to a patient's fears, to be reassuring, to show that you care, has worth that cannot be measured. No one can take away the fear and loss that goes along with sick children, nor can we always prevent bad outcomes; but the way we deal with them makes all the difference in the world. When a family feels well cared for, they can better tolerate the waiting, the uncertainty, and the grieving that we all have to face.

Remember that every family you meet has a story. Some will touch you more than others. Some you will remember better than others. But know that some member of every family will remember you, and what you say to them, and how you treat them.

You have the medical knowledge and expertise to make some children healthier, some children well. But many problems cannot be fixed. In all cases, you have the power to forge memories, good or bad, with individual patients and their families. That has an impact not only on future contacts in the health care system but also on a family's personal life and emotional well-being. It is in your hands, the doctor's hands, that parents place their children's health and sometimes their lives.

You have the potential to be known as someone who cares and listens. Added to the proper medication and surgery, it promotes healing of the body and the soul. You will always learn something by listening to your patients and their families. Sometimes it's what they don't say, sometimes it's what they don't know, but sometimes it's what they do say and know. Sometimes it's what you learn about yourself as you listen that will help you to help them.

REFERENCES

1. Selzer SC: Normal psychological development: theories and concepts. In *Behavioral Pediatrics*. Greydanus DE, Wolraich ML, eds. New York, Springer-Verlag, 1992.
2. Kessen W: The development of behavior. In *Developmental-Behavioral Pediatrics*. Levine MB, Carey WB, Crocker AC, eds. Philadelphia, WB Saunders, 1999.
3. Cruikshank BM, Cooper LJ: Common behavioral problems. In *Behavioral Pediatrics*. Greydanus DE, Wolraich ML, eds. New York, Springer-Verlag, 1992.
4. Still GF: Some abnormal psychiatric conditions in children. *Lancet* 1:1008, 1902.
5. Morgan AM: Attention-deficit/hyperactivity disorder. *Pediatr Clin North Am* 46, 1999.
6. Williams C, Wright B, Partridge I: Attention deficit hyperactivity disorder—a review. *Br J Gen Pract* 49:563, 1999.
7. Lin-Dyken DC, Wolraich ML: Attention deficit hyperactivity disorder. In *Behavioral Pediatrics*. Greydanus DE, Wolraich ML, eds. New York, Springer-Verlag, 1992.
8. American Psychiatric Association: *Diagnostic and Statistical Manual of Mental Disorders*, 4th ed. Washington, DC, American Psychiatric Association, 1994.
9. Greenhill LL, Halperin JM, Abikoff H: Stimulant medications. *J Am Acad Child Adolesc Psychiatry* 38:503, 1999.
10. Conner DF, Fletcher KE, Swanson JM: A meta-analysis of clonidine for symptoms of attention-deficit hyperactivity disorder. *J Am Acad Child Adolesc Psychiatry* 38:1551, 1999.
11. Kolko DJ, Bukstein OG, Barron J: Methylphenidate and behavior modification in children with ADHD and comorbid ODD or CD: main and incremental effects across settings. *J Am Acad Child Adolesc Psychiatry* 38:578, 1999.
12. Beitchman JH, Young AR: Learning disorders with a special emphasis on reading disorders: a review of the past 10 years. *J Am Acad Child Adolesc Psychiatry* 36:1020, 1997.
13. Mauk JE: Autism and pervasive developmental disorders. *Pediatr Clin North Am* 40:567, 1993.
14. Charman T: Autism and the pervasive developmental disorders. *Curr Opin Neurol* 12:155, 1999.
15. Hamdan-Allen G, Vilda B, Scott-Miller D: Infantile autism. In *Behavioral Pediatrics*. Greydanus DE, Wolraich ML, eds. New York, Springer-Verlag, 1992.
16. Rapin I: Current concepts: autism. *N Engl J Med* 337:97, 1997.
17. Feldman HM, Kolmen BK, Gonzaga AM: Naltrexone and communication skills in young children with autism. *J Am Acad Child Adolesc Psychiatry* 38:587, 1999.

CHAPTER 6 / PROVIDING CARE FOR THE CHILD, PARENT, AND FAMILY

18. Riddle MA, Bernstein GA, Cook EH, et al: Anxiolysis, adrenergic agents and naltrexone. *J Am Acad Child Adolesc Psychiatry* 38:546, 1999.
19. Goldson E: The behavioral aspects of chronic illness. In *Behavioral Pediatrics*. Greydanus DE, Wolraich ML, eds. New York, Springer-Verlag, 1992.
20. Perrin JM, Thyen U: Chronic illness. In *Developmental–Behavioral Pediatrics*. Levine MB, Carey WB, Crocker AC, eds. Philadelphia, WB Saunders, 1999.
21. Perrin EC: Hospitalization, surgery, and medical procedures. In *Developmental–Behavioral Pediatrics*. Levine MB, Carey WB, Crocker AC, eds. Philadelphia, WB Saunders, 1999.
22. Aylward GP: Behavioral and developmental disorders of the infant and young child: assessment and management. In *Behavioral Pediatrics*. Greydanus DE, Wolraich ML, eds. New York, Springer-Verlag, 1992.
23. Wolke D: Psychological development of prematurely born children. *Arch Dis Child* 78:567, 1998.
24. Ellerbeck KA, Smith ML, Holden EW, et al: Neurodevelopmental outcomes in children surviving d-transposition of the great arteries. *Dev Behav Pediatr* 19:335, 1998.
25. Wolraich ML: Communicating with patients and parents. In *Behavioral Pediatrics*. Greydanus DE, Wolraich ML, eds. New York, Springer-Verlag, 1992.
26. Kagan J: The role of parents in children's psychological development. *Pediatrics* 104:164, 1999.
27. Schulman JL, Foley JM, Vernon MA, Allan D: A study of the effect of the mother's presence during anesthesia induction. *Pediatrics* 39:111, 1967.
28. Hannallah RS, Rosales JK: Experience with parents' presence during anaesthesia induction in children. *Can Anaesth Soc J* 30:286, 1983.
29. Yemen TA, Nelson W: Parental presence at induction: do the parents make a difference? *Anesthesiology* 77:A1167, 1992.
30. Bevan JC, Johnson C, Haig MJ, et al: Preoperative parental anxiety predicts behavioural and emotional responses to induction of anaesthesia in children. *Can J Anaesth* 37:177, 1990.
31. Kain ZN, Mayes LC, Caramico LA, et al: Parental presence during induction of anesthesia: a randomized controlled trial. *Anesthesiology* 84:1060, 1996.
32. Kain ZN, Mayes LC, Wang S, et al: Parental presence during induction of anesthesia versus sedative premedication: which intervention is more effective? *Anesthesiology* 89:1147, 1998.
33. Kain ZN, Mayes LC, Wang S, et al: Parental presence and a sedative premedicant for children undergoing surgery: a hierarchical study. *Anesthesiology* 92:939, 2000.
34. Ryder IG, Spargo PM: Parents in the anaesthetic room: a questionnaire survey of parents' reactions. *Anaesthesia* 46:977, 1991.
35. Vessey JA, Bogetz MS, Caserza CL, et al: Parental upset associated with induction of anaesthesia in children. *Can J Anaesth* 41:276, 1994.
36. Kain ZN, Ferris CA, Mayes LC, et al: Parental presence during induction of anaesthesia: practice differences between the United States and Great Britain. *Pediatr Anaesth* 6:187, 1996.
37. McCormick ASM, Spargo PM: Parents in the anaesthetic room: a questionnaire survey of departments of anaesthesia. *Pediatr Anaesth* 6:183, 1996.
38. Roman DEM, Barker I: Anaesthetists' attitudes to parental presence at induction of general anaesthesia in children. *Anaesthesia* 48:338, 1993.
39. Hannallah RS, Abramowitz MD, Oh TH, et al: Residents' attitudes toward parents' presence during anaesthesia induction in children: does experience make a difference? *Anesthesiology* 60:598, 1984.
40. Lewyn MJ: Should parents be present while their children receive anesthesia? *Anesth Malpract Protect* 23:56, 1993.
41. Remen RN: Kitchen table wisdom: stories that heal. New York, Riverhead Books, 1996.

7 | The Child With Respiratory Problems

Jennifer E. O'Flaherty, MD, MPH
Terrance A. Yemen, MD

The child with a respiratory disease is a common problem in pediatric anesthesia. A thorough and practical knowledge of the variety of respiratory diseases and their anesthetic management is one of the cornerstones to successful pediatric anesthesia. This chapter reviews those respiratory problems most commonly encountered in our pediatric practice. Apnea of the premature and ex-premature infant and the child with an anterior mediastinal mass are covered in detail in accompanying chapters in this textbook. The goal of this chapter is to educate the reader in the pathophysiology of the disorder and its current anesthetic management. Particular effort has been made to give the reader our personal approach to these problems based on our clinical experience and our reading of the relevant literature.

THE CHILD WITH AN UPPER RESPIRATORY TRACT INFECTION

The approach to the child with a runny nose is probably the most common clinical dilemma facing the practitioner who anesthetizes children. Upper respiratory tract infection (URI) is the number one reason for cancellation of elective pediatric surgical cases. The primary problem is that URIs generally present on the day of surgery and are rarely present at the preoperative visit when the elective surgical procedure can be more easily postponed. Unfortunately, URIs are extremely common in young children. Children age 1 to 5 years are expected to have three to eight URIs per year. If we canceled surgery in every child with a runny nose, we would infrequently perform elective surgery in children.

A URI implies involvement of the airway above the vocal cords, i.e., a nasopharyngitis. It is viral in origin, and the two most common offending viruses are rhinovirus and adenovirus. Neither virus readily infects the lower airways, although certain abnormalities of the lower airways usually accompany a URI.

The gold standard for diagnosing a URI is a viral culture with acute and chronic antibody titers. Obviously this is not practical in clinical practice. In 1987, Tait and Knight proposed a way to define URIs with the use of clinical signs and symptoms, chiefly for the purpose of clinical study.[1] The criteria are listed in Table 7-1. At least two of the criteria must be met, with 1 + 2, 3 + 4, 4 + 6, and 5 + 6 requiring one additional symptom. These criteria have been adopted by many investigators, thereby allowing different clinical studies to be comparable. Although currently the best criteria in existence, these criteria are imperfect. The criteria do a good job of excluding lower respiratory tract infections but, in our experience, are likely to include other things that are not URIs, particularly allergic rhinitis.

The differential diagnosis of URI includes a foreign body in the nasal passages or airway, exanthema, lower respiratory tract infection, vasomotor rhinitis (crying), allergic rhinitis, asthma, influenza, laryngotracheobronchitis (croup), and bacterial infections such as sinusitis, streptococcal pharyngitis, and rarely epiglottitis, orbital/buccal cellulitis, and pneumonia. Allergic

TABLE 7–1 Clinical Criteria Used to Diagnose an Upper Respiratory Tract Infection

1. Sore or scatchy throat
2. Malaise
3. Sneezing
4. Rhinorrhea
5. Congestion
6. Nonproductive cough
7. Fever < 101°F (38.5°C)
8. Laryngitis

Note: At least two of the criteria must be met. Combinations of 1 + 2, 3 + 4, 4 + 6, or 5 + 6 require one additional symptom.
Source: Tait AR, Knight PR: The effects of general anesthesia on upper respiratory tract infections in children. *Anesthesiology* 67:930, 1987.

rhinitis is the most difficult condition to distinguish from a URI. Allergic rhinitis is very common in children. It is usually benign, although it may indicate a tendency toward reactive airway disease (see The Child With Asthma). The patient's parent or guardian is essential in distinguishing allergic rhinitis from a URI; they can tell you whether their child is "this way all the time."

As we learn more about the pathophysiologic changes that accompany airway infections, it is clear that the upper and lower respiratory tracts are not entirely discrete. Although viruses that cause URIs seem clinically to be restricted to the upper respiratory tract, it is becoming more and more evident that they affect the lower respiratory tract in causing abnormalities in the peripheral airways that result in alterations in airflow and distribution. Upper respiratory infections are accompanied by peripheral airway abnormalities, airway hyperreactivity, and alterations in airway secretions. It is clear from many studies that these impairments in respiratory function persist for 5 to 6 weeks after a viral URI.[2,3]

Peripheral airway abnormalities include decreases in forced expiratory volume in 1 s (FEV_1), vital capacity, and forced vital capacity (FVC). Closing volume is increased, which predisposes to intrapulmonary shunting and hypoxemia. Diffusion capacity is decreased secondary to inflammation. There is impairment of hypoxic pulmonary vasoconstriction, which also contributes to the risk of hypoxemia. Interestingly, there also appears to be some increase in oxygen uptake by the lungs themselves secondary to the inflammatory response to the acute infection. This increased oxygen need by the lungs also contributes to the risk of hypoxemia.

Increased airway reactivity is observed with direct touch (e.g., the endotracheal tube) and chemical stimulation (e.g., volatile anesthetic agents). The etiology of this hyperreactivity does not appear to be an intrinsic abnormality of the smooth muscle of the airways. Airway smooth muscle taken from animals with experimental viral infections contracts and relaxes normally in vitro. Increased airway reactivity may be due in part to direct irritation of inflamed airway mucosa through a variety of immunologic and inflammatory reactions, most of which release histamine. However, most cases of airway hyperreactivity appear to be vagally mediated. Patients with URI experience an increase in vagally mediated reflex bronchoconstriction. Of significance to practitioners, it has been shown that airway hyperreactivity seen with viral URIs in humans can be blocked with anticholinergic medications such as atropine and glycopyrrolate.[4]

Viral infections alter the quality and character of airway secretions. The increase in volume may be due to an increase in tachykinin and acetylcholine activity, both of which stimulate airway submucosal gland secretion. There is also an increase in airway debris secondary to desquamation of epithelial cells that have been destroyed or damaged by the infection. Mucus clearance is impaired because of damage to the ciliated cells, which normally clear the airways, with destruction of the epithelial border, leading to disruption of the normal micro-osmolar gradient.

Potential perioperative complications of URIs include laryngospasm, bronchospasm, coughing, endotracheal tube obstruction, breath-holding, apnea, atelectasis, hypoxemia, and rarely cardiovascular collapse secondary to viral myocarditis. A recent case-control study by Schreiner et al. found that pediatric patients who developed laryngospasm intraoperatively were over two times more likely to have an active URI. Endotracheal tube obstruction may occur secondary to increased secretions.[5] Atelectasis may occur when secretions and debris in the airway cause mucus plugging and alveolar collapse. Hypoxemia can be the result of changes in the peripheral airways or atelectasis. Viral URIs may be associated with an asthma exacerbation. Croup and pneumonia are known complications of URIs. There may be edema of the tracheal and nasal mucosa leading to stridor or nasal airway obstruction. Patients with URIs may have a stormy induction, thereby increasing the risk of regurgitation and aspiration, or a stormy emergence, thereby possibly increasing the risk of postobstructive pulmonary edema.

It has traditionally been assumed that the presence of a URI leads to increased perioperative risk.[6,7] Initially, evidence to this effect was strictly anecdotal, in the form of case reports. For instance, in 1979 McGill et al. published a retrospective case series of 11 patients who developed respiratory complications immediately after induction.[8] The only thing that these patients appeared to have in common was a URI in the preceding month. Although case reports may point to potential problems, they do not determine the incidence of a problem or delineate cause and effect. This is a very difficult area to study, particularly in any randomized fashion. The definitions of URI and increased perioperative risk used in the literature have been highly variable. A few retrospective clinical studies have been performed and seem to indicate an increased risk of respiratory complications including laryngospasm, bronchospasm, and desaturation in patients with active or resolving URIs. An inherent limitation of retrospective studies is an unclear relation between cause and effect. Further, none of the retrospective studies have shown any difference in outcome.

In 1987, Tait and Knight published the first well-conducted prospective study to address the safety of general anesthesia in children with URI.[1] They studied 243 children, aged 1 to 12 years, undergoing positron emission tomographic placement and found no increase in morbidity for patients with URI. Clearly this study is limited in scope as those patients were undergoing minor surgery lasting less than 15 min and without endotracheal intubation. In 1988, DeSoto et al. carried out a prospective study of the intraoperative and postoperative courses of 25 normal control subjects and 25 children with acute symptoms of a URI (as defined by Tait and Knight's criteria).[9] All patients underwent otolaryngologic procedures and 74% (equal numbers from each group) were intubated. They found that 20% of the URI group had SpO2 below 95% in the postanesthesia care unit, whereas none of the patients in the control group had SpO2 below 95% in the postanesthesia care unit. SpO2 quickly improved with the use of supplemental oxygen and patients were easily weaned from supplemental oxygen (maintaining SpO2 > 95%) by the time they had met their other discharge criteria (Table 7-2). The investigators concluded that children with URIs "manifest transient desaturation early in the recovery period, [which] may be related to the inability to manage secretions following general anesthesia." They recommend that patients with URI "be given supplemental oxygen and have their oxygen saturation monitored in the recovery room and during transport." In 1992, Levy et al. prospectively studied 130 children scheduled for positron emission tomographic placement and not requiring tracheal intubation.[10] They found no significant difference in intraoperative respiratory complications between the acute URI group, the recent URI group, and an asymptomatic group. However, they found that the incidence of hypoxemia (SpO2 < 93%) was significantly greater in the acute and recent URI groups during transfer to the postanesthesia care unit and in the acute URI group during the postanesthesia care unit stay. Supplemental oxygen resulted in a rapid rise in the SpO2. They concluded that "children with an acute or recent upper respiratory infection have an increased likelihood of transient hypoxaemia in the perioperative period, which responds promptly to supplemental oxygen therapy." Rolf and Cote in 1992 prospectively studied 402 pediatric patients, 30 of whom had URI with the Tait and Knight criteria. Half of each patient group was intubated.[11] The investigators found no differences in the incidence of major desaturations or other respiratory complications in patients with URI versus those without URI. They did, however, find a higher incidence of minor desaturations in patients with URI (Figure 7-1).

In 1995, Tait et al. published the results of a survey sent to 400 members of the Society for Pediatric Anesthesia.[12] Those results indicated that there is a wide range of opinions and approaches to the child with URI. The practice of canceling elective surgery for children with URI seem to be changing over time because younger anesthesiologists tend to cancel less often than do older anesthesiologists.

Because there are no clear-cut guidelines for when to proceed with elective surgery in a child with URI, a judgment is required on the part of the anesthesiologist.[13] Factors that influence our decision as to whether or not to proceed include:

1. *Nature and urgency of the surgery.* Obviously emergent cases must be done. Superficial cases requiring a quick mask general anesthetic we are most inclined to do. We also take into consideration that it may necessary to do the case to clear up the source of recurrent infection (e.g., tonsillectomy). We consider postponing cases where postoperative coughing is a serious concern (e.g., breakage of abdominal sutures, vitreous bleeding).

TABLE 7–2 Number of Patients Who Had SaO2 < 95% While Breathing Room Air in the Recovery Room*

	Control group (*n* = 25)	URI group (*n* = 25)
SaO2 ≥ 95%	25	20
SaO2 ≤ 95%	0	5

URI, upper respiratory tract infection.
*$p < 0.03$.
Source: Modified from DeSoto H, Patel RI, Soliman IE, Hannallah RS: Changes in oxygen saturation following general anesthesia in children with upper respiratory infection signs and symptoms undergoing otolaryngological procedures. *Anesthesiology* 68:276, 1988.

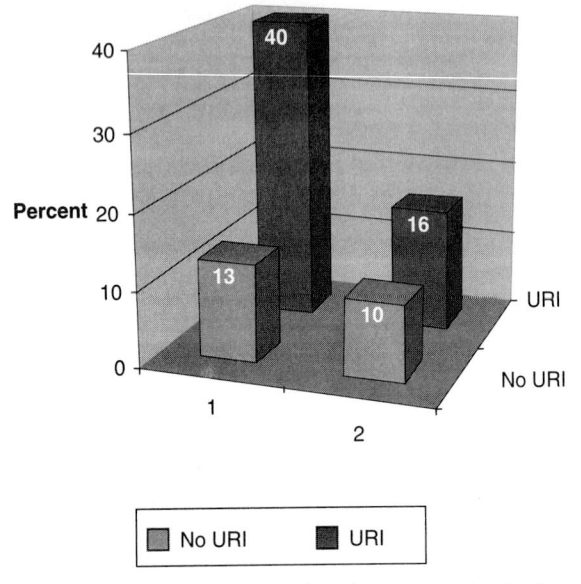

FIG. 7-1 Frequency of episodes of major oxygen desaturation (SpO2 ≤ 85% for at least 30 sec) and minor oxygen desaturation (SpO2 ≤ 95% for at least 60 sec) in patients with and without URIs. 1, minor desaturations; 2, major desaturations; URI, upper respiratory infections. *(Modified from Rolf N, Cote CJ: Frequency and severity of desaturation events during general anesthesia in children with and without upper respiratory infections.* J Clin Anesth 4:200, 1992.)

2. *American Society of Anesthetists Physical Status (ASA PS).* Evidence of serious comorbid disease, particularly asthma, makes us more inclined to postpone an elective case in a patient with URI.
3. *Nature and severity of the URI.* If the URI is severe or just starting (and it is unclear how severe it may become), then we are likely to postpone elective surgery. If the patient has a high fever, lower respiratory tract symptoms, decreased appetite, a change in activity level, a change in sleeping habits, or irritability, we postpone the surgery.
4. *Patient's age.* We are more inclined to postpone surgery for patients who are younger than 1 year.
5. *Predicted difficult airway.* We are more inclined to postpone elective surgery in a patient with a potentially difficult airway because of the compound risk of perioperative airway complications.
6. *Evidence of other infection, particularly lower respiratory tract infection.* A productive cough, rales, wheezing, decreased breath sounds, increased work of breathing, and/or tachypnea will almost certainly cause us to postpone the surgery. Purulent rhinorrhea, pharyngeal ulcers, and/or frank tonsillitis usually will lead us to postpone the surgery.
7. *Experience and confidence of the anesthesiologist.* This factor was considered very important by the respondents to Tait and Knight's questionnaire.
8. *Practical considerations.* These are of lesser importance but may play a role. We might consider previous cancellation (which is not an unusual

occurrence, as the patient may have another URI the next time around), parents' stress level, and parents' travel time.
9. *Financial considerations.* These are of lesser importance but may play a role. Parental finances (time off work) and institutional finances (use and cost of resources: operating room time, anesthesia time, surgical time) may play roles in the decision to postpone elective surgery.

There are no preoperative laboratory tests routinely in children with URI. Viral cultures are impractical and too expensive to be employed in anything but a research setting. Although the white blood cell count may be low in children with viral URI, it is usually normal and not predictive of anesthetic risk. A chest x-ray is helpful only if there are specific findings on the x-ray. The x-ray is nondiagnostic if it is normal. Further, a chest x-ray is indicated only in children with signs of lower respiratory tract infection, who are likely to be canceled for an elective procedure irrespective of the x-ray findings.

If the decision is made to proceed with surgery in a child with URI, then the anesthesiologist must be mindful of the potential complications and take precautions to avoid or remedy them. Local or regional anesthesia should be used wherever possible. Although amantidine may shorten and mitigate the clinical course of a URI, it probably does not affect the degree or duration of airway hyperreactivity. Use of amantidine perioperatively is not routinely indicated. We strongly recommend the use of an anticholinergic premedication. A major component of bronchial hyperreactivity during a URI is vagally mediated, and anticholinergic medications block this airway hyperresponsiveness and decrease the risk of coughing and bronchospasm. Anticholinergics also decrease the quantity of secretions. Atropine (0.02 mg/kg, minimum 0.1 mg, maximum 0.4 mg, intramuscularly or intravenously) or glycopyrrolate (0.01 mg/kg, minimum 0.1 mg, maximum, 0.4 mg intramuscularly or intravenously) may be used. Although premedication with nebulized lidocaine (4%) may attenuate the airway hyperreactivity associated with URI, administration of nebulized medication in an already anxious child usually results in little of the medication being delivered and a more agitated child with more airway secretions. We always have a β_2-selective agonist bronchodilator immediately available.

Our preference for induction is a slow mask induction with the use of a volatile anesthetic agent such as sevoflurane or halothane; both are minimally irritating to the airways and bronchodilatory. Alternatively, an intravenous induction can be done using propofol, which is also bronchodilatory. Ketamine is not indicated because this drug will further increase airway secretions. Barbiturates are not indicated because they have been associated with an increased risk of laryngospasm.[14] If the patient does not already have an intravenous line, it is important to insert one shortly after induction. To avoid laryngospasm, it is important to achieve sufficient depth of anesthesia before attempting to insert an oral airway or an instrument into the airway. Sometimes we administer a muscle relaxant to assist with airway control and decrease the risk of laryngospasm.

Intraoperatively we are careful to take measures to avoid atelectasis, such as ensuring adequate tidal volumes, ensuring adequate hydration, and using low gas flows with gas humidification to avoid drying of secretions, which may lead to atelectasis. We might use spontaneous or controlled ventilation, depending on the nature of the surgical case, but have found that manual expansion of the lungs may be necessary if the patient desaturates. We administer a β_2-selective agonist bronchodilator (e.g. albuterol, two to four puffs from a metered dose inhaler via the anesthesia circuit) if the patient develops bronchospasm. Intraoperatively, we might not use nitrous oxide because it can cause acute problems in the patient whose URI has led to a blocked Eustachian tube or reduced drainage from the paranasal sinuses.

At emergence we are prepared for the same potential problems as with induction: secretions and an irritable airway may lead to coughing, laryngospasm, breathholding, and apnea. We have found that a dose of intravenous lidocaine (1.0 to 1.5 mg/kg) shortly before emergence will significantly smooth emergence. Alternatively, a dose of lidocaine (3.0 to 5.0 mg/kg) applied directly to the vocal cords on induction can significantly decrease upper airway irritability by the end of the case. We are less inclined to apply lidocaine to the vocal cords in patients with URI because the act of squirting the cords with medication often causes laryngospasm. To decrease the risk of laryngospasm on emergence, we extubate these patients when they are deeply anesthetized or very awake. Because an increased likelihood of hypoxemia is clearly associated with URIs,[9–11,15] we usually plan to use supplemental oxygen and a pulse oximeter for transport to the postanesthesia care unit and in the early phase of recovery. Pain must be treated adequately because it can exacerbate an irritable airway, increase secretions, and increase the patient's oxygen requirement, thereby contributing to the potential for hypoxemia. Balanced with that, it is important to minimize postoperative sedation and respiratory depression so that the patient's airway reflexes, in particular the ability to cough up secretions, recover quickly.

Until recently, the endotracheal tube has been the only routine alternative to the face mask for intraoperative management of a patient's airway. The introduction of the laryngeal mask airway (LMA) has given clinicians another option. Endotracheal tubes are a major risk factor for the precipitation of respiratory complications such as coughing, laryngospasm, bronchospasm, and atelectasis. On the one hand, LMAs, because they are less invasive to the airway, may be less likely to precipitate these complications. Also, unlike endotracheal tubes, LMAs do not have the potential to introduce pathogens into the lower respiratory tract. Further, the incidence of postoperative sore throat is lower with the use of LMAs. On the other hand, although the trachea is not stimulated by the LMA, the epiglottis may be stimulated, which can lead to laryngospasm, bronchospasm, coughing, and breath-holding. If any of these complications were to occur, the LMA would not be as reliable an airway as an endotracheal tube. The role of LMAs in children with URIs has just begun to be studied. Tait et al. published a study in 1998 which looked at LMA use in children with URIs.[16] They studied 82 ASA PS 1 and 2 patients with URIs, 3 months to 16 years of age, scheduled for outpatient elective surgery, randomized to receive an LMA or an endotracheal tube. Although all respiratory complications were easily managed in both groups, the total number of respiratory complications (coughing, laryngospasm, bronchospasm, breath-holding, excessive secretions, oxygen desaturation) was significantly greater in the endotracheal tube group (35 vs. 19, $p < 0.05$). In addition, at 24 h, there was twice the incidence of sore throat in the endotracheal tube group as in the LMA group (25.6% vs. 13.5%). In our practices, we use a face mask or an LMA whenever practical in a patient with a URI and are always prepared to urgently replace the LMA with an endotracheal tube if a serious airway complication occurs.

In conclusion, when considering the anesthetic plan for a patient with URI, we first take a careful history and perform a thorough physical examination. Patients with clear rhinorrhea, nonproductive cough, sneezing, congestion, and/or low fever (<38.5°C) are probably fit for anesthesia and surgery. Patients with high fever, decreased appetite, a change in sleeping habits or activity level, irritability, or evidence of a lower respiratory tract infection will likely need to have their elective surgeries postponed, even though surgery may be necessary to control the source of the patient's recurrent symptoms. We discuss the risk with the parents to the extent of our current knowledge, namely that there may be an increased risk of perioperative respiratory complications that are easily managed and do not appear to pose any alteration in the outcome of the surgery or the anesthesia. We premedicate with glycopyrrolate and always have a β_2-selective agonist bronchodilator immediately available. We plan to mask ventilate or insert an LMA without clear evidence that an endotracheal tube is more appropriate for a particular surgery. Because the most likely untoward event perioperatively is mild hypoxemia, we plan to monitor the oxygen saturation and provide supplemental oxygen for transport and in the early recovery period in the postanesthesia care unit.

THE CHILD WITH CYSTIC FIBROSIS

Cystic fibrosis (CF) is an autosomal recessive disease with an incidence in people of European descent of 1 in 2000 to 1 in 5000, which makes it the most common autosomal recessive disorder in that population. One in 20 to 25 persons of European descent is a carrier of the CF gene. This disease is characterized by copious viscid mucous production that affects multiple organ systems, in particular the lungs and the exocrine pancreas. In 1938, after carefully reviewing the clinical histories and performing a number of autopsies on infants and children with the disease, Anderson published a remarkably accurate description of the disease and its end organ effects. Because of the unique microscopic changes she observed in the pancreas, she designated this disease "cystic fibrosis of the pancreas."[17] Over the next several decades therapeutic strategies for patients with CF slowly improved, with advancements in airway clearance, nutrition, and treatment of infection with antibiotics.[18,19] In the early 20th century, CF was uniformly fatal in infancy or early childhood. By 1969 8% of CF patients reached adulthood, and today most CF patients reach adulthood. In fact, the median survival age is now 28 to 30 years.[20] Because of the improved survival, anesthesiologists are seeing patients with CF in the operating suite more and more frequently for surgeries related to their disease and unrelated surgeries. Surgeries related to CF include diagnostic studies (computed tomography, esophagoscopy, bronchoscopy), surgery to secure venous access, placement of an enteral feeding tube, ENT surgery (functional endoscopic sinus surgery, nasal polypectomy), and lung transplantation. In addition, most CF patients lead an ordinary active life and may come to the operating room for surgery unrelated to their disease.

In 1985 the CF gene was isolated on the long arm of chromosome 7.[21] The gene product, which functions as a chloride channel, has been termed the cystic fibrosis transmembrane conductance regulator (CFTR). In isolating the CF gene, investigators also identified the mutation that appears to account for approximately 70% of CF cases. That mutation is known as the δ-F508 mutation because it results in the deletion of phenylalanine at position 508. More than 500 other gene mutations that can lead to CF have been identified worldwide, most of which are extremely rare. Only 20 mutations occur with any frequency worldwide. The CFTR protein appears in all organs that contain epithelial cells, including sweat glands. Reabsorption of chloride ions is impaired in the sweat glands. This forms the basis of the sweat chloride test, which is positive when a sweat chloride concentration greater than 60 mmol/L is obtained.

Cystic fibrosis is a multisystem disease. The major systemic aberrations of concern to the anesthesiologist are pulmonary compromise, sinus disease, glucose intolerance, and gastroesophageal reflux disease.[22,23] Greater than 90% of the mortality in patients with CF is secondary to pulmonary disease. CF patients exhibit decreased chloride secretion through CFTR channels and excessive sodium absorption, leading to dehydration of lumenal fluids. Relative dehydration of secretions in the respiratory tree leads to more viscous mucus and impaired mucociliary clearance and ultimately to the growth of bacterial pathogens. Colonization of the lower respiratory tract stimulates airway inflammatory responses with recruitment of neutrophils and release of cellular debris, which accumulates in the endobronchial lumen. Chronic infection and inflammation lead to bronchiectasis. Airway hyperreactivity is common and contributes to airway obstruction. Pulmonary exacerbations occur frequently, especially after viral infections. Infections with *Staphylococcus aureus*, *Streptococcus pneumoniae*, and *Haemophilus influenzae* predominate in younger patients, and the establishment of chronic *Pseudomonas aeruginosa* infection usually occurs by adolescence. *Pseudomonas aeruginosa* is not directly pathogenic to the normal lower respiratory tract. However, over time, *P. aeruginosa* may transform to a mucoid form. Mucoid *P. aeruginosa* interferes with normal opsonization and phagocytosis of bacteria. Eventually, chronic infection with *Pseudomonas cepacia* can occur and is often associated with severe lung disease. Colonization with *Aspergillus fumigatus* and atypical mycobacteria occur with very high frequency. In addition to progressive lung damage, CF patients may develop pneumothoraces, hemoptysis, and/or empyemas. Pneumothoraces are usually caused by the rupture of a subpleural bleb. Although pneumothoraces are rare in children with CF, the incidence increases in adolescence, and pneumothoraces occur in up to 20% of adults. Survival after the onset of a pneumothorax is typically 30 months. The recurrence rate is 50% to 70%.[24] Unfortunately, surgical amelioration with pleurectomy or pleurodesis may increase the technical difficulty of subsequent lung transplantation. Hemoptysis is common after age 10 years and usually results from erosion of the bronchial arteries that supply the chronically infected lung. Major bleeds may require arterial embolization and often are associated with pulmonary exacerbations requiring intravenous antibiotics. Occasionally, a chronic pulmonary infection will develop into an empyema.

Abnormal sinus mucus leads to mechanical obstruction of the sinus ostia, mucosal edema, and ciliary dysfunction. Sinus opacification is virtually universal among patients with CF. The maxillary and ethmoid sinuses may be involved as early as age 8 months, and the frontal sinuses often fail to develop. Pansinusitis and nasal polyps are common in late childhood and adolescence. Patients with persistent nasal symptoms or infections and patients preparing for lung transplantation usually require functional endoscopic sinus surgery and/or nasal polypectomy.[25] Endocrine pancreatic insufficiency is common in patients with CF by late adolescence or early adulthood. Thirty percent to 60% of patients manifest glucose intolerance and 10% to 20% develop overt diabetes. Other abnormalities of concern to the anesthesiologist include excessive dehydration, electrolyte abnormalities, hypochloremic metabolic alkalosis, and a high incidence of gastroesophageal reflux disease. In addition, patients with CF have exocrine pancreatic insufficiency leading to dietary malabsorption, with fatty stools and fat-soluble vitamin (A, D, E, K) deficiencies. Patients with CF also have a high incidence of cholelithiasis, male sterility, decreased fertility in females, recurrent constipation, and rectal prolapse.

Because the most common cause of mortality in patients with CF is respiratory failure (95% die of respiratory failure after the neonatal period), therapy for CF is focused on the respiratory system, particularly perioperatively. Pulmonary therapy for CF consists of postural drainage (which helps loosen and remove tenacious pulmonary secretions), exercise therapy, antibiotic therapy (intravenous and nebulized) to treat infectious exacerbations, bronchodilators, anticholinergics, mucolytics (N-acetylcysteine), and inhaled DNAse (which degrades neutrophil DNA and decreases the viscosity of secretions). There may be a role for corticosteroids and/or high-dose ibuprofen. High-dose ibuprofen, when taken chronically, has slowed the progression of mild pulmonary disease in some patients with CF, presumably through its anti-inflammatory effects.[26] Of interest to the anesthesiologist is that there is no evidence that acute ingestion of nonsteroidal anti-inflammatory drugs (NSAIDS) has any beneficial effect. In the not-so-distant future, gene therapy may be a realistic therapeutic option.

Preoperative evaluation for elective surgery is focused on excluding active infection, defining the extent of pulmonary disease, and maximizing the patient's condition. To exclude active pulmonary infection, it may be necessary to obtain a complete white blood cell count, a chest x-ray, and sputum cultures with sensitivities, which can then be used to guide the choice of perioperative antibiotics. Preoperatively, consideration should be given to evaluating room air oxygen saturation (with pulse oximetry), obtaining an arterial blood gas, obtaining a chest x-ray (which can identify areas of atelectasis and bullae and serve as a baseline), and/or conducting pulmonary function testing. Most patients will have variable obstructive pulmonary disease secondary to mucus plugging and airway hyperreactivity and eventually develop restrictive disease secondary to chronic lung destruction. Kerem et al. found that patients with an FEV_1 less than 30% of predicted, a partial pressure of oxygen, arterial, less than 55 mmHg, or a partial pressure of carbon dioxide, arterial, greater than 50 mmHg had a 2-year mortality rate of greater than 50%.[27] Patients with this level of disease should be evaluated for lung transplantation. In rare cases of advanced pulmonary failure, it may be advisable to obtain an echocardiogram to evaluate the patient for evidence of *cor pulmonale*.

Intraoperatively, the anesthesiologist's greatest concerns will be the management of copious secretions and bronchial hyperreactivity. The airway will require frequent suctioning. Continuous clearance of the viscous respiratory secretions is key to the success of a general anesthetic in patients with CF. Elective surgery should be performed at a time of optimal function when sputum production is at a minimum and should be avoided during a time of exacerbation. Elective procedures should be performed early in the week so that the full complement of physiotherapists and nurses is available in the early postoperative period. Surgery should be scheduled for mid-morning to maximize clearance of secretions that may have accumulated during sleep. Chest percussion therapy should continue until the patient comes to the operating room. Premedication with an anticholinergic medication to reduce respiratory secretions is controversial. The use of anticholinergics paradoxically may result in inspissated secretions, which are actually more difficult to clear. Inhaled bronchodilators and mucolytics should be taken on schedule on the morning of surgery. It is important to note that bronchodilators do not reliably improve airflow in all patients with CF and in some patients may even exacerbate airway obstruction by causing airway instability during expiration secondary to smooth muscle relaxation. Heavy sedative premedication should be avoided because it may impair clearance of pulmonary secretions. Pretreatment with H_2 blockers, antacid, or metoclopramide may be useful in patients with severe gastroesophageal reflux disease.

Because general anesthesia is associated with at least a temporary decline in pulmonary function postoperatively, regional anesthesia is the technique of choice whenever practical. Most children, however, will require a general anesthetic, in which case induction should be preceded by adequate preoxygenation. An intravenous induction using 2.0 to 3.0 mg/kg of propofol is our preference. A rapid sequence induction is usually indicated because of the high incidence of gastroesophageal reflux disease. Propofol is a good choice as an induction agent because of its rapid recovery characteristics and the absence of histamine release. Ketamine is relatively contraindicated for use in patients with CF because of its tendency to further increase secretions. Alternatively, an inhalational induction (using sevoflurane or halothane) may be used. Inhalational induction may be prolonged because of slow uptake secondary to ventilation: perfusion mismatching. Halothane is the traditional volatile agent of choice because it is bronchodilatory, but sevoflurane is probably clinically just as bronchodilatory and even less irritating to the airways on induction. Some clinicians will apply lidocaine (3.0 to 5.0 mg/kg) on the vocal cords at the beginning of the case to facilitate extubation without coughing at the end of the case. We have found that intravenous lidocaine (1.0 to 1.5 mg/kg) administered just before extubation will accomplish the same objective. Laryngospasm and coughing at induction are common. The high incidence of nasal polyps is a relative contraindication to nasal intubation. For short cases only, the LMA is a feasible alternative to the endotracheal tube and allows avoidance of the intratracheal stimulatory effects of the endotracheal tube. Disadvantages to using an LMA include the risk of laryngospasm, the risk of aspiration, and especially the inability to suction the airway. In many situations, in particular longer cases, it will be necessary to have an endotracheal tube in place for purposes of a pulmonary toilet. Typically, the airway will require frequent suctioning. Inspired gases ought to be humidified to minimize the incidence of inspissated secretions. Patients may be maintained on spontaneous, assisted, or controlled ventilation. We prefer spontaneous or assisted ventilation and avoid the use of muscle relaxants whenever possible. Positive pressure ventilation should be avoided particularly in patients with histories of recent pulmonary hemorrhage because it may lead to rebleeding of the bronchial arteries. Succinylcholine may cause myalgias that interfere with optimal chest percussion therapy postoperatively. Intermediate and long-acting muscle relaxants must be adequately reversed at the end of the procedure so that the patient's respiratory function is optimized and regain the ability to cough and clear secretions. It is important to keep in mind that aminoglycoside antibiotics, commonly used in patients with CF, can prolong the action of nondepolarizing muscle relaxants. The threshold for suspicion of a pneumothorax must be low. Nitrous oxide ought to be avoided in patients who have bullae visible on chest x-ray, who require high ventilator pressures, or who are otherwise at high risk of developing a pneumothorax. Some patients depend on hypoxic pulmonary drive and may hypoventilate when receiving supplemental oxygen. If at all possible, we extubate the patient at the end of the surgical procedure because prolonged ventilation increases the risk of infection, atelectasis, and pneumothorax. Perioperative glucose control may be an issue in patients with glucose intolerance. Because most patients with CF are relatively malnourished and thin, extra care must be taken intraoperatively to guard against heat loss. Malnutrition may make extubation difficult in some patients. Patients with CF frequently develop drug-resistant organisms because of repeated exposure to antibiotics. Strict isolation procedures must be followed and reusable equipment must be carefully sterilized after each use in these patients.

Postoperatively, adequate pain control is essential. Patients must be comfortable enough to breathe deeply and cough, thus optimizing their respiratory function. They also must be comfortable enough to tolerate chest percussion therapy. Adequate analgesia must be accomplished with minimal respiratory depression. Therefore, alternatives to opioids such as NSAIDS, local anesthesia, and regional anesthesia should be used whenever possible. Patients must receive rigorous postoperative nursing care and physiotherapy, which may be best provided in an intensive care setting.

In conclusion, when considering the patient with CF for elective surgery and anesthesia, it is crucial to have that patient's clinical condition maximized preoperatively and avoid performing elective surgery during an episode of pulmonary exacerbation. Regional anesthesia, used alone or in combination with general anesthesia, may be invaluable. The success of the general anesthetic is related directly to the success of handling the secretions. In general, our approach to patients with CF is "intubate and extubate": intubate the patient intraoperatively (to assist in handling secretions) and then extubate the patient as soon as possible postoperatively.

THE CHILD WITH ASTHMA

Asthma is a very common disorder of childhood, occurring in up to 19% of the pediatric population. It is currently the most common chronic disease in children in the United States. Asthma is characterized by airway hyperreactivity, overproduction of mucus, and chronic intermittent airway obstruction. Mucus plugging, with associated atelectasis, is common. Patients with asthma frequently exhibit other forms of atopy such as allergic rhinitis, eczema, and food intolerance. Asthma is most prevalent in young children, and most patients who develop asthma will develop it before the age of 8 years. The vast majority of patients with "mild" asthma during childhood will outgrow it by adulthood, such that fewer than 5% of adults have asthma. There is wide clinical variability in childhood asthma, ranging from mild short episodes to severe long episodes. Often, the airway obstruction can be partly or fully reversed with pharmacologic intervention. Rarely, the airway obstruction is severe and not reversed with intervention: a condition termed *status asthmaticus*. Interestingly, the incidence of asthma, in particular severe asthma requiring hospital admission, has been increasing steadily over the past several decades, possibly related to an increase in pollution and/or tobacco smoke exposure. Most disturbingly, the mortality from asthma also has been increasing.[28–30] This increase in mortality may be related to an increase in asthma severity, underusage of corticosteroids, poor patient education and compliance with respect to medication use, and/or β-agonist overusage with a consequent risk of rebound bronchoconstriction, ventricular tachycardia, or myocardial ischemia.

Young patients are especially likely to have an asthma exacerbation accompanying an upper or lower respiratory tract infection. In most patients, exercise or cold exposure will cause an exacerbation because cooling of the airways causes release of mediators and ultimately reflex bronchoconstriction. Some patients will have exclusively exercise- or cold-induced asthma. A significant percentage of patients will have the so-called allergic triad: asthma, nasal polyps, and aspirin (and other NSAID) sensitivity. Seven percent to 15% of patients with asthma have nasal polyps, which must be considered when using a nasal airway or a nasogastric tube. Aspirin-induced wheezing may be secondary to increased production of prostaglandins and leukotrienes.

Mast cell dysfunction plays a central role in the pathophysiology of asthma. Mast cell degranulation results in the release of chemical mediators of airway hyperreactivity, mucus secretion, and airway edema. These mediators include histamine, platelet-activating factor, leukotrienes, bradykinins, and adenosine. Defective autonomic control also plays an important role in the generation of airway hyperreactivity. β_2-Adrenergic hyporeactivity, α-adrenergic hyperreactivity, and/or cholinergic hyperreactivity can lead to airway hyperresponsiveness. When stimulated, β_2-adrenergic receptors release cyclic adenosine monophosphate (cAMP) intracellularly. Increased intracellular cAMP decreases airway smooth muscle tone and inhibits the release of mediators from mast cells and basophils. Decreased activity at the β_2-adrenergic receptors have the opposite effect. α-Adrenergic stimulation leads to a slight increase in airway smooth muscle tone. Cholinergic stimulation (via the vagal nerve) causes release of intracellular cyclic guanosine monophosphate. Intracellular cyclic guanosine monophosphate increases airway smooth muscle tone and promotes the release of mediators from mast cells and basophils. Vagal innervation primarily involves the central airways, the larynx and the large bronchi, with the afferent pathway being the irritant receptors in the central airways. The result is that foreign body stimulation (e.g., an endotracheal tube) may quickly result in reflex laryngospasm and bronchospasm.

Airway hyperreactivity, mucus secretion, and airway edema lead to airway obstruction and increased work of breathing. In severe asthma exacerbations, there is air trapping, hyperinflation, ventilation: perfusion mismatching, and hypoxemia. Hypoxemia may result from ventilation:perfusion mismatching secondary to bronchospasm, air trapping, or atelectasis. In unresolved episodes, diaphragmatic fatigue, hypercapnia, and respiratory failure may occur. Patients with severe chronic asthma may develop increases in pulmonary artery pressure, and chronic pulmonary hypertension may lead to *cor pulmonale*, although this is rare in childhood. Physiologic differences between children and adults are important in the pathophysiology of asthma. In children, 50% of total airway resistance is in the peripheral airways, whereas in adults, only 20% of total resistance is in the peripheral airways. As a result, small changes in the caliber of the peripheral airways in children will lead to significant changes in the total airway resistance. In addition, closing volume is relatively larger in children than in adults because of increased chest wall compliance and decreased lung compliance. When lung volumes fall, children are more likely than adults to have early airway closure (with closing volumes greater than functional residual capacity), ventilation:perfusion mismatching, intrapulmonary shunting, and hypoxemia. Significant air trapping will lead to increased lung volumes and reduced lung compliance, which will increase the work of breathing. Clinically, patients become tachypneic and recruit the accessory muscles of respiration. Infants are particularly prone to hypoxemia and respiratory failure because they have the least respiratory reserve. Their accessory muscles of respiration are not fully developed and their diaphragm may fatigue more rapidly.

Bronchodilators continue to be the mainstay of therapy for asthmatics. Most bronchodilators activate cAMP, thereby causing airway smooth muscle relaxation (bronchodilation) and prevention of mediator release (prevention of bronchoconstriction). The most common bronchodilators in use are the β-agonists. Selective $β_2$-agonists are preferable because they are responsible for smooth muscle relaxation in the lung, decreased histamine release, and increased mucociliary clearance. $β_1$-Agonist effects are best minimized because they cause increases in heart rate, heart contractility, and lypolysis. $β_2$-selective adrenergic agonists include metaproterenol (Alupent), terbutaline (Brethine), albuterol (Proventil, Ventolin), salmeterol (Serevent), and Isoetharine (Bronkosol). Side effects of the β-agonists include tremor, headache, nausea, and anorexia. These medications are delivered most frequently by the inhaled route in liquid form delivered by a jet nebulizer or by a pressurized aerosol metered dose inhaler (MDI). The jet nebulizer requires a special machine in the patient's home, but that may be preferable because MDIs are notoriously difficult for small children to manage, with most of the drug being delivered to the oropharynx or being exhaled. Success of the MDI can be improved in children with the use of a spacer. Because MDIs contain fluorocarbons, which are detrimental to the ozone, they are being replaced by negative pressure–activated powder canisters, which may be even more difficult for children to use properly.

Theophylline is a bronchodilator of less interest to the anesthesiologist because it has no role in the acute therapy of asthma. Theophylline is a methylxanthine that produces bronchodilation by inhibition of adenosine-mediated bronchconstriction. The effects of theophylline may be synergistic with the $β_2$-selective agonists. Theophylline has a very narrow therapeutic window. Therapeutic concentrations are in the range of 10 to 20 μg/mL. Toxicity may occur at concentrations above 20 μg/mL and is manifested by vomiting, central nervous system stimulation (headache, irritability, tremors, seizures), and arrhythmias. Of interest to anesthesiologists is the fact theophylline antagonizes the action of nondepolarizing muscle relaxants at the neuromuscular junction. Theophylline clearance is reduced in patients who are also receiving cimetidine, propranolol, erythromycin, and macrolide antibiotics. These patients may reach toxic levels of theophylline more quickly. Perioperatively, patients who are on theophylline therapy chronically may have their oral therapy converted to intravenous therapy. An infusion rate in the range of 0.2 to 0.6 mg/(kg · h) is usually appropriate, but serum levels of theophylline must be followed.

More recent therapy has concentrated on the role of the inflammatory response in asthma, although corticosteroids remain second-line therapy for asthmatics because of their myriad side effects. Corticosteroids are used when first-line therapy is inadequate or entails too many side effects, during acute exacerbations, for *status asthmaticus*, and for chronic severe asthma (usually on an every-other-day schedule to minimize adrenal suppression). Corticosteroids potentiate the β-adrenergic system and inhibit release of the mediators of inflammation and edema because they have a potent anti-inflammatory effect on the airways. The regular use of inhaled steroids controls symptoms, preserves lung function, reduces airway inflammation, and decreases total airway reactivity. Inhaled steroids minimize the risk of systemic toxicity. Adrenal suppression is exceedingly rare with the use of inhaled steroids and occurs only at very high doses, so stress dose steroids are rarely indicated perioperatively. The most common inhalational steroid is beclomethasone. The most common oral steroid for asthmatics is prednisone, which comes in pills or liquid form. Parenteral corticosteroids include hydrocortisone (short acting) or methylprednisolone. Oral and parenteral forms are best for acute exacerbations that are not responsive to β_2-selective agonists. Specific concerns for the anesthesiologist include the potential for adrenal suppression, osteoporosis, and cushingoid symptoms in patients who are taking steroids chronically.

Cromolyn sodium is used for chronic (prophylactic) asthma therapy. It inhibits mediator release from mast cells. It is for inhalation use only because it is not absorbed well from the gastrointestinal tract. Because cromolyn sodium is of no use after the mediators have been released, it is not useful for acute therapy and has little or no role in the perioperative period. Rare side effects include hoarseness, hyperventilation, dry mouth, and nasal congestion.

Anticholinergic medications decrease bronchial smooth muscle tone and decrease mucus gland secretion and can be useful as adjunctive therapy in asthmatics.[4] Anticholinergic medications can be administered intramuscularly or intravenously (atropine, glycopyrrolate less often) or inhaled (ipratropium bromide, glycopyrrolate less often). Side effects, which are more common with parenteral use and less common with inhalational use, include dry mouth, tachycardia, restlessness, constipation, urinary retention, hot dry skin, delirium, coma, and arrhythmias.

When evaluating a patient with asthma preoperatively, the historical data are crucial. Initially, it is important to determine the potential severity of the patient's disease. The severity of the disease correlates with the risk of respiratory complications intraoperatively. We ask about the age of onset, frequency, a typical attack, and about any attacks that required steroids, hospitalization, intubation, or care in the intensive care unit. It is important to be aware of any coexisting lung disease, such as bronchopulmonary dysplasia, a history of prematurity, or CF. We evaluate the patient's previous experiences with general anesthesia and review the intraoperative records, if possible. In each patient it is important to establish what the precipitants to an exacerbation may be, such as exercise, cold air, dry air, upper or lower respiratory tract infection, smoke, or gastroesophageal reflux. Also, it is essential to determine the patient's most recent exacerbation and whether the patient is currently experiencing an exacerbation or a respiratory tract infection. Perioperative airway hyperreactivity, mucosal edema, and airway plugging should be expected if the patient has had an asthma exacerbation or a respiratory tract infection within the preceding 4 to 6 weeks. It is important to determine whether the patient's therapy is maximized. Usually the patient and/or the parents will know if the patient is "the best that they can be." We always note the doses and effectiveness of the medications that the patient is currently taking. In addition, we note supplemental medications the patient takes during an exacerbation.

The physical examination is necessarily focused on the respiratory system. Patients with severe disease or a current exacerbation may have a prolonged expiratory phase and/or wheezing on auscultation. Lack of wheezing during an exacerbation may be due to severe bronchospasm with consequently little or no air movement. We also note any increased work of breathing such as nasal flaring, accessory muscle use, and tachypnea. Rare patients with severe disease and recurrent hypoxia may have signs of right heart failure such as jugular venous distention, hepatomegaly, peripheral edema, and pleural effusion.

No laboratory studies are routinely indicated for patients with asthma. In severe disease accompanied by chronic hypoxia, the hematocrit may be elevated. Arterial blood gases are usually normal in mild asthma without exacerbation. There may be mild hypoxemia and hypocapnea on room air in association with a mild asthma attack. Hypoxemia, hypercapnia, and respiratory acidosis may occur in a severe asthma attack and may indicate impending respiratory failure. A chest x-ray may show hyperinflation, increased lung markings (peribronchial cuffing), and atelectasis, but has not been shown to be helpful in preoperative screening. Chest x-rays are most likely to be useful if specific pulmonary pathology is suspected, such as pneumonia, pleural effusion, or pneumothorax, in which case elective surgery is likely to have been canceled. Pulmonary function testing usually is limited in children secondary to lack of cooperation. Most often, only spirometry can be performed, which usually shows an obstructive pattern with increases in lung volumes [residual volume (RV), functional residual capacity (FRC), total lung capacity] and decreases in flow rates (FEV_1, FVC). If the patient has *cor pulmonale*, prominent pulmonary arteries may be visible on the chest x-ray and right ventricular hypertrophy or a *cor pulmonale* pattern may be visible on electrocardiography.

Preoperative management of the child with asthma for elective surgery assumes that the child's therapy is maximized.[31,32] If this is not the case, the elective procedure should be postponed. It is important to note that maximizing the patient's therapy does not mean that all patients will lack evidence of airway obstruction. We may choose to proceed with an elective surgery in one child who is wheezing and cancel an elective surgery in another child who is wheezing. If the procedure is emergent and the child's condition is not maximized, then acute therapy for asthma begins immediately and the procedure is undertaken. On the morning of surgery, the patient should take the oral or inhaled bronchodilators, even if there is no evidence of bronchoconstriction. Preoperatively, we like to obtain a baseline room air oxygen saturation. We plan to premedicate these children with an anxiolytic only if anxiety or hyperventilation is precipitating an exacerbation of asthma. Our choice for anxiolysis is 0.5 to 1.0 mg/kg midazolam orally. We give these children intravenous glycopyrrolate (0.01 mg/kg, minimum 0.1 mg, maximum 0.4mg) or atropine (0.02 mg/kg, minimum 0.1 mg, maximum 0.4mg) preoperatively or as soon as the intravenous line is established and avoid intramuscular medication whenever possible. The stress of surgery may require a two- to seven-fold increase in adrenal steroid production. Patients who have received exogenous corticosteroids may not be able to raise steroid production to that level. They may develop a relative adrenal insufficiency, with a consequent risk of hypotension and cardiovascular collapse perioperatively. Patients who are currently taking oral or intravenous corticosteroids or who are at risk for adrenal suppression (three courses of oral or intravenous steroids in the previous year or one course in the previous 4 to 6 months) should receive 1 mg/kg intravenous hydrocortisone preoperatively and every 8 h during the initial postoperative period. In most patients, the corticosteroid dose can be reduced to the patient's maintenance dose within 48 h of the surgery.

Regional anesthesia is an option for some older pediatric patients and can be used in the asthmatic patient as long as there is no associated decrease in vital capacity, which is important for adequate deep breathing and coughing perioperatively. Most pediatric patients will require a general anesthetic. A smooth anesthetic induction is particularly important in children with asthma. Coughing, breath-holding, and laryngospasm on induction are potential precipitants of bronchospasm. All of the volatile agents block the afferent irritant vagal pathways and act as bronchodilators, so they prevent and treat bronchospasm. Conversely, the inhaled anesthetics are also potential airway irritants. Halothane and sevoflurane are used most commonly for induction in children because these agents are least irritating to the airways. Halothane has been associated with cardiac arrhythmias, which may be of particular concern in patients with toxic or even high therapeutic levels of theophylline. Sevoflurane, with its low incidence of coughing, breath-holding, laryngospasm on induction, and arrhythmias, might be the best choice. Our choice for an intravenous induction agent is propofol because it suppresses airway reflexes (better than sodium pentothal) and is mildly bronchodilatory.[33] Although ketamine relaxes airway smooth muscle by activating the sympathetic nervous system and depresses afferent irritant vagal pathways, it is associated with an increase in airway secretions, which can exacerbate airway problems in an asthmatic. Whatever the choice for intravenous induction agent, it is important to give a sufficient dose to blunt the airway responses, particularly if one is not planning to give a muscle relaxant to facilitate intubation. Whenever practical, we avoid endotracheal intubation because the presence of a foreign body in the trachea stimulates irritant receptors and can trigger bronchospasm, even in nonasthmatics. Mask anesthesia is least likely to directly precipitate bronchospasm. The laryngeal mask airway provides an alternative to the mask[34] but may on occasion irritate the upper airway. Any manipulation of the larynx can be a precipitant to bronchospasm.

Intraoperatively, we use humidified gases, which help keep airway secretions from becoming inspissated. Also, dry gas can be an airway irritant and provoke bronchospasm. Morphine, curare, succinylcholine, metocurine, atracurium, and mivacurium release histamine, which may precipitate bronchospasm and should be used with caution. Fentanyl probably does not release significant quantities of histamine. Lidocaine is a very important drug for prophylaxis of bronchospasm because it blocks the afferent irritant vagal pathways and may directly relax airway smooth muscle. It may be given intravenously in a dose of 1.0 to 1.5 mg/kg or intratracheally in a dose of 3.0 to 5.0 mg/kg. When compatible with the nature of the surgery and the anatomy of the airway, the patient should be extubated deep. Before extubation, particularly in a patient who will not be extubated deep, we prophylactically administer intravenous lidocaine 1.0 to 1.5 mg/kg and sometimes add an inhaled β_2-selective agonist. It is important that the neuromuscular blockade be completely reversed before emergence so that the patient can effectively breathe deeply and cough at the end of the anesthetic. For this same reason, pain should be well controlled postoperatively. Regional anesthesia as an adjunct to general anesthesia can be extremely helpful in this regard. The patient should receive humidified oxygen in the postanesthesia care unit for as long as supplemental oxygen is required. Aerosolized β_2-selective agonists should be immediately available in the postanesthesia care unit.

Intraoperative bronchospasm is one of the most difficult situations that an anesthesiologist must handle. Bronchospasm usually is heralded by ventilatory difficulty. Initially other causes of ventilatory difficulty must be ruled out or corrected, such as light anesthesia, a kinked endotracheal tube, endobronchial intubation, increased airway secretions, airway foreign body, pulmonary edema, pulmonary embolus, and aspiration. The management of intraoperative bronchospasm begins with assisted ventilation using 100% oxygen to prevent hypoxia and hypercarbia. The anesthetic should be deepened with one of the volatile agents, which are bronchodilatory. A bronchodilator (albuterol, terbutaline, epinephrine) should be administered through the endotracheal tube or intravenously. Intravenous lidocaine (1.0 to 1.5 mg/kg), intravenous glycopyrrolate (0.01 mg/kg, minimum 0.1 mg, maximum 0.4 mg) or atropine (0.02 mg/kg, minimum 0.1 mg, maximum 0.4 mg), and antihistamines (if histamine release is a likely precipitant) also may be helpful. Although they do not work immediately, intravenous corticosteroids should be administered. Intraoperatively, it is important to recognize that muscle relaxants do not generally affect the smooth muscle in the airways and therefore do not reliably reverse bronchospasm.

In conclusion, when formulating the anesthetic plan for a patient with asthma we first determine the potential severity of the patient's disease. Second, we ensure that the patient's therapeutic regimen is maximized, and that the patient is "the best that they can be." This means canceling elective surgery when the patient is having an exacerbation of asthma or is experiencing a respiratory tract infection. We pretreat with inhaled albuterol (nebulized or MDI, according to the patient's routine) and glycopyrrolate. We are liberal with the use of lidocaine. We also have a low threshold for the administration of stress doses of steroids because adrenal insufficiency can be catastrophic perioperatively and additional steroids may be beneficial in preventing an exacerbation of asthma. We prefer an inhalational induction and avoid endotracheal intubation whenever possible. We always have albuterol immediately available perioperatively. We take every opportunity to supplement general anesthesia with regional anesthesia (e.g., caudal anesthesia).

THE CHILD WITH PNEUMONIA OR BRONCHIOLITIS

Pneumonia is relatively common in young children, particularly between the ages of 6 months and 5 years. The patient's age and the season help determine the most likely causative organism. Newborns are most likely to be infected with group B streptococcus, *Klebsiella pneumoniae*, *Escherichia coli*, or *Listeria*. Between the ages of 1 month and 5 years, the cause of a bacterial pneumonia is likely to be *Streptococcus pneumoniae* or *Haemophilus influenzae (H. flu)*, although *H. flu* disease is now much less common since the introduction of the *H. flu* vaccine. Children older than 5 years with bacterial pneumonia are likely to be infected with *S. pneumoniae* or *Mycoplasma pneumoniae*. Patients with an immunodeficiency may have other causes of pneumonia, such as *Pneumocystis carinii*. Although bacterial pneumonia can occur year round, viral pneumonia is more likely to occur in the winter months and in epidemics. The most common cause of pneumonia is viral, especially respiratory syncytial virus (RSV); other common causes are influenza, parainfluenza, and adenovirus. Respiratory syncytial virus is an important cause of bronchiolitis and bronchopneumonia in children, especially children younger than 3 years. Fifty percent of children have had an RSV infection by their first birthdays. By the time they reach age 3 years, most children have been infected. Reinfection is possible but rarely as serious as the primary infection. Involvement of the lower respiratory tract decreases with advancing age and recurrent infection. Older children and adults usually have illness of just the upper respiratory tract. Even in younger children, RSV starts with URI signs such as cough, nasal stuffiness, and occasionally a low-grade fever. Subsequently the cough worsens and is accompanied by tachypnea, fever, increased work of breathing (WOB), chest hyperinflation, prolongation of the expiratory phase, wheezing, and occasionally rales. Up to 40% of patients with RSV will wheeze. This does not lead to an increased risk of subsequently developing asthma, except in severe cases of RSV associated with respiratory failure and mechanical ventilation. Many children who develop severe disease requiring hospitalization have significant coexisting disease, in particular congenital heart disease. These patients have a mortality risk of up to 4%. Luckily, the acute RSV infection is short-lived and begins to resolve after 2 to 3 days. However, it takes up to 6 weeks for the lungs to heal and for lung function to normalize, which must be taken into account when rescheduling a child's elective surgery.[2,3] Most children with an RSV infection have mild disease and do not need to be hospitalized unless they are anesthetized during their illness.

The most important issue in a child with pneumonia or bronchiolitis is for the anesthesiologist to recognize the illness and then cancel any elective surgical procedure. Pneumonia or bronchiolitis may masquerade as URI or allergic rhinitis but usually can be distinguished from those illnesses by the presence of fever and/or lower respiratory signs and symptoms, including a productive cough, rales, wheezing, dyspnea, and increased work of breathing. Pneumonia usually can be confirmed by chest x-ray, although a confirmatory chest x-ray is not needed to postpone an elective surgery. The chest x-ray in bronchiolitis typically shows hyperinflation. General anesthesia should be avoided in a child with pneumonia or bronchiolitis except in emergent situations or when the surgery is necessary to treat the condition. For example, the child may need surgical drainage of an empyema, bronchoscopy, or a lung biopsy to identify the causative organism in an immunocompromised host. Although halogenated anesthetics inhibit bacterial growth and viral replication in vitro, this effect is unlikely to be clinically significant. Regional anesthesia should be used as an alternative to general anesthesia whenever possible.

In patients with pneumonia or bronchiolitis who must undergo a general anesthetic, expected complications include excessive airway debris and secretions, airway plugging, atelectasis, periodic breathing, apnea (in small babies), hypoxemia, bronchospasm, and, not uncommonly, respiratory failure. Respiratory failure should be anticipated if the respiratory rate is greater than 60 per minute and/or the partial pressure of carbon dioxide, arterial is greater than 50 mmHg. Hypoxemia is very common and primarily the result of a mismatch between ventilation and perfusion. A baseline oxygen saturation should be obtained before induction.

In conclusion, the most important point about the child with pneumonia or bronchiolitis is that the anesthesiologist must recognize the condition before induction. Any elective surgical procedure in a child with pneumonia or bronchiolitis ought to be canceled. Surgery that is emergent or necessary to treat the condition must proceed, and the parents, surgeon, and anesthesiologist must accept the increased risk of perioperative respiratory complications including respiratory failure. Perioperatively, it is best to treat these patients similarly to patients with URI and/or bronchospasm (see above).

THE CHILD WITH BRONCHOPULMONARY DYSPLASIA

Mortality in premature infants has significantly decreased in the past two decades due to improved supportive care, improved ventilation, administration of maternal and neonatal steroids, and the availability of exogenous surfactant. Accompanying the decrease in mortality, however, has been an increase in morbidity as more and more of the younger premature infants survive. Chronic lung disease in the ex-premature infant may be due to congenital lung hypoplasia, recurrent aspiration, sepsis or pneumonia, or as a result of prematurity. Bronchopulmonary dysplasia was originally defined as oxygen dependence at 4 weeks of age. As premature infants began surviving at younger ages, the definition of bronchopulmonary dysplasia evolved into a requirement for ventilatory support or supplemental oxygen beyond 36 weeks postmenstrual age.[35] This definition is based on clinical symptomatology and not on the underlying pathophysiologic disorder, which is often not known. Exogenous surfactant therapy has significantly decreased the severity of respiratory distress syndrome and consequently the severity and possibly the incidence of bronchopulmonary dysplasia. However, 20% of infants with respiratory distress syndrome develop chronic lung disease.[36]

Bronchopulmonary dysplasia is a disease of lung parenchyma and small airways, a consequence of lung immaturity and lung damage secondary to oxygen therapy and mechanical ventilation (barotrauma). Fibrotic changes in the parenchyma may lead to hypoxemia, carbon dioxide retention, pulmonary hypertension, and *cor pulmonale*. Small airway disease may lead to airway hyperreactivity and air trapping. Patients with bronchopulmonary dysplasia have increased airway resistance, decreased airway conductance, decreased lung volumes, a relatively low functional residual capacity, airway obstruction, a decreased FEV_1, and lung hyperinflation. These patients often have reactive airways disease and are particularly likely to wheeze when they have URI. Increased airway reactivity may persist for 4 to 6 weeks after a URI (see above). Many patients will show improvement after bronchodilator therapy. Patients with bronchopulmonary dysplasia may be on supplemental oxygen, bronchodilators, and/or diuretics (which reduce extravascular lung fluid).

The pulmonary abnormalities seen in ex-premature infants are most evident in the first 3 years of life. By age 5 to 8 years there is evidence of improvement in lung function, suggesting lung healing. Recent longitudinal studies of school-age children histories of prematurity have associated the neonatal administration of surfactant with improved lung function parameters.[37] School-age children with histories of bronchopulmonary dysplasia have exercise tolerance similar to children without histories of chronic lung disease. However, they use more of their ventilatory reserve during exercise and have an increased risk of oxygen desaturation.[38] Even ex-premature infants without bronchopulmonary dysplasia probably have some degree of chronic lung disease and a mild degree of obstructive airway disease until the age of 4 or 5 years.[39] This may have implications for the perioperative period. Children with histories of prematurity, even if not currently receiving supplemental oxygen therapy, may require supplemental oxygen perioperatively.

There is a high incidence of coexisting disease in patients with bronchopulmonary dysplasia. Premature infants have a higher incidence of a variety of congenital abnormalities, the congenital abnormality often being a contributing factor to the prematurity. Premature infants are at risk for intracranial bleeding and subsequent hydrocephalus, which may have long-term neurodevelopmental consequences. In addition, hypoxemia over time may lead to neurodevelopmental delay. Chronic hypoxemia also may lead to pulmonary hypertension. Many ex-premature infants have feeding difficulties and are at increased risk for gastroesophageal reflux. Caloric needs in patients with bronchopulmonary dysplasia are increased because of the increased work of breathing. This must be taken into account when providing perioperative nutritional therapy.

The symptomatic patient with bronchopulmonary dysplasia (tachypnea, increased work of breathing, wheezing, oxygen dependence) needs a careful preoperative evaluation, which may include a baseline oxygen saturation, arterial blood gas (to document the level of hypoxemia and/or carbon dioxide retention), and a chest x-ray. Elective surgery should be undertaken only if the surgery cannot be delayed until the child is older. Preoperatively, the patient's condition must be maximized. The child's parents or guardians usually will have a very accurate assessment of the patient's condition as compared to his or her norm. There should be no history of URI in the preceding 4 to 6 weeks. The patient should be on an optimum drug regimen, which may mean a course of bronchodilator therapy and/or steroids perioperatively. The apparently asymptomatic patient (the former premature infant with no history of lung disease; the now asymptomatic school-age child with a history of bronchopulmonary dysplasia) may be at risk for perioperative bronchospasm and hypoxemia because these patients may have persistent subtle abnormalities in lung volumes, airway resistance, and airway reactivity.

Intraoperatively, airway hyperreactivity is the primary difficulty. Laryngospasm, coughing, breath-holding, bronchospasm, and hypoxemia are common. In fact, these events are so predictable in this population of patients when undergoing general anesthesia that many pediatric anesthesiologists have adopted (often uncomplimentary) terms for such episodes (we call them "stupid premie tricks"). Most patients respond well when treated like asthmatics (see above). Patients with histories of prolonged intubation may have developed subglottic stenosis and/or tracheomalacia. A smaller than expected endotracheal tube may be indicated for patients with subglottic stenosis. Baseline oxygen saturation is likely to be normal, but there is an increased risk of perioperative hypoxemia. Oxygen saturation must be monitored closely, and supplemental oxygen administered appropriately. Failure to thrive may indicate chronic hypoxemia. Perioperative fluid management must be well controlled because excessive extravascular lung fluid may exacerbate pulmonary problems. Patients taking diuretic medication chronically may have abnormalities of serum electrolytes.

In conclusion, although the incidence and severity appear to be decreasing, bronchopulmonary dysplasia is still a significant problem for the anesthesiologist because so many former premature infants will require surgery. Elective surgery should be delayed as long as possible to maximize lung healing and minimize the risk of perioperative apnea. The patient with bronchopulmonary dysplasia should have lung function maximized preoperatively. "Stupid premie tricks" such as laryngospasm, coughing, breath-holding, bronchospasm, and hypoxemia should be anticipated. In addition, the anesthesiologist must remain wary of the apparently asymptomatic patient (the former premature infant with no history of lung disease; the now asymptomatic school-age child with a history of bronchopulmonary dysplasia) who may exhibit decreased ventilatory reserve and/or require supplemental oxygen perioperatively.

OBSTRUCTIVE SLEEP APNEA

Obstructive sleep apnea (OSA) is a member of a diverse group of breathing problems in children referred to as "sleep-related breathing disorders in children." For the purposes of this chapter, OSA is considered the most significant of these commonly encountered disorders.

With improvements in microbiologic care, the incidence of chronic tonsillitis and, as a result, adenotonsillectomy has declined. However, adenotonsillectomy has become increasingly popular as a surgical remedy for children with OSA. As such, it is important that anesthesiologists are familiar with the pathophysiology of this disorder and its medical and surgical management.

Certainly, many children have mild airway obstruction during sleep. In fact, this mild form of airway obstruction, or snoring, is never more prevalent than in children during the first few weeks of life.[40] Mild snoring is not abnormal. Healthy children commonly snore and sleep polysomnography in these selected children have shown no evidence of disturbed sleep patterns, apnea, or oxygen desaturation. However, there are children who have moderate to severe airway obstruction associated with apnea and hypoxia. These children often appear normal in all other regards, with the OSA being an isolated finding. In some children, the diagnosis of OSA is part of a greater pathophysiologic process. Such children have cerebral palsy (especially spastic quadraparesis), hemifacial microsomia, and Down's, Apert's, Cruzon's, and Pierre–Robin syndromes. In addition, certain populations (African American vs. Hispanic) seem to have a higher incidence of OSA than the combined general population.[41,42]

Unlike adults, OSA correlates poorly with obesity, at least until children reach their teenage years. Males and females are equally affected. The degree, or severity, of OSA does not directly correlate with the size of the adenotonsils in children, despite the improvement of the condition when tonsils are removed. It is hypothesized that children with OSA have an unnoticeable predisposing facial dysmorphology but that the neural control of the oral pharyngeal muscles is just as important or more so.[43] Interestingly, children with true OSA are at their best early during their sleep; the number and severity of obstructive-related sleep events increase as the night goes on. This may be explained in part by the fatigue of the oral pharyngeal muscles trying to compensate for the obstruction and then failing.

OSA, as a chronic ailment, has a number of significant and diverse pathophysiologic consequences. Studies have shown that children with OSA have altered and depressed responses to hypoxia and hypercarbia.[44] The effects of inhalational and intravenous anesthetic drugs further aggravate this response. It is thought that this effect further predisposes OSA children to obstructive events during, and especially immediately after, an anesthetic or the administration of sedative drugs. The chronic hypoxic events lead to increased levels of endogenous catecholamines, hypoxic vasoconstriction of the pulmonary artery, and thus pulmonary hypertension. Left untreated, the pulmonary hypertension results in *cor pulmonale,* with right ventricular hypertrophy. This chain of events can lead to a life-threatening event requiring the emergent relief of airway obstruction and cardiopulmonary support. Several case reports of sudden cardiac failure and death secondary to OSA have been reported over the years.

In addition to the cardiorepiratory consequences of OSA, a number of other more subtle changes have been noted. Severe OSA disrupts rapid eye movement sleep. This disruption is associated with learning impairment of preschool and school-age children. Depression, anxiety, and aggression also have been associated with these patients. Decreased levels of insulin-related growth hormone have been documented in OSA patients, with values returning to normal after adenotonsillectomy.

The diagnosis of OSA is based on parental observations, clinical suspicion and examination, and the use of polysomnography. There is considerable debate over the value of polysomnography.[45] Current opinion seems to support the selective use of polysomnography, especially in patients with marginal findings. Certainly the severity of OSA is underestimated in some children and overestimated in others when studied by polysomnography. However, as clinicians, it has to be acknowledged that polysomnography is not without its problems and is far from 100% accurate. As such, it seems prudent to investigate any child whose history is questionable or to establish a baseline from which to follow treatment success or failure. Some children have mild OSA, as measured by polysomnography, and improve without treatment as they grow older.[46] However, in some cases, the history, family background, and associated conditions greatly predispose the child to moderate or severe OSA. These children should not be denied aggressive care while they wait for a sleep study and interpretation, which is not available in many centers. Clinical judgment is especially important in these cases.

A few anesthetic points should be made, but we acknowledge that the studies correlating anesthetic and surgical outcome with OSA are lacking. Most treatment studies have focused on the success or failure of a given surgical option. Studies assessing anesthetic techniques and management in relation to OSA are nonexistent. Most information is from the "school of hard knocks" tempered by a reasonable understanding of the issues involved with OSA.

Children with OSA may present for surgery that is unrelated to this diagnosis. This is most common in children with syndromes and hemifacial disorders. In these cases it is important that all caregivers be familiar with the association of OSA and the associated problems. Failure to do so can result in catastrophic results secondary to insufficient monitoring and inappropriate use of sedatives or narcotics postoperatively.[47] Commonly, although the actual surgery does not necessitate it, these children will require a monitored care bed such as the pediatric intensive care ward or a stay overnight in the recovery room. The use of continuous positive pressure, nasal airways (which are better tolerated than the oral versions), or delayed endotracheal extubation should be considered postoperatively. Regional anesthetic techniques and the use of NSAIDs that reduce or eliminate the use of sedatives or narcotics are preferred. Personal experience with this approach has been highly favorable. Many of these OSA patients obviously make poor outpatients, which emphasizes the fact that the medical condition of the child is just as important in selecting the outpatient as is the nature of the surgery.

Adenotonsillectomy is commonly used as a surgical therapy to ameliorate, or resolve, OSA in children. It is, undoubtedly, the most common encounter we have with children affected by OSA. Some of these children do very well with their anesthesia and postoperative care and others do not. At present, there are no studies predicting which child can or cannot tolerate a tonsillectomy for OSA without complications. Extreme caution is advised when dealing with hemifacial and syndrome-affected children.

The best choices of anesthetic technique or medication have not yet been identified. Whether these children benefit from local infiltration of the tonsillar bed at the completion of surgery remains a subject of considerable controversy. In children who are otherwise healthy, the decision to admit them to a monitored care bed or a regular bed, or schedule them as outpatients is often very difficult. This decision requires a great deal of experience and cooperation between the surgeon and the anesthesiologist.

We favor planned admission of all children scheduled for a tonsillectomy secondary to OSA (the insurance companies are not always cooperative in this venture; they readily acknowledge the condition of OSA in adults but question its validity in children). We as anesthesiologists and the attending surgeon observe these children in the recovery room for at least 2 h and then make the decision to admit or discharge patients based on their condition at that time. Only children who live in the immediate area of the hospital are considered for discharge. Future studies on this issue might identify the best course of care and eliminate the guesswork currently used. At present, *caution* is the operative word!

In conclusion, OSA children form a diverse group of patients. Children with OSA who are otherwise healthy and scheduled for tonsillectomy are commonly encountered. A number of significant secondary pathophysiologic concerns should be addressed when dealing with children diagnosed with OSA. It is important to appreciate that children with syndromes often have associated OSA and how commonly they are scheduled for surgery unrelated to OSA. Making the appropriate postoperative provisions is paramount in the care of OSA patients.

POSTOBSTRUCTIVE PULMONARY EDEMA

Postobstructive pulmonary edema may not be a common problem in pediatric anesthesia, but it is more common than we like to admit. It is certainly important that everyone practicing pediatric anesthesia understand the situations in which this disorder is seen, its diagnosis, and its appropriate management. Although there are many unanswered questions about the pathophysiology of postobstructive pulmonary edema, we discuss the current understanding of those points we do know and open the door to further discussion of this unusual problem.

Pulmonary edema after airway obstruction has been observed by anesthesiologists for years.[48] This complication is probably more common than thought. Undoubtedly, confusion arises in distinguishing this complication from the more commonly diagnosed aspiration syndrome, an often misdiagnosed and misunderstood disorder.

Postobstructive pulmonary edema commonly occurs after laryngospasm in healthy children with or without an anesthetic.[49] It has been described as a sequela of severe croup and epiglottitis or some entity that produces airway obstruction.[50] More than 60 years ago, it was described in the radiology literature as a sequela to reinflation of chronically collapsed lungs.

Postobstructive pulmonary edema classically presents with the rapid onset of pulmonary edema and the production of copious amounts of pink frothy sputum, which is evident immediately after establishment of an airway. Its presentation may be in a delayed and gradual manner, with progressive tachycardia, tachypnea, dyspnea, and hypoxia as late as 6 h after the inciting airway obstruction.

The pathophysiology of postobstructive pulmonary edema is unclear. Most commonly, those not familiar with this problem attribute it to fluid overload. Yet most published reports show no evidence supporting inappropriate fluid management. Although commonly unavailable, when performed, measurements of cardiac filling pressures have been normal.[51] In the past, many believed that the marked negative pressures generated in the thorax, by effort against a closed glottis, favor transudation of fluid into the alveoli. Animal studies, in an attempt to reproduce this effect, have failed to reproduce pulmonary edema. However, if the animal is made hypoxic at the same time, the result is pulmonary edema.[52,53] Current research and experience suggest that multiple factors are at play in producing postobstructive pulmonary edema. Negative pressures generated in the chest cavity in response to the obstructed airway increase the blood volume in the pulmonary arteries and veins. In addition, afterload is increased, affecting the right and left ventricles. Hypoxia produces pulmonary arterial and venous vasoconstriction and myocardial depression.[54] Hypoxia also may be a contributing factor in the disruption of the normal capillary membrane. When these factors are combined, the resultant effect is pulmonary edema.

Effective treatment results from understanding the clinical circumstances in which postobstructive pulmonary edema occurs and the resultant pathophysiology. First, and most important, a patent airway must be established and adequate oxygen delivery assured. Steroids, aminophylline, digoxin, oxygen, and positive pressure ventilation, with or without positive end expiratory pressure, have been used. Recently, it has been appreciated that only supportive care and adequate oxygenation are necessary.[54] In some patients, with only mild pulmonary edema and hypoxia, supplemental oxygen is all that is necessary, with resolution occurring over a period of hours. In the case of fulminant pulmonary edema, positive pressure airway support is required, commonly with continuous positive pressure or positive end expiratory pressure. Most young children will require intubation for a short period. Because fluid overload and abnormal filling pressures are not factors, the use of furosemide and/or cardiac inotropes is unnecessary. Resolution of severe postobstructive pulmonary edema occurs usually over a day, with marked improvement in a matter of minutes or hours. Children should be sedated only to make them comfortable; it is not therapeutic.

When treating postobstructive pulmonary edema, one must distinguish it from other causes of pulmonary edema. In those situations the treatment may more appropriately be directed at fluid balance. A careful history is the single most important factor in making the correct diagnosis. The absence of an obstructed airway and hypoxia makes the diagnosis unlikely. Aspiration is commonly considered in the differential diagnosis of dyspnea, with subsequent radiologic changes. Aspiration does not require the presence of an obstructed airway or hypoxia, although it may produce both as a result. Fortunately, in most cases the treatment of aspiration pneumonia is the same as that of postobstructive pulmonary edema.

REFERENCES

1. Tait AR, Knight PR: The effects of general anesthesia on upper respiratory tract infections in children. *Anesthesiology* 67:930, 1987.
2. Empey DW, Laitinen LA, Jacobs L, et al: Mechanisms of bronchial hyperreactivity in normal subjects after upper respiratory tract infection. *Am Rev Respir Dis* 113:131, 1976.
3. Wald ER, Guerra N, Byers C: Upper respiratory tract infections in young children: duration of and frequency of complications. *Pediatrics* 87:129, 1991.
4. Gal TJ: Bronchial hyperresponsiveness and anesthesia: physiologic and therapeutic perspectives. *Anesth Analg* 78:559, 1994.
5. Schreiner MS, O'Hara I, Markakis DA, Politis GD: Do children who experience laryngospasm have an increased risk of upper respiratory tract infection? *Anesthesiology* 85:475, 1996.
6. Jacoby DB, Hirshman CA: General anesthesia in patients with viral respiratory infections: an unsound sleep? [editorial; comment]. *Anesthesiology* 74:969, 1991.

7. Hinkle AJ: What wisdom is there in administering elective general anesthesia to children with active upper respiratory tract infection? [letter]. *Anesth Analg* 68:414, 1989.
8. McGill WA, Coveler LA, Epstein BS: Subacute upper respiratory infection in small children. *Anesth Analg* 58:331, 1979.
9. DeSoto H, Patel RI, Soliman IE, Hannallah RS: Changes in oxygen saturation following general anesthesia in children with upper respiratory infection signs and symptoms undergoing otolaryngological procedures. *Anesthesiology* 68:276, 1988.
10. Levy L, Pandit UA, Randel GI, et al: Upper respiratory tract infections and general anaesthesia in children. Peri-operative complications and oxygen saturation. *Anaesthesia* 47:678, 1992.
11. Rolf N, Cote CJ: Frequency and severity of desaturation events during general anesthesia in children with and without upper respiratory infections. *J Clin Anesth* 4:200, 1992.
12. Tait AR, Reynolds PI, Gutstein HB: Factors that influence an anesthesiologist's decision to cancel elective surgery for the child with an upper respiratory tract infection. *J Clin Anesth* 7:491, 1995.
13. Cohen MM, Cameron CB: Should you cancel the operation when a child has an upper respiratory tract infection? [see comments]. *Anesth Analg* 72:282, 1991.
14. Olsson GL, Hallen B: Laryngospasm during anaesthesia. A computer-aided incidence study in 136,929 patients. *Acta Anaesthesiol Scand* 28:567, 1984.
15. Kinouchi K, Tanigami H, Tashiro C, et al: Duration of apnea in anesthetized infants and children required for desaturation of hemoglobin to 95%. The influence of upper respiratory infection. *Anesthesiology* 77:1105, 1992.
16. Tait AR, Pandit UA, Voepel-Lewis T, et al: Use of the laryngeal mask airway in children with upper respiratory tract infections: a comparison with endotracheal intubation [see comments]. *Anesth Analg* 86:706, 1998.
17. Anderson D: Cystic fibrosis of the pancreas and its relation to celiac disease: clinical and pathological study. *Am J Dis Child* 56:344, 1938.
18. Webb AK, David TJ: Clinical management of children and adults with cystic fibrosis. *BMJ* 308:459, 1994.
19. Fiel SB: Clinical management of pulmonary disease in cystic fibrosis. *Lancet* 341:1070, 1993.
20. Elborn JS, Shale DJ, Britton JR: Cystic fibrosis: current survival and population estimates to the year 2000 [see comments]. *Thorax* 46:881, 1991. (Erratum: *Thorax* 47:139, 1992.)
21. Tsui LC, Buchwald M, Barker D, et al: Cystic fibrosis locus defined by a genetically linked polymorphic DNA marker. *Science* 230:1054, 1985.
22. Lamberty JM, Rubin BK: The management of anaesthesia for patients with cystic fibrosis. *Anaesthesia* 40:448, 1985.
23. Weeks AM, Buckland MR: Anaesthesia for adults with cystic fibrosis. *Anaesth Intens Care* 23:332, 1995.
24. Walsh TS, Young CH: Anaesthesia and cystic fibrosis. *Anaesthesia* 50:614, 1995.
25. Hui Y, Gaffney R, Crysdale WS: Sinusitis in patients with cystic fibrosis. *Eur Arch Oto-Rhino-Laryngol* 252:191, 1995.
26. Konstan MW, Byard PJ, Hoppel CL, Davis PB: Effect of high-dose ibuprofen in patients with cystic fibrosis [see comments]. *N Engl J Med* 332:848, 1995.
27. Kerem E, Reisman J, Corey M, et al: Prediction of mortality in patients with cystic fibrosis [see comments]. *N Engl J Med* 326:1187, 1992.
28. Yunginger JW, Reed CE, O'Connell EJ, et al: A community-based study of the epidemiology of asthma. Incidence rates, 1964–1983 [see comments]. *Am Rev Respir Dis* 146:888, 1992.
29. Silverstein MD, Reed CE, O'Connell EJ, et al: Long-term survival of a cohort of community residents with asthma [see comments]. *N Engl J Med* 331:1537, 1994.
30. Weiss KB, Wagener DK: Changing patterns of asthma mortality. Identifying target populations at high risk [see comments]. *JAMA* 264:1683, 1990.
31. Bishop MJ, Cheney FW: Anesthesia for patients with asthma. Low risk but not no risk [editorial; comment]. *Anesthesiology* 85:455, 1996.

32. Warner DO, Warner MA, Barnes RD, et al: Perioperative respiratory complications in patients with asthma [see comments]. *Anesthesiology* 85:460, 1996.
33. Brown RH, Wagner EM: Mechanisms of bronchoprotection by anesthetic induction agents: propofol versus ketamine. *Anesthesiology* 90:822, 1999.
34. Kim ES, Bishop MJ: Endotracheal intubation, but not laryngeal mask airway insertion, produces reversible bronchoconstriction. *Anesthesiology* 90:391, 1999.
35. Ballard R, Banks B: Definition of bronchopulmonary dysplasia. In reply. *Pediatrics* 103:533, 1999.
36. Lenoir S, Grandjean H, Leloup M, et al: [Short and mid-term outcome of a cohort of 1157 newborn infants with respiratory distress syndrome]. *Arch Pediatr* 1:1004, 1994.
37. Pelkonen AS, Hakulinen AL, Turpeinen M, Hallman M: Effect of neonatal surfactant therapy on lung function at school age in children born very preterm. *Pediatr Pulmonol* 25:182, 1998.
38. Jacob SV, Lands LC, Coates AL, et al: Exercise ability in survivors of severe bronchopulmonary dysplasia. *Am J Respir Crit Care Med* 155:1925, 1997.
39. Koumbourlis AC, Motoyama EK, Mutich RL, et al: Longitudinal follow-up of lung function from childhood to adolescence in prematurely born patients with neonatal chronic lung disease. *Pediatr Pulmonol* 21:28, 1996.
40. Kato I, Franco P, Groswasser J, et al: Frequency of obstructive and mixed sleep apneas in 1,023 infants. *Sleep* 23:487, 2000.
41. Stepanski E, Zayyad A, Nigro C, et al: Sleep-disordered breathing in a predominantly African-American pediatric population. *J Sleep Res* 8:65, 1999.
42. Hoeve HL, Joosten KF, van den Berg S: Management of obstructive sleep apnea syndrome in children with craniofacial malformation. *Int J Pediatr Otorhinolaryngol* 1:S59, 1999.
43. Finkelstein Y, Wexler D, Berger G, et al: Anatomical basis of sleep-related breathing abnormalities in children with nasal obstruction. *Arch Otolaryngol Head Neck Surg* 126:593, 2000.
44. Strauss SG, Lynn AM, Bratton SL, et al: Ventilatory response to CO_2 in children with obstructive sleep apnea from adenotonsillar hypertrophy. *Anesth Analg* 89:328, 1999.
45. Messner AH: Evaluation of obstructive sleep apnea by polysomnography prior to pediatric adenotonsillectomy. *Arch Otolaryngol Head Neck Surg* 125:353, 1999.
46. Nieminen P, Tolonen U, Lopponen H, et al: Snoring and obstructive sleep apnea in children: a 6-month follow-up study. *Arch Otolaryngol Head Neck Surg* 126:481, 2000.
47. Pena M, Choi S, Boyajian M, Zalzal G: Perioperative airway complications following pharyngeal flap palatoplasty. *Ann Otol Rhinol Laryngol* 109:808, 2000.
48. Oswalt CE, Gates GA, Holmstrom MG: Pulmonary edema as a complication of acute airway obstruction. *JAMA* 238:1833, 1977.
49. Lee KW, Downes JJ: Pulmonary edema secondary to laryngospasm in children. *Anesthesiology* 59:347, 1983.
50. Rothstein P, Lister G: Epiglottitis: Duration of intubation and fever. *Anesth Analg* 62:785, 1983.
51. Spiekerman BF, Reikersdorfer CG, Yemen TA, et al: Unexplained transient postoperative myocardial dysfunction in a previously healthy child. *Anesth Analg* 82:419, 1996.
52. Newton-John H: Pulmonary oedema in upper airway obstruction. *Lancet* 2:510, 1977.
53. Bressack MA, Bland RD: Alveolar hypoxia increases lung fluid filtration in unanesthetized newborn lambs. *Circ Res* 46:111, 1980.
54. Lang SA, Duncan PG, Shephard DAE, et al: Pulmonary oedema associated with airway obstruction. *Can J Anaesth* 37:210, 1990.

8 | The Child With Stridor

Andrew M. Woods, MD
Terrance A. Yemen, MD

Stridor is the sound caused by air movement through a partially obstructed airway. The sound is harsh, vibratory, and high-pitched. Stridor is always abnormal and every child with stridor has a pathologic process. The challenge to the clinician is to correctly identify the etiology of stridor, assess the significance and severity of the obstruction, and, with knowledge of the expected clinical progression of the lesion, make proper management decisions.

The single fact of paramount importance regarding stridor is that it may, suddenly and unexpectedly, and in the worst environments and situations, herald impending total airway obstruction and death. Thus, stridor stands as the sentinel marker for the single most critical clinical situation—loss of an airway—that anesthesiologists who care for children can expect to confront.

Airway management is still the single most defining skill that separates anesthesiologists from other clinicians and practitioners who administer most of the same drugs (potent inhalational agents excluded) as anesthesiologists. *We* are the airway experts, and stridor is the clarion call for our airway expertise. On occasion stridor may turn out to be transient and inconsequential, but such an assumption must never be made in the setting of new or acute onset stridor. Until proven otherwise, stridor is a desperate cry for help from a child. This is the moment when what you do may be life-saving for a child. Alternatively, it is the moment in which improper diagnosis and/or management may precipitate a chaotic crisis in which the end is the death of a child. The failure to properly manage a *reversible* airway lesion is surely one of the worst failures that an anesthesiologist can experience.

To the extent possible, this chapter presents stridor within the context of the different clinical scenarios and locations in which it is encountered. It is designed to help clinicians rapidly integrate the signs and symptoms of airway obstruction with the information available from basic and essential monitoring equipment—capnographs, pulse oximeters, airway pressure manometers—and correctly diagnose and manage the situation. It is somewhat different from the usual reviews and chapters on stridor in that it is weighted toward stridor arising in the perioperative period rather than presenting a differential diagnosis of all the etiologies for stridor in newborns and children.

THE SOUND OF STRIDOR

Stridor is a harsh, musical sound with a harmonious frequency and pitch acoustically similar to a "wheeze." However, stridor and wheezes are not the same thing and they do not have the same clinical significance. Wheezes are high-pitched, musical, mewing sounds that emanate from medium-size airways and are primarily expiratory in nature, whereas stridor is predominantly inspiratory. Stridor is usually heard best over the larynx, whereas wheezes are heard best over the involved lung fields. However, since there is a continuum of the airway column from the interface with the atmosphere (mouth and nose) to the alveoli, there is a continuum of sounds associated with obstruction of the airways; for the most part, as one goes more distally in the airway, the sounds of obstruction become progressively higher pitched.

The anatomic location of the airway obstruction determines the timing of the stridor in relation to the respiratory cycle; airway obstruction at or above the level of the vocal cords typically produces inspiratory stridor that is high pitched. Obstruction of the airway between the vocal cords and the thoracic inlet is associated with intermediate pitch biphasic stridor, i.e., affecting inspiration and expiration. Airway obstruction within the thorax primarily results in stridor during expiration, although fixed circumferential tracheal and bronchial lesions can produce biphasic stridor. Stridor produced by obstruction in the trachea or bronchus is typically less harsh than that produced by more proximal obstruction. However, in cases of fixed circumferential lesions of the trachea or bronchus, the pitch of the biphasic stridor may reflect the degree of narrowing.

Stridor is not snoring. *Stertor* is the term used to describe the noise that results from soft tissue obstruction of the supraglottic airway. Snoring is coarse, low pitched, and vibratory. Even total airway occlusion, as in patients with obstructive sleep apnea, does not produce the high-pitched sound of stridor when the etiology is from soft tissue extrinsic to the larynx.

Stridor also must be differentiated from rhonchi. Secretions in the airway produce coarse, moist, vibratory sounds of lower pitch than stridor. Rhonchi are a marker for excessive airway secretions that may, particularly in neonates and infants, totally occlude endotracheal tubes and produce complete obstruction of the airway.

It should be clear by now that there is a great deal to be gained by an attentive awareness of the airway sounds of patients. However, there is a steady trend in the field of anesthesiology to intraoperatively listen directly to the patients less and less and to more and more rely on the excellent monitoring devices available to us. The consequence of this reliance on electronic monitoring is that the first response to disturbing information from a monitor (i.e., abrupt decrease in oxygen saturation, blood pressure, or expired level of carbon dioxide) is too often to query the monitor rather than the patient.

The inconvenient habit of being intimately connected to the anesthetized child through an earpiece that allows breath-to-breath monitoring of ventilation and beat-to-beat monitoring of heart rate represents a critical link to the most sophisticated monitor in the room—the brain and nervous system of the anesthesiologist. Our raison d'être is diminished when our ears are tuned to music coming from the operating room compact disk player rather than the critical organs of the patient. To hear stridor before it is audible to everyone else in the room, one must be attentive and vigilant.

PHYSICAL PRINCIPLES AND PATHOPHYSIOLOGY OF STRIDOR

Gas Flow Through Tubes

More than most clinicians, anesthesiologists are aware of the physical principles governing the movement of gases through tubes and have a working familiarity with the concept of *resistance*. Although it is not essential to recall a mathematical equation to manage stridor in a child, an understanding of the physical principles involved and the pathophysiologic abnormalities that arise when airflow is obstructed enhance one's mental schematic. An understanding of these principles increases the likelihood of correct decision-making when there is uncertainty of diagnosis in a child with stridor and respiratory distress.

Normal flow of air through the airways is laminar and laminar flow is silent. It is governed by the Hagen–Poisseuille equation:

$$V = P(\pi r^4/8\eta l), \tag{8-1}$$

where V is the gas flow rate, P is the pressure gradient, r is the tube radius, η is the coefficient of viscosity of the gas mixture, and l is the length of the tube.

When the ordered laminar flow of airway gas is shred asunder by violation of the absolute requirement of a straight tube of constant caliber, whether it is a kink, a curve, a bifurcation, a bulge, or a foreign body, turbulence is created. The noise of stridor is the noise of turbulent airflow, and it is governed by the following equation:

$$V^2 = P(4\pi^2 r^5/\mu l f), \tag{8-2}$$

where V is the gas flow rate, P is the pressure gradient, r is the tube radius, μ is the density of the gas mixture, l is the length of the tube, and f is the coefficient of wall friction.

When there is stridor and, hence, turbulent flow, the physiochemistry of the airway gases interacts with the hydraulic principles of flow through tubes to produce physiologic consequences, none of which are good. However, an understanding of these interactions may, on occasion, allow noninvasive, minimalist interventions that are beneficial to the patient.

It is perhaps overly stressed in anesthesia texts and training programs that laminar flow is proportional to the fourth power of the radius of the tube, which means that a small decrease in airway caliber causes a dramatic decrease in airflow at constant pressures. However, this has very little bearing when one is dealing with stridor, for by definition the flow is not laminar but turbulent. Under laminar flow conditions, flow and pressure are linearly related (see Equation 8-1); i.e., once the resistance is determined by the radius and length of the tube and the viscosity of the gases flowing through the tube, a two-fold increase in pressure produces a two-fold increase in flow (within the limits of the system). This is in contrast to the disordered state of turbulent flow, in which it is the *square* of the flow rate that is proportional to the pressure. This results in an *exponential* rather than a linear relationship and *redefines resistance at each flow rate*. Under conditions of turbulent flow, increasing the flow rate increases the resistance of the system, with no change in the dimensions of the tube. Thus, increases in turbulent flow require increases in pressure that are the sum of the pressure that would be needed in the laminar flow state plus the pressure that is needed to overcome the increased resistance associated with the higher flow rates. The exponential nature of turbulent flow creates states in which, as the tube radius gets very small, the length gets very long, or the density or wall friction coefficient gets very high; further increases in pressure produce no appreciable increase in flow. Thus, it is understandable why stridulous patients have increased work of breathing.

Because the formula for turbulent flow has the radius raised to the fifth power, it has been simplistically explained that turbulent flow is more adversely affected by decreases in tube radius than in laminar flow, in which the formula contains the radius raised only to the forth power (mea culpa, circa 1986). Turbulent flow is actually proportional to the *square root of the fifth power* of the radius of the conducting tube, which is only a power of 2.5. The zinger is that, unlike in the laminar state (where flow and pressure are linearly related), turbulent flow is proportional to the square root of the pressure. Therefore, an exponential, not linear, increase in pressure is needed for an increase in flow.

Another difference between laminar and turbulent flows is a function of the physiochemical properties of the gas mixtures in motion. Laminar flow is proportional to the viscosity of a gas or liquid, whereas turbulent flow is proportional to the density.

In terms of managing a child with stridor, these formulas matter. For example, these principles provide the basis for physicians urging agitated patients with stridor and upper airway obstruction to "try to slow your breathing down." Slower flow rates of gas movement produce *exponential decreases in resistance* and the *work of breathing*. As airway experts, anesthesiologists can give narcotics (in controlled situations) to people in severe respiratory distress and, in many cases, improve their clinical status by decreasing their anxiety and agitation. This allows a better clinical environment for making decisions regarding the level or degree of intervention. In such situations, there are sound principles of physical chemistry, hydraulics, and pharmacology providing the scientific rationale for behavior that violates many a textbook nostrum regarding the use of narcotics in respiratory distress.

A clinical situation that takes advantage of the relation between viscosity and density involves the in-hospital treatment of infectious croup in certain children. Croup causes a narrowing of the upper trachea in the subglottic region, and children have audible inspiratory stridor and a "barky" cough. The child must exert high inspiratory pressures to overcome the resistance of the narrowed upper trachea. The stridor ("croup") that is heard indicates that there is turbulent flow; this results in less air movement per unit of respiratory work done by the child and may lead to respiratory failure and the requirement for tracheal intubation.

By administering a mixture of helium and oxygen (Heliox), clinicians can take advantage of the principle that the lower density of helium in relation to oxygen allows for more flow through areas of turbulence and may decrease work of breathing. However, this therapeutic option is somewhat limited by the fact that, once the obstruction has passed and laminar flow is restored, the Heliox mixture is more viscous than oxygen or air plus oxygen and thus moves down the airways somewhat more slowly. Also, the benefits of helium require oxygen concentrations in the range of 30% or less. In hypoxic children, this may not provide sufficient oxygen delivery. The use of Heliox in expiratory obstructive diseases (asthma) may be more beneficial than in inspiratory diseases such as croup. Despite almost 70 years of availability, there are no good double-blinded controlled studies that address the efficacy of Heliox. Its use is still supported by clinical reports of "we were ready to intubate the patient, but then we gave Heliox and things got better." This is just one example of the complexities involved in the physiochemistry of stridor and subsequent clinical decisions.

Airway Patency

During inspiration and expiration, there is a continuous column of gas that extends from the atmosphere to the oral and nasal cavities to the pharynx to the larynx to the trachea to the bronchi to the distal bronchi to the bronchioles to the terminal bronchioles to the alveoli. When there is linear movement of airway gases, the pressure exerted increases in the forward vector and is maximal in the center of the airway. The law of energy conservation requires a commensurate decrease in pressure somewhere along the air column, and this decrease occurs perpendicular to the forward flow vector (i.e., the *lateral pressure* decreases). At rest, the lateral pressure is a distending pressure that serves to maintain the patency of a nonrigid tube. When gas passes through a tube, the lateral pressure that has held the tube open can decrease precipitously and cause the lumen to close. This phenomenon of decreased intraluminal pressure is known as the *Venturi principle*.

Think of a child's balloon that is partly inflated, with the seal maintained by finger pressure; the pinched end of the balloon forms a hollow tube between the fingers and the round balloon that is distended by the pressure within the balloon (lateral pressure). When the balloon is released, air suddenly rushes from the balloon. However, the distended balloon neck collapses, and there is a fluttering sound as the gas in the balloon escapes through that narrow orifice. This is not an intuitive concept, and it would seem that the pressure in the balloon should sustain the patency of the open end. It does not.

Thus, at all times when there is linear movement of gases through the nonrigid tubes of the airway, the intralumenal forces favor tube collapse. This collapse is prevented by a combination of factors at different levels of the airway.

Within the thorax, the rigidity conferred by the cartilaginous U-shaped tracheal rings prevent collapse during expiration, when the increased intrathoracic pressure surrounding the trachea is added to the lateral pressure—forces that favor tube closure. Also, if the walls of the bronchi were not very thick relative to the size of the bronchial lumen, these structures also would collapse under the centripetal lateral pressures exerted during expiratory gas flow.

As the airways branch and divide distally and their walls become progressively thinner, the surrounding stromal structure of the lung parenchyma becomes the tethering cord that maintains patency and prevents airway collapse. However, at certain intrathoracic pressures, even these forces are overcome and the airways close on forced exhalation. This is what produces the "effort independent" portion of the flow–volume loop used in pulmonary function studies.

When the muscles of the diaphragm contract to initiate normal inspiration, there is a small decrease (~2 cm H_2O) in the pressure within the chest cavity (intrathoracic pressure). This pressure change is sufficient to overcome the forces of inertia and resistance, accelerate the gas column remaining in the airways at the end of exhalation (dead space gases), and draw in gas from the atmosphere or anesthesia circuit. The negative intrathoracic pressure opposes the centripetal effects on lateral pressure caused by gas movement in the airway and the intrathoracic airways remain open and are slightly increased in caliber.

Anywhere along the airway, anatomic abnormalities can impair the mechanisms of airway patency. When this occurs, the rapid opening and closing (partial or complete) of the airway in the region of the pathologic segment produces audible sounds that may be heard as rales, wheezes, rhonchi, or stridor. These vibrations often can be felt and heard.

Dynamic obstructing intrathoracic lesions cause expiratory stridor, or wheezing, and may prolong exhalation. Extrathoracic dynamic lesions cause inspiratory stridor and tend to prolong inspiration. These lesions are dynamic because the degree of obstruction is a function of the pressure state on both sides of the airway wall.

Fixed circumferential lesions are not dynamic and are associated with biphasic stridor. They may prolong inspiration and expiration. Biphasic stridor indicates that there is increased work of breathing associated with inspiration and expiration. Biphasic stridor in the setting of significant respiratory distress may be an ominous sign and herald respiratory failure.

PRESENTATIONS OF STRIDOR

When children with stridor electively present to the anesthesiologist, it is usually with a diagnosis or at least a high index of suspicion. However, this does not obviate the need for the anesthesiologist to review the history and perform a physical examination, thereby verifying that the clinical findings are consistent with the diagnosis. Because the anesthetic management will depend on the diagnosis, actions based on an incorrect diagnosis can convert a partly obstructed airway into a totally obstructed airway. Thus, *proper diagnosis is the key element* in the management of stridor in children.

Usually, there is a single cause and, hence, only one correct diagnosis, with the exception of congenital lesions and children with syndromes. In the vast majority of cases, the correct diagnosis is based on a focused history and physical examination. Diagnostic imaging studies (x-ray, computed tomography, magnetic resonance imaging [MRI]) and endoscopic examinations are most often confirmatory and helpful in the assessment of the extent of the lesion causing airflow obstruction. *Imaging is rarely helpful in a crisis situation, whereas ongoing physical assessment is essential at such a time.*

Etiologies of Stridor

The most common etiologies of stridor in the newborn period are laryngomalacia, subglottic stenosis, vocal cord paralysis, and vascular rings. Subglottic stenosis may be iatrogenic as a consequence of endotracheal intubation; vocal cord paralysis also may be iatrogenic due to birth trauma or recurrent laryngeal nerve injury during surgery in the newborn (usually for ligation of a ductus arteriosus).

Stridor appearing beyond the newborn period may still be due to iatrogenic causes; subglottic stenosis may not manifest until there is a concurrent airway tract illness, and distal tracheal stenosis may be silent until the child is older and more active. However, stridor beyond the newborn period should make one think of infectious causes (croup, supraglottitis, bacterial tracheitis); if there is a history of surgery, then consider iatrogenic causes (subglottic stenosis, vocal cord injury, injury to the recurrent laryngeal nerve).

Foreign bodies in the larynx or trachea may present at any time but are most common in toddlers. Stridor after a coughing or choking episode with food or other objects in the mouth may be caused by a laryngeal or tracheal foreign body; less frequently, esophageal foreign bodies may cause extrinsic compression of the airway and produce stridor.

Benign and malignant neoplasms can cause stridor, and the mechanisms run the gamut (see Chap. 15).

History

The first question to consider in an infant with stridor, who is not *in extremis* is, "Has this been present since birth or shortly afterwards?" Congenital stridor may not be evident in the first few weeks of life due to the reduced metabolic state of the newborn. Congenital stridor, as distinct from acquired lesions, is more likely to be associated with other airway abnormalities and other organ system abnormalities, particularly of the cardiovascular system.

In addition to the timing of the onset, it is important to know the setting of onset. Was there trauma? Coughing? Also, what is the quality of the child's cry? A normal cry excludes vocal cord abnormalities. Is there any relation of stridor to feeding? Is there evidence of reflux or aspiration? Is there any position that makes the stridor better or worse, and how is the stridor affected by activity? Was there anything unusual at the time of birth? And, is there a history of prematurity, tracheal intubation, or prior chest or neck surgery?

Physical Examination

The clinical examination involves careful observation and auscultation using both the ear and the stethoscope. In localizing the site of obstruction in infants and children, it is often helpful to remove the head from the stethoscope and apply just the hollow tube to various regions of the neck. *However, the critical question is whether there is gas exchange occurring and whether the patient is in distress.* The assessment and management of stridor are elements in an ongoing physical examination. Because there is already some degree of airway compromise, there is a decreased margin for error, especially in consideration of any intervention that may further compromise the airway. Not surprisingly, this is frequently the case when anesthesiologists, airway endoscopists or surgeons, and a child with stridor get together.

MANAGEMENT OF STRIDOR

The key issues in the management of stridor are assessment of the degree of respiratory distress and assessment of the potential for the progression of obstruction. In some cases stridor will herald the rapid onset of total airway obstruction; in another situation, the identical sounds will be caused by a relatively benign condition that will resolve without medical or surgical intervention. Continuous observation becomes an essential element of verification; there are almost no situations where the new onset of stridor in a child should not be directly observed by a health professional, with the possible exception of infectious croup.

Croup has a slow onset and the child is obviously ill but not toxic. This is a viral illness that is frequently managed over the telephone by pediatricians and family practitioners. The disadvantage of this practice is that croup can arise from a laryngeal foreign body such as a piece of a plastic toy; the fever that may be present could be from a subsequent bacterial infection at the site of lodging. Thus, in all cases of stridor, regardless of the presumptive diagnosis, someone must observe the child and report the symptoms to a health professional. In the rare, but real, case of a laryngeal foreign body, one hopes that it will be recognized and that proper action will be taken before there is total occlusion of the upper airway due to edema or infection.

Assessment of Airway Distress

In cases of *mild* airway distress, stridor can be heard with a stethoscope or felt with a hand on the child's thorax or neck. The respiratory rate may or may not be increased, and one phase of respiration may or may not be prolonged. The child's color is normal. If dyspnea is present, it does not seem to bother the child. There may be flaring of the nasal alae on inspiration. It should be noted that the compliant chest wall of the young child greatly exaggerates the degree of retractions and dyspnea compared with similar lesions in older patients.

Moderate airway distress may include any or all of the mild symptoms. However, audible stridor is almost always a marker for moderate distress, and a stethoscope is not needed. There are moderate retractions and dyspnea.

The patient is anxious and may be mildly cyanotic if not receiving supplemental oxygen. A certain posture may be required to maximize airflow. The phase of respiration during which stridor is heard is prolonged.

Severe respiratory distress will include any or all of the symptoms of moderate distress plus cyanosis (often despite supplemental oxygen), obtundation, extreme agitation, and progressive respiratory fatigue. The volume (noisiness) and pitch of the stridor will diminish as progressive exhaustion of the respiratory musculature impairs respiratory effort.

As stated by a management colleague, "The greatest error made in the differential diagnosis of respiratory distress is not in the differential diagnosis but in the assessment of the degree of compromise." It is vitally important that this assessment be performed before the blood gas is drawn or the x-ray is obtained. Observing the child for several minutes, counting the respiratory rate and determining the degree of effort, position preference, color, level of consciousness, presence or absence of drooling, the appearance of toxicity, and the degree of fatigue are much more informative than an arterial partial pressure of carbon dioxide (PCO_2) or lateral neck findings on a radiograph. This period of observation also can give the physician time to ask relevant historical questions that, coupled with observations, are better guides to further investigations and management than any laboratory studies. It matters little whether the distress or obstruction is caused by croup rather than by epiglottitis if the child experiences a respiratory arrest in the radiology suite.

Progression of the Airway Obstruction

Lesions causing stridor are static or progressive in their physiologic presentation. Even with a nonprogressive lesion, the patient may deteriorate over time due to a vicious cycle of increased metabolic demands secondary to increased work of breathing and eventually malnutrition as a result of impaired feeding during the period of respiratory compromise. As an example, consider the case of a 6-month-old with *severe* laryngomalacia and failure to thrive. The collapse and closure of the upper airway on inspiration can be expected to resolve by the age of 2 years. In such a case, a gastostomy for feeding may allow for an improvement in the patient's status without airway intervention; a gastrostomy in a 6 month old carries considerably less morbidity than a tracheostomy. Similarly, a circumferential scarring of the subglottic region in a toddler may be fixed and, absent a comorbid insult, nonprogressive. However, the clinical status of the child may deteriorate over time as the growth of the child, and the resultant increased gas exchange necessary to support the increased metabolic demands of growth render the lesion increasingly severe. In this sense, any fixed obstruction of a young child's airway may become progressive in terms of severity. However, in most situations, the issue is *rapid* progression: Will the degree of obstruction change at such a rate as to put the child at risk unless prompt intervention is undertaken?

Table 8-1 presents a suggested classification scheme based on the potential for progression of an airway lesion *in relation* to the degree of respiratory distress exhibited by the patient.

Figures 8-1 and 8-2 make the general point that it is the *combination* of the factors of *progression* and *distress* that determine the need for intervention. A diagonal of the same-shade rectangles connects the various equivalent combinations of lesion progression and distress. Combinations along the same diagonal tend to require the same management. Thus, all the categories indicated by rectangles in the grid that are any color except white in Figure 8–1

TABLE 8–1 Evaluation of Stridor Based on Progression and Degree of Respiratory Distress

	Signs and symptoms of respiratory distress		
Progression of the lesion	Minimal	Mild–Moderate	Severe
Nonprogressive	RD-1/NP	RD-2/NP	RD-3/NP
Potentially progressive	RD-1/PP	RD-2/PP	RD-3/PP
Rapidly progressive	RD-1/RP	RD-2/RP	RD-3/RP

NP, nonprogressive; PP, potentially progressive; RP, rapidly progressive; RD-1, respiratory distress minimal; RD-2, respiratory distress mild to moderate; RD-3, respiratory distress severe.

(RD-1/RP, RD-2/PP, and RD-3/NP) usually require that the airway be secured by tracheal intubation or, at a minimum, that the patient be monitored with a high level or airway expertise available. However, categories along the light gray central diagonal (RD-1/NP, RD-2/PP; RD-3/NP in Figure 8–1) usually allow time for this to be accomplished in a controlled environment.

ILLUSTRATIVE CASE SCENARIOS BASED ON STRIDOR STATUS

RD-1/NP: Minimal Signs and Symptoms of Respiratory Distress and a Nonprogressive Lesion

A 4-year-old child underwent a left thoracotomy 2 months previously for coartation of the aorta. Her hospital course was complicated by development of left lobar pneumonia, persistent atelectasis, and a prolonged intubation of her trachea (5 days). She was discharged with a painless persistent hoarseness. The nursing staff told her father that the hoarseness was due to the endotracheal tube being in place for 5 days. His response was that his greatest fear was that his daughter would be paralyzed by the aortic surgery and that a "froggy"-sounding voice was a small price to pay.

The child was seen in a preoperative clinic at the same institution 2 months later for surgical exploration of her previous chest tube site that had persistent nonpurulent drainage. Her history showed that she had developed noisy breathing with exertion that had never been noted before surgery. Her activity level appeared normal, which meant she tried to keep up with her two older brothers in outdoor activities. Her father stated that as soon as she got home from the hospital after her major surgery, she was out running around and would not "take it easy" like the doctor and nurses had requested. However, he insisted that there had been no change in her "wheezes," the term he used to describe her stridor, over the previous 2 months.

An aunt who was a public health nurse thought that the child had developed "exercise-induced asthma," and a neighbor thought that the child's noisy breathing was caused by being outdoors and breathing the air from a nearby coal-burning power plant. The child was eating well and had no physical complaints.

On physical examination the child exhibited inspiratory stridor, which changed with the degree of exertion. The stridor localized to the thyrohyoid region of the neck in the midline. An ultrasound examination showed that the left vocal cord did not move with respiration. There was also moderately restricted motion of the right vocal cord. The subglottic region appeared normal on anterior–posterior neck radiographs. The thoracic surgeon was quick to point out that, if the stridor was due to recurrent laryngeal nerve damage from the coarctation surgery, the right vocal cord should not be affected. A

	Signs and symptoms of respiratory distress		
Progression of the lesion	Minimal	Mild–moderate	Severe
Nonprogressive			
Potentially progressive			
Rapidly progressive			

FIG. 8-1 Common patterns of progression and distress.

| No intervention required, follow up if change in symptoms |
| Diagnostic study usually required, often can be done electively |
| Airway must be secured, usually adequate time for controlled intubation of trachea |
| Respiratory failure or total airway obstruction may rapidly ensue unless airflow improves |
| Severe airway obstruction already present and ability to establish an airway uncertain |

FIG. 8-2 Likely intervention and outcome based on stridor status.

flexible fiber-optic laryngoscopy was carried out under topical anesthesia and sedation. A synechia was noted at the apex of the vocal cords such that the right vocal cord was tethered to the left cord.

Subsequently, and before the thoracotomy, anesthesia was induced with a mask induction; with the aid of suspension laryngoscopy, the synechia was excised with a carbon dioxide laser. Afterward, the right vocal cord moved freely, but the left was fixed in midposition. The remainder of the case (chest tube wound exploration) was carried out under mask anesthesia to avoid additional trauma to the vocal cords.

Discussion

RD-1/PA–type lesions are classic iatrogenic lesions resulting from possible vocal cord trauma, subglottic injury, or recurrent laryngeal nerve injury. The child usually will have a history of tracheal intubation, and this may occasionally obscure the exact etiology. However, office endoscopy by a skilled pediatric practitioner with a flexible fiber-optic laryngoscope can almost always immediately establish the correct diagnosis.

RD-1/PB: Minimal Signs and Symptoms of Respiratory Distress and a Moderately Progressive Lesion

A 1-year-old boy presented with new onset stridor after breakfast with his family. He appeared to choke while eating cereal. Subsequently, he had a croupy cough and inspiratory stridor. The mother called her family physician. After hearing the symptoms he suggested that she put the boy in the bathroom, turn on the hot water spigot, and have the boy breath the warm, humid air to help with his croup. After 1 h, she called back to say that he was worse and was told to take the child to an emergency room.

Anterior–posterior and lateral neck radiographs were taken and the diagnosis of acute epiglottitis was made. The mother insisted that the child had been given a vaccine that was supposed to prevent this disease. The child was afebrile and did not seem to prefer any position. He did not drool. There was audible inspiratory stridor heard best over the upper larynx, but there was also expiratory stridor that was readily heard through a stethoscope. There were no retractions and the child did not appear overly anxious. He periodically had spasms of coughing that were "barky." Based on the radiographic findings, despite an atypical presentation, the hospital's acute epiglottitis protocol was set in motion.

While the child was being observed in the emergency department and awaiting the arrival of the pediatric otolaryngologist, the anesthesiologist noted that the quality of the stridor was slowly changing and becoming somewhat less high pitched and more stertorous. Soon thereafter, the child was taken to the operating room and anesthesia was induced by mask with sevoflurane in oxygen, an intravenous cannula was placed, and, after a deep plane of anesthesia was attained, direct laryngoscopy was performed. Topical application of local anesthetic to the airway was not used before direct visualization of the airway. The epiglottis was normal, but there was marked edema of the arytenoid cartilages and vocal folds bilaterally. A fragment of purple plastic (later identified as Major Marvel's left arm) was impacted in the airway just above the true vocal cords.

While maintaining a fairly deep level of anesthesia, topical anesthesia and a vasoconstrictor, neosynephrine, were applied to the edematous vocal folds that were partly encasing the toy fragment. An angled forceps was used to grasp the fragment and gently removed it intact from the larynx. A rigid pediatric bronchoscope was then passed to inspect the right and left bronchial airways. No additional fragments were seen.

Discussion

Obstructions at the level of the vocal cords can cause a disproportionate amount of stridor for the amount of airway compromise produced because the turbulent flow, which results in the stridor, occurs over a very short segment of the airway. In turbulent flow states, the flow is related to the square root of the *inverse* of the length (see Equation 8-2). As the constricted segment of a tube becomes shorter, the deleterious effects on flow decrease in an exponential manner. Thus, one may hear stridor as gas moves through a narrow segment at the vocal cords, and there may be a certain amount of supraglottic stridor produced by a Venturi effect as the patient makes a moderate increase in respiratory effort, but the inspiratory time will not be significantly increased. There may be no obvious increase in work of breathing.

RD-1/PP: Minimal Signs and Symptoms of Respiratory Distress and a Rapidly Progressive Lesion

The rescue squad brought in a 7-year-old child from a house fire that had occurred 20 min before his arrival in the emergency department. The details of the event were sketchy, but the child was apparently home alone and turned on the gas burners of the stove for heat but the pilot light was out. He had then tried to start a fire in the fireplace, and there had been a gas explosion when he struck a match. The outer layer of a jacket he was wearing had been burned away in several places and the plastic buttons were melted. He was awake, seemed somewhat indifferent to his burns, but was concerned about his pet tree frog that had been in his bedroom. There were second- and third-degree burns on his face and neck, and his eyelids and nose hair were singed away. The child's voice was slightly hoarse. There were soot particles in his nostrils and, with visual inspection, in the back of his mouth. His breath sounds were clear.

Discussion

The hoarseness in this child's voice is a precursor to likely extreme stridor and airway obstruction. Recall the relation of airflow to airway size in children. The edema that occurs after thermal and chemical injury to the airway is delayed but progressive. As important as the edema is the fact that the cilia of the airway are destroyed. Thus, enhanced secretions from injury, inhaled debris and soot, and the desquamated airway endothelium accumulate in the airway, thus obstructing it and causing further irritation and edema. Prompt tracheal intubation can bypass the upper portion of this process, down to the region just proximal to the carina; most thermal burns do not extend far beyond the carina. Also, early intubation in such a situation provides a safety margin because the supraglottic structures have not yet become severely edematous and the child's pulmonary function has not yet become as impaired as it will. Judicious bronchoscopic lavage after tracheal intubation can decrease the pathologic consequences of inhalation injury as it affects the bronchi and smaller airways.

A carboxyhemoglobin level obtained on arrival in the emergency department was reported as 35%. The level of carboxyhemoglobin is of minimal management consequence at this stage of care. The history and clinical presentation of this child dictate prompt securing of the airway, and a laboratory value that may be indicative of long-term outcome is of little value at this point. An extremely low value could be laboratory error and would not warrant withholding prompt airway intervention. Likewise, one must assume that a closed space fire involves carbon monoxide poisoning, and the pulse oximetry may give a poor assessment of the degree of intracellular hypoxia due to abnormal binding of oxygen by carboxyhemoglobin.

Children who have evidence of an airway burn need their airways secured immediately. Waiting until they become progressively symptomatic is often met with disastrous results; intubation may be impossible secondary to massive edema and swelling subsequent to fluid resuscitation. Commonly these children's faces are unrecognizable within 6 to 12 h postresuscitation; the change is dramatic.

RD-2/NP: Moderate Signs and Symptoms of Respiratory Distress and a Nonprogressive Lesion

A 12-week-old infant was scheduled for upper airway endoscopy to evaluate expiratory stridor. It had developed when she was 2 to 3 weeks of age and had not changed since that time. A barium swallow was performed in a community hospital near the infant's home and reported as normal.

The child had been born at 34 weeks' gestation and had not required intubation initially; at age 4 days, she had developed apnea and was eventually diagnosed with sepsis. She required tracheal intubation and cardiovascular support with dopamine. Her trachea was extubated after 7 days, and her subsequent course was uneventful.

The mother reported that the stridor did not appear to change with position but got worse during breast feeding. At these times, the child appeared to become dusky. The baby's growth was not keeping up with the growth chart, and her pediatrician had advised the mother to stop breast feeding.

The child had audible expiratory stridor at rest, and it was auscultated best at the suprasternal notch. The stridor worsened with crying.

An MRI scan performed while the child was under intravenous sedation showed a collapse of the mid-trachea, that was approximately 25% of the cross-sectional diameter.

Rigid bronchoscopy under general anesthesia was performed to evaluate the area of abnormality. There was no evidence of granulation tissue intruding into the tracheal lumen. There was a moderate degree of scarring along the anterior tracheal wall at the level of the lowest three tracheal rings; on spontaneous exhalation, the tracheal lumen narrowed to a slit-like lumen.

The infant was managed conservatively at home with nasal continuous positive airway pressure. This treatment appeared to particularly benefit the infant during nursing. The infant's nutrition was supplemented with gavage feeding of breast milk through orogastric tubes. At the age of 5 years, the child had a modest degree of exercise limitation, but her parents declined procedures to address that problem.

Discussion

Tracheomalacia often is associated with prematurity and tracheal intubation, and the risk of ischemic injury to the trachea and tracheal cartilage likely is increased by the same factors that prolong tracheal intubation: hypoxemia, hypotension, and the intracellular hypoxia of sepsis. *Congenital tracheomalacia is due most frequently to extrinsic compression of the trachea by vascular abnormalities of the mediastinum.* These aberrant vascular structures are readily identified on MRI scans.

Such lesions are usually of minimal consequence to the anesthesiologist *who understands the pathophysiology of the lesion*. Vigorous coughing at the end of a case, as might follow tracheal extubation, may produce distal air trapping, decreased venous return to the heart due to increased intrathoracic pressure, hypotension, and hypoxemia. Judicious airway management is advised and should be as noninvasive as safety allows—the liberal use of "good" airway drugs such as fentanyl, lidocaine, sevoflurane, and propofol (rather than thiopental and halothane) and use of laryngeal mask airways (LMAs) rather than endotracheal tubes. Continuous positive airway pressure is very beneficial in the management of the airway during anesthesia, just as it is at home in children with tracheomalacia.

Another important point is that one should not add insult to injury by using an endotracheal cuff at the site of the tracheal lesion during anesthesia. Do not let the tip of an uncuffed tube remain at the injury site. Do not use a stiff suction catheter through the endotracheal tube during the case. There is a fine line between the child who "outgrows" his tracheomalacia and the child who eventually has tracheal surgery(s), an approach that carries a significant morbidity and mortality. What is learned in medical school about the pancreas in adults is analogous to the trachea in young children, and the risk increases as the size of the patient decreases.

RD-2/PP: Moderate Signs and Symptoms of Respiratory Distress and a Moderately Progressive Lesion

Acute supraglottitis is considerably less common in the West since the advent of immunization of children for *Haemophilus influenzae*, but not necessarily so for children in other countries or immigrants from developing countries.

An American couple adopted a 3-year-old child refugee from Romania. Six months after his arrival in the United States, the child developed a fever. He appeared pale and refused his breakfast. A couple of hours later, the mother noted the child had a harsh cough. His fever increased. Their family physician was contacted and they were advised to bring the child to the physician's office that morning. While driving to the office the child appeared more lethargic and began to drool slightly. Upon arrival at the doctor's office, the child was sitting upright, appeared toxic, and was constantly drooling. The doctor called 911 and preparations to emergently transfer the child to the hospital were made.

During the transfer the child exhibited marked stridor, agitation, and appeared dusky. Humidified oxygen was administered by face mask. Upon arrival to the hospital the child suffered a respiratory arrest. The emergency personnel made several attempts to intubate the child but were unable to visualize the vocal cords due to massive edema of the supraglottic area. A complete cardiovascular arrest ensued.

Upon arrival of the pediatric anesthesia and otolaryngology physicians, all attempts at intubation were discontinued. Cardiopulmonary resuscitation was continued, an intravenous line was inserted, and the child was managed by mask ventilation with 100 % oxygen. The child's color improved dramatically and his heart rate and blood pressure stabilized. Subsequently the child was taken to the operating room. With the child stable and under sevoforane anesthesia, an oral endotracheal tube was inserted by following the trail of air bubbles emanating from the obscured vocal cords. A throat swab and blood cultures were obtained. The oral endotracheal tube was changed to a nasal tube to ease the management and security of the tube. Arms splints were applied and the child was given intravenous sedation and transferred to the pediatric intensive care unit. Intravenous antibiotics were given. Twenty-four hours later a leak was noted around the uncuffed endotracheal tube and the child appeared nontoxic and was afebrile. The child was extubated under close supervision the following day and made a complete recovery.

Discussion

This real case illustrates the dramatic progression of acute epiglottitis. Not uncommonly children appear well at one moment, only to appear toxic and in severe respiratory distress a few hours later. Arguably, these children could be classified as RD-2/RP (moderate respiratory distress, rapidly progressive). It depends on the presentation and illustrates how easily patients may move from one category to another more critical one. In this case the true severity of the child's condition was not appreciated until the child was *in extremis*. It cannot be overstated that, when moderate or rapidly progressive lesions are suspected, someone capable of managing the airway must observe the child. *These children can never be left unattended, anywhere, especially in the radiology suites or preoperative areas.*

This case also illustrates that ventilation is more important than intubation. Too often, considerable time and effort are wasted trying to intubate a patient rather than making alternative attempts at ventilation. In the case of acute epiglottis, even in the worst of conditions, it is worth attempting ventilation by mask and oxygen. Such efforts are usually life saving.

All hospitals caring for children should have an acute epiglottitis protocol for children and adults. Learn what your hospital protocol is. Make sure that you and it are updated. Do not underestimate the importance of the team ap-

CHAPTER 8 / THE CHILD WITH STRIDOR 121

proach involving the emergency room, operating room, pediatric anesthesia, and otolaryngology personnel.

It is important to appreciate the systemic nature of this disease. Although the airway usually is the presenting feature, these children are at best bacteremic and more often in sepsis. Throat and blood cultures are critical for the proper selection of antibiotics. We have, unfortunately, seen children who survived the respiratory presentation only to develop cerebral infections and abscesses.

RD-2/RP: Moderate Signs and Symptoms of Respiratory Distress and a Rapidly Progressive Lesion

This category is illustrated best as a child who is quickly getting worse but is not yet *in extremis;* there is time to do the right thing. Thus, these patients may go from a RD-1 to a RD-3 status over a very brief period.

A 16-year-old male was scheduled for thorascopic biopsy of a large mediastinal mass that had been detected the previous day on a plain radiograph at an outside hospital. His chief complaint had been fever and malaise, and he had no respiratory symptoms at the time. He was a star tackle on the state championship football team and weighed 275 lb.

When he arrived at the preoperative clinic the following day, an anesthesigologist was urgently called to see him. He was sitting on the side of the examining table and having difficulty breathing. He was agitated, had inspiratory and expiratory stridor, and the nurses were unable to get an oximeter probe on his finger to measure his oxygen saturation. He did not have an intravenous catheter in place.

The anesthesiologist could not obtain a good history. The boy's mother was screaming and pleading frantically for a "doctor to help Ricky!" She could not be calmed and was unable to respond to questions. The anesthesiologist requested a STAT page for the anesthesia code team and an otolaryngology (ENT) surgeon. Meanwhile, the anesthesiologist instructed the clinic nurse to prepare for a possible cricothyroidotomy. While several people tried to restrain the patient, the anesthesiologist gave him an intramuscular injection of fentanyl (250 µg).

Within 45 s, the young man stopped struggling and his respiratory rate slowed to two to three breaths per minute. However, improved gas movement was noted, and the patient was able to identify himself and state that he had suddenly become short of breath. His mother was visibly relieved.

Lest you think that, during the period this future National Football League player was thrashing about, possibly risking injury to himself and others, an intramuscular injection of ketamine and succinylcholine would be easy to administer, the editor of this text (TAY) did that very thing to a similarly sized, aggressive young man with Down's syndrome during his early years of practice. His patient subsequently threw off his five "handlers" like rag dolls and dashed into a nearby bathroom and locked the door (a fire door) behind himself, thus answering the question, How far can a really strong kid go with a 3 mg/kg dose of succinylcholine in his deltoid muscle? Fortunately, the child recovered uneventfully despite the care.

The patient had a firm mass extending cephalad through his thoracic inlet. His normal neck circumference was distended an additional 7 in. After a short discussion, he was taken to the operating room with the full emergency team in tow. An intravenous catheter was placed, and additional fentanyl was injected to prepare the patient for an "awake" nasotracheal intubation.

Immediately after a generous application of neosynephrine and topical lidocaine jelly to his right nostril, an 8.5-cm endotracheal tube was advanced over a flexible fiber-optic laryngoscope and guided *into the hypopharynx*. Oxygen saturation by oximetry was 98%.

The trachea was extrinsically compressed 3 cm below the vocal cords. Audible inspiratory and expiratory stridor was still present but decreased by the delivery of oxygen into the trachea through the bronchoscope.

Topical anesthesia was administered into the trachea directly as a nebulized spray, with minimal response from the patient. After evaluating and anesthetizing the trachea, an endotracheal tube was advanced over the bronchoscope and correct placement was confirmed by identification of the carina just distal to the end of the tube.

There was an acceptable expired CO_2 trace on the capnograph, and breath sounds were heard over both lung fields. The inspiratory stridor was no longer present, and the expiratory stridor had greatly diminished. The patient was still awake, not coughing, and gave a "thumbs up" sign to indicate that he was doing much better. He was then given 200 mg intravenous propofol, 8 mg rocuronium, and 4% sevoflurane in 100% oxygen through the anesthesia circuit. Within minutes, his end-tidal CO_2 became nondetectable.

There was no apparent disconnect of the patient or circuit, and a suction catheter readily passed through the endotracheal tube. Laryngoscopy confirmed that the endotracheal tube was still passing through the vocal cords. The patient at this time was ashen, and the oximeter had ceased functioning at an oxygen saturation of 60%. He was given two ampoules of epinephrine (1:1000) and cardiopulmonary resuscitation commenced.

At this point, a second anesthesiologist assessed the situation and said, "Roll him over and reverse the muscle relaxant!" Then he said, "Let the boy breathe on his own!" The relaxant was reversed, the patient began to breathe spontaneously, and everything got better, albeit upside down.

Discussion

Anterior mediastinal masses can be deadly, even when benign, due to their ability to compress airway and, equally important, cardiac structures. Lymphomas are particularly troublesome because some have doubling times of 24 h. When all this is happening in the anterior mediastinum, it is only a matter of time until disaster strikes.

Obviously, the response of the anesthesiologist to someone with pending airway obstruction is to establish an artificial airway, almost always by tracheal intubation. However, mediastinal masses have a notorious habit of obstructing more than the airway. They may obstruct blood vessels such as the superior vena cava and the pulmonary veins returning blood to the left atrium from the lungs. This tendency is exacerbated by general anesthesia and with neuromuscular blockade for reasons that are clearly understood.

Cardiopulmonary resuscitation on a 275-lb patient in the prone (face down) position who has *some* pulmonary blood flow is vastly superior to conventional cardiopulmonary resuscitation with no pulmonary blood flow and, hence, very poor delivery of oxygenated blood to the coronary circulation. How can one tell whether there is pulmonary blood flow? If there is a significant and repetitious amount of CO_2 measured as end-tidal gas, it can come only from tissue metabolism and reach the alveoli only through the pulmonary circulation. The only way that significant amounts of CO_2 can get to the lungs is by cardiac output.

A drastic decrease in cardiac output, from an intrinsically obstructed pulmonary artery (embolus), constricted vessels (extreme pulmonary hypertension), or extrinsic compression (pericardial mass causing tamponade and pulmonary outflow tract obstruction), has the same effect—a marked decrease in expired CO_2. The patient's arterial partial pressure of *oxygen* had not decreased initially. However, gas delivery to the alveoli was significantly impaired, and the dead space problem thus created is one of classic situations of ventilation and perfusion mismatching. *Anesthetic management of mediastinal masses may mislead the unsuspecting to be concerned about ventilation and airway patency when in fact perfusion is compromised.*

A state-of-the-art capnograph is permanently attached to our departmental code 12 box. More than any other, the capnograph provides data about the adequacy of ventilation *and* perfusion, and it is an essential monitor.

Previous management of aggressive mediastinal lymphomas argued for early radiation therapy to decrease the airway hazards. However, this practice made adequate histologic diagnosis difficult and compromised disease treatment; Bedford and Ferrari showed that, given an awareness of the ways in which these patients can be compromised during anesthesia, it is possible to safely obtain mediastinal biopsies under general anesthesia before tumor shrinkage using radiation. An additional discussion of this problem is included in Chapter 15.

RD-3/NP: Severe Signs and Symptoms of Respiratory Distress and a Nonprogressive Lesion

A young woman, with minimal prenatal care, presented to the emergency room while she was 8 months pregnant. An ultrasonic examination showed a singleton fetus with a heart rate of 40 to 60 bpm. She was rushed to the obstetric operating suite for an emergency cesarian section.

After general anesthesia, a small-for-gestational-age baby boy was delivered. The child had an obvious lumbar meningomylocele. The child made gasping respiratory efforts with significant chest wall retractions. His heart rate was slower than 100 beats per minute and he was grossly cyanotic.

The neonatal care team immediately intubated his trachea. He was easily ventilated and his condition improved dramatically. No other abnormalities were noted and he was transported to the neonatal intensive care unit. Several hours later, with no further cardiorespiratory distress, it was decided to extubate the infant. Immediately after extubation, the child had marked respiratory stridor, agitation, and quickly became cyanotic. The trachea was immediately reintubated and his condition improved quickly.

The following day he was scheduled for bronchoscopy. Under general anesthesia, with the infant breathing spontaneously, the endotracheal tube was removed and direct laryngoscopy quickly showed no movement of either vocal cord. The rest of the examination was negative and a diagnosis of bilateral vocal cord paralysis, secondary to the child's Arnold–Chiari defect, was made. The child was subsequently scheduled for a tracheotomy after further discussion with the parents.

Discussion

This case is a simple illustration of a child with severe life-threatening stridor and a fixed anatomic lesion. Such cases are generally straightforward. These children require an immediate solution. The important aspect of such cases is that treatment not be withheld while a diagnosis is sought. The lesions are stable but the children are not!

RD-3/PP: Severe Signs and Symptoms of Respiratory Distress and a Moderately Progressive Lesion

A 4-month-old female infant presented to the emergency room with a 2-day history of a low-grade fever and cough. Examination of the child showed a tired, agitated child with a rapid respiratory rate, sinus tachycardia, and a harsh barking or "seal-like" cough. The child was admitted to the pediatric intensive care unit for observation. Upon admission the child's oxygen saturation was 89% breathing room air.

The child was placed in a crib and given cold humidified oxygen to breath by face tent. Her respiratory rate continued at 50 breaths per minute. A healstick capillary blood gas showed a Pco_2 of 60 mmHg. One dose of racemic epinephrine was administered. The child was given a small amount of sedation rectally, and her condition improved slightly. During the night the child's condition remained unchanged, although the infant slept from time to time. The following day the infant's condition improved and she was discharged 1 day later without sequelae.

Discussion

Children with severe croup present a unique challenge for pediatric caregivers. This case illustrates the effective use of sedation in certain appropriate circumstances. In this case the use of sedation reduced the amount of turbulent airflow in the cricoid region. Slower, smaller breaths are more likely to produce laminar airflow through the restricted subglottic area, thereby reducing airway resistance and reducing the work of breathing. Fatigue can be a significant factor in children with croup. Therapeutic measures, cold humidified oxygen to reduce airway edema and improve oxygenation, and sedation to promote laminar airflow reduce fatigue and impending respiratory failure. Giving sedation to a child with a Pco_2 of 60 mmHg seems inappropriate to many. However, used sparingly, in a properly monitored setting and with the correct diagnosis, sedation can be a useful adjunct. Racemic epinephrine is best reserved for the child *in extremis* who then should be closely monitored. Not infrequently, rebound edema occurs. If one dose does not improve the child's condition, several more will only risk complications of the therapy.

Why not intubate this child? We would in so many other circumstances; why not in this case? These infants should be intubated only as a last resort, when hypoxia persists despite the conservative measures previously mentioned. When these children are intubated, they often remain so for several days. *They are not easily extubated.* Despite its presentation, croup usually responds to conservative treatment and resolves over a period of hours; intubation should be reserved for the worst of cases and/or a child *in extremis*.

RD-3/PC: Severe Signs and Symptoms of Respiratory Distress and a Rapidly Progressive Lesion

A 3-year-old child was having a general anesthetic to facilitate MRI of the head. The child had had a craniopharyngioma resected the year before. The child had recovered remarkably and the examination was for the purpose of follow-up. An LMA had been placed into the child's mouth at induction and she was spontaneously breathing sevoflurane. At the mid-point of the examination the radiologist decided that radiographic contrast medium would enhance imaging of the area of interest. An intravenous catheter was inserted into her arm and the contrast given. All anesthesia and radiology personnel returned to the MRI control area and the scan continued.

A change in the shape of the end-tidal CO_2 trace and a small drop in the oximeter reading were noted about 3 minutes later. Her blood pressure monitor did not register a pressure. Within less than a minute, her oximeter readings dropped below 80% and there was no end-tidal CO_2 trace.

The examination was immediately discontinued. The anesthesia team ran into the MRI room and pulled the child into view. She appeared ashen but was making some respiratory effort. The LMA was in good position. By this point her heart rate dropped below 50 beats per minute and her pulse was barely palpable. The LMA was removed and direct laryngoscopy showed marked edema of the entire supraglottic structures and the vocal cords. An endotracheal tube was inserted with moderate difficulty. Ventilation through the endotracheal tube was commenced and 100 µg epinephrine was given through the intravenous line. Airway resistance decreased subsequent to the epinephrine. Her blood pressure and heart rate also were restored. Physical examination showed that bilateral rhonchi were audible.

The MRI examination was canceled and the child was taken to the pediatric intensive care unit for further management and observation. Shortly after arrival in the intensive care her condition again deteriorated, but again she responded favorably to a small dose of epinephrine. She required repeated doses of epinephrine throughout the evening. She was sedated and ventilated throughout the night.

The following day her condition had improved immensely and, after discontinuation of sedation, she was extubated without difficulty. She was discharged the following day.

Discussion

Anaphylactic reactions are commonly severe and progress rapidly. Fortunately, this child was closely monitored and attended before her reaction. If this event had occurred in a more casual setting, the result might have been much different. Anaphylaxis causes rapid swelling of the entire airway, upper and lower. These patients require an endotracheal tube to bypass the swelling of the glottis and aggressive respiratory support as a result of lower airway reactivity. There is little time to respond in such circumstances. In this case it was imperative that the LMA be removed immediately, followed by intubation. Although epinephrine is the drug of choice in such situations, it will do little if the "A" of the "ABCs" is not established quickly.

PERIOPERATIVE STRIDOR AND LARYNGOSPASM

The practice of anesthesia has changed in no small way secondary to the use of new drugs. Sevoflurane is one of those drugs. Laryngospasm during induction and emergence, so common with halothane, currently is a much more uncommon event during induction . . . even at fairly light levels of sevoflurane anesthesia (all things being relative!). When laryngospasm does occur with sevoflurane, it is usually readily managed by the gentle application of positive pressure by mask and continuing with the induction. Rarely does one need to emergently give a muscle relaxant or some other intervention. The noted exceptions to this are young infants with upper respiratory infections and premature infants. *Respect* and *caution* are the operative words with these patients. Their management is discussed in detail in Chapter 7.

With experience, it is not unreasonable to think that laryngospasm, however mild, is an expected routine, even with today's current drugs; albeit less so with intravenous than with inhalational induction. However, the capable management of laryngospasm is the hallmark of the good pediatric anesthesiologist. Unfortunately for the reader, this skill is learned by experience, not from a textbook. Children are most prone to this common complication when their levels of anesthesia are light and unstable. Laryngospasm rarely occurs at 1.5 minimum alveolar concentration (MAC). Knowing the patients' depth of anesthesia and what can and cannot be done comes from experience.

Laryngospasm after induction with sevoflurane usually occurs because the operator is struggling with laryngoscopy and cannot intubate the trachea. It is unclear what the role of topical lidocaine is in this scenario. Many practitioners habitually deposit liquid lidocaine directly on the vocal cords and surrounding laryngeal tissues immediately before insertion of the endotracheal tube into the trachea. If the anesthetic depth of the patient is insufficient, this may provoke various protective airway reflexes, such as cough and/or laryngospasm. Other practitioners eschew the delay and airway provocation associated with topical lidocaine and pass the endotracheal tube as expeditiously as possible once laryngoscopy is initiated. Speed matters with this approach!

Stridor after insertion of LMAs in children generally is the result of the epiglottis being displaced posteriorly and caudally such that it overlies the glottic inlet. Laryngospasm usually is not the culprit. The displaced epiglottis obstructs gas inflow during spontaneous ventilation (Venturi effect) but usually does not block egress of airway gases during exhalation.

Stridor during administration of a general anesthetic requires the rapid identification of the site of obstruction and correction of the problem. The etiology tends depends on the type of airway (mask, LMA, endotracheal tube).

During mask anesthesia, stridor is very uncommon once an adequate depth has been attained. One may have stertor (a snoring noise) due to partial soft tissue obstruction, but stridor should make one check the expired gas concentration and the level of anesthetic liquid in the vaporizer because this may be a patient on the verge of arousal. A second but unusual possibility is reflux of gastric contents into the hypopharynx and reflex closure of the vocal folds. Either diagnosis is readily established with the most cursory of observations.

Stridor with an LMA in place and properly seated is usually due to subsequent rotation of the LMA caused by the torque exerted by the anesthetic gas hoses. The laryngeal mask becomes a pharyngeal foreign body partly obstructing the larynx. This usually is associated with a change in the CO_2 waveform; a decrease in the area under the curve results from a decrease in tidal volume. If repositioning of the LMA does not promptly relieve the obstruction, it should be removed and replaced with a facemask. If this does not correct the stridor, laryngoscopy should be performed to visualize the upper airway and intubate the trachea.

In intubated patients under general anesthesia, new onset stridor is a potentially ominous sign. It requires a rapid assessment of the patient (is the chest wall moving, are respirations labored, is there an obvious etiology from events in the surgical field?).

Kinking of the endotracheal tube—at the back of the throat, at the teeth, and at the attachment of the breathing circuit—is a common source of obstruction and/or stridor. In addition, obstruction of the distal endotracheal tube by secretions occurs more commonly than realized, especially in preschool children. Commonly, the presentation is one of increasing stridor, respiratory effort, and an increasing end-tidal CO_2. Hypoxia is a much less common presenting feature. The surgeon may complain that the child is moving a lot, referring to the increased breathing activity. The ability to pass a suction catheter through the endotracheal tube means nothing. We have seen suction catheters pass through tubes full of thick secretions. If there is any question that the tube is obstructed distally in this scenario, then replace it.

Laryngospasm at the end of anesthesia is not infrequent. The problem is related to the depth of anesthesia. How the extubation is managed depends on the surgery and the child's condition. *For general purposes, extubate the trachea while the patient is deeply anesthetized or awake; in between is always a mistake.* Deep extubations are most successful at 1.5 MAC or deeper. For awake extubations, our best sign is furrowing of the brow. Scrunching the eyebrows is a sign of higher cortical function and not a crude reflex response to painful stimulation; it is more reliable than a cough, which is the result of tracheal irritation and unrelated to successful extubation.

Laryngospasm in the recovery room is most commonly related to light planes of anesthesia (or sedation) *and* secretions, blood, or gastric contents annoying the vocal cords. In the case of the child posttonsillectomy, always consider that a blood clot may have been inhaled during emergence. These need to be removed. Succinylcholine does not dissolve blood clots! On several occasions and at different institutions, we have found the source of stridor after extubation to be a retained throat pack (despite a correct count in the operating room).

When laryngospasm does not resolve with the conservative management of deepening the level of anesthesia or gentle positive pressure with oxygen by mask, then more definitive treatment is warranted. Once the child becomes hypoxic and/or bradycardic, the use of a muscle relaxant is appropriate and necessary. Succinylcholine is the drug of choice in all but a few uncommon situations (muscular dystrophy, malignant hyperthermia [MH] susceptibility, hyperkalemia, etc.). During the anxiety of treating this problem, unreasonable doses of succinylcholine are commonly given. A full dose is appropriate only if one plans to reintubate the child and one is prepared to wait several minutes for the drug to wear off. Otherwise, laryngospasm can be resolved by using only 0.1 mg/kg succinylcholine intravenously (1–3 mg/kg if given intramuscularly). We usually give 10 µg/kg atropine at the same time; by the time succinylcholine is needed, the patient's bradycardia needs to be treated as well.

CROUP IN THE RECOVERY ROOM

Postextubation croup has decreased over the years. Although a rate of 1% is traditionally taught, our experience suggests that it is less common than previously reported.

The incidence of postextubation croup is related to young infants, lack of leak around the endotracheal tube, pre-existing respiratory infections, multiple attempts at intubation or bronchoscopy, pre-existing tracheal stenosis, movement of the head and neck during the surgery, and unknown causes. Clearly, careful attention to the placement and use of appropriately sized endotracheal tubes is important in limiting this complication. Whether the endotracheal tube has a cuff matters less than the appropriate size and inflation of that cuff. Cuffs should be inflated only if necessary, if there is a leak around the deflated cuff, and to produce a seal at 20 cm of water pressure or less. An uncuffed endotracheal tube that does not leak, even at high airway pressures, does significant damage, even during short cases.

Postextubation croup is rarely noted at the time of extubation. More commonly, the child sounds fine at the time of extubation, and the recovery room nurses, or parents, may notice a harsh cough and eventually stridor over the next 20 to 30 min.

Management consists of reassuring parents and nurses, cold humidified oxygen (its value may be questioned, but you at least are doing something), and sedation. A crying or screaming child only makes croup worse. In 99.9% of cases, the croup will dissipate within the hour. Postextubation croup is usually worst within 2 h of onset. If a child is better within 1 h, then the issue is resolving and the child may be discharged from the recovery room with confidence. Nonetheless, we tell parents what to watch for, in the case of pediatric outpatients, and provide appropriate instructions and contacts.

We have found that postextubation croup does not require more aggressive therapy; if so, then other causes should be considered. The use of steroids is not beneficial in the acute situation. Their value as a prophylaxis is still questionable and their effect may be delayed up to 2 h after administration. However, steroids are still used in children at risk until more substantial evidence indicates otherwise.

The use of racemic epinephrine should be reserved for those children who are severely affected and/or in extremis. The effect is short lived, rebound edema of the airway is the rule, and children usually will get better in spite of it. Children receiving racemic epinephrine should be observed for at least 2 h after the last administration to avoid missing reoccurrence of the croup or rebound edema.

CONCLUSION

Stridor is a symptom, the result of a constellation of disorders. The management of stridor is important, complex, and requires considerable skill and experience for success. Practitioners who want to obtain these skills need to understand the physics behind the etiologies. Proper diagnosis is based on clinical acumen. Without a proper diagnosis and differential, management is difficult, often inappropriate and dangerous.

Children with stridor need hands-on care. They cannot be managed remotely. They must be seen, listened to, and touched. Hi-tech equipment is an aid to the physician, not a substitute. Most importantly, we hope that readers of this chapter have learned that stridor has many presentations. Its time course can be short or long, the condition mild or severe, and each can progress from the benign to the disastrous with or without the wrong management.

REFERENCES

1. Rittichier KK, Ledwith CA: Outpatient treatment of moderate croup with dexamethasone: intramuscular versus oral dosing. *Pediatrics* 106:1344, 2000.
2. Elphick HE, Sherlock P, Foxall G, et al: Survey of respiratory sounds in infants. *Arch Dis Child* 84:35, 2001.
3. Bent JP III, Miller DA, Kim JW, et al: Pediatric exercise-induced laryngomalacia. *Ann Otol Rhinol Laryngol* 105:169, 1996.
4. Gay BB Jr, Atkinson GO, Vanderzalm T, et al: Subglottic foreign bodies in pediatric patients. *Am J Dis Child* 140:165, 1986.
5. McLaughlin RB Jr, Wetmore RF, Tavill MA, et al: Vascular anomalies causing symptomatic tracheobronchial compression. *Laryngoscope* 109(2 Pt 1):312, 1999.

6. Olney DR, Greinwald JH Jr, Smith RJ, Bauman NM: Laryngomalacia and its treatment. *Laryngoscope* 109:1770, 1999.
7. Davis L, Ross N: Bilateral vocal cord palsy after ventricular drainage in a child. *Anesth Analg* 92:358, 2001.
8. Rizk SS, Kacker A, Komisar A: Need for tracheotomy is rare in patients with acute supraglottitis: findings of a retrospective study. *Ear Nose Throat J* 79:952, 2000.
9. Botma M, Kishore A, Kubba H, Geddes N: The role of fibreoptic laryngoscopy in infants with stridor. *Int J Pediatr Otorhinolaryngol* 55:17, 2000.
10. Massie RJ, Robertson CF, Berkowitz RG: Long-term outcome of surgically treated acquired subglottic stenosis in infancy. *Pediatr Pulmonol* 30:125, 2000.
11. Sandhu RS, Pasquale MD, Miller K, Wasser TE: Measurement of endotracheal tube cuff leak to predict postextubation stridor and need for reintubation. *J Am Coll Surg* 190:682, 2000.
12. Markovitz BP, Randolph AG: Corticosteroids for the prevention and treatment of post-extubation stridor in neonates, children and adults [computer file]. *Cochrane Database System Rev* 2:CD001000, 2000.
13. de Jong AL, Kuppersmith RB, Sulek M, Friedman EM: Vocal cord paralysis in infants and children. *Otolaryngol Clin North Am* 33:131, 2000.
14. Cohen LF: Stridor and upper airway obstruction in children. *Pediatr Rev* 21:4, 2000.
15. Goodman TR, McHugh K: The role of radiology in the evaluation of stridor. *Arch Dis Child* 81:456, 1999.
16. Damm M, Eckel HE, Jungehulsing M, Roth B: Management of acute inflammatory childhood stridor. *Otolaryngol Head Neck Surg* 121:633, 1999.
17. Whitelock-Jones L, Bass DH, Millar AJ, Rode H: Inhalation burns in children. *Pediatr Surg Int* 15:50, 1999.
18. Silva AB, Muntz HR, Clary R: Utility of conventional radiography in the diagnosis and management of pediatric airway foreign bodies. *Ann Otol Rhinol Laryngol* 107(10 Pt 1):834, 1998.
19. Rizos JD, DiGravio BE, Sehl MJ, Tallon JM: The disposition of children with croup treated with racemic epinephrine and dexamethasone in the emergency department. *J Emerg Med* 16:535, 1998.
20. Holzki J, Laschat M, Stratmann C: Stridor in the neonate and infant. Implications for the paediatric anaesthetist. Prospective description of 155 patients with congenital and acquired stridor in early infancy. *Paediatr Anaesth* 8:221, 1998.
21. Lesperance MM, Zalzal GH. Laryngotracheal stenosis in children. *Eur Arch Oto-Rhino-Laryngol* 255:12, 1998.
22. Koc C, Kocaman F, Aygenc E, et al: The use of preoperative lidocaine to prevent stridor and laryngospasm after tonsillectomy and adenoidectomy. *Otolaryngol Head Neck Surg* 118:880, 1998.
23. Wiel E, Vilette B, Darras JA, et al: Laryngotracheal stenosis in children after intubation. Report of five cases. *Paediatr Anaesth* 7:415, 1997.
24. Lesperance MM, Zalzal GH: Assessment and management of laryngotracheal stenosis. *Pediatr Clin North Am* 43:1413, 1996.
25. Mancuso RF: Stridor in neonates. *Pediatr Clin North Am* 43:1339, 1996.
26. Kucera CM, Silverstein MD, Jacobson RM, et al: Epiglottitis in adults and children in Olmsted County, Minnesota, 1976 through 1990. *Mayo Clin Proc* 71:1155, 1996.
27. Brodsky L: Congenital stridor. *Pediatr Rev* 17:408, 1996.
28. Bent JP, Miller DA, Kim JW, et al: Pediatric exercise-induced laryngomalacia. *Ann Otol Rhinol Laryngol* 105:169, 1996.
29. Mayo-Smith MF, Spinale JW, Donskey CJ, et al: Acute epiglottitis. An 18-year experience in Rhode Island. *Chest* 108:1640, 1995.

9 | Perioperative Management of the Former Preterm Infant

Leila G. Welborn, MD

Respiratory function in preterm infants (gestational age less than 37 weeks) is a major concern because of their immature organ systems. Therefore, they represent a significant operative risk. The incidence of apneic episodes in the preterm infant is inversely related to postconceptual age (gestational age plus postnatal age). Given this increased risk, it is prudent to consider delaying elective surgery when possible in these patients. If surgery cannot be delayed, a number of special precautions should be taken with respect to anesthetic management.

RESPIRATORY FUNCTION IN THE NEONATE

Neonates and premature infants show a biphasic response to hypoxemia. When exposed to a hypoxic gas mixture, they exhibit an initial hyperventilatory response that is followed by a sustained decrease in ventilation. By the time the infant is 3 weeks old, hypoxemia induces a sustained hyperventilatory response similar to that of the adult. The reason for the lack of a sustained response in the premature infant is unknown. The immediate change in ventilation indicates that the peripheral chemoreceptors are intact and that biphasic depression therefore may be due to depression of central respiratory responsiveness.

Response to hypercapnia is also limited in the neonate. The neonate can increase ventilation by only three to four times the baseline values; in contrast, older infants and adults can increase ventilation by 10- to 20-fold. The slope of the CO_2 response curve increases (indicating increased ventilatory response to CO_2) with advancing gestational and postnatal age and, unlike the response to hypoxia, is independent of postconceptual age.

EFFECTS OF ANESTHETICS ON RESPIRATORY MECHANICS AND CONTROL

Anesthetics produce dose-dependent and drug-specific changes in the mechanics and central control of the respiratory system. The inhaled anesthetics produce a decrease in muscle tone in the airways, chest wall, and diaphragm. Inhaled anesthetics may induce apnea in neonates by augmenting central respiratory responsiveness to inhibitory afferents and decreasing central respiratory responsiveness to ventilatory stimulants. Inhaled anesthetics also alter the ventilatory response to CO_2 and the pattern of breathing. They produce a dose-dependent decrease in slope and rightward shift of the CO_2 response curve. Inhaled anesthetics increase the apneic threshold (i.e., the maximal arterial partial pressure of CO_2 that does not initiate spontaneous breathing). This decrease in ventilation is a direct effect on the medullary respiratory centers. The ventilatory response to hypoxemia is significantly attenuated by inhaled anesthetics.

Intravenous anesthetics also alter respiratory function. Opioids produce a dose-dependent depression of medullary respiratory centers, which leads to decreased responsiveness to arterial partial pressure of CO_2, which is characterized by a shift to the right of the CO_2 response curve with no decrease in slope. Ketamine causes respiratory depression, and the slope of the CO_2 response curve decreases. Barbiturates decrease the ventilatory response to CO_2.

PERIOPERATIVE COMPLICATIONS IN THE FORMER PRETERM INFANT

Former preterm infants are more likely than full-term infants to develop perioperative complications. Apnea, periodic breathing (PB), and bradycardia are the most common complications.

In a retrospective chart review of healthy infants undergoing herniorrhaphy, Steward[1] concluded that preterm infants undergoing surgery in the first months of life are more likely than full-term infants to develop respiratory complications during and after anesthesia. Twelve percent of the preterm infants had apnea during anesthesia. None required postoperative mechanical ventilation.

Lui et al.[2] prospectively studied 41 preterm infants undergoing minor and major surgical procedures. Narcotics and barbiturates were given to some of those infants. Eighteen infants, all of whom were younger than 41 weeks' postconceptual age, had postoperative apnea, required postoperative mechanical ventilation, or both. None of the infants older than 46 weeks' postconceptual age developed prolonged postoperative apnea. They concluded that infants younger than 46 weeks' postconceptual age are at risk for postoperative apnea and should not undergo outpatient surgery. They should be hospitalized and monitored for 24 h after surgery.

My colleagues and I[3] conducted a prospective study to identify those infants undergoing inguinal hernia repair under general anesthesia who might develop perioperative complications. Preoperative and postoperative impedance pneumographies were used to determine the incidence of postoperative apnea, PB, and bradycardia in these infants, all of whom were younger than 1 year. The pneumograms were analyzed by a pulmonologist for evidence of apnea, PB, and bradycardia.

Brief apnea was defined as a respiratory pause of less than 15 s not associated with bradycardia. Prolonged apnea was a respiratory pause of 15 s, or less than 15 s if accompanied by bradycardia. Periodic breathing was three or more periods of 3 to 15 s, separated by fewer than 20 s of normal respiration. Bradycardia was a heart rate of fewer than 100 beats per minute for at least 5 s.

Eighty-six infants (38 premature, 48 full term) were studied. Seven of the 48 full-term infants were at least 44 weeks' postconceptual age. No full-term infants had a preoperative history of apnea or other risk factor, and none developed postoperative prolonged apnea or PB (Table 9-1). Sixteen of the 38 premature infants were 44 weeks' or younger postconceptual age at the time of surgery. Although 12 had preoperative histories of apnea, none developed preoperative or postoperative prolonged apnea or PB. Eighteen of the 22 preterm infants younger than 44 weeks' postconceptual age had histories of apnea; none experienced preoperative prolonged apnea or PB. There were no episodes of postoperative prolonged apnea in that group. Periodic breathing was noted in 14 former preterm infants with postconceptual ages of 44 weeks or younger. Two of those 14 patients showed PB as late as 5 h postopera-

TABLE 9-1 Comparison of Age, Incidence of Apnea, Periodic Breathing, and Postoperative Ventilation in Premature and Full-Term Infants

	Premature infants* (n = 38)		Full-term infants (n = 48)[†]	
	≤44 (34–44)	>44 (45–77)	≤44 (41–44)	>44 (46–88)
Postconceptual age in weeks (range)				
Range of gestational age in weeks	26–37	26–36	38–40	38–42
n Patients	22	16	7	41
With history of apnea	18	12	0	0
Postoperative periodic breathing	14[‡]	0	0	0
Postoperative intubation	0	0	0	0

*Gestational age ≤37 weeks.
[†]Gestational age >37 weeks.
[‡]$p < 0.001$, Fisher's exact test.

tively. None of the patients with a postconceptual age older than 44 weeks developed PB ($p < 0.001$, Fisher's exact test). None of the patients required endotracheal intubation or controlled ventilation postoperatively.

We concluded that outpatient herniorrhaphy can be safely performed in term infants 44 weeks' postconceptual age or older who do not have major respiratory, cardiac, neurologic, endocrine, or metabolic diseases. Conversely, preterm infants younger than 44 weeks' postconceptual age are at risk for postoperative ventilatory dysfunction.

Kurth et al.[4] in a prospective study using pneumography reported a 37% incidence of prolonged apnea after anesthesia in a group of former preterm infants whose postconceptual ages ranged from 32 to 55 weeks. The initial episode of apnea occurred as late as 12 h after anesthesia. Some of the infants in that study had more complicated medical histories than did those in our study; included were infants with histories of necrotizing enterocolitis and others undergoing placement of ventriculoperitoneal shunts. They concluded that former preterm infants younger than 60 weeks' postconceptual age should be monitored for at least 12 h postoperatively.

Malviya et al.[5] attempted to define the postconceptual age beyond which apnea is less likely to occur. They prospectively looked at 91 infants younger than 60 weeks' postconceptual age undergoing minor and major surgical procedures under general anesthesia. Patients were induced with thiopental, and opioids and nondepolarizing muscle relaxants were administered when indicated. Postoperative pneumography was initiated at arrival in the postanesthesia recovery unit. Thirty-five infants were younger than 44 weeks' postconceptual age. Nine of those infants developed postoperative apnea that did not resolve spontaneously. Fifty-six infants were at least 44 weeks' postconceptual age. One of those infants developed apnea postoperatively, but that infant had neurologic problems. Seven infants developed bradycardia without apnea and that resolved spontaneously.

They concluded that former preterm infants younger than 44 weeks' postconceptual age are at greater risk for developing apnea after general anesthesia than infants older than 44 weeks' postconceptual age and that the maximum risk for postoperative complications is 5% with 95% confidence.

This brief summary emphasizes the difficulty of interpreting and objectively comparing much of the existing data. Each study has limitations. Many of the data were derived from retrospective reviews of complications or from patients with pre-existing disease who underwent complex surgical procedures. There are many other predisposing factors in the development of prolonged apnea in premature infants. These include hypoglycemia, hypoxia, hyperoxia, sepsis, anemia, hypocalcemia, and environmental temperature changes. Institutional differences regarding patient selection, caring for the premature infant, assignment of gestational age, type of surgery, type of anesthetic management, number of patients studied, and the method and duration of recording and monitoring apnea also can influence the results and conclusions in this type of study. None of the studies have a large series of American Society of Anesthetists Physical Status 1 and 2 patients undergoing the same operative procedures with the same anesthesiologist, the same surgeon, or under the same operating room conditions. Therefore, it is difficult to make definitive statements that can be applied to all conditions. However, one can say that infants with histories of prematurity must be observed very carefully for episodes of postoperative apnea. The age at which the premature infant attains physiologic maturity and no longer presents an increased risk must be considered individually, with attention given to growth and development.

The problem of postoperative apnea and PB in the former preterm infant can be avoided by deferring elective operations until the infant is older than 44 to 46 weeks' postconceptual age, if possible, and monitoring postoperative respirations and electrocardiograms in infants 44 weeks' postconceptual age or younger.

MANAGEMENT OF THE FORMER PRETERM INFANT

Having established these general guidelines for the management of former preterm infants requiring surgery, there are special considerations concerning this patient population: (1) the perioperative use of caffeine, (2) the use of spinal versus general anesthesia, and (3) anemia as a complicating factor in apnea and PB.

Perioperative Use of Caffeine

Theophylline and caffeine have been used widely by neonatologists as respiratory stimulants in premature infants and have gained acceptance in the management of neonatal apnea in intensive care nurseries.

Kuzemko and Paala[6] were the first to report that aminophylline significantly decreases the frequency of apneic episodes in newborns. Since then, a number of other investigators have reported successful treatment of neonatal apnea with various theophylline preparations. Aranda et al.[7] described similar findings with caffeine.

Bory[8] reported that theophylline is biotransformed to caffeine by premature newborns and found that a significant amount of theophylline's respirogenic effect is due to caffeine. In adults and children, theophylline undergoes extensive demethylation and oxidation. In contrast, demethylation and oxidation pathways are markedly deficient in neonates who instead tend to methylate theophylline to produce caffeine. Although theophylline and caffeine share several pharmacologic actions of therapeutic interest, caffeine is a more potent central nervous system and respiratory stimulant and possesses fewer cardiac side effects than does theophylline. Other advantages of caffeine are greater therapeutic index, ease of administration, less fluctuation in plasma concentrations, less need for therapeutic drug level monitoring, and fewer peripheral effects.

Aranda et al.[9] showed that caffeine concentrations as low as 3 to 5 mg/L can eliminate apneic spells in neonates, but plasma concentrations of 8 to 20 mg/L are required for an optimal response. No toxicity has been observed with concentrations as high as 50 mg/L. This is in contrast to theophylline, which can cause cardiovascular toxicity at plasma concentrations of only 13 to 32 mg/L.

The mechanism underlying this respirogenic effect of caffeine and other methylxanthines is not well established. They may increase the sensitivity of the medullary respiratory center to CO_2 because minute ventilation is increased.

The elimination rate of all methylxanthines is significantly decreased in the newborn infant. In adults, the half-lives of caffeine and theophylline are 6 and 9 h, respectively; in newborns, the half-lives are prolonged (caffeine: 37 to 231 h, theophylline: 12 to 64 h). In a study of the maturation of caffeine elimination, Aranda et al.[9] found that the half-life of caffeine decreases with age and reaches adult values by about 4 months of age.

There have been no studies of the effects of caffeine administration in patients undergoing surgical operations. Therefore, we[10] designed a prospective, double blind, randomized study to examine the possible efficacy of caffeine in the prevention of apnea after anesthesia and surgery in former premature infants.

Twenty otherwise healthy premature infants born at 37 weeks' gestational age or younger and undergoing general anesthesia for inguinal hernia repair were studied. All were no older than 44 weeks' postconceptual age at the time of surgery. Infants with pre-existing cardiac, neurologic, or metabolic diseases and those already receiving methylxanthines were excluded. We found that the administration of 5 mg/kg intravenous caffeine given slowly immediately after the induction of anesthesia in one single dose significantly reduces the incidence of prolonged postoperative apnea over that observed in the control group (Tables 9-2 and 9-3). However, it did not totally abolish all types of ventilatory dysfunction. Although the dose of caffeine that we selected (5 mg/kg) was effective in other studies in patients who were not anesthetized,[10] the resulting caffeine concentration (5 to 8.6 mg/L) was on the low side of the ideal therapeutic range (8 to 20 mg/L).

A second prospective, double blind, randomized study[11] examined the efficacy of a higher dose of intravenous caffeine in the control of all types of postoperative apnea in a population of former premature infants identical to the first group (Tables 9-4 and 9-5).

Thirty-two former preterm infants (≤44 weeks postconceptual age) undergoing inguinal hernia repair were prospectively studied. General inhalational anesthesia with neuromuscular blockade was used. No barbiturates or opioids were given. Infants were assigned randomly to two groups. Group 1 received caffeine 10 mg/kg intravenously immediately after induction of anesthesia. Group 2 received intravenous saline. Respiratory pattern, heart rate, and hemoglobin oxygen saturation (SpO_2) were monitored with an impedance pneumograph and a pulse oximeter, respectively, for at least 12 h postoperatively. Tracings were analyzed for evidence of apnea, PB, and bradycardia by a pulmonologist blinded to the drug given. None of the patients who received caffeine developed postoperative bradycardia, prolonged apnea, or PB, and none had a postoperative SpO_2 of less than 90%. In the control group, 13 (81%) developed prolonged apnea 4 to 6 h postoperatively. Fifty percent of the patients had a SpO_2 of less than 90% at the time.

It was concluded that 10 mg/kg intravneous caffeine completely eliminates brief and prolonged apnea in this group of infants. The caffeine concentration achieved (15 to 19 mg/L) with this dose is well within the recommended therapeutic range for this drug and required one single intravenous administration. We recommend the use of 10 mg/kg caffeine in addi-

TABLE 9–2 Perioperative Data of Study Patients (n = 20)

	Caffeine group (5 mg/kg; n = 9)	Control group (n = 11)
Gestational age (wk)		
Mean ± SD	29.8 ± 3	31.6 ± 3
Range	25–35	26–36
Postconceptual age (wk)		
Mean ± SD	40.6 ± 2	40.6 ± 2
Range	38–44	25–44
History of preoperative apnea, n (%)	8 (89)*	5 (45)

*p <0.001, Fisher's exact test.

TABLE 9–3 Incidence of Postoperative Apnea and Periodic Breathing

	Caffeine group (5 mg/kg; $n = 9$)	Control group ($n = 11$)
Postoperative prolonged apnea with bradycardia (%)	0	8 (73)*
Postoperative periodic breathing >1% (%)	0	2 (18)
Postoperative apnea <15s, no bradycardia (%)	8 (89)	1 (9)
Postoperative intubation	0	0
Postoperative caffeine level (mg/L)	5–8.6	0

*p <0.001, Fisher's exact test.

tion to monitoring for apnea and bradycardia in all infants at risk for postoperative apnea after general anesthesia.

Caffeine Preparations

Caffeine base is only slightly soluble in water. Various synthetic mixtures of caffeine have been prepared to increase its solubility. The only commercial preparation available for intravenous use is caffeine sodium benzoate. This preparation is not recommended for use in infants because the sodium benzoate component has been reported to potentially contribute to kernicterus in neonates by uncoupling albumin-bilirubin binding.

Caffeine citrate is available in powder form only. Twenty milligrams per kilogram of caffeine citrate or benzoate is equivalent to 10 mg/kg of caffeine base. There is no readily available commercial preparation of caffeine base for intravenous use in neonates; however, it can be prepared from caffeine citrate powder by the hospital pharmacist.

Spinal Versus General Anesthesia

Several investigators have described the use of spinal anesthesia in former preterm infants. In a retrospective study of 36 premature infants undergoing a variety of operative procedures under spinal anesthesia, Abajian[12] reported that 31 blocks were successful after the first attempt and that 5 required a second attempt. Six patients who had successful spinal anesthetics required intravenous narcotic or nitrous oxide supplementation. There were no episodes of hypotension or bradycardia. No intraoperative or postoperative complications occurred. Harnik[13] studied 20 infants who underwent inguinal hernia repair under spinal anesthesia. Eleven of the infants were younger than 44 weeks' postconceptual age, and eight weighed less than 2500 g. Spinal anesthesia was supplemented with general anesthesia, intravenous ketamine, or local anesthesia in several patients. The sole reported intraoper-

TABLE 9–4 Perioperative Data of Study Patients ($n = 32$)

	Caffeine group (10 mg/kg; $n = 16$)	Control group ($n = 16$)
Mean (range) gestational age (wk)	30 (24–35)	30.4 (25–36)
Mean (range) postconceptual age (wk)	40.9 (37–44)	40.5 (37–44)
History of preoperative apnea, n (%)	10 (63)	8 (50)

TABLE 9–5 Incidence of Postoperative Apnea Periodic Breathing and Desaturation

	Caffeine group (10 mg/kg; n = 16)	Control group (n = 16)
Postoperative prolonged apnea with bradycardia (%)	0	13 (81)*
Postoperative periodic breathing >1% (%)	0	4 (25)
Postoperative desaturation <90% (%)	0	8 (50)*
Postoperative intubation	0	0
Postoperative caffeine level (mg/L)	15–19	0

*p <0.05, Fisher's exact test.

ative complications were apnea and bradycardia, which developed in one infant after injection of the local anesthetic, tetracaine. The infant had a history of frequent apnea. Postoperative apnea developed in one patient 8 h after the procedure, when the patient became hypothermic (temperature 34.2°C). No child demonstrated cardiovascular instability. Harnik concluded that spinal anesthesia is a satisfactory alternative to general anesthesia for selected preterm infants and suggested that it might avoid the postoperative respiratory complications associated with general anesthesia.

The observations that high-risk infants are less likely to develop apnea or bradycardia when spinal as opposed to general anesthesia is used has not been demonstrated in a controlled, randomized, prospective manner with the use of postoperative pneumography. To address this question, we[14] designed a prospective, double-blind, randomized study using pneumography to compare the effects of spinal and general anesthesia on the incidence of postoperative apnea, bradycardia, and PB in former preterm infants.

Included in the study were 36 otherwise healthy former preterm infants undergoing inguinal hernia repair. All were 51 weeks' postconceptual age or younger at the time of surgery. Patients were assigned randomly to three groups. Group 1 received general inhalation anesthesia with neuromuscular blockade. Group 2 received spinal anesthesia using 0.6 to 0.8 mg/kg 1% tetracaine in conjunction with an equal volume of 10% dextrose and 0.02 mL epinephrine, 1:1000 (Tables 9-6 and 9-7). Group 2 was subdivided into subgroups A and B. Group 2A included those patients enrolled in the early phases of the study who received adjunct sedation with 1 to 2 mg/kg ketamine intramuscularly before the spinal anesthetic. Infants in Group 2B, who were entered at a later date, did not receive ketamine sedation. Respiratory pattern and heart rate were continuously monitored using impedance pneumography for at least 12 h postoperatively. Tracings were analyzed for evidence of apnea, PB, and bradycardia by a pulmonologist who was unaware of group assignment. None of the patients who received spinal anesthesia without ketamine sedation developed postoperative prolonged apnea, PB, or bradycardia. Eight of nine infants who received spinal anesthesia and adjunct intraoperative sedation with ketamine developed prolonged apnea with bradycardia; two of those eight infants had no prior history of apnea. Only 5 of the 16 patients who received general anesthesia developed prolonged apnea with bradycardia; two of those five infants had no prior history of apnea. This study showed that spinal anesthesia without ketamine sedation is not associated with any episodes of life-threatening apnea and appears to be

TABLE 9–6 Perioperative Data of Study Patients (n = 36)

	Group 1 (n = 16)*	Group 2A (n = 9)†	Group 2B (n = 11)‡
Mean (range) gestational age (wk)	31.8 (25–36)	31.4 (28–36)	31.3 (26–35)
Mean (range) postconceptual age (wk)	43.3 (38–51)	41.2 (36–46)	40.5 (35–45)
History of preoperative apnea (n)	6	6	3

*Group 1 received general inhalation anesthesia with neuromuscular blockade.
†Group 2A received spinal anesthesia using 0.6 to 0.8 mk/kg 1% tetracaine in conjunction with an equal volume of 10% dextrose and 0.02 mL epinephrine (1:1000). This group also received adjunct sedation with 1 to 2 mg/kg ketamine intramuscularly before the spinal anesthetic.
‡Group 2B received spinal anesthesia using 0.6 to 0.8 mk/kg 1% tetracaine in conjunction with an equal volume of 10% dextrose and 0.02 mL epinephrine (1:1000). This group did not receive ketamine.

better tolerated by former preterm infants than general anesthesia or spinal anesthesia with ketamine sedation.

Krane et al.[15] also compared spinal and general anesthesia in former preterm infants and looked at the incidence of postoperative complications. They assigned 18 former preterm infants younger than 51 weeks' postconceptual age to receive spinal or general anesthesia. All infants were scheduled to have inguinal hernia repair. Preoperative and postoperative pneumography and O_2 saturation monitoring were done. They found that infants in the general anesthesia group had lower O_2 saturation and lower heart rate in the postoperative period than did infants in the spinal anesthesia group. They concluded that spinal anesthesia reduces postoperative oxygen desaturation and bradycardia in the former preterm infants undergoing inguinal hernia repair.

TABLE 9–7 Incidence of Postoperative Apnea and Periodic Breathing

	Group 1 (n = 16)*	Group 2A (n = 9)†	Group 2B (n = 11)‡
Prolonged apnea with bradycardia (%)§	5 (31)	8 (89)	0
Periodic breathing >1%	1	2	0
Postoperative intubation	0	0	0

*Group 1 received general inhalation anesthesia with neuromuscular blockade.
†Group 2A received spinal anesthesia using 0.6 to 0.8 mk/kg 1% tetracaine in conjunction with an equal volume of 10% dextrose and 0.02 mL epinephrine (1:1000). This group also received adjunct sedation with 1 to 2 mg/kg ketamine intramuscularly before the spinal anesthetic.
‡Group 2B received spinal anesthesia using 0.6 to 0.8 mk/kg 1% tetracaine in conjunction with an equal volume of 10% dextrose and 0.02 mL epinephrine (1:1000). This group did not receive ketamine.
§Fischer's exact test: $p < 0.015$, 1 versus 2A; $p < 0.0001$, 2A versus 2B; $p < 0.06$, 1 versus 2B.

ANEMIA AND PERIOPERATIVE RISK

As the relation between postconceptual age and operative risk becomes clearer, other factors that place former preterm infants at higher risk for respiratory and cardiac complications require attention. Among these is anemia. In the human fetus, fetal hemoglobin (HbF) constitutes the major hemoglobin (Hb) fraction. It reaches a peak of 95% at 10 weeks' gestation, remains at this high level until 30 weeks, and then declines to 80% at term. Postnatally, HbF gradually disappears; it constitutes 50% of the total Hb at age 1 to 2 months and 5% at age 6 months. Infants born prematurely have higher HbF fractions than term infants and experience a fall of Hb concentration that exceeds that in term infants. Hemoglobin concentrations reach their lowest levels at 1 to 3 months of age, when values as low as 7 to 8 g/dL are commonplace. Erythropoiesis is active at birth, as reflected by high Hb concentrations, reticulocyte counts commonly above 5%, and occasional nucleated red blood cells. Once separated from the hypoxic intrauterine environment, the premature baby enters a quiescent stage of red cell production. The reticulocyte counts fall to 2% or less, and the Hb concentration decreases. When the Hb concentration falls below 10 g/dL, erythropoiesis is stimulated, and reticulocytes increase to between 5% and 15% over a 2-week period, followed by correction of anemia. This phenomenon, which is relatively benign and self-limiting, has been termed the *physiologic anemia of prematurity*. It has little apparent effect on the infant's overall well-being.

Red blood cell transfusions have been shown in some studies to decrease the incidence of apnea and PB in premature infants. In contrast, other studies have found no clinical benefit from red blood cell transfusion.

The high Hb-O_2 affinity of the preterm infant's blood also may impair the release of O_2 to the tissues. If the fall in Hb concentration were an isolated phenomenon, it would diminish the availability of O_2 to the tissues. While Hb concentration is decreasing, however, there are changes that lead to a progressive rightward shift of the Hb-O_2 equilibrium curve that permits more O_2 to be extracted from saturated Hb. The rightward shift, or increase, in the P50 is due to an increase in the proportion of adult Hb relative to HbF and to an increase in the concentration of 2,3-diphosphoglycerate (2,3-DPG).

Although specific postoperative complications have been identified in the former preterm infant, it is not known whether anemia, decreased oxygen-carrying capacity, or both contribute to the frequency of complications. The definition of anemia in preterm infants is not precise. The need for preoperative correction of anemia by blood transfusion in infants undergoing the stress of anesthesia and surgery has not been studied.

We conducted a prospective study[16] to determine whether a relation exists between preoperative hematocrit (Hct) and the incidence of postoperative apnea, PB, and bradycardia and to evaluate other factors that might affect oxygen availability in former preterm infants. Twenty-four former preterm infants undergoing inguinal hernia repair, all of whom were younger than 60 weeks' postconceptual age at the time of operation, were studied. Hemoglobin and Hct concentrations were measured preoperatively. A preoperative Hct of at least 25% was required for study participation. General endotracheal inhalational anesthesia, supplemented with neuromuscular blockade and controlled ventilation, was used. No barbiturates or narcotics were administered. After the induction of anesthesia, reticulocyte count, percentage of fetal hemoglobin (HbF%), 2,3-DPG, and adenosine triphosphate (ATP) levels were measured. Respiratory pattern and heart rate were recorded using impedance pneumography for at least 12 h postoperatively. Tracings were analyzed for apnea, PB, and bradycardia by a pulmonologist who was unaware of the hematologic profile of the infant.

Nineteen infants had Hcts of 30% or greater (group 1), and five infants had Hcts less than 30% (group 2). The reticulocyte and HbF levels of infants in group 2 were significantly higher than those of infants in group 1; however, the ATP and 2,3-DPG concentrations of infants in group 2 were lower than those of infants in group 1. Infants in group 2 showed a significantly higher incidence of postoperative prolonged apnea than those in group 1. Four infants of the 19 in group 1 developed postoperative prolonged apnea, only one of whom had a prior history of apnea; in contrast, four of the five infants in group 2 developed postoperative prolonged apnea and bradycardia, and none had a prior history of apnea. Two of the infants had postconceptual ages of 47 and 51 weeks (Tables 9-8 through 9-10); this is a concern because most institutions would consider sending an otherwise healthy former preterm infant with a postconceptual age of 47 to 50 weeks home without postoperative monitoring after minor surgical procedures. We concluded that anemia in former preterm infants is associated with an increased incidence of postoperative apnea. Many anemic infants had high HbF percentages and low 2,3-DPG concentrations, which shifts the oxygen dissociation curve to the left and decreases the amount of oxygen available to the tissues.

Red cell transfusions have many potential complications and cannot be recommended or justified for the correction of an otherwise medically treatable condition. It seems preferable to delay elective surgery until the Hct is above 30% by supplementing the feeds with iron. If surgery cannot be deferred, anemic infants must be observed and monitored very carefully in the postoperative period.

Cote et al.[17] subjected the original prospective studies on perioperative complications in the former preterm infant to a combined analysis. Only patients undergoing inguinal hernia repair under general anesthesia were included in the study. They were looking for the postconceptual age after which the risk decreases to less than 1% with 95% statistical confidence for developing postoperative complications.

This complicated statistical analysis has its limitations: with the small number of patients, they assumed that their statistical model is equally valid over the full range of ages, and there was considerable variation in the dura-

TABLE 9–8 Comparison of Age and History of Apnea in the Two Study Groups

	Hematocrit ≥30% (n = 19)	Hematocrit <30% (n = 9)	p
Gestational age (wk)			
Mean ± SD	33.5 ± 2.7	32.4 ± 3.3	>0.1*
Range	28–36	28–36	
Postconceptual age (wk)			
Mean ± SD	45.5 ± 4.6	43.6 ± 5.5	>0.1*
Range	40–45	34–51	
History of apnea, n (%)	4 (21)	1 (20)	>0.99†

*Mann–Whitney test.
†Fisher's exact test.

TABLE 9–9 Comparison of Hematologic Profile in the Two Study Groups

Hematologic profile	Hematocrit ≥30% (n = 19)	Hematocrit <30% (n = 5)	p
Hematocrit (%)	32.7–39.1	27.6–29.7	
Reticulocyte (%)	2.32 ± 1.34	4.42 ± 2.49	<0.05*
Fetal hemoglobin (%)	36.7 ± 15	61.2 ± 33.8	<0.03†
Adenosine triphosphate (μm/dL)	50.8 ± 5.6	43 ± 3.3	<0.008†
2,3-Diphosphoglycerate (μm/dL)	1.55 ± 0.28	1.27 ± 0.21	>0.07†

*Mann–Whitney test.
†Fisher's exact test.

tion and type of monitoring, definitions of apnea, and availability of historical information. They concluded that the risk of apnea in nonanemic infants is less than 5% with 95% statistical confidence at 48 weeks' postconceptual age with 35 weeks' gestational age and 1% at 56 weeks' postconceptual age with 32 weeks' gestational age. Older infants with anemia should be monitored postoperatively. Given the limitations of this combined analysis, each physician and institution must decide what is acceptable risk for postoperative apnea.

CONCLUSION

Former preterm infants younger than 44 weeks' postconceptual are at increased risk for developing postoperative complications in the form of apnea, PB, and bradycardia. When surgery cannot be deferred until the infant is developmentally more mature, several measures should be taken to minimize the risk of ventilatory dysfunction. First, outpatient surgery is not advisable for infants younger than 44 weeks' postconceptual age. All infants should be admitted to the hospital and monitored for apnea and bradycardia for at least 12 to 18 h postoperatively. Second, I recommend the use of 10/ mg/kg intravenous caffeine base in all infants at risk for postoperative apnea after general anesthesia or a spinal anesthetic without sedation. Infants with anemia of prematurity, generally a benign condition, are at increased risk for postoperative apnea. Thus, it is preferable to delay elective surgery and supplement the feeds with iron until the Hct is above 30%. It is still recommended that monitoring for apnea and bradycardia is performed in all infants at risk for postoperative apnea after all types of anesthesia.

TABLE 9–10 Comparison of Postoperative Complications in the Two Study Groups

	Hematocrit ≥30% (n = 19)	Hematocrit <30% (n = 5)	p
Brief apnea	0	0	
Periodic breathing >1%	0	1 (20%)	>0.2*
Prolonged apnea	4 (21%)	4 (80%)	<0.03*
Bradycardia	0	1 (20%)	>0.2*

*Fisher's exact test.

REFERENCES

1. Steward DJ: Preterm infants are more prone to complications following minor surgery than are full-term infants. *Anesthesiology* 56:304, 1982.
2. Liu LMP, Cote CJ, Goudsouzian NG, et al: Life-threatening apnea in infants recovering from anesthesia. *Anesthesiology* 59:506, 1983.
3. Welborn LG, Ramirez N, Oh TH, et al: Postanesthetic apnea and periodic breathing in infants. *Anesthesiology* 65:656, 1986.
4. Kurth CD, Hutchison AA, Caton DG, et al: Postoperative apnea in preterm infants. *Anesthesiology* 66:483, 1987.
5. Malviya S, Swartz J, Lerman J: Are all preterm infants younger than 60 weeks postconceptual age at risk for postanesthetic apnea? *Anesthesiology* 78:1076, 1993.
6. Kuzemko JA, Paala J: Apnoeic attacks in the newborn treated with aminophylline. *Arch Dis Child* 48:404, 1973.
7. Aranda JV, Grondin D, Sasyniuk BI: Pharmacologic considerations in the therapy of neonatal apnea. *Pediatr Clin North Am* 28:113, 1981.
8. Bory C, Baltassat P, Porthault M: Metabolism of theophylline to caffeine in premature newborn infants. *Pediatrics* 94:988, 1978.
9. Aranda JV, Gorman W, et al: Efficacy of caffeine in the treatment of apnea in the low-birth-weight infant. *J Pediatr* 90:467, 1977.
10. Welborn LG, DeSoto H, Hannallah RS, et al: The use of caffeine in the control of postanesthetic apnea in former premature infants. *Anesthesiology* 68:796, 1988.
11. Welborn LG, Hannallah RS, Fink R, et al: High dose caffeine suppresses postoperative apnea in former preterm infants. *Anesthesiology* 71:347, 1989.
12. Abajian JC, Mellish PRW, Browne AF et al: Spinal anesthesia for surgery in the high-risk infant. *Anesth Analg* 63:359, 1984.
13. Harnik EV, Hoy GR, Potolicchio S, et al: Spinal anesthesia in premature infants recovering from respiratory distress syndrome. *Anesthesiology* 64:95, 1986.
14. Welborn LG, Rice LJ, Broadman LM, et al: Postoperative apnea in former pretem infants: Prospective comparison of spinal and general anesthesia. *Anesthesiology* 72:838, 1990.
15. Krane EJ, Haberkern CM, Jacobson LE: Postoperative apnea, bradycardia, and oxygen desaturation in formerly premature infants: Prospective comparison of spinal and general anesthesia. *Anesth Analg* 80:7, 1995.
16. Welborn LG, Hannallah RS, Luban NL, et al: Anemia and postoperative apnea in former preterm infants. *Anesthesiology* 74:1003, 1991.
17. Cote CJ, Zaslavsky A, Downes JJ, et al: Postoperative apnea informer preterm infants after inguinal herniorrhaphy. A combined analysis [see comments]. *Anesthesiology* 82:809, 1995.

10 | Management of the Child With a Difficult Airway

Barbara A. Castro, MD
Frederic A. Berry, MD

Regardless of the training and experience of the anesthesiologist, the child with the difficult airway remains one of the foremost challenges in pediatric anesthesia. The reasons are many. First, infants and children can desaturate rapidly. This is often attributed to their relatively high rate of oxygen consumption (7 to 9 mL/[kg·min]) compared with that of adults (2 to 3 mL/[kg·min]) and the relative ease with which obstruction can occur. Second, pediatric patients range in size from the very-low-birthweight premature infant to the adult-size teenager. This in turn requires a large array of equipment, which varies greatly in size. The smallest fiberoptic bronchoscopes, for example, are very fragile and expensive and require significant experience for successful use. Third, an awake fiber-optic intubation is rarely an option in the pediatric population. The anesthesiologist therefore must be familiar with a variety of other airway management techniques.

The difficult airway presents in one of two ways: (1) the expected difficult airway (by history or physical examination) or (2) the unexpected difficult airway. Fortunately, both presentations are relatively rare occurrences in the day-to-day practice of anesthesia. Because anesthesiologists experience such a high rate of success with their daily practice, airway management and intubation of patients becomes so automatic and routine that, over time, the ability to recognize the difficult airway and the technical skills required to manage it may become a bit rusty. Therefore, it is key that anesthesiologists maintain a high level of expertise in the preanesthetic evaluation of pediatric airways (which is based on an awareness of the basic anatomic factors in evaluation) and the ability to secure the airway. Even in the best of hands the difficult airway cannot always be identified preoperatively. Anesthesiologists must be able to quickly discern when they are having difficulty with mask ventilation, the placement of a laryngeal mask airway (LMA), or intubation and then identify the exact nature of the problem. They must then quickly apply this knowledge to alternative techniques of airway management. All airway management is based on these principles.

The objective of this chapter is to assist the anesthesiologist in identifying the difficult airway perioperatively and in developing management strategies for intraoperative care. The algorithm for this management is taken primarily from the American Society of Anesthesiologists (ASA) difficult airway algorithm (Figure 10-1).[1]

Preanesthetic Evaluation

Information about the pediatric airway will come from three major sources: the history obtained from the parents or guardian and patient, the physical examination of the child, and the history of previous anesthesia.

One must obtain a thorough history from the parents or guardians and patient whenever possible. A history of prolonged intubation during infancy or

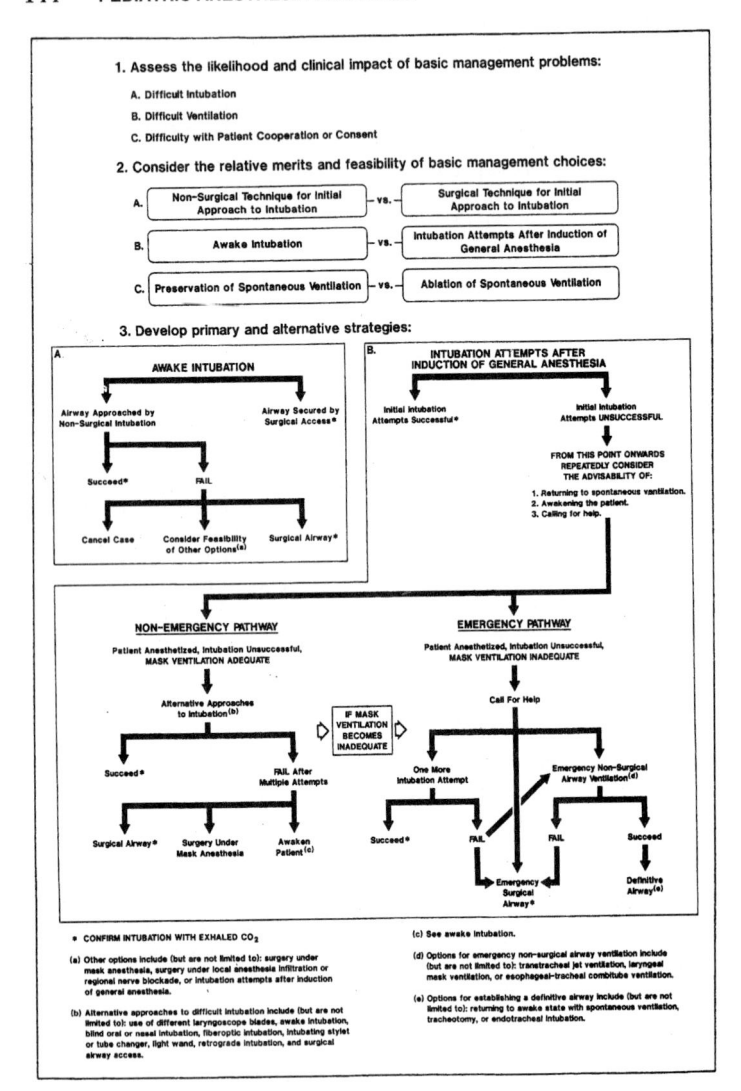

FIG. 10-1 American Society of Anesthesiologists difficult airway algorithm. *(Reproduced with permission from Practice guidelines for management of the difficult airway. Anesthesiology 78:597, 1993.)*

recurrent episodes of croup with upper respiratory infections may alert the anesthesiologist to the possibility of subglottic stenosis. In the United States the incidence of subglottic stenosis in children with a history of prolonged intubation is approximately 50%. Noisy breathing with feeding, positional changes, or agitation may signal a more dynamic process such as laryngomalacia. A history of inspiratory stridor or recurrent aspiration may raise suspicion of vocal cord pathology. Older children should be questioned about changes in the quality of their voices and dyspnea on exertion, which may indicate an obstructive process.

There is no single method or system of anatomic evaluation of the airway that absolutely predicts which airway will be simple and which will not. Airways that are normal in appearance in fact may be difficult for reasons that are not fully understood. Most clinicians are aware of the Mallampati et al. classification system (Figure 10-2), which is the use of clinical signs to predict the potential for difficult laryngoscopy.[2] This system was developed for adults and is not as reliable in the infant and young child. Moreover, physical examination of a child is not always easily accomplished.

The anesthesiologist should focus on three major anatomic features: the mouth, the mandible, and the neck. When assessing a child's mouth, the ability to open the mouth and the size of the tongue are crucial factors. The ability to open the mouth often is best assessed when the child is crying or feeding; parents often can relay this information if the child is being uncooperative. In some patients macroglossia is obvious, as in Beckwith–Wiedeman syndrome (Figure 10-3),[3] whereas in others the tongue may be large relative to the size of the mouth, as in Trisomy 21.[4]

Mandibular hypoplasia is seen in a variety of congenital malformation syndromes including Pierre–Robin, Treacher–Collins, and Goldenhar's syndromes. Sometimes the anatomic problems are very subtle. Children with mild Treacher–Collins syndrome or Goldenhar's syndrome may appear, superficially, to have relatively normal anatomy. However, knowledge of the "anatomy of intubation" will assist the anesthesiologist in recognizing how

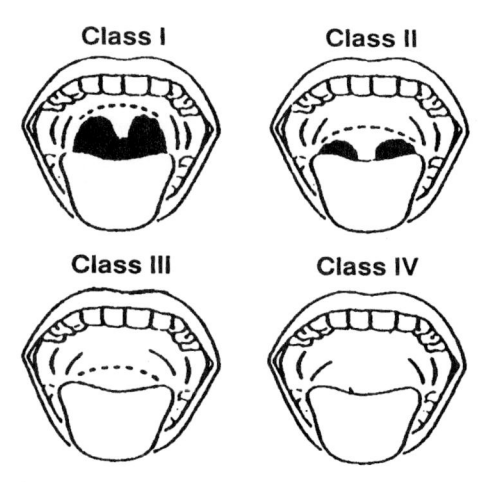

FIG. 10-2 Mallampati classification system. *(Reproduced from Stoelting RK, Miller RD:* Basics of Anesthesia, *3rd ed. New York, Churchill Livingstone, 1994.)*

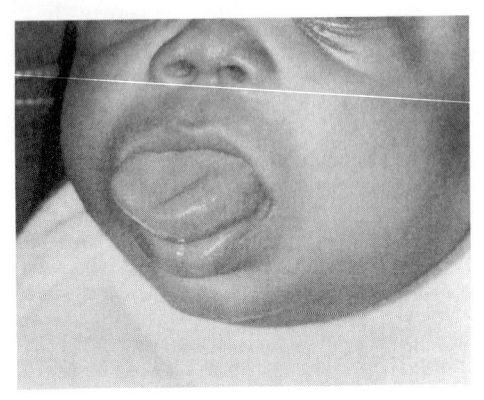

FIG. 10-3 Macroglossia in a child with Beckwith–Wiedeman syndrome. *(Reproduced from Myer CM, Cotton RT, Shott SR: The Pediatric Airway: An Interdisciplinary Approach. Philadelphia, JB Lippincott, 1995.)*

important it is to feel the area under the mandible. This will be discussed later.

Goldenhar's syndrome and Treacher–Collins syndrome fit into a category of malformations known as hemifacial microsomia (HFM) (Figure 10-4).[3,5] There is a wide spectrum of physical abnormalities in these patients, which include microtia, varying degrees of mandibular hypoplasia, ophthalmic abnormalities, and vertebral abnormalities. This type of defect is categorized as the first and second branchial arch developmental syndrome. Developments of the ear and the airway are part of the first and second branchial arches. Even if the anesthesiologist does not recognize the mandibular abnormalities in a child, other abnormalities, such as microtia, should alert the anesthesiologist to the potential for trouble. Most cases of HFM are unilateral but bilateral defects do occur. Hemifacial microsomia also may be associated with cardiac, pulmonary, skeletal, and other anomalies.

Nargozian et al. published a very comprehensive and excellent review of HFM.[6] Patients were categorized by using a radiographic assessment of the mandible and classified as type I (minor; mini mandible), type II (moderate; abnormal condylar size and shape), and type III (severe; absent ramus condyle and temporomandibular joint). Table 10-1 shows an evaluation of airway difficulty according to the mandible classification and Table 10-2 presents airway difficulty characterizations in 20 cases of bilateral facial microsomia according to the mandible classification. One of the surprising elements of this review was that, although mandibular surgery was done on a large number of children and even though they may have had some improvement in appearance, there was increased difficulty with direct rigid laryngoscopy for subsequent anesthesia due to scarring. As will be discussed later, it is the degree of mandibular involvement that correlates best with the degree of difficulty of airway management.

An evaluation of the neck is essential. Certain abnormalities such as cystic hygroma may be evident by visual inspection. However, the degree of involvement may be misleading. It may be necessary to review the radiologic, computed tomographic, or magnetic resonance imaging studies to truly appreciate the extent of disease. Some congenital malformation syndromes

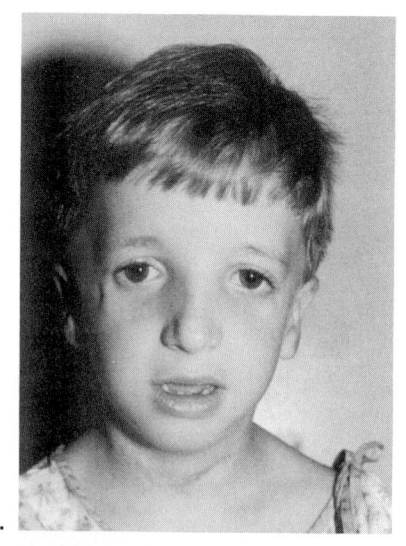

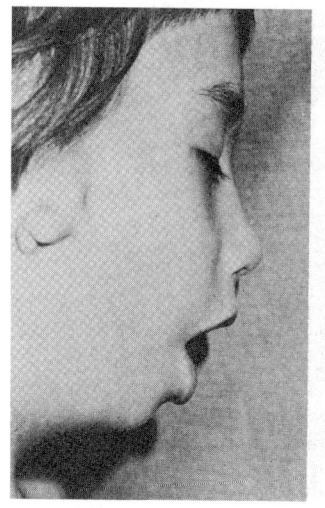

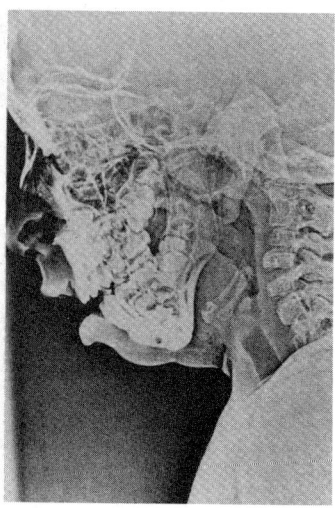

FIG. 10-4 Hemifacial microsomia in children with **(A)** Treacher–Collins and **(B)** Goldenhar's syndromes. (**A** *reproduced from Myer CM, Cotton RT, Shott SR:* The Pediatric Airway: An Interdisciplinary Approach. *Philadelphia, JB Lippincott, 1995;* **B** *reproduced from Berry FA, ed:* Anesthetic Management of Difficult and Routine Pediatric Patients. *New York, Churchill Livingstone, 1990.)*

may be associated with limited range of motion of the neck. For example, Klippel–Feil sequence (Figure 10-5) is most commonly characterized by a short neck, low posterior hairline, and limited mobility of cervical spine due to vertebral anomalies, most commonly fusion of cervical vertebrae.[7] However, some patients with this sequence have hypermobility of the cervical spine and are at risk of neurologic impairment during intubation.

TABLE 10-1 Ease of Laryngoscopy According to Mandibular Classification

Type*	Easy	Difficult	Very difficult
I (%)	28 (90)	3 (10)	0 (0)
II (%)	20 (65)	8 (26)	3 (9)
III (%)	9 (45)	6 (30)	5 (25)
Total (%)	57 (70)	17 (21)	8 (9)

Intubation[†]

*Mandible classification: I, minor (mini-mandible); II, moderate (abnormal condylar size and shape); III, severe (absent ramus, condyle, and temporomandibular joint).
[†]Grading of intubation: A, easy (one or two attempts with good view); B, difficult (three or four attempts with poor view or larynx deviated significantly with difficult visualization); C, very difficult (four or more attempts and/or inability to intubate under direct vision).
Source: Modified with permission from Nargozian C, et al: Hemifacial microsomia: anatomical prediction of difficult intubation. *Paediatr Anaesth* 9:393, 1999.

The history of a difficult intubation is the best indicator of the difficult airway. Unfortunately, it is often difficult to obtain old charts and previous anesthetic records. When available, a review of previous anesthetic records can prove invaluable. The ASA's Task Force on the Difficult Airway strongly recommends that the anesthesiologist provide the patient with a descriptive letter of the difficult intubation.[1] The patient, or family, then has information to give subsequent anesthesiologists concerning the anesthetic difficulties and the techniques of management, which worked or failed. One of the other issues regarding communication with patients after a difficult airway encounter is what information should be provided to assist the patient in the immediate postoperative period, especially concerning potential complications. For example, there are no case reports in the literature concerning esophageal rupture with mediastinitis; however, for older patients and those who are chronically ill, this certainly is a potential problem and it might be appropriate to discuss this with the patient or the patient's family. Outpatients in particular should be warned about this possibility and the signs and symptoms of trouble, such as shortness of breath, fever, and pharyngeal pain.[8,9] Other more common problems, particularly in smaller children, are

TABLE 10-2 Bilateral Facial Microsomia and Airway Difficulty (*n* = 20)

Type*	Easy	Difficult	Very difficult
I	6	2	1
II	0	5	2
III	0	0	4
Total	6 (30)	7 (35)	7 (35)

Intubation[†]

*Mandible classification: I, minor (mini-mandible); II, moderate (abnormal condylar size and shape); III, severe (absent ramus, condyle, and temporomandibular joint).
[†]Grading of intubation: A, easy (one or two attempts with good view); B, difficult (three to four attempts with poor view or larynx deviated significantly with difficult visualization); C, very difficult (four or more attempts or inability to intubate under direct vision).
Source: Modified with permission from Nargozian C, et al: Hemifacial microsomia: anatomical prediction of difficult intubation. *Paediatr Anaesth* 9:393, 1999.

CHAPTER 10 / MANAGEMENT OF THE CHILD WITH A DIFFICULT AIRWAY 149

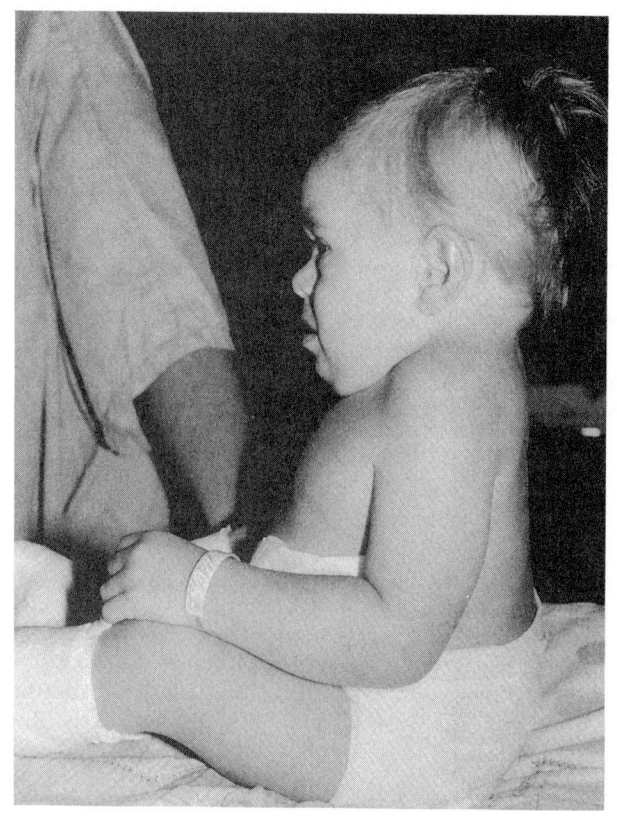

FIG. 10-5 Klippel–Feil sequence. Note the short neck, with the head resting on the shoulders. *(Reproduced from Gregory GA: Pediatric Anesthesia, 3rd ed. New York, Churchill Livingstone, 1994.)*

croup and vocal cord damage. Parents should be told to expect a change in the quality of the child's voice and cry initially, but that it should resolve in time. If the change persists, they should have the child evaluated for laryngeal damage.

Informed Consent

After the potentially difficult airway is identified by a history of a previous difficult intubation or the current physical examination, the anesthesiologist must share this information with the parents and surgeon. It is probably best to begin with the surgeon. The very first decision is whether or not an elective tracheotomy would provide a safer airway, not only for the purposes of the surgery but also for the immediate postoperative recovery period. One important factor that may influence this decision is the anticipated number of surgical procedures the child is facing. The second issue that needs to be addressed is the urgency of the surgical procedure. If a satisfactory airway cannot be established, the surgeon should be prepared to proceed with a tracheotomy to perform the surgical procedure or the child might be awakened and the need for surgery reconsidered. In the event of total loss of control of the airway, an emergent cricothyrotomy or tracheotomy is unavoidable.

Once the anesthesiologist and surgeon have established a plan, the information is shared with the parents or guardians and the patient. They must be informed of the potentially difficult airway and all significant risks, including the possible need for an elective or emergent tracheotomy.

CLINICAL MANAGEMENT OF THE DIFFICULT AIRWAY

Preoperative Preparation

Once the difficult airway has been identified or suspected, the strategies for establishing the airway must be considered according to the age of the child and the experience and training of the anesthesiologist. Additional information often can be obtained by consultation with colleagues, reliable Internet sources, or the medical literature (as in the case of known congenital problems such as Goldenhar's syndrome or Treacher–Collins syndrome).

The availability and familiarity of equipment are crucial in these situations. As a result, most anesthesia departments have developed a difficult airway cart that includes: (1) different-size oral airways, endotracheal tubes, and laryngoscope blades, (2) fiber-optic equipment, (3) LMAs of different sizes, and (4) a transtracheal jet ventilator (Figure 10-6).

The anesthesiologist also should be familiar with the algorithm of the difficult airway, as described by the ASA (Figure 10-1).[1] There are several important concepts from the algorithm. The most important are to get help and to get out, i.e., awaken the patient and return another day, if the situation is deteriorating. When intubating a patient with a known difficult airway, attempts should be made to have another colleague present. Unfortunately, there are times such as emergencies and manpower shortages when this is not possible. One also may choose to have an otolaryngologist or pediatric surgeon on standby to provide an emergent surgical airway, if necessary. Looking to them after the fact is of limited value!

Premedication

Premedication is given to pediatric patients for two major reasons: sedation and the reduction of oral and tracheal secretions. The decision to use a sedative premedication is made on an individual basis with regard to the experience of the anesthesiologist, the potential risk of airway obstruction, and the anxiety level of the patient or family. The best rule to follow is that if there is a serious concern about airway obstruction due to sedation, then premedication should be avoided. Conversely, if the patient is extremely anxious and the appropriate monitoring is available, a sedative premedication may help smooth the induction period. Oral midazolam is the most commonly used sedative premedication. The advantages include anxiolysis, amnesia, and low risk of apnea. It is best to avoid heavy sedatives, such as rectal methohexital, and narcotics, such as transmucosal fentanyl, in children with suspected difficult airways due to the risk of airway obstruction or apnea. The goal is to have a relaxed, cooperative child who can maintain a natural airway on separation from the parents.

CHAPTER 10 / MANAGEMENT OF THE CHILD WITH A DIFFICULT AIRWAY 151

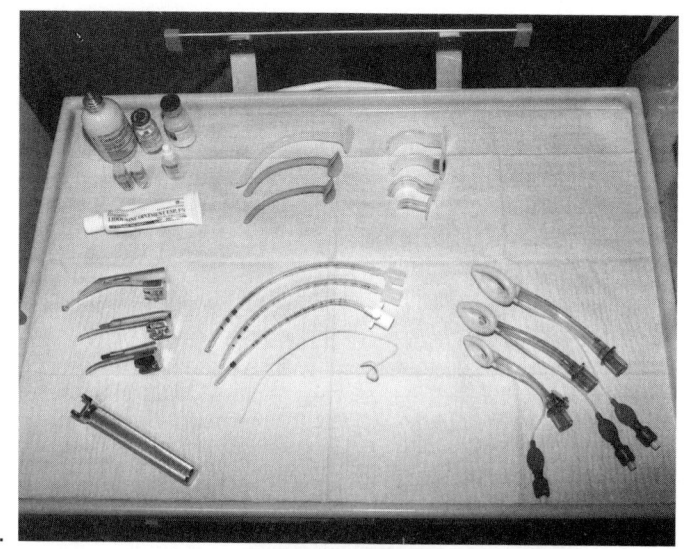

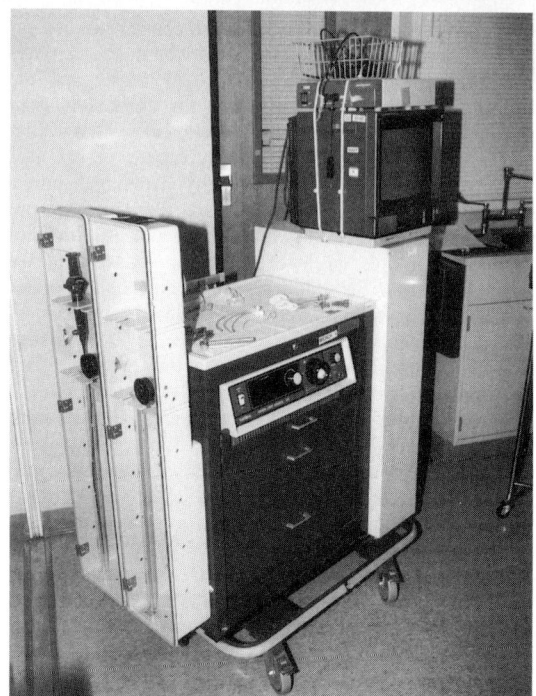

FIG. 10-6 Difficult airway cart. *(A)* Selection of airways, tubes, laryngoscopes, and medications. *(B)* Airway cart with fiberoptic capabilities and video.

In the management of a child with a difficult airway, secretions can be very troublesome. Excessive oropharyngeal secretions increase the risk of laryngospasm during inhalational inductions, obstruct the view of the airway during laryngoscopy, and interfere with the effectiveness of topical anesthetics. The anticholinergics atropine and glycopyrrolate are effective antisialagogues when given preoperatively. Dosage, preparation and route of administration are outlined in Table 10-3. They (atropine more so than glycopyrrolate) also have a vagolytic effect that may be helpful if repeated prolonged attempts at laryngoscopy are necessary.

Induction of Anesthesia

One of the most controversial topics in pediatric anesthesia today is parental presence for induction. Inductions with parents present often are done in separate induction rooms and then the child is moved to the operating room. However, in a child with a suspected difficult airway, it would seem more appropriate to induce anesthesia in the operating room, where the equipment and personnel necessary to establish an airway emergently are located. In this situation parents can be dressed and taken to the operating room for the induction with the understanding that, if difficulties arise, they will have to leave immediately. As soon as the child loses consciousness, the parents should be escorted from the operating room. If the anesthesiologist is at all uncomfortable with the parents being present for normal inductions, then certainly this is not the time for the parents to be present and increase the stress level at a time when the airway is critical. Certainly, the decision to have parents present should err on the side of safety, with the priority being the child and the airway.

Induction of anesthesia can be achieved by inhalational, intravenous, or intramuscular routes. Inhalational induction has the advantage of maintaining spontaneous ventilation in the child with a potential difficult airway. Sevoflurane has become the agent of choice for inhalational induction of anesthesia in the children. Sevoflurane's low blood/gas solubility (0.68 vs. 2.4 for halothane) allows for rapid induction of anesthesia. It is also less irritating to the airway then halothane, leading to a lower incidence of laryngospasm and breath-holding on induction. Another advantage is that it has relatively minimal effect on the cardiovascular system (i.e., decreased contractility or cardiac output as seen with halothane), and it does not sensitize the myocardium to catecholamines. As a result, hypotension and arrhythmias are less likely to occur. Because of the nonirritating nature of sevoflurane, induction can begin with high flow nitrous oxide and oxygen (4 L nitrous

TABLE 10-3 Antisialogogues*

	Atropine	Glycopyrrolate
Dosage (mg/kg)	0.02 PO	0.01 PO
	0.015–0.02 IM	0.01 IM
	0.01–0.015 IV	0.01 IV
Onset (min)	30–60 PO	30–60 PO
	15–30 IM	15–30 IM
	3–5 IV	3–5 IV
Duration (min)	60–120	240–360

IM, intramuscular; IV, intravenous; PO, per oral.
*Refers to antisialogogue, not vagolytic, characteristics.

oxide and 2 L oxygen) and 8% sevoflurane. Alternatively, high flow nitrous oxide can be given for a minute or so and then increasing increments of sevoflurane added, similar to the halothane induction.

Intravenous induction may be necessary in the child at high risk for aspiration or with a known difficult mask airway. The advantage of an intravenous induction is the rapid onset of maximal relaxation for the initial attempt at intubation, which is usually the best attempt. The disadvantage is the need to support a difficult airway, if the attempt at intubation is unsuccessful. In any case, establishing intravenous access early on, even before an inhalational induction, is a good idea because one cannot always predict the need for emergency drugs. There are no studies demonstrating the safety of intravenous versus inhalational induction in the child with a difficult airway.

Intramuscular inductions are reserved for the extremely uncooperative child. These are most often children with congenital syndromes associated with some degree of developmental delay and requiring multiple surgical procedures. The most commonly used drug is ketamine. Ketamine has the advantage of inducing anesthesia and preserving respirations. However, the major disadvantage is the increase in secretions, making an antisialogue essential.

Laryngoscopy and Intubation

Anatomy of Intubation

All airway maneuvers begin with the appropriate alignment of the oral, pharyngeal, and laryngeal airway axes (Figure 10-7). As with adults, positioning is important. Infants and children are somewhat different than adults because of the relatively larger occiput. If a pillow is placed under the head, such as is done in older children and adults, rather than extending the airway in the sniffing position and assisting in aligning the airway axes, the airway can be compromised because the large occiput, on a pillow, causes the head to flex onto the chest. The proper placement of a pillow or a pad in the small infant and child is at the base of the neck so that the head can be allowed to extend comfortably.

The next step after positioning is the actual laryngoscopy. Laryngoscopy involves displacement of the soft tissues of the oropharynx (Figure 10-8). This allows for a line of vision from the mandibular alveolar ridge to the epiglottis and then, as the epiglottis is lifted with a Macintosh or Miller blade, to the larynx. This is accomplished by placing the blade slightly to the right of midline, following the tongue to the epiglottis as the laryngoscope is lifted toward the ceiling. The soft tissue of the tongue and submandibular area is displaced into a potential space that is encompassed and therefore potentially restricted by an incomplete bony ring bound posteriorly by the hyoid bone, laterally by the rami of the mandible, and anteriorly by the mentum of the mandible.

Any increase in the amount of soft tissue such as occurs with macroglossia or cystic hygroma (Figure 10-9) interferes with laryngoscopy because there is excessive soft tissue to be displaced into the potential displacement area. Also, if there is any alteration in the shape or size of the bony structures such as occurs in HFM and the Pierre–Robin syndrome (Figure 10-10), there is a great decrease in this potential displacement area so that visualization of the epiglottis is difficult and in some cases impossible. The use of muscle relaxants will maximize the potential displacement space; however, even with maximum relaxation, if the anatomic area is not sufficiently large to accept

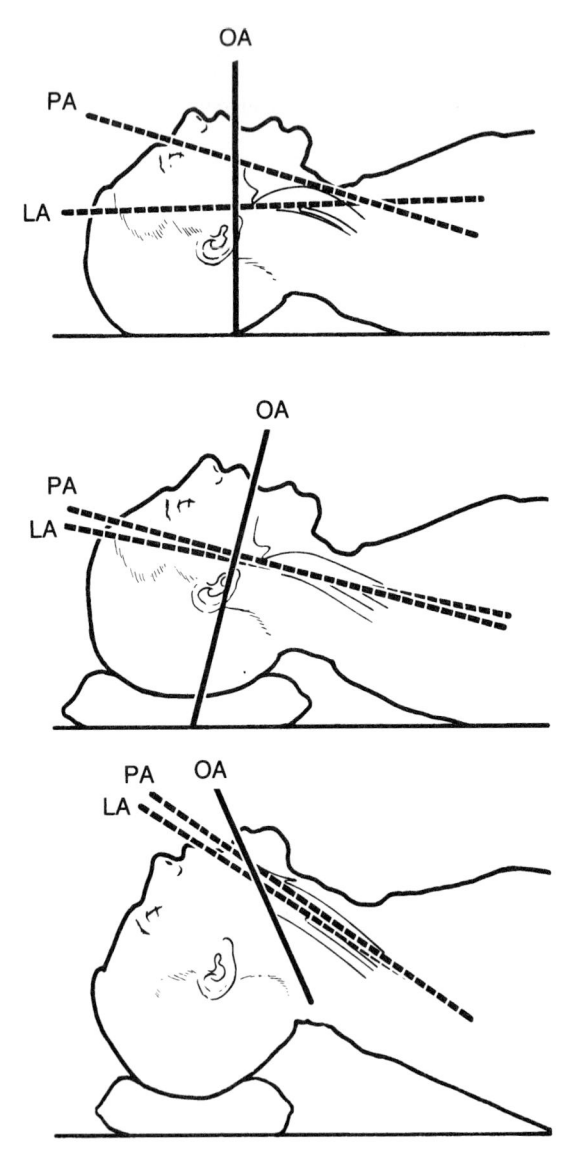

FIG. 10-7 Alignment of axes for intubation. *(Reproduced from Stoelting RK, Miller RD:* Basics of Anesthesia, *3rd ed. New York, Churchill Livingstone, 1994.)*

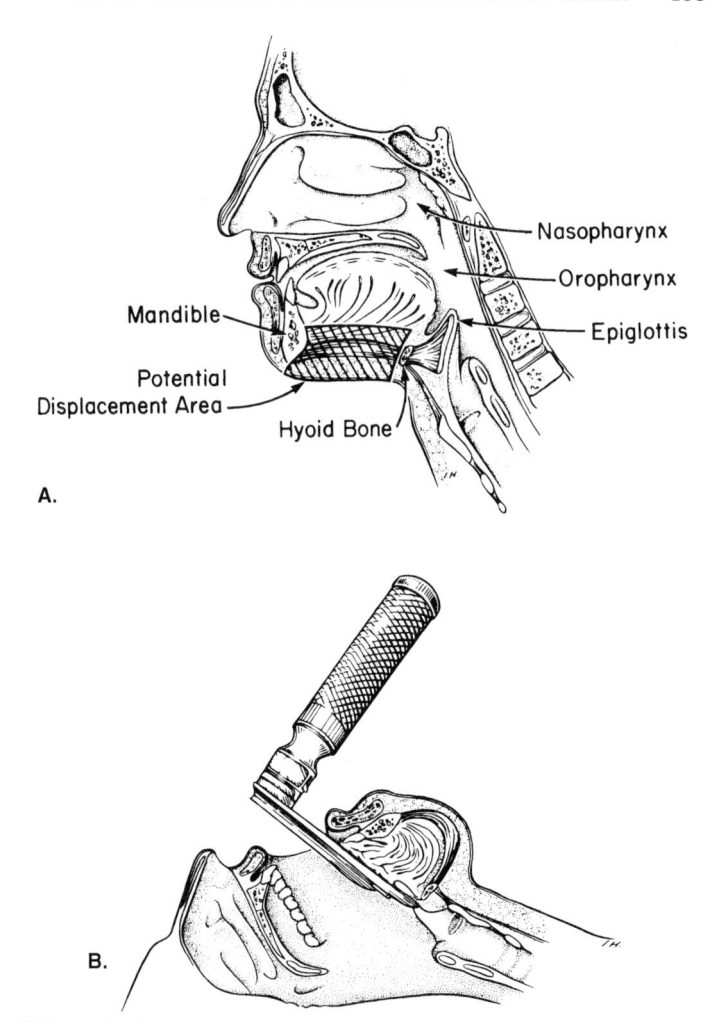

FIG. 10-8 Displacement of tongue and soft tissues into potential displacement area during laryngoscopy. **(A)** Potential displacement area. **(B)** Laryngoscopy with displacement of tongue and tissue into potential displacement area. *(Reproduced with permission from Berry FA, ed: Anesthetic Management of Difficult and Routine Pediatric Patients. New York, Churchill Livingstone, 1990.)*

the displacement of the soft tissue, laryngoscopy may not result in visualization of the epiglottis.

Preoperative assessment of this submandibular region provides information about the adequacy of the potential displacement area. Measurement of the anterior–posterior distance from the middle of the inside of the mentum of the mandible to the hyoid bone is one method for assessing the potential space for laryngoscopy. In the cooperative patient this distance can be measured easily by gently placing the examining fingers in this space. In infants

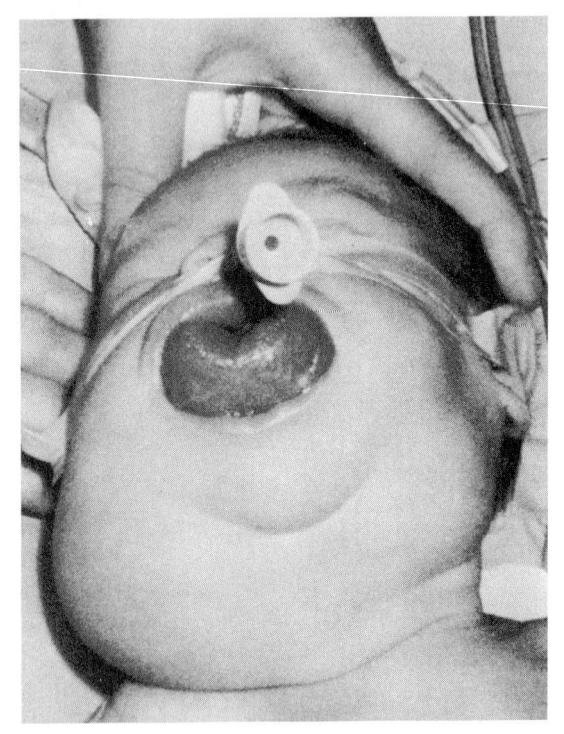

FIG. 10-9 Child with massive cystic hygroma. *(Reproduced with permission from Berry FA, ed:* Anesthetic Management of Difficult and Routine Pediatric Patients. *New York, Churchill Livingstone, 1990.)*

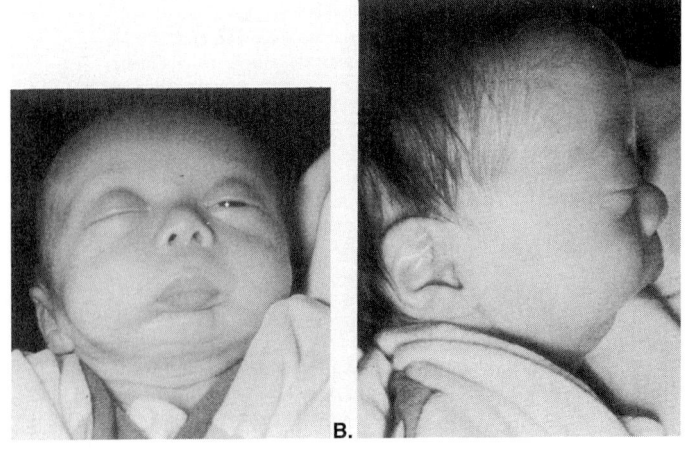

FIG. 10-10 Micrognathia in infant with Pierre–Robin sequence. **(A)** Anterior view. **(B)** Lateral view. *(Reproduced from Myer CM, Cotton RT, Shott SR:* The Pediatric Airway: An Interdisciplinary Approach. *Philadelphia, JB Lippincott, 1995.)*

and small children two fingers usually fit quite comfortably in this space; in the older child and adult the minimum distance for normal airway is about two and a half to three fingers.

Inability to visualize all or part of the epiglottis and, hence, the larynx is often referred to as an *anterior larynx*. Anatomically speaking, the larynx is no more anterior in these patients than in any patient. However, it is anterior to the line of vision because of the inability to displace the soft tissue into this potential displacement area. This problem can be greatly magnified by factors such as the patient's inability to open the mouth or extend the neck.

Topicalization

Topicalizing the airway may prove highly beneficial in the management of a difficult airway. In the infant younger than 6 months, topicalization may be achieved by spreading 5% lidocaine paste in the hypopharynx with one's fingertip. Laryngoscopy then can be attempted with the infant awake or minimally sedated. In the older infant and child, topicalization may be achieved by spraying the larynx with 4% lidocaine (4 to 5 mg/kg) during laryngoscopy. However, if the larynx cannot be visualized, the hypopharynx can be sprayed and anterior pressure applied to the larynx, thus bringing it in contact with the topical anesthetic.

Direct Laryngoscopy

If the technique of spontaneous ventilation and deep anesthesia has been chosen as the technique of choice, which we prefer because it preserves spontaneous respirations and allows for continuous oxygenation via insufflation, certain conditions must be present for the laryngoscopy to be successful. It is obvious that the child has to be anesthetized deeply so that the protective reflexes of coughing or swallowing have been suspended. Breath-holding, coughing, and swallowing during attempted laryngoscopy are obvious signs of a light plane of anesthesia. Assessment of the depth of anesthesia may be difficult; however, feeling the abdominal musculature and the degree of relaxation of the jaw will assist the clinician in determining an adequate depth. The depth of anesthesia necessary for laryngoscopy and tracheal intubation is at least 2 minimum alveolar concentration (MAC). It is important to realize that some patients, neonates in particular, may not be able to tolerate this level of anesthesia from a cardiovascular standpoint. Topicalization of the larynx often is beneficial for deep laryngoscopy and may be very useful in these situations.

If any part of the airway can be visualized by direct laryngoscopy, meaning the epiglottis or the arytenoids, there is an excellent chance that intubation can be accomplished with the use of a stylet in the endotracheal tube. If only the epiglottis is seen, then attempts can be made to lift the epiglottis with the laryngoscope blade. This may be very difficult to accomplish. If the epiglottis cannot be lifted, then consider using the Miller blade as a Macintosh blade, with the tip of the blade in the vallecula. The styletted endotracheal tube is advanced slowly, in the midline, toward the laryngeal opening. The styletted endotracheal tube can then be used to gently lift the epiglottis to visualize the arytenoids or vocal cords. If visualized, the endotracheal tube can be advanced gently. However, if the laryngoscopist cannot visualize any part of the airway, the styletted endotracheal tube can be advanced in a blind fashion. After recognizing the anatomic relation of the larynx to the epiglottis, the tube is advanced under the epiglottis while listening for breath sounds or watching for condensation within the endotracheal tube as the child exhales. Another "clinical trick" is to place the end-tidal CO_2 aspirating tubing at the end of the endotracheal tube and watch for end-tidal CO_2. When the tip of the endotracheal tube is thought to be through the vocal cords, the endotracheal tube should be advanced off the stylet. The tube and stylet should never be forced blindly!

One of the major keys to the ASA algorithm is to secure help. It is better if the help is an anesthesiologist or a health care professional with at least some experience in airway management. Most clinicians recognize that, with the laryngoscope in the left hand and the patient in an ideal position, they can use the right hand to manipulate the larynx and often bring the tip of the epiglottis or the arytenoids into view with downward pressure on the larynx. The technique for improving the view during laryngoscopy with external pressure has been given several names. One of these is *optimal external laryngeal manipulation* and another is *backward upward right pressure.* The problem is that, when the pressure to intubate is released, the view often disappears. It is the ability to secure a better view through this downward pressure on the larynx that makes the second person very useful. While the primary laryngoscopist presses down on the larynx and secures a view of either the epiglottis or the arytenoids, the second person comes over the right shoulder and passes the endotracheal tube while the primary laryngoscopist holds position and visualization. This is referred to as the *two-person laryngoscopy technique* (R. E. Creighton, personal communication).

At times the mid-line approach to laryngoscopy proves to be impossible, so it is worthwhile to attempt a left lateral approach to the airway. In this technique, the laryngoscope is placed on the left lateral aspect of the patient's mouth, external laryngeal manipulation is performed, and a styletted endotracheal tube is introduced into the right corner of the mouth and directed into the larynx if laryngeal structures can be identified.[10]

The Bullard laryngoscope is an indirect oral laryngoscope that uses a combination of fiber optics and mirrors to provide visualization of the larynx. Its major advantage is that the oral, pharyngeal, and tracheal axes do not need to be aligned to visualize the larynx. Therefore, it is possible to easily visualize the larynx in patients with micrognathia or limited neck mobility. Its disadvantage is that, despite visualizing the cords, it is often technically difficult to pass the endotracheal tube. Common problems include right aryepiglottic fold contact and anterior vocal cord contact. The Bullard laryngoscope is available in two sizes for pediatric patients, the pediatric short (newborn to 2 years) and the pediatric long (children up to 10 years). Experience is crucial and it is highly recommended that the anesthesiologist gain experience with this airway device on normal airways before using it for difficult airways.[11]

Muscle Relaxants

For the child with the difficult airway, most techniques involve some form of deep inhalational anesthesia with spontaneous ventilation; the alternative is to paralyze the child after the induction of the anesthesia. In certain situations muscle relaxation may offer the best conditions for endotracheal intubation. The muscle relaxant of choice for rapidly securing the difficult airway is succinylcholine because it has a rapid onset, profound muscle relaxation, and a relatively rapid offset. For routine intubation, in male children younger than 7 or 8 years, many anesthesiologists, for fear of the relatively rare situation in which the male child may have an unrecognized muscular dystrophy, have avoided succinylcholine. The administration of succinylcholine to these children can result in life-threatening hyperkalemia. Despite this concern, succinylcholine remains the drug of choice for rapid onset muscle relaxation in an emergent situation. The benefits of establishing an emergent airway and avoiding severe hypoxia outweigh the relatively rare risk of inducing severe hyperkalemia.

If a decision is made to use a nondepolarizing muscle relaxant instead of succinylcholine, the anesthesiologist must appreciate the pharmacokinetics of such drugs (Table 10-4), particularly their duration of action. The approximate time to recovery for succinylcholine is 5 to 8 min; even with the newest nondepolarizing muscle relaxant rapacuronium, the time to recovery may be 15 min. With the other nondepolarizing muscle relaxants, the time to recovery may well be 30 min. Because oxygenation and ventilation will need to be supported during this period, it is essential to establish that the airway can be managed before administering these drugs.

Alternative Intubating Techniques

Unfortunately, even the most experienced anesthesiologist will be confronted with a situation in which the surgical procedure requires that the patient be intubated but this cannot be successfully achieved with direct laryngoscopy. When ideal techniques of laryngoscopy fail, the anesthesiologist should reassess the situation and use alternative techniques rather than persist in multiple, unsuccessful laryngoscopies that may lead to trauma, edema, and laryngospasm. Several options are available: (1) fiber-optic intubation, (2) intubation via an LMA, (3) blind oral or blind nasal intubation, or (4) retrograde intubation. The choice of technique will depend on the experience of the anesthesiologist and the availability of equipment. The ASA difficult algorithm strongly suggests that, if no progress is being made or there is difficulty in maintaining the airway, the anesthetic should be discontinued and the patient awakened.

Fiberoptic Intubation

When a difficult airway is identified in the adult population, an awake, fiber-optic intubation is immediately considered. The technique of fiber-optic intubation is limited in the pediatric population by the availability of equipment and the technical skill required to use such equipment. As in many other areas of pediatric anesthesia, the development of equipment has lagged behind that which was available for the larger child and adult. It took

TABLE 10-4 Nondepolarizing Muscle Relaxants

	ED_{95} (mg/kg)	Intubating dose (mg/kg)	Onset of maximum twitch depression (min)	T_{25} Recovery to 25% of control twitch height (min)
Mivacurium	0.07	0.15–0.25	2.5–4	12–20
Rapacuronium	1.03	2.0–3.0	0.75–1.5	15–20
Rocuronium	0.3	0.6–0.12	1–2	20–35
Cisatracurium	0.05	0.1	3–5	20–35
Vecuronium	0.05	0.1	3–5	25–40
Pancuronium	0.05	0.1	3–5	60–90

Note: Comparison of dose, onset time, and duration of commonly used nondepolarizing muscle relaxants.
ED_{95}, effective dose95.

160 PEDIATRIC ANESTHESIA HANDBOOK

a long time to develop a fiber-optic bronchoscope that would fit into small endotracheal tubes and provide good visualization and a suction channel. This equipment is available today (Figure 10-11). The good news about intubation in pediatric patients is that it is rare to have a patient who cannot be intubated with standard techniques. The bad news is that, because of the rarity of this occasion, it is difficult for clinicians to secure adequate experience and training to maintain these skills. Therefore, the anesthesiologist must look for cases in which fiber-optic intubation can be considered a useful adjunct or technique.[12] The situation that lends itself to the continued use and practice of fiber-optic intubation is nasal intubation for dental surgery. As a matter of fact, any nasal intubation lends itself to the use of fiber-optic intubation for maintaining the skills necessary for fiber-optic intubation.

There are many techniques for fiber-optic intubation, but several principles are mentioned here.[13] Adequate patient preparation is essential. In most situations, the pediatric patient will be deeply sedated or under general anesthesia before attempts at fiber-optic intubation. Only the most mature teenager will tolerate an attempt at awake fiber-optic intubation. Premedication with an antisialagogue to decrease secretions and topicalization of the larynx will greatly enhance the success rate of fiber-optic intubation. Preparation of and familiarity with the equipment is crucial. For example, the suction channel of the bronchoscope may be used not only for suction but also for insufflating oxygen and administering local anesthetic.

Knowledge of the appropriate-size endotracheal tube for a given patient and the ability to pass it over the bronchoscope are also crucial (Table 10-5). If fiber-optic intubation is going to be used because of the difficulty with laryngoscopy, it should be done early because repeated unsuccessful attempts at laryngoscopy will cause edema and bleeding, which will interfere with the visualization through the bronchoscope.

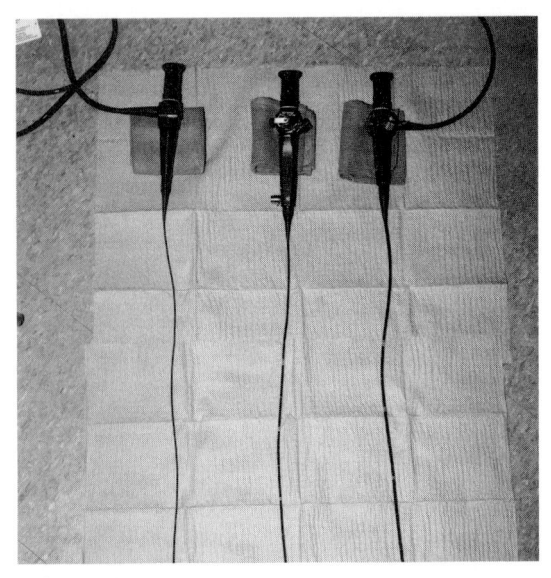

FIG. 10-11   Pediatric fiberoptic bronchoscopes.

TABLE 10-5 Pediatric Fiber-optic Bronchoscopes

	Length* (mm)	Working channel[†]	OD (mm)[‡]	Smallest ETT ID (mm)[§]
Olympus				
BF-3C30	550	Yes	3.6	4.0
LF-2	600	Yes	4.0	4.5
LF-P	600	No	2.2	2.5
Pentax				
FB-10X	600	Yes	3.5	4.0
F1-10P	600	Yes	3.5	4.0

*Length of insertion tube.
[†]Presence of working channel for insufflation or topicalization.
[‡]Outer diameter (OD) of insertion tube.
[§]Internal diameter (ID) of smallest endotracheal tube (ETT) that fits over the insertion tube.

Intubation via an LMA

The LMA, first introduced in the United States in 1991, has been an enormous boon to the entire field of anesthesia and critical care.[14] It has been used safely and effectively in more than 30 million patients worldwide. With the introduction of different sizes, the LMA has gained popularity in the pediatric population for conducting anesthesia, for neonatal resuscitation, for establishing an airway in trauma victims, and for maintaining an airway during bronchoscopy.[15,16] The LMA has limitations in newborn resuscitation because, when the alveoli are still filled with amniotic fluid, the first breath requires approximately 50 cm of water pressure to expand the alveoli and develop a normal functional residual capacity (FRC) and tidal volume. In resuscitative efforts, the LMA can achieve pressures up to 40 cm H_2O. In the infant who is attempting to breathe but having difficulty because of an obstructed airway, as in Treacher–Collins syndrome, the LMA has been used successfully for resuscitation.[17]

However, an important advantage of the LMA is its use as a conduit for tracheal intubation in the patient with a difficult airway. A successfully placed LMA sits just above the glottic inlet, thereby allowing easy access to the larynx. As a result, an endotracheal tube may be passed blindly or with the aid of a fiber-optic bronchoscope. Multiple techniques have been reported in the literature, including passing an endotracheal tube over the bronchoscope or introducing an intubating stylet such as a guidewire or Fogerty catheter alongside the bronchoscope and then passing the endotracheal tube over the stylet. Once intubation is accomplished, removing the LMA without dislodging the endotracheal tube can be tricky. There are reports of using a second endotracheal tube as a stabilizer or grasping the endotracheal tube in the shaft of the LMA with a long forceps and backing the LMA out over the forceps (Figure 10-12). Of course if the LMA is not in the surgical field and the surgery is relatively short, both the LMA and the endotracheal tube can be left in place.[18–23]

Blind Oral and Blind Nasal Intubation

The major requirements for blind intubation techniques are (1) anatomic knowledge of the path that the endotracheal tube must take to pass through the hypopharynx in the larynx, (2) adequate anesthesia to prevent the protective airway reflexes from becoming activated, and (3) spontaneous ventila-

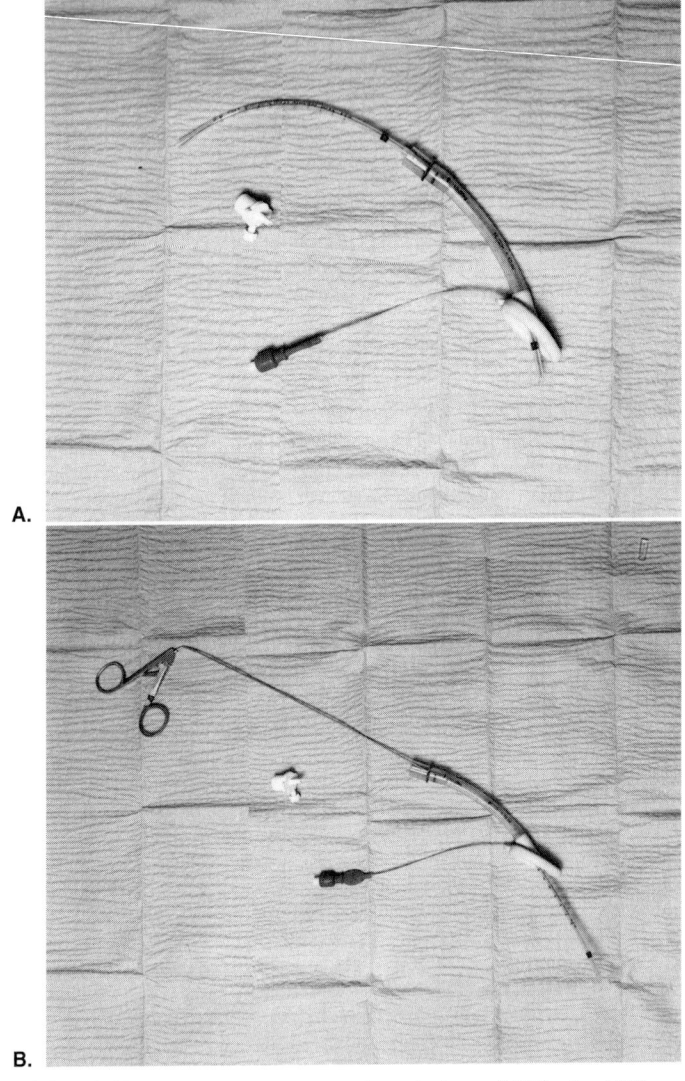

FIG. 10-12 Retrieving the laryngeal mask airway (LMA) after LMA-assisted endotracheal intubation. **(A)** Two endotracheal tubes joined end to end. **(B)** Withdrawing the LMA over a rigid forceps.

tion. The major reason for failure of blind intubation is inadequate anesthesia. The use of topical anesthesia is very useful in blind techniques.

The technique for blind oral intubation was briefly described earlier. A few points deserve emphasis. First, in doing blind oral intubations, attempts should not be made to visualize the airway because, most likely, previous attempts have proven unsuccessful. A laryngoscope blade, Macintosh or Miller, placed in the vallecula will aid in lifting the epiglottis and displacing the tongue to facilitate passage of the endotracheal tube, but it is not intended to provide visualization. In some patients it may be necessary to pull the tongue forward with a forceps or towel clip to facilitate passage of the endotracheal tube. Second, the endotracheal tube and stylet need to be introduced in the configuration of the anticipated anatomy of the patient's airway. For some patients this means a J or hockey-stick shape to the end of the endotracheal tube. Third, the endotracheal tube must be advanced slowly and gently while listening for breath sounds, watching for condensation of expired gases, and monitoring for end-tidal CO_2. The endotracheal tube should never be forced against resistance because this may lead to trauma, edema, and bleeding. If the patient moves or coughs during attempts at blind intubation, the attempt should be aborted until adequate anesthesia is achieved.

The technique for blind nasal intubations follows the same principles as those for blind oral intubations. However, one additional requirement is preparation of the nasopharynx. Adequate preparation requires vasoconstriction and topicalization. The vasoconstrictor increases the size of the nasal airway by vasoconstricting the mucosa. This allows the endotracheal tube to be passed in a manner that produces less trauma and bleeding. It should be kept in mind that children between the ages of 2 to 8 years may have hypertrophied adenoid tissue that may bleed despite vasoconstriction. Oral intubation is preferred in this age group. Topicalization of the nasal mucosa may be achieved by local anesthetic spray or inserting a nasal airway coated with local anesthetic. A significant problem with blind nasal intubations is that the tongue deflects the endotracheal tube into the esophagus. However, having an assistant manually displace the tongue forward, as in blind oral intubations, may prove beneficial. Visualizing the neck around the larynx enables the anesthesiologist to see whether the endotracheal tube is in the piriform sinus area and can help direct the tube in the midline. In addition, gentle downward pressure on the larynx may well bring the larynx into the path of the nasotracheal tube.[5]

Retrograde Tracheal Intubation

The technique of retrograde tracheal intubation, first described in adults in 1960, has been successfully applied to the pediatric population. Three basic steps are involved: 1) entering the trachea at the level of the cricothyroid membrane, (2) passing a stylet through the cricothyroid membrane in a retrograde direction into the oropharynx, and (3) advancing an endotracheal tube antegrade over the stylet into the trachea. Multiple modifications of the original technique have been described.[24–26] The cricothyroid membrane can be punctured with a Tuohy needle, as originally described, or with an angiocatheter, which is believed to be less traumatic. The retrograde stylet may be a guidewire, an epidural catheter, or a tracheal tube exchanger (Figure 10-13). The endotracheal tube may be advanced over the stylet into the trachea blindly or with fiber-optic guidance. Neither the retrograde stylet nor the endotracheal tube should be forced against resistance because this could lead to laryngeal trauma or bleeding.

This technique can be performed in the awake or anesthetized patient. Topicalization of the oropharynx and trachea of the awake patient is critical. The trachea is anesthetized by transtracheal injection of lidocaine or local anesthetic nebulization. The oropharynx is anesthetized with local anesthetic

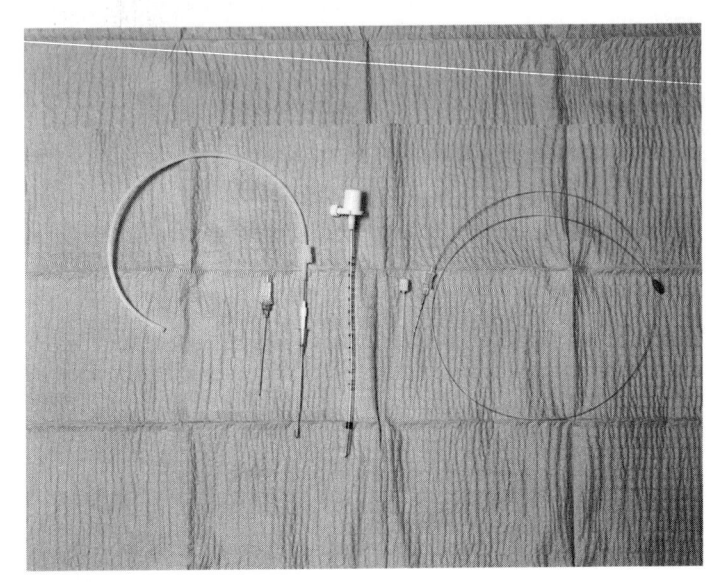

FIG. 10-13 Equipment for retrograde intubation.

spray. Contraindications to this technique are coagulopathy, infection at the site of the cricothyroid membrane, and lesions that obstruct the upper airway.

Miscellaneous Considerations

Elective Tracheotomy

There are three approaches to the management of the airway for elective tracheotomy. The preferred technique is to perform the tracheotomy with an endotracheal tube in place. The second option is to establish an airway with an LMA before performing the tracheotomy. This option is usually chosen in the child who could not be tracheally intubated but will require a secure airway for the procedure or postoperative period. The third option is to perform the tracheotomy under local anesthesia in the awake patient. Although this technique is common in adult patients, the feasibility in the pediatric population is obviously limited.

The Unsuspected Difficult Airway

Regardless of the skill and expertise of the anesthesiologist, there are the rare but ever-present, unsuspected difficult airways. Even after adequate evaluation of the airway, this situation may present itself and never at an opportune moment. As anesthesiologists fine-tune their practice and become more familiar with the various congenital and acquired airway problems, there will be fewer and fewer unsuspected difficult airways but they will be present. This is the reason it is important to understand the associated anatomic problems in children who have difficult airways such as the microtia that is associated with Treacher–Collins and Goldenhar's syndromes.

The goal of all anesthesiologists should be that their initial laryngoscopy is their best laryngoscopy. At times, changing laryngoscope blades and using sufficient posterior pressure can accomplish a successful laryngoscopy and intubation. However, multiple repeated laryngoscopies may be of little benefit and may actually convert a difficult airway into an impossible airway secondary to edema and bleeding. Therefore, when anesthesiologists are confronted with an unsuspected difficult airway, they should (1) call for help, (2) consider alternative airway techniques early, and (3) consider awakening the patient and proceeding at a different time with a different plan.

Steroids

One of the empirical adjuncts to the traumatized airway is the use of steroids to prevent or reduce inflammation and swelling. Although there are no outcome studies that clearly support the use of steroids for patients with difficult airways, this is a frequent empiric practice. The most frequently used drug is dexamethasone at 0.5 to 1.0 mg/kg.

Emergence and Extubation

The choice of anesthetic technique for the child with a difficult airway should be determined by the fact that the child will need to be fully awake for extubation. Narcotics should be used cautiously because they may delay awakening. Alternative techniques for pain control are regional blocks, non-steroidal anti-inflammatory drugs, and the preemptive ketamine–magnesium combination. Volatile agents should be discontinued early and muscle relaxants fully reversed. Lidocaine, 1.5 mg/kg intravenously, may be administered at the completion of surgery to help smooth emergence. In addition, suctioning of the oropharynx should be accomplished before recovery of the airway reflexes to allow for a peaceful awakening.

The "awake" state implies recovery of airway reflexes and purposeful movement. Older children, like adults, should be able to follow commands. However, in infants and younger children, one will need to assess their level of consciousness by looking for signs such as eye opening, attempts to cry, reaching for the endotracheal tube, furrowing of the forehead, or drawing up the lower extremities. Patience is crucial because premature extubation may lead to laryngospasm or upper airway obstruction. Regardless of whether the extubation is to be accomplished in the operating room, the recovery room, or the intensive care unit, the equipment and personnel required to re-establish an airway must be immediately available should the need arise.

Post Case Analysis

The ASA Task Force on the Difficult Airway specifically addressed the issue of communicating to the patient or the family that the patient has a difficult airway. This should be done with a simple, concise letter to the patient that outlines in sufficient detail the issues and techniques used so that subsequent anesthesia providers can determine the nature of the difficulty and the techniques used to establish an airway.

REFERENCES

1. Practice guidelines for management of the difficult airway. *Anesthesiology* 78:597, 1993.
2. Stoelting RK, Miller RD: *Basics of Anesthesia,* 3rd ed. New York, Churchill Livingstone, 1994.

3. Myer CM, Cotton RT, Shott SR: *The Pediatric Airway: An Interdisciplinary Approach.* Philadelphia, JB Lippincott, 1995.
4. Frei FJ, Ummenhofer W: Difficult intubation in paediatrics. *Paediatr Anaesth* 6:251, 1996.
5. Berry FA, ed: *Anesthetic Management of Difficult and Routine Pediatric Patients.* New York, Churchill Livingstone, 1990.
6. Nargozian C, Ririe DG, Bennun RD, Mulliken JB: Hemifacial microsomia: anatomical prediction of difficult intubation. *Paediatr Anaesth* 9:393, 1999.
7. Gregory GA: *Pediatric Anesthesia,* 3rd ed. New York, Churchill Livingstone, 1994.
8. Domino KB, Posner KL, Caplan RA, Cheney FW: Airway injury during anesthesia. *Anesthesiology* 91:1703, 1999.
9. Herlich A: Complications from securing the difficult airway. *Int Anesth Clin* 35:13, 1997.
10. Yamamoto K, Tsubokawa T, Ohmura S, et al: Left-molar approach improves laryngeal view in patients with difficult laryngoscope. *Anesthesiology* 92:70, 2000.
11. Boreland LM, Casselbrant M: The Bullard laryngoscope: a new indirect oral laryngoscope (pediatric version). *Anesth Analg* 70:105, 1990.
12. Erb T, Marsch SCU, Hampl KF, Frei FJ: Teaching the use of fiber-optic intubation for children older than two years of age. *Anesth Analg* 85:1037, 1997.
13. Wheeler M, Ovassapian A: Pediatric fiberoptic intubation. In *Fiberoptic endoscopy and the difficult airway.* Ovassapian A, ed. Philadelphia, Lippincott-Raven, 1996, p. 105.
14. Benumof JL: Laryngeal mask airway and the ASA difficult airway algorithm. *Anesthesiology* 84:686, 1996.
15. Boehringer LA, Bennie RE: Laryngeal mask airway and the pediatric patient. *Int Anesth Clin* 36:45, 1999.
16. Boehringer LA, Bennie RE: Laryngeal mask airway and the pediatric patient. *Int Anesth Clin* 36:45, 1999.
17. Bandla HPR, Smith DE, Kiernan MP: Laryngeal mask airway facilitated fiber-optic bronchoscopy in infants. *Can J Anaesth* 44:1242, 1997.
18. Walker RWM: The laryngeal mask airway in the difficult paediatric airways: an assessment of positioning and use in fiberoptic intubation. *Paediatr Anaesth* 10:53, 2000.
19. Bahk J-H, Han S-M, Kim S-D: Management of difficult airways with a laryngeal mask airway under propofol anaesthesia. *Paediatr Anaesth* 9:163, 1999.
20. Ellis DS, Potluri PK, O'Flaherty JE, Baum VC: Difficult airway management in the neonate: a simple method of intubating through a laryngeal mask airway. *Paediatr Anaesth* 9:460, 1999.
21. Osses H, Poblete M, Asenjo F: Laryngeal mask for difficult intubation in children. *Paediatr Anaesth* 9:399, 1999.
22. Heard CMB, Caldicott LD, Fletcher JE, Selsby DS: Fiberoptic-guided endotracheal via the laryngeal mask airway in pediatric patients: a report of a series of cases. *Anesth Analg* 82:1287, 1996.
23. Arndt GA, Topp H, Hannah J, et al: Intubation via the LMA using a Cook retrograde intubation kit. *Can J Anaesth* 45:257, 1998.
24. Hung OR, Al-Qatari M: Light-guided retrograde intubation. *Can J Anaesth* 44:877, 1997.
25. Harvey SC. Retrograde intubation through a laryngeal mask airway. *Anesthesiology* 85:1503, 1996.
26. Przybylo HJ, Stevenson GW, Vicari FA, et al: Retrograde fiberoptic intubation in a child with Nager's syndrome. *Can J Anaesth* 43:697, 1996.

11 | The Child With Congenital Heart Disease

Victor C. Baum, MD

Congenital heart disease is not uncommon, with an incidence of approximately 0.8%. Although many children will have physiologically trivial or even self-limiting lesions, such as the ventricular septal defect that spontaneously closes, any anesthesiologist who cares for children will have the occasion to care for children with potentially significant congenital heart disease. Many children with congenital heart disease can be managed appropriately in a general hospital setting. Additional information about the patient with congenital heart disease is available from a variety of sources[1-3] and the large anesthesia textbooks.

The first issues to be addressed by the anesthesiologist are anatomy and, more importantly, physiology. Lesions superficially gathered under one rubric may have vastly differing physiologies. For example, the anesthetic implications of the 4 year old with an almost closed ventricular septal defect leaving only a murmur but almost no shunting of blood differs from those of a 4 month old with a very large ventricular septal defect and congestive heart failure, as it does from the 14 year old who was lost to follow-up and whose large ventricular septal defect has resulted in Eisenmenger physiology with fixed pulmonary arterial hypertension and right-to-left shunting with cyanosis.

The most important first step after ascertaining the presence of congenital heart disease is to review the most recent physiologic data. On the one hand, this may require personally reviewing the results of cardiac catheterizations, chest radiographs, electrocardiograms, and echocardiograms. On the other hand, it may require only a call to the pediatric cardiologist's office, whence a fax of the most recent office visit will suffice. It should go without saying that, if such children are encountered on the morning of surgery without background data having been obtained, one will be working at a distinct disadvantage.

The key to understanding physiology, particularly of complex anatomy, is often just drawing a simple box diagram rather than trying to conceptualize the problem as a list of lesions in text format. The physiologic sequelae of abnormal valves, septal defects, etc., will be much more readily apparent. For example, consider the patient shown in Figure 11-1A who has D-transposition of the great arteries, tricuspid atresia, atrial septal defect, ventricular septal defect, and valvar pulmonic stenosis. In this example, it becomes immediately apparent (Figure 11-1B) that there is obligate right-to-left shunting with the risk of paradoxical emboli and that the left ventricle has an obstruction imposed by pulmonary stenosis, so any pharmacologic manipulation of pulmonary vascular resistance is likely to be unproductive, whereas modifications of systemic vascular resistance can have significant effects on blood flow and shunt.

Congenital heart disease does not exist in a vacuum. Surgery is the point where the patient, cardiac lesion, prior cardiac surgery, non-cardiac lesions, anesthesiologist, and surgeon intersect. All must be taken into account. When considering a patient with a congenital cardiac lesion, the following factors should be considered:

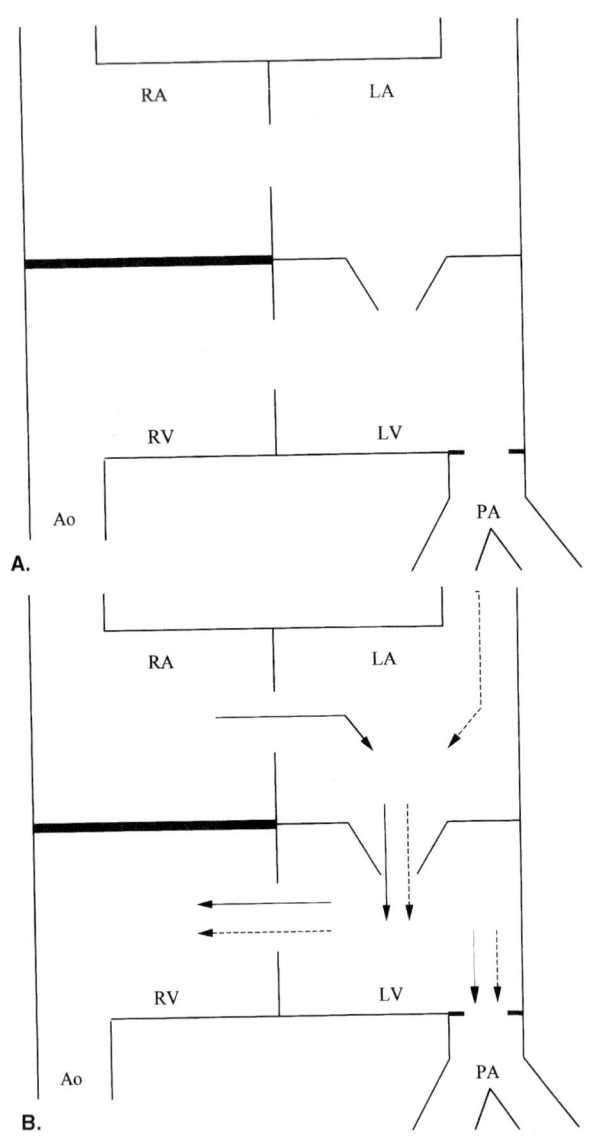

FIG. 11-1 *(A, B)* Examples of the utility of drawing a simple box diagram in understanding complex structural disease. Ao, aorta; LA, left atrium; LV, left ventricle; PA, pulmonary artery; RA, right atrium; RV, right ventricle. Solid arrows represent systemic venous return. Dashed arrows represent pulmonary venous return.

1. Has the patient been adequately managed preoperatively? What is the ratio of risk to emergency? Except in truly emergent situations or in medically underserved populations, this usually is not a problem.
2. Is there obstructed flow (i.e., stenosis) and is obstruction to flow fixed (e.g., a stenotic valve) or dynamic (severity changes with cardiac physiology, such as muscular obstruction with tetralogy of Fallot or hypertrophic obstructive cardiomyopathy)?
3. Is there valve incompetence?
4. Is there abnormal shunting of blood?
5. Severity of the lesion: In general, exercise tolerance is a good guide to the overall severity of the cardiac disease, as it is in adults.
6. Is the severity of the disease adequate to affect a safe anesthetic, or are the induction and maintenance of anesthesia likely to adversely affect cardiac physiology? If so, which of the components of abnormal physiology can be addressed?
7. Are there noncardiac manifestations of congenital heart disease? These are numerous and summarized in Tables 11-1 through 11-4. These are discussed in greater detail in other sources.[1,2]
8. Is congenital heart disease only one component of a multiorgan genetic or dysmorphic syndrome? Are there issues associated with these syndromes that might affect airway management or anesthesia?

HISTORY AND PHYSICAL EXAMINATION

The history and physical examination will confirm the presence of cardiac disease. However, the physical examination can offer additional information about the severity of the disease. Infants who develop heart failure often will have a history of diaphoresis. Normal babies can have sweating of the head. Infants with diaphoresis sweat all over. Tachypnea is another early sign of heart failure in infants. Children with significant increases in pulmonary blood flow may have audible wheezes from impingement of bronchioles and small airways (known in the past as "cardiac asthma"). This may be partly reversible with bronchodilators. Infants who are failing to thrive from heart failure will fall off the growth curve for weight and then for length; only when extremely ill will they fall off the growth curve for head circumfer-

TABLE 11–1 Potential Pulmonary Interactions Associated With Congenital Heart Disease

---

Decreased lung compliance in lesions with increased pulmonary blood flow (i.e., left-to-right shunting); may require higher airway pressure for ventilation

Compression of airways by enlarged, hypertensive vascular structures

Scoliosis (up to 19% of patients; more common with cyanotic lesions; may present in adolescence, years after corrective cardiac surgery; rarely severe enough to impair pulmonary function)

Hemoptysis (in end-stage Eisenmenger's syndrome)

Phrenic nerve injury (from prior surgery)

Recurrent laryngeal nerve injury (from prior surgery or an enlarged hypertensive pulmonary artery)

Normal ventilatory response to hypercarbia

Cyanotic patients have blunted ventilatory responses to hypoxemia that normalize after surgical repair

TABLE 11–2 Hematologic Problems Associated
With Congenital Heart Disease

Symptomatic hyperviscosity with hematocrit above ~65% (or lower if iron deficient; see Table 11-3)

Falsely elevated hematocrit of erythrocytotic blood if done manually (use of hematocrit tubes with erythrocytotic blood causes plasma trapping and false elevation of the hematocrit; this is not a problem with automated methods)

Bleeding diathesis (abnormalities of different factors have been described in cyanotic patients, none consistently)

In addition, elevated central venous pressure may cause increased operative bleeding, as may prior thoracic surgery during repeat thoracic procedures

Artifactually elevated prothrombin and partial thromboplastin times (erythrocytotic blood has less plasma per milliliter of whole blood; the fixed amount of anticoagulant in the tube may be excessive, as it assumes a normal amount of plasma; the clinical laboratory can prepare an appropriate tube for patients with an elevated hematocrit if informed about it in advance)

Gallstones (calcium bilirubinate stones from increased heme turnover in cyanotic disease; may not become symptomatic until years later)

---

ence. Children with cyanotic disease tend to grow and develop normally but may have diminished exercise tolerance. Children with heart failure tend to grow poorly, and children with lesions resulting in cyanosis and heart failure tend to have very poor appetites and severe failure to thrive.

In infants and young children, short fat necks will obscure the jugular veins but the liver is the window to the central venous pressure. The liver normally is palpable 1 to 2 cm below the right costal margin in infants and young children, and it will descend farther in direct relation to worsening heart failure and increases in central venous pressure. Worsening failure also will be manifested early by tachypnea and later by pulmonary crackles. Peripheral edema as a sign of congestive failure is much less common in children than in adults.

All young infants may develop some degree of perioral cyanosis with crying. Infants with cyanotic heart disease will have central cyanosis. Children with borderline desaturated states will have almost a dusky, venous plethora look rather than frank cyanosis. Cyanosis depends on an absolute level of desaturated hemoglobin (3 to 5 g/dL) and not a relative amount (percentage of saturation). Thus a patient who is very anemic may never become visibly cyanotic, whereas a patient with a high hematocrit may be visibly cyanotic at a higher level of oxygen saturation than normal. Also, because of a shift in the oxygen–hemoglobin saturation curve of fetal hemoglobin, neonates may not be visibly cyanotic until oxygen saturation is lower than that resulting in visible cyanosis in older children.

TABLE 11–3 Symptoms of Hyperviscosity Due to Elevated Hematocrit

---
Headache
Faintness, dizziness, light-headedness
Blurred or double vision
Fatigue
Myalgias, muscle weakness
Paresthesias of fingers, toes, or lips
Depressed mentation, a feeling of dissociation

TABLE 11–4 Neurologic Problems Associated With Congenital Heart Disease

Paradoxical emboli to central nervous system
Brain abscess in patients with right-to-left shunts
Cerebral thrombosis (in erythrocytotic children but not in adults)
Compression of nerve by vascular structure (recurrent laryngeal)
Nerve injury during prior surgery (recurrent laryngeal, phrenic, sympathetic chain), particularly after surgery at the apices of the thorax, such as PDA ligation, coarctation repair, or Blalock–Taussig shunt

PDA, Patent Ductus Arteriosus.

PREOPERATIVE CONSIDERATIONS

Preoperative fasting should be limited in patients with cyanosis and erythrocytosis (to avoid further increasing the hematocrit and blood viscosity from dehydration) and in young infants with congestive failure and failure to thrive, who may have limited glycogen reserves. Young infants with failure should take glucose-containing intravenous fluid intraoperatively and until able to take fluids orally. Dehydration from a protracted preoperative fast is not a problem with the less restrictive fasting guidelines that have emerged over the past few years. In children with these characteristics who sleep through the night, it is helpful to awaken and feed them with clear liquids 2 to 4 h preoperatively. Generally speaking, cardiac medications can be continued until the time of surgery, although the last dose of diuretic can be held to avoid any relative hypovolemia before induction of anesthesia. There is no contraindication to appropriate preoperative medication of individuals with congenital heart disease in normal doses, relative to those without congenital heart disease. This is true for cyanotic and acyanotic patients. Patients with dynamic obstruction to blood flow (e.g., tetralogy of Fallot or IHSS) and those with pulmonary vascular disease will particularly benefit from appropriate preoperative anxiolysis. I have not found routine use of preoperative anticholinergics or intramuscular premedication necessary. With the exception of a baseline hematocrit in cyanotic patients (to exclude a dangerously high hematocrit or provide a baseline for surgery with potential significant blood loss) or a serum potassium and bicarbonate in patients receiving high doses of diuretics, patients with congenital heart disease do not require preoperative laboratory tests in excess of the general population. Presumably cardiac-related evaluations, such as electrocardiograms, would have been obtained as appropriate on an ongoing basis by the pediatric cardiologist and are available for review.

Almost all patients with congenital heart disease will require perioperative antibiotics for endocarditis prophylaxis for appropriate surgical procedures.[4] Current recommendations are listed in Tables 11-5 and 11-6. Not all patients with congenital heart disease require endocarditis prophylaxis (Table 11-7). Surgical procedures that do not require endocarditis prophylaxis are listed in Table 11-8.

INDUCTION AND MAINTENANCE OF ANESTHESIA

Although much is made of which specific agent to use, it must be remembered that the most important factor in anesthetizing children with congenital heart disease is maintaining the airway[5] (Table 11-9). Cyanotic infants in particular begin with decreased oxygen saturation and may rapidly desaturate with a transient inability to ventilate. General approaches to the different types of pathophysiology are summarized in Table 11-10. A complete delin-

TABLE 11–5 Endocarditis Prophylaxis Regimens for Dental, Oral, Respiratory Tract, and Esophageal Procedures

Situation	Agent	Regimen*
Standard general prophylaxis	Amoxicillin	50 mg/kg orally 1 h before procedure (adults: 2 g)
Unable to take orally	Ampicillin	50 mg/kg IM or IV within 30 min of procedure (adults: 2 g)
Allergic to penicillin	Clindamycin *or*	20 mg/kg orally 1 h before procedure (adults: 600 mg)
	Cephalexin or cefadroxil *or*	50 mg/kg orally 1 h before procedure (adults: 2 g)
	Azithromycin or clarithromycin	15 mg/kg orally 1 h before procedure (adults: 500 mg)
Allergic to penicillin and unable to take orally	Clindamycin *or*	20 mg/kg IV within 30 min of procedure (adults: 600 mg)
	Cefazolin	25 mg/kg IM or IV within 30 min of procedure (adults: 1 g)

IM, intramuscularly; IV, intravenously.
*Children's dose should not exceed adult dose.
Source: Modified from Dajani AS, Taubert KA, Wilson W, et al: Prevention of bacterial endocarditis. Recommendations by the American Heart Association. *JAMA* 277:1794, 1997.

TABLE 11–6 Endocarditis Prophylaxis Regimens for Genitourinary and Gastrointestinal (Excluding Esophageal) Procedures

Situation	Agent	Regimen[†]
High-risk patients*	Ampicillin + gentamicin	Ampicillin 50 mg/kg IM or IV + gentamicin 1.5 mg/kg within 30 min of procedure; 6 hr later, ampicillin 25 mg/kg IM or IV or amoxicillin 25 mg/kg orally (adults: ampicillin 2 g + gentamicin 1.5 mg/kg, up to 120 mg; 6 h later, ampicillin 1 g IM or IV or amoxicillin 1 g orally)
High-risk patients* allergic to penicillin	Vancomycin + gentamicin	Vancomycin 20 mg/kg by slow IV infusion + gentamicin 1.5 mg/kg IM or IV to be completed within 30 min of starting procedure (adults: vancomycin 1 g, gentamicin 1.5 mg/kg, up to 120 mg)
Moderate-risk patients*	Amoxicillin or ampicillin	Amoxicillin 50 mg/kg orally 1 h before procedure or ampicillin 50 mg/kg IM or IV within 30 min of starting procedure (adults: amoxicillin 2 g, ampicillin 2 g)
Moderate-risk patients* allergic to ampicillin or amoxicillin	Vancomycin	Vancomycin 20 mg/kg by slow IV infusion, completed within 30 min of procedure (adults: 1 g)

IM, intramuscularly; IV, intravenously.
*See Table 11–7 for definitions of medium- and high-risk groups.
[†]Children's dose should not exceed adult dose.
Source: Modified from Dajani AS, Taubert KA, Wilson W, et al: Prevention of bacterial endocarditis. Recommendations by the American Heart Association. *JAMA* 277:1794, 1997.

TABLE 11-7 Cardiac Conditions Requiring Endocarditis Prophylaxis

Prophylaxis recommended
- Prosthetic valves (bioprosthetic and homograft)*
- Previous bacterial endocarditis*
- Complex cyanotic heart disease*
- Systemic pulmonary shunts (e.g., Blalock-Taussig)*
- Most cardiac structural abnormalities, not delineated above or below[†]
- Acquired valve dysfunction (e.g., rheumatic)[†]
- Hypertrophic cardiomyopathy[†]
- Mitral valve prolapse with insufficiency[†]

Prophylaxis *not* required (endocarditis risk no higher than for the general population)
- Isolated secundum atrial septal defect
- Surgical repair beyond 6 months without residua of secundum atrial septal defect, ventricular defect or patent ductus arteriosus
- Mitral valve prolapse without insufficiency
- Cardiac pacemaker (intravenous and epicardial)
- Functional murmur

*High risk.
[†]Moderate risk.
Source: Modified from Dajani AS, Taubert KA, Wilson W, et al: Prevention of bacterial endocarditis. Recommendations by the American Heart Association. *JAMA* 277:1794, 1997.

eation of the approaches to the numerous cardiac malformations with subtypes and the variety of palliative and corrective repairs is impossible in the space allowed. Several investigators have popularized the use of a "cardiac grid" to summarize the physiologic manipulations required for a cardiac lesion and other noncardiac problems. Examples of entries for several cardiac malformations are given in Table 11-11.

Differences in induction times with intravenous and volatile agents in lesions with right-to-left and left-to-right shunts are common issues raised

TABLE 11-8 Procedures Where Endocarditis Prophylaxis Is Not Recommended

Orotracheal intubation
Injection of intraoral anesthetics
Tympanostomy tube placement
Flexible bronchoscopy with or without biopsy*
Cardiac catheterization
Endoscopy with or without biopsy* (includes transesophageal echocardiography)
Casarean section
In the absence of infection: urethral catheterization, dilatation and curettage, uncomplicated vaginal delivery,* therapeutic abortion, sterilization procedures, insertion or removal of intrauterine devices
Cardiac catheterization
Implanted pacemakers
Incision or biopsy of surgically scrubbed skin
Circumcision

*Prophylaxis optional in high-risk group (see Table 11-7 for delineation of high-risk patients).
Source: Modified from Dajani AS, Taubert KA, Wilson W, et al: Prevention of bacterial endocarditis. Recommendations by the American Heart Association. *JAMA* 277:1794, 1997.

TABLE 11–9 The Six Important Factors in Anesthetizing Children With Congenital Heart Disease

Airway
Airway
Airway
Alterations in vascular resistance
Alterations in vascular resistance
Everything else

when studying for examinations.[6] In clinical practice and with the modern inhalational agents of intermediate solubility, differences are clinically trivial. Inhalational inductions may be slightly slower in children with right-to-left shunts. The effect on inductions with sevoflurane, whose low solubility should have a more pronounced effect, has not been documented. If the circuit is overpressurized to hasten induction, this may be a problem if there is an overdose of anesthetic because it will take longer to lower airway concentrations. The circulation time is short enough in children so that any shortening of induction time with intravenous inductions in children with right-to-left shunts is not likely to be appreciated. Small to moderate left-to-right shunts are unlikely to have noticeable effects. Any changes based on shunting also may be affected by a variety of other influences, including differences in cardiac output and blood volume.

A wide variety of anesthetics has been used to induce and maintain anesthesia in these children. It is axiomatic that agents with significant myocardial depressant activity should be avoided in children with poor ventricular function; however, for the vast majority of children with congenital heart disease, any otherwise appropriate technique can be used. It is impressive that the onset of anesthesia is uniformly accompanied by an increase in oxygen saturation in cyanotic patients, independent of the anesthetic agent or technique (intravenous or inhalational) used.[7] This can be explained in part by the fact that, in addition to a high fraction of inspired oxygen, with induction

TABLE 11–10 General Approaches to Congenital Heart Disease Physiology

Right-to-left shunts
  Avoid intravenous air
  Intravascular volume will generally improve pulmonary blood flow by increasing oxygen saturation, particularly for atrial level shunts
  Minimize pulmonary vascular resistance (rarely helpful because pulmonary vascular resistance is already low)
  Increase systemic vascular resistance to increase pulmonary blood flow and increase systemic oxygen saturation, particularly for ventricular and great vessel level shunts; most helpful acutely: phenylephrine (diluted to 10 µg/mL) 1–4 µg/kg
Left-to-right shunts
  For large shunts, keeping pulmonary vascular resistance relatively high will limit shunting
  For dynamic (muscular) obstruction
    Decrease inotropy
    Avoid pharmacologic inotropes
    Intravenous volume
    Regional anesthesia (which lowers systemic vascular resistance) with care

TABLE 11–11 Desired Hemodynamic Changes for a Variety of Cardiac Defects

Defect	Preload	SVR	PVR	Rate	Contracility
ASD	↑	↓	↑	–	–
VSD (L → R)	↑	↓	↑	–	–
VSD (R → L)	–	↑*	↓	–	–
Patent ductus arteriosus	↑	↓	↑	–	–
Tetralogy of Fallot (with inf. PS)	↑	↑*	0	– to ↓*	– to ↓*
Tetralogy of Fallot (with shunt)	↑	↑*	↓ or 0	–	–
Transposition	–	– to ↑	↓	↑	–
Transposition after switch or Rastelli repair	–	–	–	–	–
Tricuspid atresia (↑PBF)	–	↓	– to ↑	–	–
Tricuspid atresia (↓PBF)	–	↑	↓ or 0	–	–
After Fontan procedure	↑	–	↓*	–	–
Unrepaired AV canal	↑	↓	↑	–	–
Valvar pulmonic stenosis	↑	–	0	– to ↓	–

AV, atrioventricular canal; inf. PS, infundibular pulmonic stenosis; L → R, left-to-right shunt; PBF, pulmonary blood flow; R → L, right-to-left shunt; SD, atrial septal defect; shunt, aortopulmonary shunt such as Blalock–Taussig or central shunts; VSD, ventricular septal defect; –, normal; *, particularly important; 0, modifications unlikely to have an effect (e.g., pulmonary vasculature already likely maximally dilated or effects of PVR not seen in the face of pulmonary stenosis).

Source: Modified from Moore RA: Anesthesia for the pediatric congenital heart patient for noncardiac surgery. *Anesth Rev* 8:23, 1981; Salem MR, Hall SC, Motoyama EK: Anesthesia for thoracic and cardiovascular surgery. In S*mith's Anesthesia for Infants and Children,* 5th ed. Motoyama EK, Davis PJ, eds. St. Louis, CV Mosby, 1990, p. 463.

of anesthesia oxygen consumption decreases, and the saturation of venous blood that is shunted to the left side is increased, thus increasing the saturation of arterial blood. Patients with dynamic obstruction and good cardiac function might benefit from the use of halothane or enflurane, which have relatively greater myocardial depression.

Nitrous oxide is a mild myocardial depressant and in adult patients increases pulmonary vascular resistance, particularly in patients in whom it is already elevated. In children no significant increase in pulmonary vascular resistance has been observed with 50% nitrous oxide regardless of the pre-existing pulmonary vascular resistance.[8] Nitrous oxide is routinely used as part of an inhalational induction in these children without detriment,[7,9] including those who are particularly sensitive to elevated pulmonary vascular resistance, such as children after a Glenn or Fontan procedure who lack a subpulmonary ventricle. Although the use of nitrous oxide precludes the use of 100% oxygen, these children are quite used to only 21% oxygen. A cautionary note is that nitrous oxide may increase the size of an intravascular air embolism and so should be used cautiously, if at all, in children with right-to-left shunts who are having surgery with risk of introducing intravascular air.

Modifications in right-to-left shunting at the atrial level are addressed primarily by increasing intravascular volume. Modifications in shunting at the ventricular and great vessel levels are modulated primarily by changes in pulmonary and systemic vascular resistance (Table 11-12). For patients with any variety of large left-to-right shunts at the ventricular or great vessel level, moderate hypercarbia and as low a fraction of inspired oxygen as tolerated will increase pulmonary vascular resistance, thereby decreasing the shunt and in turn decreasing left ventricular diastolic volume and improving the ventricular oxygen supply–demand relationship. In patients who have developed Eisenmenger physiology with increased pulmonary vascular resistance and decreasing left-to-right shunt or even reversal of the shunt such that it is now right-to-left, attempts should be made to minimize pulmonary vascular resistance. These attempts include moderate hypocarbia, 100% oxygen, and the avoidance of endogenous or exogenous catecholamines, cold, acidosis, or hypoxia. If pulmonary vascular resistance has become fixed, these efforts likely will be useless.

Vascular access and intraoperative monitors may be affected by the presence of congenital heart disease. Cyanotic patients and patients with elevated central venous pressure in particular are at risk for increased perioperative blood loss and require adequate intravenous access. All cyanotic patients require that intravenous lines be kept scrupulously clear of air bubbles, but it should be remembered that there can be small amounts of right-to-left shunting during the cardiac cycle even with lesions thought of as left-to-right shunting lesions. Thus, it is prudent to be very aware of small air bubbles in all children with any shunting lesion. Stopcocks are a common place for air to hide. Other issues regarding vascular access are listed in Table 11-13. Congenital heart dis-

TABLE 11–12 Modulators of Vascular Resistance

Increase systemic vascular resistance
  Light anesthesia
  α-Adrenergic agents (particularly phenylephrine diluted to 10 µg/mL for smaller children, dose 1–4 µg/kg)
Decrease systemic vascular resistance (rarely needed)
  Nitroprusside
Increase pulmonary vascular resistance
  Hypoxia
  Hypercarbia
  Low fraction of inspired oxygen
  Acidosis
  High mean airway pressure
  α-Adrenergic agents
  Hypervolemia
  Lung collapse or loss of functional residual capacity
Decrease pulmonary vascular resistance
  Hypocarbia
  β-Adrenergic agents
  Nitroglycerine
  Nitric oxide
  Prostaglandin E_1

TABLE 11–13 Vascular Access Considerations

Femoral vein thrombosis or ligation from prior cardiac catheterization
Anatomic discontinuity of inferior vena cava and right atrium (particularly with polysplenia syndrome)
Reduced lower extremity blood pressure with coarctation (left arm is variable)
Discontinuity of subclavian artery with classic Blalock–Taussig anastomosis or stenosis of subclavian artery after modified Blalock–Taussig anastomosis
Artifactually elevated right arm blood pressure with supravalvar aortic stenosis

---

ease, even cyanotic congenital heart disease, is not an indication for invasive arterial or central venous monitoring.

Measures of end-tidal CO_2 correlate well with those of arterial partial pressure of carbon dioxide (P_{CO_2}) in acyanotic patients. However, in children and adults with cyanotic congenital heart disease, end-tidal P_{CO_2} tends to underestimate arterial P_{CO_2} in patients with normal, decreased, or increased total pulmonary blood flow.[10]

It would be uncommon these days to encounter a patient with uncorrected, unpalliated tetralogy of Fallot requiring noncardiac surgery. These children should have had some type of surgical repair, either total correction or an aortopulmonary shunt such as a Blalock-Taussig (subclavian artery to ipsilateral pulmonary artery) or a central (ascending aorta to main pulmonary artery) shunt, as soon as there was evidence of pulmonary stenosis. Nevertheless, hypercyanotic "tet" spells are a dangerous and potentially fatal complication of anesthesia in these patients, and even the first spell has the potential to be very severe. The treatment of these patients is delineated in Table 11-14.

POSTOPERATIVE CARE

Patients with congenital heart disease clearly need close observation in the postanesthesia care unit (PACU). The specific period of observation depends on the patient and the surgical procedure and cannot be generalized. Patients with good hemodynamic function who undergo relatively minor noncardiac surgery are not specifically excluded from ambulatory surgery.

Patients with cyanotic disease, it must be remembered, have little increase in systemic oxygen saturation in response to supplemental oxygen. Similarly, their oxygen saturation will not be markedly decreased by removing supplemental oxygen (other causes for postoperative hypoxemia being absent). Those caring for these children in the PACU should be aware of this, lest the PACU stay be needlessly prolonged for fear of removing supplemental oxygen in the face of a lower than normal oxygen saturation, which may be the baseline for these patients.

TABLE 11–14 Treatment of Hypercyanotic "Tet" Spells

100% oxygen (O_2 alone will have little effect)
Phenylephrine 1–4 µg/kg
Esmolol 100–200 µg/(kg · min) or propranolol 0.1 mg/kg
Aortic compression to increase systemic vascular resistance (raising knees to knee-to-chest position)
Parenteral sedation or deepen anesthesia with nonvasodilating anesthetic (halothane, ketamine)
Emergent aortopulmonary shunt or definitive repair as last resort

Hypovolemia, not infrequently encountered postoperatively, may worsen right-to-left shunting in cyanotic patients and should be rapidly corrected. The onset of hypovolemia may be insidious if it is due to gradual oozing from surgical drains. Cyanotic patients should have hematocrit levels measured serially after surgery, especially after significant blood loss. They may require a higher than normal hematocrit level. In general, they should be maintained at a level similar to the preoperative hematocrit level.

Congenital heart disease does not contraindicate good postoperative pain relief. In fact, good analgesia may be particularly important. Even cyanotic patients have a normal, ventilatory response to hypercarbia and will respond appropriately to appropriate doses of parenteral, intrathecal, or epidural opiates. Patients with labile pulmonary arterial hypertension in particular benefit from good postoperative analgesia. Patients who have had a Glenn or Fontan procedure are dependent on low pulmonary vascular resistance, and, if such patients should require postoperative ventilation, pulmonary vascular resistance should be minimized by limiting positive inspiratory pressure and using low levels of PEEP to optimize functional residual capacity, which in turn lowers pulmonary vascular resistance.

Children with elevations in pulmonary vascular resistance and hypertrophy of the pulmonary vascular musculature may develop life-threatening episodes of acute pulmonary vasoconstriction or pulmonary hypertensive crises. These are much more common after cardiac surgery. An in-depth discussion of postoperative ventilation of children with congenital heart disease can be found elsewhere.[11]

REFERENCES

1. Baum VC, Perloff JK: Anesthetic implications of adults with congenital heart disease. *Anesth Analg* 76:1342, 1993.
2. Baum VC: The adult patient with congenital heart disease. *J Cardiothorac Vasc Anesth* 10:261, 1996.
3. Frankville DD: Anesthesia for noncardiac surgery in children and adults with congenital heart disease. In *Pediatric Cardiac Anesthesia,* 3rd ed. Lake CL, ed. Stamford, Appleton & Lange, 1998, p 601.
4. Dajani AS, Taubert KA, Wilson W, et al: Prevention of bacterial endocarditis. Recommendations by the American Heart Association. *JAMA* 277:1794, 1997.
5. Strafford MA, Henderson KH: Anesthetic morbidity in congenital heart disease patients undergoing non-cardiac surgery [abstract]. *Anesthesiology* 75:A1056, 1991.
6. Tanner GE, Angers DG, Barash PG, et al: Effect of left-to-right, mixed left-to-right, and right-to-left shunts on inhalational anesthetic induction in children: a computer model. *Anesth Analg* 64:101, 1985.
7. Laishley RS, Burrows FA, Lerman J, et al: Effect of anesthetic induction regimens on oxygen saturation in cyanotic congenital heart disease. *Anesthesiology* 65:673, 1986.
8. Hickey PR, Hansen DD, Strafford M, et al: Pulmonary and systemic hemodynamic effects of nitrous oxide in infants with normal and elevated pulmonary vascular resistance. *Anesthesiology* 65:374, 1986.
9. Greeley WJ, Bushman GA, Davis DP, et al.: Comparative effects of halothane and ketamine on systemic arterial oxygen saturation in children with cyanotic heart disease. *Anesthesiology* 65:666, 1986.
10. Burrows FA: Physiologic dead space, venous admixture, and the arterial to end-tidal carbon dioxide difference in infants and children undergoing cardiac surgery. *Anesthesiology* 70:219, 1989.
11. Willson DF, Baum VC: Postoperative respiratory function and its management. In Pediatric Cardiac Anesthesia, 3rd ed. Lake CL, ed. Stamford, Appleton & Lange, 1998, p 577.

12 | Dysrhythmias in the Pediatric Patient

Denise Joffe, MD

Dysrhythmias are rare in the pediatric population. Dysrhythmias in pediatric patients may be secondary to congenital or acquired diseases or occur in patients with normal hearts. The most frequent cause of intraoperative rhythm disturbances in children is related to anesthetic technique. However, with advances in the surgical management of children with congenital heart disease, more pediatric cardiac patients with arrhythmias will present for noncardiac surgery. Fortunately, many of these patients have had early neonatal repair of their heart disease. This is thought to decrease the risk of some arrhythmias by reducing the time the heart in the pediatric cardiac patient is exposed to pressure, volume overload, and cyanosis.[1,2] In addition, new techniques are being used to treat intractable arrhythmias and it is important to be familiar with related complications of the underlying arrhythmia and the treatments used.

In general, the types of rhythm disturbances are similar in pediatric and adult patients, although their prevalence differs.[3] For example, ventricular arrhythmias, ventricular fibrillation in particular, are uncommon in very young patients. In addition, atrial fibrillation is uncommon in small children because the small atrial size cannot support the electrophysiologic requirements for atrial fibrillation. Further, pediatric patients are more likely than adult patients to tolerate the hemodynamic effects from prolonged episodes of tachycardia. However, the cumulative effects of tachyarrhythmias often lead to the development of secondary cardiomyopathies.[4,5]

DYSRHYTHMIAS IN PATIENTS WITH CONGENITAL HEART DISEASE

Dysrhythmias in patients with congenital heart disease can develop as a result of inverted cardiac looping, interruption of the conduction system, or abnormal coronary blood flow patterns. These factors alter the normal conduction characteristics of the heart. The most common rhythm disturbances are first-, second-, and third-degree atrioventricular (AV) block, pre-excitation syndromes, or sinoatrial and AV node dysfunctions.[3] Dysrhythmias also can occur after surgical repair of congenital heart disease. Although there is a large spectrum of complex lesions, some are quite common (Table 12-1).[6] In these cases, it is often the method of surgical repair that causes the dysrhythmia.

Understanding which postoperative dysrhythmias are induced often allows one to extrapolate whether a given procedure is likely to result in a problem. Atrial manipulation and cannulation during cardiopulmonary bypass for any repair may lead to sinus node damage and result in sinus node dysfunction. Although most patients recover function, some do not and require pacemaker implantation. Incisions or sutures can interrupt normal conduction pathways. Incisions also might isolate areas of myocardium and create a nidus for re-entry, which is a precursor for the development of arrhythmias.[7]

These dysrhythmias do not always occur immediately postoperatively. Distention, scarring, and suture interruption of conduction tissue can lead to

TABLE 12–1 Incidence of Various Congenital Heart Defects at Boston Children's Hospital Over a 14-Year Period*

Diagnosis (1973–1987)	n Patients
Ventricular septal defect	3322
Pulmonary valve abnormality	1500
Tetralogy of Fallot	1403
Aortic valve abnormality	1060
Secundum atrial septal defect	891
Patent ductus arteriosus	866
Coarctation of the aorta	826
D-loop transposition	755
Endocardial cushion defect	717
Ventricular dysfunction	369
Malposition (heterotaxy)	335
Mitral valve abnormality	296
Hypoplastic left ventricle	287
Double-outlet right ventricle	224
Single ventricle	192
Tricuspid atresia	154
Pulmonary hypertension	135
Total anomalous pulmonary venous return	118
Pericardial abnormality	111
Truncus arteriosus	107
Rheumatic fever or rheumatic heart disease	102
L-loop transposition	90
Pulmonary atresia and intact ventricular septum	83
Systemic hypertension	76
Tricuspid valve abnormality	76
Ebstein's disease	75
Systemic artery anomaly	70
Systemic arteriovenous fistula	34
Cardiac tumor	32
Anomalous coronary artery from pulmonary artery	29
Aortopulmonary window	19
Origin of right pulmonary artery from aorta	10
Aneurysm, artery	13
Primary arrhythmia	883
Bicuspid aortic valve	71
Mitral valve prolapse	367
Patent foramen ovale	65
Questionable heart disease	63
No significant heart disease	6743
Noncardiac anomaly	577
No data[†]	466
Total	23,612

*Each patient listed once.
[†]A file was begun but no data entered.
Source: Reproduced with permission from Fyler DC: Trends. In *Nadas' Pediatric Cardiology.* Fyler DC, ed. Philadelphia, Hanley & Belfus, 1992.

the development of late dysrhythmias via mechanisms similar to those described above. After surgery, areas of myocardium may become fibrotic and generate foci of irritable tissue. Patients with suboptimal repairs are also at increased risk of developing arrhythmias because of factors such as poor myocardial function, persistent volume and pressure overload, cyanosis, and ischemia. In some patients, acute changes in cardiac filling or medications given during an anesthetic may induce rhythm disturbances.

ACQUIRED DYSRHYTHMIAS IN THE PEDIATRIC PATIENT

Acquired dysrhythmias in pediatric patients are often drug induced or related to metabolic or hemodynamic derangements. Other less common etiologies include endocrinologic problems (pheochromocytomas, thyroid disease), neoplasm, and infectious (myocarditis) and intracranial pathologies.

The most common acquired dysrhythmias seen in the operating room are induced by anesthetic technique or surgical manipulation. They are the direct result of medications or physiologic changes and abnormalities that are induced by administration of anesthesia. Pediatric patients are particularly sensitive to parasympathetic stimulation because of the minimal contribution the sympathetic nervous system makes to their autonomic control.

Almost all the agents commonly administered during anesthesia have been reported to cause rhythm disturbances.

Inhaled agents such as enflurane, halothane, and isoflurane exert a direct negative chronotropic effect on the sinoatrial and AV nodes.[8,9] Halothane has been reported to cause bradycardia in 0.16% to 30% of cases.[10] Isoflurane has less of an effect on the node than enflurane or halothane.[8] Sevoflurane and desflurane share many hemodynamic similarities with isoflurane and probably have a similar effect on the sinoatrial node. The routine administration of intravenous atropine to prevent untoward effects of the inhaled agents at induction of anesthesia probably is not necessary in healthy pediatric patients, especially in view of the marked increase in use of sevoflurane. A survey conducted in Australia suggests that most anesthesiologists no longer regularly administer atropine to most pediatric patients younger than 1 year, although approximately 55% give atropine to neonates.[11] The inhaled agents also alter the conduction characteristics of the myocardium, thus setting up conditions required for re-entrant ventricular dysrhythmias. All of the inhaled agents have been reported to cause premature ventricular contractions (PVCs), ventricular tachycardia, and ventricular fibrillation.[8,12,13]

Hypercarbia exacerbates the arrythmogenic effects of halothane.[14] The inhaled anesthetics, in particular halothane, have been shown to sensitize the myocardium to epinephrine.[15,16] Atrioventricular dysrhythmias (junctional rhythms) also occur with all the inhaled agents. The incidence of ventricular arrhythmias (extrasystoles, bigeminy, and ventricular tachycardia) induced by inhaled agents is up to 40%.[13]

Local anesthetics, especially bupivacaine, have been implicated in causing ventricular fibrillation that is resistant to conventional treatment. Bretylium is reported to be the antiarrhythmic agent of choice in treating bupivacaine toxicity.[17] Other studies have shown that amiodarone also may have a role in the management of bupivacaine-induced arrhythmias.[18] The recent introduction of ropivacaine may decrease the toxicity risk of local anesthetics in the pediatric population. In some cases, the epinephrine that is often used with the local agent to prolong the effect of anesthesia and serve as a marker of intravascular injection has been implicated in causing life-threatening ventricular dysrhythmias after accidental intravenous injection.[19] Paradoxically, it has also been reported to cause relative bradycardia.[20] Of note, the doses of epinephrine used with the local anesthetics are, if given intravenously, about 50 times what one would administer clinically for inotropic support.

Succinylcholine has been reported to cause bradycardia, especially after a second dose. In the past, it was standard practice to pretreat pediatric patients with atropine because of their propensity to develop bradycardia even after a single dose of succinylcholine. However, a study of 41 healthy patients ages 1 to 12 years suggests it is probably unnecessary to administer atropine if only a single dose of succinylcholine is given.[21] Of course, succinylcholine has resulted in hyperkalemic arrests when administered to patients with underlying myopathies.[22] Its use also has been implicated in causing sinus tachycardia and ventricular arrhythmias, including ventricular tachycardia.[23,24]

During an anesthetic, it is important to view ectopy as a warning sign. The adequacy of oxygenation and ventilation are foremost on the checklist. An inadequate depth of anesthesia in addition to the type and quantity of surgical stimuli also should be evaluated. Pharmacologic therapy should always be suspect. A review of the patient's history and underlying medical problems is also crucial to the appropriate diagnosis and management of intraoperative rhythm disturbances.

COMMON DYSRHYTHMIAS IN THE PEDIATRIC POPULATION

Although any rhythm disturbance can be seen in the adult and pediatric populations, there are some that are more prevalent in the pediatric population, mostly because of cardiac developmental issues. Many will not be common in the intraoperative setting but will be presented briefly because of their uniqueness to the pediatric patient.

Atrial Dysrhythmias

Premature Atrial Contractions

Isolated premature atrial contractions are most common in infants and young children. They are usually benign but should be investigated if they are complex (originate from multiple foci) or symptomatic. Premature atrial contractions are often the initiating impulse for atrial tachycardias.[3]

Junctional Ectopic Tachycardia

This rhythm is seen almost exclusively in the postoperative cardiac patient, particularly those with procedures performed near the AV junction. It results from increased automaticity of the AV node or proximal His-Purkinje system (Figures 12-1 and 12-2A). Junctional ectopic tachycardia can be very difficult to treat and often causes severe cardiac compromise in these patients. However, it is a transient phenomenon and does not recur after the immediate postoperative period.[2,3]

Ectopic Atrial Tachycardia

This rhythm accounts for 5% to 20% of atrial tachycardias. It is thought to result from abnormal automaticity in a single nonsinus atrial focus (Figure 12-2B). Rates are usually between 100 and 280 beats per minute and the electrocardiogram is characterized by an abnormal p-wave morphology. This rhythm is often incessant and results in the development of ventricular dysfunction. It does not respond well to antiarrythmic therapy, electric car-

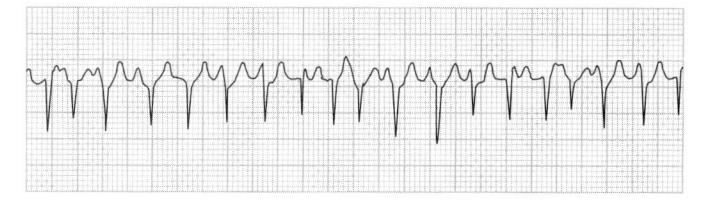

FIG. 12-1 Electrocardiogram from a patient with junctional ectopic tachycardia. The ventricular rate is faster than the atrial rate (*arrows* indicate atrial activity). *(Reproduced with permission from Walsh EP, Saul JP: Cardiac arrythmias. In* Nadas' Pediatric Cardiology. *Fyler DC, ed. Philadelphia, Hanley & Belfus, 1992.)*

dioversion, or surgery. Catheter ablation has been the most successful intervention for the treatment of this rhythm.[3,25]

Paroxysmal Supraventricular Atrial Tachycardia (PSVT)

The most common etiologies of PSVT in children are preexcitation syndromes secondary to an accessory pathway or AV nodal re-entrant tachycardias. Ninety percent of episodes of infant PSVT are related to an accessory pathway, in contrast to the adolescent, in whom the etiology of PSVT is AV node re-entry in up to 30% of patients.[25,26] The mechanism of AV node re-entry is similar to that in the adult patient. It involves two discrete conduction pathways in the AV node (or in close proximity to the node), with different conduction velocities and refractory periods. An appropriately timed premature beat can start circular conduction in the node that perpetuates a tachycardia (Figure 12-2F).

Tachycardia in patients with preexcitation syndromes are often referred to as AV reciprocating tachycardias. They are also described according to the direction of conduction through the accessory pathway during a tachycardia: orthodromic reciprocating tachycardia implies retrograde conduction through the accessory pathway, and antidromic reciprocating tachycardia implies antegrade conduction through the accessory pathway. In both cases, the other limb of the "circuit" is the AV node (Figures 12-2C and 12-2D). The mechanism is the same as that for AV node re-entry but the circuit is longer. The most common preexcitation syndromes are Wolff–Parkinson–White (WPW), concealed accessory pathways and Lown–Ganong–Levine.[3] They are due to one or more accessory pathways. Although accessory pathways are not unique to the pediatric population, many patients with congenital heart disease are at increased risk of having them. Patients with Ebstein's malformation, congenitally corrected transposition of the great arteries, AV canal defects, and tricuspid atresia have an incidence of accessory pathways up to 9%.[3] Patients with structurally normal hearts also may have bypass tracts. The conduction characteristics of the accessory pathway determines the pathophysiologic response to supraventricular tachycardias. Although infants usually have anterograde and retrograde conduction through their tracts, in 40% of cases, anterograde conduction disappears by age 1 year. Other patients have complete regression of bypass conduction in any direction altogether.[27] Regression of bypass conduction is supported by the clinical presentation of many patients. Patients with PSVT who present during infancy have a greater than 50% chance of being arrhythmia free after their first year of life. In contrast, patients who present later

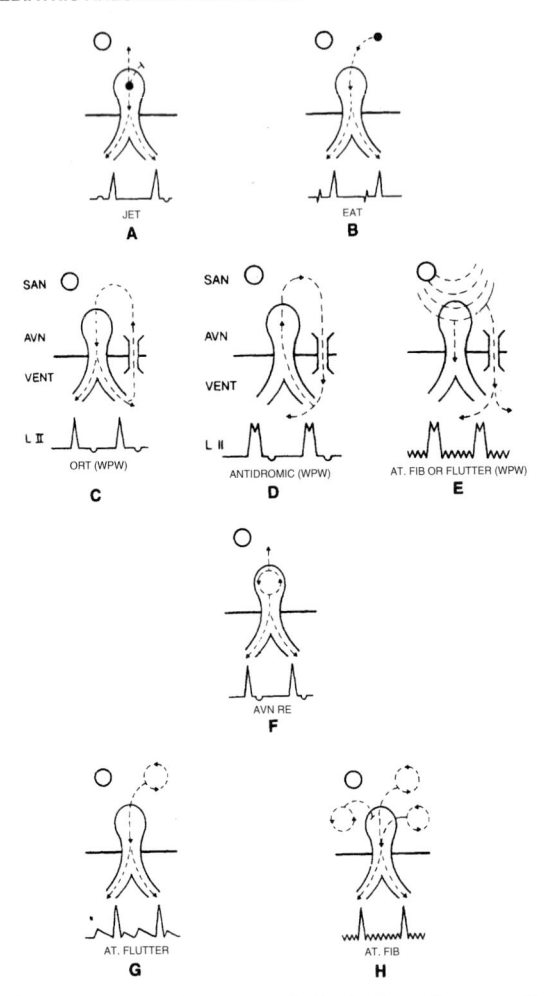

FIG. 12-2 Mechanisms of supraventricular tachycardia generation. JET, junctional ectopic tachycardia; EAT, ectopic atrial tachycardia; ORT, orthodromic reciprocating tachycardia in Wolf–Parkinson–White syndrome; AT FIB, atrial fibrillation; AT Flutter, atrial flutter; AVN REAV node re-entrant tachycardia. *(Reproduced with permission from Walsh EP, Saul JP: Cardiac arrythmias. In Nadas' Pediatric Cardiology. Fyler DC, ed. Philadelphia, Hanley & Belfus, 1992.)*

in life (after age 5 years) have a 78% incidence of recurrent episodes of PSVT.[27]

Older patients may have changing modes of conduction during sinus rhythm and tachycardias. Anterograde conduction in patients with WPW produces wide QRS complexes and in sinus rhythm also has the classic short PR interval and δ-wave (Figure 12-3). Approximately 0.2% to 0.3%[28] of the

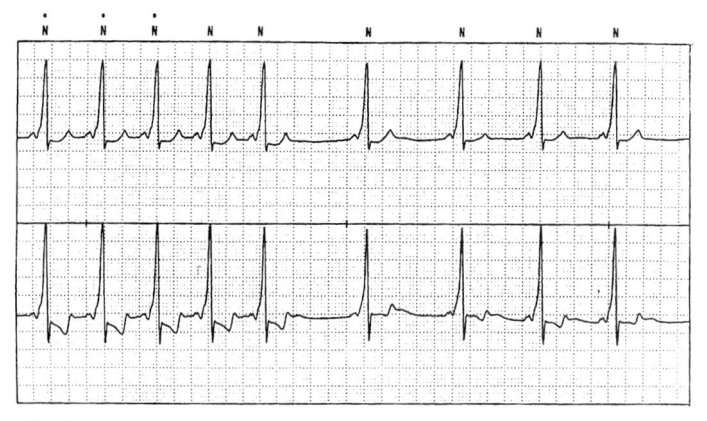

FIG. 12-3 Electrocardiogram in a patient with Wolf–Parkinson–White syndrome. Note the short PR interval, the δ-wave, and the wide QRS complex.

normal population have bypass tracts diagnosed by electrocardiography, although patients who have retrograde-only conduction (concealed accessory pathway) cannot be diagnosed by electrocardiography. Only 5% of patients develop anterograde conduction via the accessory pathway during an episode of tachycardia (antidromic AV reciprocating tachycardia)[26] (Figure 12-4). In these patients, retrograde conduction through the AV node completes the circuit and promulgates the dysrhythmia. In most patients, conduction occurs normally, or antegrade, through the AV node and retrograde through the bypass tract (orthodromic AV reciprocating tachycardia).

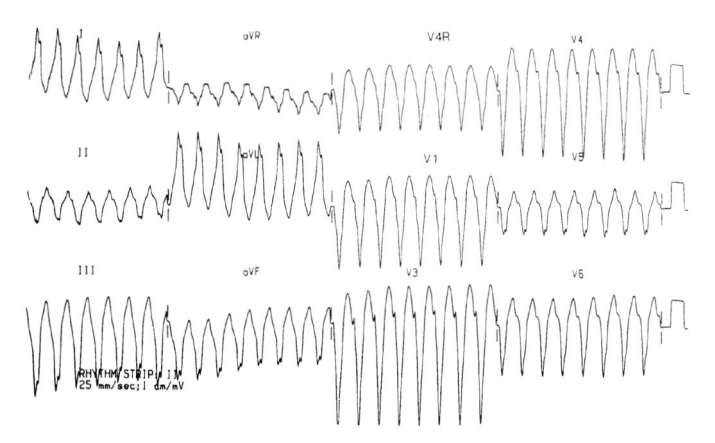

FIG. 12-4 Electrocardiogram from a patient with Wolf–Parkinson–White syndrome and antidromic reciprocating tachycardia. The QRS complexes are wide and similar in morphology to the patient's complexes in sinus rhythm. Patients may conduct differently during sinus rhythm than during tachycardias.

Patients who have the capacity for rapid anterograde conduction through an accessory pathway are at risk of developing malignant dysrhythmias (ventricular tachycardia and ventricular fibrillation) during episodes of atrial fibrillation and flutter because of the likelihood of 1:1 conduction through the tract. During atrial flutter or fibrillation, the accessory pathway and the AV node are "bombarded" with impulses. Most impulses conduct through the accessory pathway because of its greater conduction velocity. Any impulses that conduct through the AV node result in a decrease in heart rate because the AV node can slow conduction. Anterograde conduction can occur during atrial fibrillation even in patients who usually develop orthodromic tachycardias (Figure 12-2E). Except for young infants, patients with WPW are also at greater risk of developing atrial fibrillation than the general population.[29] This has critical implications for the natural history and treatment of these patients. Medications that decrease AV node conduction, such as digoxin and verapamil, increase the chance of 1:1 conduction through the accessory pathway because the AV node no longer can serve to interrupt impulses. These medications also can increase the velocity of conduction in the accessory pathway. For these reasons, they are contraindicated as chronic therapy in WPW and as acute therapy of atrial fibrillation in WPW.

Ideally, a cardiologist should be consulted when managing these patients. Many patients will have had electrophysiologic studies that can describe the conduction characteristics of their accessory pathways. The cardiologist can recommend a treatment regimen based on the results of those studies.

In general, if a patient with an accessory pathway develops a narrow complex tachycardia, the arrhythmia can be treated acutely as though a bypass tract did not exist (see treatment of PSVT).[3,25,26] Wide complex tachycardias in these patients can be treated in the same fashion because the AV node is a necessary part of the circuit.[3,25,26] However, drugs that decrease AV node conduction are contraindicated in any patient with WPW who develops atrial flutter or fibrillation. If hemodynamic compromise is present, cardioversion is used; if the patient is hemodynamically stable, procainamide is probably the most effective drug for the treatment of atrial flutter or fibrillation in the presence of WPW. A short-acting β-blocker such as esmolol also can be tried because it reduces conduction in the accessory pathway.[3,25,26] However, these treatment plans should be applied only to patients with known accessory pathways. Wide complex tachycardias always should be treated as ventricular tachycardia if the patient's history is not clear.

The management of PSVT depends on the patient's hemodynamic condition.[3,25,26] Unstable patients with acute PSVT should be cardioverted with 0.25 to 2 J/kg. Stable patients can have vagal maneuvers attempted. Ice or cold water applied to the face is successful in up to 62% of cases. Adenosine in doses of 100 µg/kg repeated up to 350 µg/kg can be used. Its mechanism of action is slowing AV conduction. Although adenosine has a 15-s half-life, it can cause serious adverse side effects in up to 10% of patients (atrial fibrillation, episodes of apnea or bronchospasm, asystole, and ventricular dysrhythmias).[30] Verapamil is an alternative therapy for PSVT termination. However, it should be used with extreme caution, if at all, in patients younger than 2 years because of reported episodes of death due to congestive heart failure.[31] Digoxin, edrophonium, esmolol, propanolol, and phenylephrine also have been used for patients of all ages with PSVT, but there are serious drawbacks to these agents.[3,25,26] Procainamide has been touted as a useful drug for these patients.[2] Some investigators have suggested that cardioversion or overdrive atrial pacing (transesophageal) should be attempted early, even in the hemodynamically stable patient, if adenosine or esmolol fail to restore normal rhythm.[2]

Long-term therapy options for treatment of recurrent PSVT include watchful waiting, medications, and radiofrequency ablation.[3,25,26] Many patients with infrequent episodes of tachycardia manage without medications and often terminate dysrhythmias on their own with vagal maneuvers. In other patients, multiple medication regimens have been tried, including amiodarone. Surgical interruption of the bypass tract and radiofrequency ablation are other options. A recent study associated radiofrequency ablation of accessory pathways with the highest success rate of ablation procedures (96%).[32] The incidence of serious complications was 1.2% and included cardiac perforation, complete heart block, ventricular dysfunction, cerebrovascular accidents, and death.

Atrial Fibrillation and Atrial Flutter

Atrial flutter is often referred to as *atrial re-entrant tachycardia*. Atrial flutter is due to a single re-entrant circuit in the atrium and atrial fibrillation is due to many small re-entrant circuits in the atrium[3] (Figures 12-2G and 12-2H). In the pediatric patient, the classic saw-tooth pattern of atrial flutter with an atrial rhythm of 300 beats per minute is often absent. Changing p-wave morphologies and atrial rates between 180 and 400 beats per minute can be observed with atrial flutter.[3] In addition, a regular atrial rate and abrupt initiation of the dysrhythmia, which are classic findings in the adult, will also be found in the child. The ventricular response can be 1:1, although it can change over time (Figure 12-5). Rapid 1:1 conduction can occur in normal patients without a bypass tract and with an intact AV node.[3,33] Atrial flutter is a common dysrhythmia in postoperative cardiac patients if the sinus node is injured. It also occurs less commonly in patients with normal hearts. In older children atrial flutter usually is associated with congenital heart disease, whereas neonates with atrial flutter often have normal hearts.[33] Diseases causing atrial dilatation and involving significant surgical manipulation of the atrium are most associated with the dysrhythmia. Atrial switch procedures (Mustard and Senning operations) and the Fontan procedure have inci-

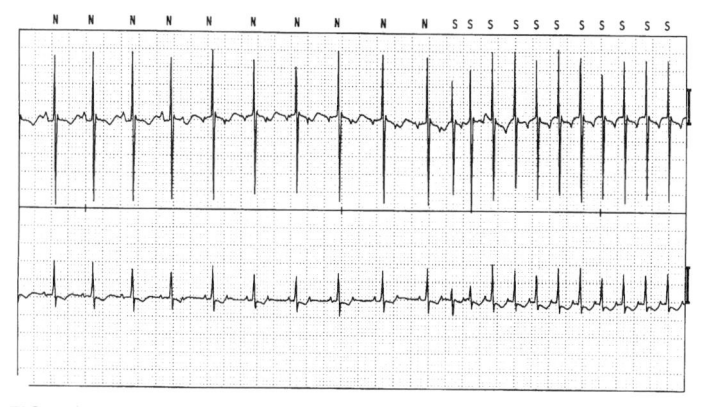

FIG. 12-5 Electrocardiogram from a patient with variable conduction during atrial flutter. It varies from 2:1 to 1:1 conduction.

dences of atrial flutter of up to 50% at 12 years.[2,3,34] Patients with different cardiomyopathies (especially hypertrophic and dilated) have an increased incidence of atrial fibrillation (about 16%).[35]

Acute termination of atrial flutter often requires cardioversion or overdrive atrial pacing because medications frequently are not successful in terminating the dysrhythmia.[2,3,25,26] Chronic therapy is considered necessary in patients with congenital heart disease because as many as 40% of them have been shown to have periods of 1:1 conduction during atrial flutter.[2] In addition, there is a four times greater incidence of sudden death in patients in whom recurrent episodes of atrial flutter could not be prevented.[36] Chronic therapy has consisted mostly of antiarrhythmic medications, despite their significant side effects. Propanolol and digoxin will at least slow AV conduction in the event of a recurrence; more recently, sotalol and amiodarone have been used to prevent recurrences.[2,25] Atrial antitachycardia pacing can be successful in some patients, although technical factors related to complex arrhythmia detection requirements often preclude its use.[37] Radiofrequency ablation has been used in patients with success and it will likely become a more common procedure because it avoids the need for long-term medication in children. However, ablation is technically difficult or impossible in patients with certain surgical repairs, such as the Fontan procedure, and ablation is associated with high recurrence rates of arrhythmias in those patients.[36] Atrial fibrillation is treated in a similar fashion to atrial flutter, except that overdrive pacing is not effective in terminating the dysrhythmia.[3,25,26]

Ventricular Dysrhythmias

Premature Ventricular Contractions

Unifocal, asymptomatic PVCs are generally considered benign especially in a patient with a heart known to be normal. When PVCs occur in a patient with congenital heart disease, are multifocal, occur in salvos of more than two, occur on the T wave (R on T), or increase with exercise, they should be investigated.[3] Extensive noninvasive evaluation should be performed in these patients to identify treatable causes. Also suspect are PVCs occurring in patients with systemic illness or electrolyte abnormalities and in patients on medications or using recreational drugs. Studies have shown that only 1% of normal infants have PVCs, whereas 50% to 60% of normal young adults and teenagers have them.[38,39] This suggests that this form of ectopy is probably less of a concern in the older child.

Ventricular Tachycardia (VT)

This dysrhythmia is much less common than supraventricular tachycardia in the pediatric patient. It is defined as three or more ventricular beats occuring at a rate of greater than 120 beats per minute. Symptomatic patients are more likely to have underlying heart disease (tetralogy of Fallot, myocarditis, and mitral valve prolapse), a ventricular rate exceeding 150 beats per minute, and an increase in the degree of ventricular dysrhythmias with exercise.[40,41] Although controversial, in one study mitral valve prolapse was reported to be the most frequent underlying condition associated with ventricular tachycardia.[40]

Ventricular tachycardia in the neonate falls into one of two categories: benign or malignant. In the benign category are accelerated idiopathic ventricular rhythm (a stable rhythm that does not require therapy) and many myocardial tumor-induced VTs (these do require therapy). In the neonate, malignant VTs are associated with myocarditis, long QT syndrome, and myocardial infarction (neonatal myocardial infarctions are usually the result of abnormalities of coronary artery development or maternal cocaine abuse).[42]

Ventricular tachycardia is frequently associated with congenital heart disease. For example, a strong association is present between ventricular tachycardia and tetralogy of Fallot and ventricular septal defect repair.[3,41] Patients with a history of left ventricular outflow tract obstruction are also at increased risk of developing postoperative VT, even after successful relief of the obstruction.[1] Left ventricular outflow tract obstruction induces left ventricular hypertrophy and chronic pressure overload, which predisposes the patient to develop ventricular arrhythmias.

Ventricular tachycardia after repair of tetralogy of Fallot occurs in 0% to 6% of patients.[43] Ventricular tachycardia may occur decades after the surgical repair. Multiple factors have been shown to increase the incidence of sudden death, including age at repair, right ventricular pressure and volume overload, a prior large systemic-to-pulmonary shunt, the presence of complex ventricular ectopy, and a transannular patch used for repair.[43] The dysrhythmias seem to be caused by macro re-entry circuits in the right ventricular outflow tract. Because this group of patients has a significant risk of developing ventricular dysrhythmias, most institutions recommend frequent (every 1 to 3 years) cardiac evaluations for life.[2,3] Although there is some controversy about which of these patients should be treated medically, there is increasing evidence that catheter ablation and internal cardioverter defibrillator placement are very effective in terminating malignant VT in this group.[2,3]

Long QT Syndrome

Long QT syndrome can be congenital or acquired, and it is characterized by an increase in the corrected QT interval.

Congenital long QT occurs in four forms. Three variants occur as an inherited disease and one variant occurs as a spontaneous mutation. In all forms, patients generally present at a young age with a history of syncope or sudden death. About 30% of patients have associated congenital deafness. When present in young patients, there is often relative bradycardia (70 to 90 beats per minute) and various forms of AV block. Any form of dysrhythmia may occur: the most common are torsade de pointes ventricular tachycardia, ventricular fibrillation, and asystole.[44] Torsade de pointes is characterized by a pattern of positive and negative oscillations of the QRS direction, which twists around the isoelectric point (Figure 12-6). It often terminates spontaneously. Often the attacks are induced by exercise or stress.[45] A group of patients may have a normal resting QT interval that increases only with stress or exercise.[45] Although the etiology of the syndrome is not certain, the most popular theory suggests that it results from asymmetric adrenergic stimulus in the heart. Recently, a large majority of these patients have also been shown to have long pauses in their cardiac cycle before the induction of torsade de pointes. These pauses are thought to provide the electrophysiologic requirements necessary for torsade.[46,47]

Untreated congenital long QT syndrome results in high mortality rates and is a primary cause of sudden death in the pediatric population. β-Adrenergic blockers are the treatment of choice, but a combination of medical therapy and pacemakers is necessary to treat some patients.[3] Calcium channel blockers, phenytoin, controlled hyperkalemia, and stellate ganglion blocks (surgical or medical) have been used with variable success.[44,46,48,49]

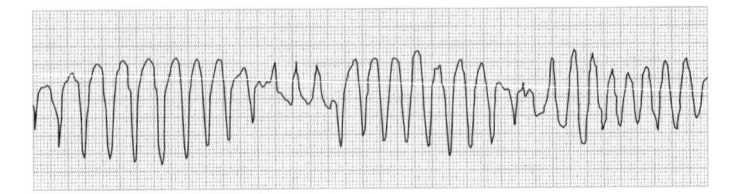

FIG. 12-6 Torsade de pointes has a distinctive appearance that must be recognized. Some antiarrythmics (especially procainamide) will lengthen the QT interval and worsen the arrhythmia. *(Reproduced with permission from Walsh EP, Saul JP: Cardiac arrythmias. In* Nadas' Pediatric Cardiology. *Fyler DC, ed. Philadelphia, Hanley & Belfus, 1992.)*

Anesthetic management of patients with congenital long QT syndrome should consist of ensuring adequate β-blockade preoperatively and preventing adrenergic stimulation. Factors that increase the QT interval such as hypothermia, electrolyte abnormalities, and some medications should be avoided. Stimulating the adrenergic nervous system with agents such as atropine, ketamine, and pancuronium presumably can induce arrhythmias. Most of the inhaled agents prolong the QT interval, although some studies suggest that halothane decreases it.[50] However, inhaled agents usually are used without complication. Treatment of intraoperative dysrhythmias consists of additional doses of β-blockers, phenytoin, or verapamil. Lidocaine and bretylium also can be used, although procainamide is contraindicated because it increases the QT interval. Discontinuing the inhaled agent should be considered. Ventricular tachycardia is treated with a precordial thump and cardioversion.[3,44]

The acquired version of the long QT syndrome can be caused by electrolyte abnormalities (hypomagnesemia or hypocalcemia), exposure to certain medications (antiarrhythmics, antipsychotics, and most recently cisapride have been shown to increase the QT interval and have caused VT[51]), neurologic and endocrine abnormalities. The electrophysiologic mechanism of VT induction in the acquired long QT syndrome is thought to be the result of pauses in the cardiac cycle, as in congenital long QT syndrome.[47]

Congenital and acquired long QT syndrome must be distinguished because their treatments differ. β-Blockers increase the QT interval in normal patients and patients with acquired long QT syndrome. Isoproterenol is used to decrease the interval in patients with acquired long QT syndrome but is contraindicated in patients with congenital long QT syndrome. Although any underlying physiologic abnormality should be corrected in patients with acquired long QT syndrome, isoproterenol, atropine, magnesium sulfate, ventricular pacing, and cardioversion may be necessary to treat unstable dysrhythmias. Recently, the use of magnesium sulfate, even in patients with normal magnesium levels, has been recommended as first-line therapy in patients with the acquired long QT syndrome. Some investigators have even suggested it may be useful in congenital long QT syndrome.[52] The recommended dosing regimen in adults is 2 g over 2 to 3 min and an infusion of 2 to 4 mg/min. Three repeat boluses of the same dose and an increase in the infusion rate to 6 to 8 mg/min is given for recurrences.[52] The dosage range for pediatric patients is not well established. One group recommends a dose of 25 mg/kg given over 15 min.[2]

Bradydysrhythmias

This category includes patients with sick sinus syndrome, sinus node dysfunction, and abnormalities in AV conduction, congenital or postoperative.[53] Conduction defects are inherent components of some congenital heart lesions such as Ebstein's anomaly and congenitally corrected transposition of the great arteries. Procedures most likely to result in postoperative sinus node dysfunction are those that require extensive atrial baffling such as the Mustard, Senning, and Fontan procedures.[2,3,7] Sick sinus syndrome is characterized by slow and irregular sinus rates with a variety of escape rhythms and episodes of atrial fibrillation and atrial flutter. Symptomatic patients may require pacemaker implantation and suppressive medical therapy for the tachydysrhythmias. Some patients may be candidates for atrial antitachycardia pacemakers.[2,3]

The etiology of congenital complete heart block includes congenital heart diseases such as AV canal and ventricular inversion. Fetal exposure to maternal antibodies as in lupus occurs in another large percentage of patients. Patients with congenital complete heart block who are symptomatic or who have prolonged pauses require pacemaker insertion. Neonates with ventricular rates less than 50 beats per minute or who develop cardiomegaly or symptoms of congestive heart failure also require pacemaker insertion.[54]

In general, postoperative cardiac patients who have not recovered from a symptomatic bradydysrhythmia after 10 to 14 days require pacing.[2,3] This category includes patients with third-degree AV block and Mobitz type II AV block. Data for other categories are less clear and electrophysiologic studies are often used to assist in decision-making.

IMPLANTABLE PACEMAKERS AND CARDIOVERTER-DEFIBRILLATORS

In the pediatric population, antitachycardia devices for the treatment of ventricular tachycardia are often limited to shock-only devices because antitachycardia pacing requires the presence of monomorphic ventricular tachycardia, a rare occurrence in children (although patients with repaired congenital heart disease are more likely to develop monomorphic VT; Figure 12-7). In addition, these devices often inappropriately shock during sinus tachycardia in children. Of greater utility in pediatrics will be the development of devices able to discriminate atrial rhythm and the AV relationship during tachycardias. Atrial defibrillators capable of atrial flutter termination by burst pacing or cardioversion may have a larger role in the management of patients with congenital heart disease.[34]

Sudden cardiac death is an uncommon disease in the pediatric population. In the otherwise healthy child, the etiology is usually hypertrophic obstructive cardiomyopathy or the long QT syndrome.[37]

The role of pacemakers and defibrillators in patients with hypertrophic obstructive cardiomyopathy is two-fold. They are used to decrease the outflow tract gradient by altering conduction and, hence, myocardial contraction patterns. They can be used to terminate supraventricular tachycardias such as atrial fibrillation, which occur more frequently in these patients. They also can terminate ventricular dysrhythmias, which occur in about 30% of patients with hypertrophic obstructive cardiomyopathy.[55]

Patients with the long QT syndrome can benefit from pacing and defibrillators in several ways. Pacing at higher heart rates can decrease the QT inter-

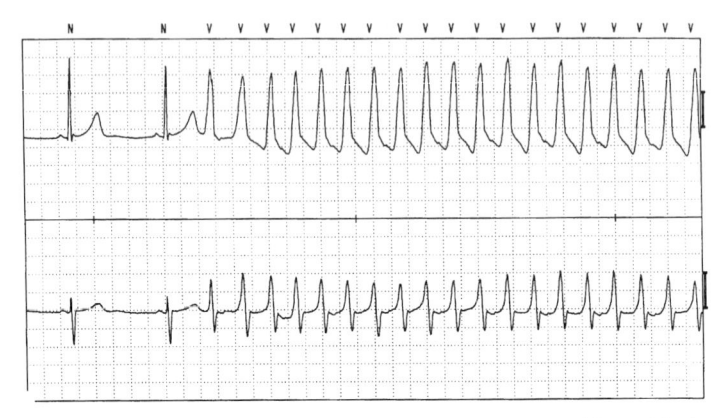

FIG. 12-7 Electrocardiogram from a patient with monomorphic ventricular tachycardia. The configuration differs from that of polymorphic ventricular tachycardia (torsade de pointes).

val. Unfortunately, the optimal heart rate is not known, and prolonged pacing at heart rates as low as 110 beats per minute has resulted in a tachycardia induced cardiomyopathy. Pacing algorithms that avoid prolonged pauses in the cardiac cycle decrease the incidence of ventricular tachycardia.[46] Although pacemakers cannot be used to cardiovert patients who have developed polymorphic VT (torsade), they can defibrillate once ventricular fibrillation has occurred.

The anesthetic considerations for the care of pediatric patients with pacemakers or cardioverter defibrillators are similar to those for the adult patient. The most important issues relate to the sensitivity of these devices to electromagnetic interference. Close cooperation with a cardiologist is necessary. Some of these devices may need to be turned off during surgery. The sophisticated programming that is involved with increasingly complex arrhythmia detection and treatment likely will need to be reassessed after the procedure to ensure that reprogramming has not occurred.

CONCLUSION

It is incumbent on the anesthesiologist caring for young patients to have some knowledge of the etiology, diagnosis, and management of arrhythmias in the pediatric surgical patient. Although the prevalence of malignant dysrhythmias in the general pediatric population is low, they are not uncommon in the increasingly large number of patients with histories of congenital heart disease.

Supraventricular tachycardias are the most common arrhythmias in children. The most frequent mechanism perpetuating the tachycardia is re-entry circus conduction through an accessory pathway and the AV node. In most cases, the acute management of these dysrhythmias in the stable patient requires suppression of conduction through the AV node. Atrial flutter and atrial fibrillation are rarely seen in the pediatric patient without congenital heart disease. These dysrhythmias usually are treated very aggressively in these patients because they can conduct 1:1 to the ventricle and create severe hemodynamic instability leading to ventricular fibrillation. Unfortunately, atrial flutter and fibrillation often recur despite therapy; however, medication is used to slow the ventricular response.

Ventricular dysrhythmias are uncommon in children with normal hearts. Unfortunately, it is often not clear which ventricular dysrhythmias should be treated in patients with congenital heart disease. Patients with the congenital long QT syndrome are at risk for the development of torsade de pointes ventricular tachycardia and they require a meticulous anesthetic plan that avoids increases in their adrenergic states or factors that increase the QT interval.

Bradydysrhythmias are often an inherent component of a heart defect or the result of the surgical correction of any cardiac lesion. Symptomatic bradydysrhythmias and some asymptomatic ones require pacemaker insertion. Left untreated, these bradycardias may be the cause of sudden cardiac death in a significant number of postoperative cardiac patients.

More symptomatic tachydysrhythmias, whether supraventricular or ventricular in origin, are being treated successfully with catheter ablation therapy. Highly programmable pacemakers and cardioverter defibrillators also may have a role in these patients. Due to the complexity of their surgical repairs, many patients with congenital heart disease are formidable technical challenges during attempts at ablation and pacemaker or cardioverter defibrillator placement. However, these treatments are well worth the effort because patients can avoid a lifetime commitment to medical therapy that often has multiple side effects including proarrhythmic activity.

There are no studies comparing anesthetic techniques in patients with various arrhythmias. However, it seems appropriate to tailor anesthetic management based on the likely interactions expected and to avoid agents associated with exacerbation or instigation of arrhythmias.

REFERENCES

1. Bockoven JR, Wemovsky G, Vetter VL, et al: Perioperative conduction and rhythm disturbances after the Ross procedure in young patients. *Ann Thorac Surg* 66:1383, 1998.
2. Castaneda AR, Jonas RA, Mayer JE, et al: *Cardiac Surgery of the Neonate and Infant.* Philadelphia, WB Saunders, 1994.
3. Walsh EP, Saul JP: Cardiac arrythmias. In *Nadas' Pediatric Cardiology.* Fyler DC, ed. Philadelphia, Hanley & Belfus, 1992, p 337.
4. Shinbane J, Wood M, Jensen N, et al: Tachycardia-induced cardiomyopathy: a review of animal models and clinical studies. *J Am Cardiol* 29:709, 1997.
5. Klein HO, Levi A, Kaplinsky E, et al: Congenital long-QT syndrome: deleterious effects of long-term high-rate ventricular pacing and definitive treatment by cardiac transplantation. *Am Heart J* 132:1079, 1996.
6. Fyler DC: Trends. In *Nadas' Pediatric Cardiology.* Fyler DC, ed. Philadelphia, Hanley & Belfus, 1992, p 277.
7. Stevenson W, Klitzner T, Perloff JK: Electrophysiologic abnormalites. In *Congenital Heart Disease in Adults.* Perloff JK, Child JC, eds. Philadelphia, WB Saunders, 1991, p 259.
8. Bosnjak ZJ, Kampine JP: Effects of halothane, enflurane, and isoflurane on the SA node. *Anesthesiology* 58:314, 1983.
9. Atlee JL, Alexander SC: Halothane effects on conductivity of the AV node and His-Purkinje system in the dog. *Anesth Analg* 56:378, 1977.
10. Keenan RL, Shapiro JH, Kane FR, et al: Bradycardia during anesthesia in infants. *Anesthesiology* 80:976, 1994.

11. Pamis SJ, Van Der Walt JH: A national survey of atropme use by Australian anesthetist. *Anaesth Intens Care* 22:61, 1994.
12. Abe K, Takada K, Yoshiya I: Intraoperative torsade de pointes ventricular tachycardia and ventricular fibrillation during sevoflurane anesthesia. *Anesth Analg* 86:701, 1998.
13. Annila P, Rorarius M, Reinikainen P, et al: Effect of pre-treatment with intravenous atropine or glycopyrrolate on cardiac arrhythmias during halothane anaesthesia for adenoidectomy in children. *Br J Anaesth* 80:756, 1998.
14. Robertson BJ, Clement JL, Knill RL: Enhancement of the arrhythmogenic effect of hypercarbia by surgical stimulation during halothane anaesthesia in man. *Can Anaesth Soc J* 28:342, 1981.
15. Johnston RR, Eger El, Wilson C: A comparative interaction of epinephrine with enflurane, isoflurane, and halothane in man. *Anesth Analg* 55:709, 1976.
16. Moore MA, Weiskopf RB, Eger EI, et al: Arrythmogenic doses of epinephrine are similar during desflurane or isoflurane anesthesia in humans. *Anesthesiology* 79:943, 1993.
17. Kasten GW, Martin ST. Bupivacaine cardiovascular toxicity comparison of treatment with bretylium and lidocaine. *Anesth Analg* 64:911, 1985.
18. Haasio J, Pitkanen MT, Kytta J, et al: Treatment of bupivacaine-induced cardiac arrhythmias in hypoxic and hypercarbic pigs with amiodarone or bretylium. *Reg Anesth Pain Med* 15:174, 1990.
19. Ved SA, Pinosky M, Nicodemus H: Ventricular tachycardia and brief cardiovascular collapse in two infants after caudal anesthesia using bupivacaine–epinephrine solution. *Anesthesiology* 79:1121, 1993.
20. Freid EB, Bailey AG, Valley RD: Electrocardiographic and hemodynamic changes associated with unintentional intravascular injection of bupivacaine with epinephrine in infants. *Anesthesiology* 79:394, 1993.
21. McAuliffe G, Bissonnette B, Boutin C: Should the routine use of atropine before succinylcholine in children be reconsidered? *Can J Anaesth* 42:724, 1995.
22. Sullivan M, Thompson WK, Hill GD: Succinylcholine-induced cardiac arrest in children with undiagnosed myopathy. *Can J Anaesth* 41:497, 1994.
23. Gibb DB: Suxamethonium—a review. *Anaesth Intens Care* 2:9, 1974.
24. Perez HR: Cardiac arrythmia after succinlycholine *Anesth Analg* 49:33, 1970.
25. Saul JP, Walsh EP, Triedman JK: Mechanisms and therapy of complex arrythmias in pediatric patients. *J Cardiovasc Electrophysiol* 6:1129, 1995.
26. Kugler JD, Danford DA: Management of infants, children and adolescents with paroxysmal supraventricular tachycardia. *J Pediatr* 129:324, 1996.
27. Perry JC, Garson A Jr. Supraventricular tachycardia due to Wolff–Parkinson–White syndrome in children: early disappearance and late recurrence. *J Am Coll Cardiol* 16:1215, 1990.
28. Chung KY, Walsh TJ, Massie E: Wolff–Parkinson–White. *Am Heart J* 69:116, 1965.
29. Paul T, Guccione P, Garson A Jr: Relation of syncope in young patients with Wolff–Parkinson–White syndrome to rapid ventricular response during atrial fibrillation. *Am J Cardiol* 65:318, 1990.
30. Wilbur SL, Marchlinski FE: Adenosine as an antiarrythmic agent. *Am J Cardiol* 79:30, 1997.
31. Epstein ML, Kiel EA, Victorica BE: Cardiac decompensation following verapamil therapy in infants with supraventricular tachycardia. *Pediatrics* 75:737, 1985.
32. Tanel RE, Walsh EP, Triedman JK, et al: Five-year experience with radiofrequency catheter ablation: implications for management of arrhythmias in pediatric and young adult patients. *J Pediatr* 131:878, 1997.
33. Gow RM: Atrial fibrillation and flutter in children and in young adults with congenital heart disease. *Can J Cardiol* 12A:45A, 1996.
34. Gelatt M, Hamilton RM, McGrindle BW, et al: Risk factors for atrial tachyarrhythmias after the Fontan operation. *J Am Coll Cardiol* 24:173 5, 1994.
35. Cecchi F, Montereggi A, Olivotto I, et al: Risk factors for atrial fibrillation in patients with hypertrophic cardiomyopathy assessed by signal averaged P wave duration. *Heart* 78:44, 1997.

36. Garson A Jr, Bink-Boelkens M, Hesslein PS, et al: Atrial flutter in the young. A collaborative study of 380 cases. *J Am Coll Cardiol* 6:871, 1985.
37. Silka MJ: Implantable cardioverter-defibrillators in children. *J Electrocardiol* 29:223, 1996.
38. Southall DP, Richards J, Mitchell P, et al: Study of cardiac rhythm in healthy newborn infants. *Br Heart J* 43:14, 1980.
39. Viitasalo MT, Kala R, Eisalo A: Ambulatory electrocardiographic findings in young athletes between 14 and 16 years of age. *Eur Heart J* 5:2, 1984.
40. Pedersen DH, Zipes DP, Foster PR, et al: Ventricular tachycardia and ventricular fibrillation in a young population. *Circulation* 60:988, 1979.
41. Rocchini AP, Chun PO, Dick M: Ventricular tachycardia in children. *Am J Cardiol* 47:1091, 1981.
42. Perry JC: Ventricular tachycardia in neonates. *Pacing Clin Electrophysiol* 20:2061, 1997.
43. Garson A Jr, Randall DC, Gillette PC, et al: Prevention of sudden death after repair of tetralogy of Fallot and treatment of ventricular arrhythmias. *J Am Coll Cardiol* 6:221, 1985.
44. Galloway PA, Glass PSA: Anesthetic implication of prolonged QT interval syndromes. *Anesth Analg* 64:612, 1985.
45. Leenhardt A, Lucet V, Denjoy I, et al: Catecholaminergic polymorphic ventricular tachycardia in children. *Circulation* 91:1512, 1995.
46. Viskin S, Fish R, Roth A, Copperman Y: Prevention of torsade de pointes in the congenital long QT syndrome: use of a pause prevention pacing algorithm. *Heart* 79:417, 1998.
47. Viskin S, Alia SR, Barren HV, et al: Mode of onset of torsade de pointes in congenital long QT syndrome. *J Am Coll Cardiol* 28:1262, 1996.
48. Tzivoni D, Banai S, Schuger C, et al: Treatment of torsade de pointes with magnesium sulfate. *Circulation* 77:392, 1988.
49. Tanel RE, Triedman JK, Walsh EP, et al: High-rate atrial pacing as an innovative bridging therapy in a neonate with congenital long QT syndrome. *J Cardiovasc Electrophysiol* 7:812, 1997.
50. Michaloudis D, Fraidakis O, Petrou A, et al: Anesthesia and the QT interval. Effects of isoflurane and halothane in unpremedicated children. *Anaesthesia* 53:435, 1998.
51. Hill SL, Evangelista JK, Pizzi AM, et al: Proarrythmia associated with cisapride in children. *Pediatrics* 101:1053, 1998.
52. Banai S, Tzivoni D: Drug therapy for torsade de pointes. *J Cardiovasc Electrophysiol* 4:206, 1993.
53. Bonatti V, Agnetti A, Squarcia U: Early and late postoperative complete heart block in pediatric patients submitted to open-heart surgery for congenital heart disease. *Pediatr Med Chir* 20:181, 1998.
54. Michaelsson M, Riesenfeld T, Jonzon A: Natural history of congenital complete atrioventricular block. *Pacing Clin Electrophysiol* 20:2098, 1997.
55. Zhu DW, Sun H, Hill R, et al: The value of electrophysiology study and prophylactic implantation of cardioverter defibrillator in patients with hypertrophic cardiomyopathy. *Pacing Clin Electrophysiol* 21:299, 1998.

13 | Anesthetic Considerations for the Child With Multiple Trauma

Aisling Conran, MD
Madelyn Kahana, MD

Trauma is the most common cause of death in childhood. Although the incidence of unintentional trauma deaths has recently declined, there is an ever-increasing epidemic of intentional violence in the United States that claims the lives of thousands of children each year. Firearms injuries alone were responsible for more than 5000 pediatric deaths in this country in 1995. In fact, firearm deaths are nearly as numerous in children as are deaths from motor vehicle accidents. Appropriate use of child-restraint devices has been crucial to the prevention of serious motor vehicle trauma. Helmet use has dramatically reduced injury to the bicyclist. Recent estimates suggest that the elimination or secure storage of handguns in the home would reduce firearm deaths by almost 50%.[1,2]

Neurologic injury is the most important determinant of outcome in the pediatric trauma victim. A serious head injury by itself or in addition to multiple trauma significantly increases a child's morbidity and mortality. During initial stabilization of the multiple trauma victim in the field, in the emergency department, and during operative care, meticulous attention to the management of the patient's head injury is crucial to the child's ultimate outcome.

FROM THE FIELD TO THE EMERGENCY DEPARTMENT

The integrity and the stability of a child's airway must be the first priority of the emergency management of the pediatric trauma patient. The airway is examined first, and it must be continually re-evaluated. Airway management may include the use of jaw thrust maneuvers, supplemental oxygen, mask ventilation, oral or nasal airways, laryngeal mask airways, or tracheal intubation. As a last resort a surgical cricothyroidotomy may be required. The airway is controlled because of respiratory compromise, hemodynamic instability, head trauma, or multiple injuries. Potential and identified cervical spine injuries demand a carefully considered approach to the airway.

Initial assessment of the patient in the field or emergency department is frequently aided by the Pediatric Trauma Score and the Glasgow Coma Score (GCS). These tools are easy to use, provide a quick overall view of the patient, and guide the choice of transport to a pediatric trauma center or a more proximate local hospital (Tables 13-1 and 13-2). Immediate intervention for severe head or multiple trauma or further evaluation of the patient with apparently minimal trauma continues at the hospital or trauma center.

Personnel involved in trauma resuscitation include the trauma surgeon, the emergency physician, the anesthesiologist, two to three emergency room nurses, a pediatric intensive care nurse, and a radiology technician. Each person on the trauma team has an assigned role. The trauma surgeon must

TABLE 13–1 Modified Glasgow Coma Score for Infants and Younger Children

Activity	Best response	Score
Eye opening	Spontaneous	4
	To speech	3
	To pain	2
	None	1
Verbal	Coos and babbles	5
	Irritable cries	4
	Cries to pain	3
	Moans to pain	2
	None	1
Motor	Normal spontaneous movements	6
	Withdraws to touch	5
	Withdraws to pain	4
	Abnormal flexion	3
	Abnormal extension	2
	None	1

organize care and ensure that the sequence of assessment, resuscitation, stabilization, and re-evaluation of the patient proceeds smoothly in a seemingly chaotic environment.

Airway management is the primary focus of the resuscitation and is the responsibility of the senior anesthesiologist. If the child was intubated in the field, then the intubation must be assessed. Bilateral breath sounds should be evaluated to ensure proper tube placement. If necessary, the endotracheal tube may be repositioned. An end-tidal CO_2 monitor may confirm tracheal location.

An unintubated, spontaneously breathing child must be examined carefully. Ideally, the child should be evaluated for the presence of facial fractures; neck and cervical spine injury; and trauma to the teeth, mouth, and oral cavity before airway instrumentation. Apneic or pulseless children and those with severe thoracic injuries, elevated intracranial pressure (ICP), or a GCS below 8 *need endotracheal intubation immediately*. A surgical airway should be considered if the child has facial or neck trauma or cervical spine injury. Endotracheal intubation may be difficult or may worsen the child's condition.

In the hemodynamically stable child, endotracheal intubation with the use of cricoid pressure, in-line cervical traction, and a rapid sequence technique are indicated if, after careful airway evaluation, no difficulties are anticipated. Awake intubation may be performed in the neonate or cooperative teenager but is otherwise quite difficult in the pediatric population.[3] Fiberoptic intubation is also problematic in children. It requires proper equipment and is often more time consuming than other methods of intubation.

TABLE 13–2 Pediatric Trauma Score

Categories	+2	+1	−1
Weight (kg)	>20	10–20	<10
Airway	Normal	Maintained	Unmaintained
Systolic blood pressure (mmHg)	>90	50–90	<50
Central nervous system function	Awake	Obtunded	Coma
Open wound	None	Minor	Major/penetrating
Skeletal trauma	None	Closed fracture	Open or multiple

Trauma patients are always "full stomach" risks. With endotracheal intubation, pulmonary aspiration is a real concern. When Bricker et al. evaluated gastric volume in 110 traumatized children, ages 1 to 14 years, who needed surgery, they found that 49% with a "nothing by mouth" (NPO; nil per os) time longer than 8 h had gastric volumes larger than 0.4 mL/kg, 12% had solid food particles aspirated from their stomachs, and 21% vomited during intubation or emergence. Clearly, this high-risk population is best served by awake or rapid sequence intubation techniques.[4]

A rapid sequence intubation technique begins with preoxygenation. Cricoid pressure is applied, intravenous sedatives and paralytic agents are administered, and the trachea is intubated. A modified rapid sequence technique may be helpful in a combative, noncooperative child who will not accept preoxygenation. In the modified technique, gentle mask ventilation is delivered while cricoid pressure is applied. Without effective preoxygenation, a modified rapid sequence intubation technique may avoid hypoxemia in a child at risk.

Choice of induction agent before intubation depends on the patient's cardiovascular stability and neurologic compromise. Ketamine (1 to 3 mg/kg) may increase intracranial pressure, an effect that may be blunted by prompt hyperventilation. Propofol (1 to 2 mg/kg) and thiopental (3 to 5 mg/kg) may result in hypotension, particularly in the hypovolemic patient. Etomidate (0.2 to 0.3 mg/kg) maintains stable hemodynamics without adversely affecting ICP and is the sedative or hypnotic of choice in this setting. After the administration of the sedative/hypnotic, succinylcholine (1 to 2 mg/kg), rocuronium (1 to 1.2 mg/kg), or rapacurium (2 mg/kg) is recommended to facilitate rapid intubation. Succinylcholine also can increase ICP, an effect well tempered by a defasciculating dose of a nondepolarizing muscle relaxant. The advantage of succinylcholine remains the rapidity of offset, a pharmacokinetic property unavailable in a nondepolarizing agent. Despite many absolute and relative contraindications for the use of succinylcholine, it is the current gold standard for the rapid control of an airway in a life-threatening situation (Table 13-3).

TABLE 13–3 Drug Recommendations for Endotracheal Intubation in the Hypovolemic Trauma Patient

Type of drug	Medication	Dose (mg/kg)	Advantages	Disadvantages
Induction agents	Ketamine	1–3	Stable hemodynamics	Raises intracranial pressure
	Thiopental	3–5		Hypotension
	Propofol	1–2		Hypotension
	Etomidate	0.2–0.3	Stable hemodynamics	
Depolarizing musle relaxant	Succcinylcholine	1–2	Rapid onset, rapid offset	Hyperkalemia, raises intracranial pressure
Non-depolarizing muscle relaxants	Rocuronium	1–1.2		Long duration
	Rapacurium	2		Histamine release, bronchospasm

Blind nasotracheal intubation has been suggested as an alternative to direct laryngoscopy and oral endotracheal tube placement. In a child, blind nasotracheal intubation is at best a difficult procedure. Maxillofacial fractures and fractures of the base of the skull are contraindications for nasal intubations of any type because the endotracheal tube may be inadvertently introduced into the cranial cavity.[5] In a study of emergent tracheal intubations in pediatric trauma patients, more than 90% of children had head injuries. Intubation was required in 63 of 605 patients. Intubation was successful at the scene of the accident in 57.1% of cases but often only after multiple attempts. Two attempts at cricothyroidotomy in the field resulted in massive subcutaneous emphysema. One child was successfully intubated at a local hospital and the second child died in transport with an unsecured airway. Complications occurred in approximately 25% of intubations and varied from relatively minor, e.g., right mainstem location with mild hypoxemia, to severe, e.g., massive aspiration. These complications were distributed fairly evenly among the three intubating locations: the field, the local hospital, and the children's hospital. Of real concern were the approximately 20% of intubations that were considered unnecessary during case review. Among them were children with GCS above 10 who were spontaneously breathing, had no airway obstruction, and were extubated within 2 days. Six of these children, approximately 30%, suffered complications because of an unnecessary intubation.[6] The most skilled manager should certainly assume the responsibility for a traumatized child's airway. The process of achieving endotracheal intubation or surgical airway control, if necessary, is fraught with risk. Ventilation should commence with 100% oxygen at an age-appropriate rate and depth as soon the airway is secure.

Concomitant with the effort to manage the airway is the need to secure intravenous access with the largest possible intravenous catheters. Blood samples should be sent for a type and cross-match, hemoglobin, hematocrit, and other laboratory tests. If peripheral access is difficult, central venous or intraosseous access can be quickly achieved. With either an 18-gauge spinal needle or a bone marrow aspirate needle, the anteromedial surface of the tibia may be accessed, 1 to 3 cm below the tibial tuberosity, at an angle of 60° to 80° directed inferiorly to the long axis of the tibia. This technique may be used emergently in patients younger than 5 years when intravenous access is difficult.[7] Femoral veins offer an option for placement of large-bore, central venous access with relative ease in infants and small children. In patients without vascular compromise to the selected lower extremity or intraabdominal vascular trauma, femoral lines are easily placed during a resuscitation. In a review of central lines, the incidence of infectious complications was lower in femoral lines than those at other sites.[8]

Resuscitation after trauma frequently involves massive fluid and blood transfusions. Volume resuscitation in pediatric patients often begins with balanced salt infusions in 20-mL/kg boluses. Crystalloid resuscitation supports physiologic end-points: adequate peripheral and central perfusion, urine output, and blood pressure (Table 13-4). Warming the fluids, which are infused in large volumes, will help maintain the patient's core temperature.[9] When blood loss is excessive, transfusion of red cells may be lifesaving. Emergency type O cells and type-specific blood can be obtained within a few minutes from the blood bank.[10] Transfusion therapy must be directed accordingly (Tables 13-5 and 13-6). Restoration of the circulating blood volume also must be directed to support physiologic end-points. Blood loss must be controlled, coagulopathy corrected, normothermia maintained, gas exchange

TABLE 13–4 Age-Appropriate Vital Signs

Age	Heart rate	Systolic blood pressure	Respiratory rate
Preterm	120–180	40–60	55–60
Newborn	95–145	50–70	35–40
6 mo	110–180	60–110	25–30
1–2 y	100–160	65–115	20–24
2–3 y	90–150	75–125	16–22
3–5 y	65–135	80–120	14–20
5–8 y	70–115	92–120	12–20
9–12 y	55–110	92–130	12–20
12–14 y	55–105	100–140	10–14

Source: Reproduced with permission from Bell C, Kain Z, eds: *The Pediatric Anesthesia Handbook,* 2nd ed. St. Louis: Mosby, 1997, p 13.

optimized, and electrolyte balance restored. Blood transfusions in children, greater than an estimated one blood volume of the patient, can be associated with hyperkalemia, hypocalcemia, hypothermia, metabolic acidosis, coagulopathy, and thrombocytopenia.[10,11] As many as 47% of pediatric patients with severe trauma suffer the complications of massive transfusion.[12] In the most severely injured child, resuscitation continues during surgical attempts to control bleeding or to treat life-threatening intracranial injuries.

STRATEGIES FOR MANAGING SPECIFIC INJURIES

Pediatric Head Trauma

Among pediatric patients with multiple trauma, 80% to 90% have head injuries. Severe head injuries in children elevate ICP and alter cerebral blood flow. Of children with head injuries brought into the emergency room for evaluation, 97% show little change in mental status. Glasgo Coma Scores and a thorough neurologic examination will rule out intracranial pathologic conditions in conscious children. If the patient cannot cooperate with a full neurologic examination, as in the case of depressed consciousness, or if the physical neurologic examination reveals a neurologic deficit, an emergent computed tomographic (CT) scan is required. Securing a child's airway before this procedure may be necessary.

Computed tomography is used to evaluate the extent of head injury. Injury may result from increased ICP because of a space-occupying lesion or generalized cellular injury and swelling. Interventions to correct ICP, altered cerebral oxygen utilization, or reductions in the cerebral perfusion pressure include modest hyperventilation, induced systemic hypertension, hyperosmolality, and barbiturate coma.[9]

Optimal cerebral perfusion (CPP) can be achieved by raising mean arterial pressure or reducing ICP. Ventilation can be enhanced to allow the partial pressure of CO_2 to decrease to 30 to 35 mmHg; this reduces cerebral blood

TABLE 13–5 Blood Volume Related to Age

Age (y)	Blood volume (mL/kg)
0–1	80
1–16	70
>16	55–60

TABLE 13–6 Blood Replacement After One or More Blood Volume Transfusions

Transfusion	Replacement	Amount/kg
One blood volume	Platelets	0.5–1 U
	Fresh frozen plasma	10–20 mL
Two blood volumes	Cryoprecipitate	0.5 U

flow and lowers ICP. Mannitol (0.25 to 1 g/kg), the osmotic agent of choice, is useful to decrease cellular edema and lower ICP. Alternatively, blood pressure can be increased with α-agonists (e.g., neosynephrine) or other vasoactive agents, and the dose is adjusted to maintain CPP above 70 mmHg. The target CPP of 70, thought to be optimal for the older pediatric child and adult, clearly must be adjusted in an age-based fashion based on age-appropriate mean arterial pressure. In addition, a percutaneous ventriculostomy can be performed to monitor and treat intracranial hypertension. The ventriculostomy monitor can be transduced as is any pressure line. Cerebrospinal fluid can be drained intermittently or constantly in response to increased ICP. In rare circumstances of refractory intracranial hypertension, barbiturates are used to lower cerebral metabolic rate. However, the profound depressant effect of barbiturates on cardiac performance and systemic vascular resistance limits their utility.

In the operating room, therapy for increased ICP must continue. Anesthetic agents affect ICP. Thiopental (4 to 7 mg/kg) decreases ICP. However, barbiturates may result in pronounced hypotension and decreased CPP in the hypovolemic child because of vasodilation and myocardial depression. Unlike thiopental, etomidate (0.2 to 0.3 mg/kg) reduces ICP without reducing mean arterial pressure, so it may be the better choice. Succinylcholine increases ICP by increasing afferent neural traffic from muscle spindle receptors. This effect begins 1 min after administration, peaks at 3 min, and is particularly problematic in those patients with CT evidence of decreased intracranial compliance. Hyperventilation, voluntary or via mask ventilation, and premedication with nondepolarizing neuromuscular relaxants will blunt the increase in ICP associated with succinylcholine.[13] Nondepolarizing muscle relaxants have little effect on ICP. Lidocaine (1.5 mg/kg) also may be given 3 to 4 min before intubation to attenuate the increase in ICP in response to laryngoscopy.[14] All inhalational anesthetics will increase cerebral blood flow and, hence, ICP. This effect is well attenuated by prior hyperventilation, making an inhalation agent a reasonable anesthetic choice[9,13](Table 13-7).

Cervical Spinal Injury

As many as 16% of children with serious head injuries in motor vehicle accidents will have cervical spinal injuries. At particular risk are children in high-speed motor vehicle accidents, those in forward-facing infant seats, and those with achondroplasia or trisomy 21 (Down's syndrome).[15] Two types of injuries occur: ligament stretching and bony fractures. The ligamentous injury is found almost exclusively in children younger than 8 years. Stretch injuries are most common at the alanto-occipital junction, the alantoaxial junction, and the level between C2 and C3. Preadolescents, teenagers, and adults acquire fractures along the entire cervical spine. High cervical injuries, which are common in young children, uniformly result in apnea and

TABLE 13-7 Anesthetic Effects on Cerebral Blood Flow

Drugs	Cerebral blood flow
Barbiturates	↓↓
Narcotics	↓ or ↔
Ketamine	↑↑↑
Propofol	↓
Sevoflurane	↑
Desflurane	↑
Isoflurane	↑
Halothane	↑↑
Enflurane	↑ or ↔
Nitrous oxide	↔

Source: Adapted from Michenfelder JD: Anesthetics and cerebral metabolism. In *27th Annual Refresher Course Lectures.* Park Ridge, American Society of Anesthesiologists, 1976, p 209; Omoigui S: *The Anesthesia Drug Handbook,* 2nd ed, St. Louis, Mosby, 1995, p 298, 361, 389.

bradycardia at the scene of the injury and are therefore often lethal. Approximately 20% of children with Down's syndrome develop alantoaxial subluxation during childhood, even without injury. This population is at risk of cord compression during hyperextension, hyperflexion, and extreme rotation of the neck. These positions may be necessary during elective or urgent endotracheal intubation of an injured child.[3,16]

The child with a cervical neck injury should be intubated only after head and neck immobilization. Immobilization and careful technique are more important to the success and safety of intubation than is the choice of a sedative or neuromuscular relaxant in a child with a normal-appearing airway. Preoxygenation, neck stabilization, and a rapid sequence technique are essential for the safe intubation of a patient with cervical neck trauma. Awake intubation and the use of fiber optics to facilitate airway control are viable options.[3,13,17] The typical position for laryngoscopy and oral endotracheal intubation with extension of the head on the cervical spine results in displacement of the upper three cervical vertebra. Fractures in small children almost always involve the very portion of the cervical spine most often displaced by maneuvers to facilitate intubation. Small children are at *very high risk.*

Multiple Trauma

In children, multiple trauma often involves severe injury to the head, abdomen, thorax, and extremities. In the abdominal cavity, the liver and spleen are the most frequently injured organs, although the duodenum and ileum may be injured in a child who was restrained by a lap seatbelt during a motor vehicle accident. Isolated splenic or hepatic injury may be managed medically if the patient is hemodynamically stable. Laparotomy is indicated if any of the following conditions are present: persistence of unstable vital signs, pneumoperitoneum, transfusion of greater than one-half of the patient's blood volume, rebound abdominal tenderness on physical examination, penetrating injury to the bladder or kidneys, or tears in the rectal mucosa.[18] The "lap belt syndrome," a combination of injuries to the intestines and the lumbar spine, is suspected after a motor vehicle accident if the victim has an abdominal or flank ecchymosis in the shape of a lap belt.

Thoracic trauma, which may not be apparent immediately, commonly accompanies abdominal injury. In the chest, the great vessels and the airway can be injured because of greater mobility of the mediastinum and heart in children.[15] Oxygenation and ventilation may be more challenging in the patient with pulmonary contusions, necessitating close attention to fluid management and ventilation. Specifically, over-resuscitation will exacerbate pulmonary dysfunction. Cardiac injuries, although unusual, clearly complicate management significantly. These children often require short-term inotropic support. Diagnosis of myocardial contusion is best made with echocardiography, which can also guide volume management.

Continued observation and diligent attention may result in a diagnosis that might have been missed on the initial survey.[3] A hemodynamically unstable child with suspected thoracoabdominal injury and a possible head injury is a clinical decision-making dilemma. It may be dangerous to waste time in transporting the child to x-ray. A surgical laparotomy may be more productive during treatment for ongoing blood loss. If there is a localizing neurologic finding, a CT scan may identify a life-threatening intracranial hematoma. In the absence of a focal neurologic deficit, the hemodynamic challenge demands direct transfer to the operating room.

FROM THE OPERATING ROOM TO THE PEDIATRIC INTENSIVE CARE UNIT

To prepare for the surgical management of the trauma victim, the operating room must be warmed and blood products must be ready. Monitors should include pulse oximetry, electrocardiogram, end-tidal CO_2, precordial stethoscope, thermometer, and a Foley catheter. Invasive monitors also may be required, such as an arterial line to monitor beat-to-beat blood pressure and obtain frequent blood gas analysis and a central venous line to evaluate volume status and the delivery of vasoactive agents. A pulmonary artery catheter rarely is required in children. Adequate vascular access is absolutely imperative, preferably large-bore, peripheral intravenous lines suitable for rapid administration of fluids and blood products. For a child with severe intraabdominal vascular injury, the lines should be placed in an upper extremity. Such placement ensures resuscitation capacity if the inferior vena cava must be occluded temporarily to control bleeding. *All fluids and blood must be warmed.*

Induction of anesthesia should proceed with the same precautions described for an emergency endotracheal intubation. In the hemodynamically unstable child, etomidate and fentanyl are the induction agents of choice. Intubation should be conducted as if there were cervical trauma without evidence to the contrary. After intubation, muscle relaxation can be achieved by any one of a number of nondepolarizing agents. Succinylcholine remains the drug of choice for rapid sequence intubation in an acute trauma setting because of its speed of onset and offset. Issues relating to the increase in ICP with succinylcholine are real, but the increase is easily tempered with hyperventilation or a defasciculating dose of a nondepolarizing muscle relaxant.

Anesthesia is maintained with inhalation agents, narcotics, benzodiazapines, or a combination, as dictated in large part by the patient's hemodynamic profile. The presence of intracranial hypertension also influences anesthetic choice. Agents are chosen because of their favorable effects on the relation between cerebral blood flow and cerebral oxygen use. Fentanyl,

TABLE 13–8 Glasgow Coma Score and Outcome

		Good outcome	Partly dependent or dependent	Died
GCS ≤5, n (%)	27	11 (40.7)	2 (7.4)	14 (51.9)
GCS >5, n (%)	70	58 (82.9)	8 (11.4)	4 (5.7)

GCS, Glasgow Coma Score.
Source: Reproduced with permission from Thakker JC, Splaingard M, Zhu J, et al: Survival and functional outcome of children requiring endotracheal intubation during therapy for severe brain injury. *Crit Care Med* 25:1396, 1997.

propofol, thiopental, lidocaine, etomidate, and isoflurane are preferred for children with known or suspected head injury (Table 13-6).

Emergence from anesthesia and postoperative pain management must be planned. After a neurosurgical procedure, it is often best to awaken the patient and re-evaluate neurologic function. In the patient with hemodynamic challenge or severe lung injury, transfer of an anesthetized child to the intensive care unit may be preferable. The use of propofol or remifentanil infusion may provide for a comfortable patient who is easily awakened. Postoperative pain management in the severely injured patient is generally achieved with intravenous opioids. Alternatively, paraspinal opiates may be useful in some patients.

CONCLUSION

Trauma management demands involvement of the anesthesiologist in the emergency department and the operating room. Securing a traumatized child's airway can be treacherous. Choice of anesthetic agents is often crucial. Proper volume resuscitation is imperative. With careful multidisciplinary care, children with life-threatening injuries can and do make good recoveries.

Several assessments over time, with an evaluation tool like the GCS, have a stronger correlation with outcome than does a single measurement. Even among children with an initial GCS no higher than 5, nearly 40% had a good long-term outcome. This emphasizes the importance of early and appropriate interventions[19] (Table 13-8).

REFERENCES

1. Rivara FP, Grossman DC: Prevention of traumatic deaths to children in the United States: how far have we come and where do we need to go? *Pediatrics* 97:791, 1996.
2. Hazinski MF, Francescutti LH, Lapidus GD, et al: Pediatric injury prevention. *Ann Emerg Med* 22:456, 1993.
3. Harris MM, Berry FA: Pediatric trauma patients. In *Textbook of Trauma Anesthesia and Critical Care.* Grande CM, ed. Chicago, Mosby, 1993, p 619.
4. Bricker SR, McLuckie A, Nightingale DA: Gastric aspirates after trauma in children. *Anaesthesia* 44:721, 1989.
5. Seebacher J, Nozik D, Mathieu A: Inadvertent intracranial introduction of a nasogastric tube, a complication of severe maxillofacial trauma. *Anesthesiology* 42:100, 1975.
6. Nakayama DK, Gardner MJ, Rowe MI: Emergency endotracheal intubation in pediatric trauma. *Ann Surg* 211:218, 1990.
7. Harte FA, Chalmers PC, Walsh RF, et al: Intraosseous fluid administration: a parenteral alternative in pediatric resuscitation. *Anesth Analg* 66:687, 1987.

8. Stenzel JP, Green TP, Fuhrman BP, et al: Percutaneous femoral venous catheterizations: a prospective study of complications. *J Pediatr* 114:411, 1989.
9. Striker TW: Anesthesia for trauma in the pediatric patient. In *Pediatric Anesthesia,* 3rd ed. Gregory GA, ed. New York, Churchill Livingstone, 1994, p 805.
10. Donaldson MD, Seaman MJ, Park GR: Massive blood transfusion. *Br J Anaesth* 69: 621, 1992.
11. Cosgriff N, Moore EE, Sauaia A, et al: Predicting life-threatening coagulopathy in the massively transfused trauma patient: hypothermia and acidosis revisited. *J Trauma* 42: 857, 1997.
12. Moront ML, Williams JA, Eichelberger MR, Wilkinson JD: The injured child: an approach to care. *Pediatr Clin North Am* 41:1201, 1994.
13. Stoelting RK: Neuromuscular blocking drugs. In *Pharmacology and Physiology in Anesthetic Practice.* Stoelting RK, ed. Philadelphia, JB Lippincott, 1991, p 183.
14. Nakayama DK, Waggoner T, Venkataraman ST, et al: The use of drugs in emergency airway management in pediatric trauma. *Ann Surg* 216:205, 1992.
15. Hendey GW, Votey SR: Injuries in restrained motor vehicle accident victims. *Ann Emerg Med* 24:77, 1994.
16. Moore RA, McNicholas KW, Warran SP: Atlantoaxial subluxation with symptomatic spinal cord compression in a child with Down's syndrome. *Anesth Analg* 66:89, 1987.
17. Chekan EM, Weber S: Intubation with or without neuromuscular blockade in trauma patients with cervical spine injury [abstract]. *Anesth Analg* 70:S54, 1990.
18. Newman KD, Bowman LM, Eichelberger MR, et al: The lap belt complex: intestinal and lumbar spine injury in children. *J Trauma* 30:1133, 1990.
19. Thakker JC, Splaingard M, Zhu J, et al: Survival and functional outcome of children requiring endotracheal intubation during therapy for severe brain injury. *Crit Care Med* 25:1396, 1997.

14 | Management of the Child With Thermal Injury

Tracy Koogler, MD

Pediatric burn patients challenge the anesthesiologist from the initial stabilization period until the final surgery, which may be years after the initial burn. Careful attention to detail during initial stabilization inevitably will lead to improved survival of these difficult patients.

THERMAL INJURY

Thermal injuries occur from scald, flame, and contact. With scald burns, the skin contacts a hot liquid such as water or grease. The temperature and the consistency of the liquid greatly affect the depth of a burn. Water at 140°F will cause a third-degree burn in 3 s; a liquid at 155°F will take only 1 s. Boiling water can easily reach 180°F and grease can reach 400°F. Thick substances like grease are more likely to adhere to the skin, which will increase the depth of the burn. Areas covered by clothing will have deeper burns because the cloth will keep the hot liquid next to the skin.

Flame burns occur from exposure to a direct flame. These burns vary in thickness based on the temperature and the length of exposure. Flame retardant or thick protective clothes may decrease the exposure, whereas petroleum-based cloth such as nylon may worsen the burn.

Contact burns occur when skin contacts hot objects, e.g., stoves, radiators, irons. The depth of the wound depends on the temperature of the object and the time of contact.

ELECTRICAL BURNS

Electrical burns can produce low-tension or high-tension injuries. Most house-related electrical injuries are low tension because house current is 110 to 120 V. Biting or chewing on electrical cords is the most common cause of low-tension injuries, followed by placing uninsulated items into electrical outlets. These children's injuries resemble contact burns with a surface burn that extends into the underlying tissues.

High-voltage injuries occur with current greater than 1000 V, such as from lightning or high-voltage outdoor wires. High-tension injuries have a surface burn at the point of entrance and exit of the electrical current. The true damage is internal, in the underlying muscle layer, because the electrical current follows the path of least resistance, usually blood vessels, nerves, and muscles. When the current reaches areas of relative resistance such as bone, large amounts of heat are generated. The direct damage to the blood vessels and muscle results in thrombosis and necrosis, which is followed by ongoing necrosis from the heat generated by the bones. The electrical current can take any path once it enters the body, including the heart, which creates fatal arrhythmias, or the brain, which creates neurologic injury. The muscle injury can produce compartment syndromes rapidly. Patients with electrical burns must be monitored for arrhythmias, rhabdomyolysis, and neurologic injury.

CHEMICAL BURNS

Chemical burns produce an injury that resembles a thermal burn; however, the mechanism is different. When a child presents to the emergency room with a chemical burn, he is likely to have active chemical on his skin, increasing the depth and extent of the burned surface. Chemical burns can be caused by acids, bases, organic, or inorganic compounds. Acid compounds decrease the pH of a substance and cause the protein structure to collapse. Bases destroy proteins by being a proton donor. Organic compounds cause direct heat production and chemical reactions that disrupt the skin. Inorganic compounds bind directly to the skin and create salts, which damage the skin's integrity. Immediate therapy includes complete disrobing of the patient to remove any ongoing source of chemicals and lavage of all affected body parts with copious amounts of water. If the airway is contaminated, the airway's patency must be examined. Intubation is necessary if there is evidence of significant injury that will cause edema and desquamation.

SKIN INJURY

Irrespective of the agent, thermal injury to the skin begins as an acute inflammatory response at the burned skin. Heat burns the skin, disrupting the epithelium and impairing the Na^+ pump. This impairment leads to the activation of platelets, macrophages, and leukocytes. These cells release interleukins, cytokines, histamine, tumor necrosis factor, and inflammatory mediators, which create capillary leak and edema formation.

In first-degree burns such as sunburns, only the epidermis is damaged. In second-degree burns, the dermis is damaged, resulting in blister formation. Beneath the blister, the skin may be pink with capillary refill, which indicates a superficial partial-thickness burn. The underlying skin is white without evidence of capillary refill. Third-degree burns extend through the dermis into the subcutaneous fat or even the periosteum in severe cases. An eschar forms from the devitalized tissue.

Thermal injury causes direct microvascular injury to the skin. This change leads to increased capillary permeability and edema formation, which is greatest in the first 6 to 8 h after injury but often continues for 24 to 48 h. The cell membrane releases collagen, thrombin, bradykinin, histamine, and oxygen free radicals as it is injured. These substances lead to arachidonic acid production, which creates leukotrienes, prostaglandins, and thromboxane. Proteins break down, causing activation of the coagulation system and complement activation. Locally, this leads to edema formation, protein and fluid loss from the wound, and erythema. The unburned skin surrounding the wound also can be affected with these changes. In the patient with greater than a 20% wound, this cascade leads to a systemic reaction known as *burn shock*.

The extent of the burn may be estimated with a rule of 9s graph in an adult patient (Figure 14-1). The Lund and Browder variation of this chart works well for the small child because it recognizes the relatively large size of the child's head in relation to the rest of his body (Figure 14-2).[1] Another method is to use the child's palm to represent 1% of his body surface area and then estimate the total burn surface area (TBSA) by this area.

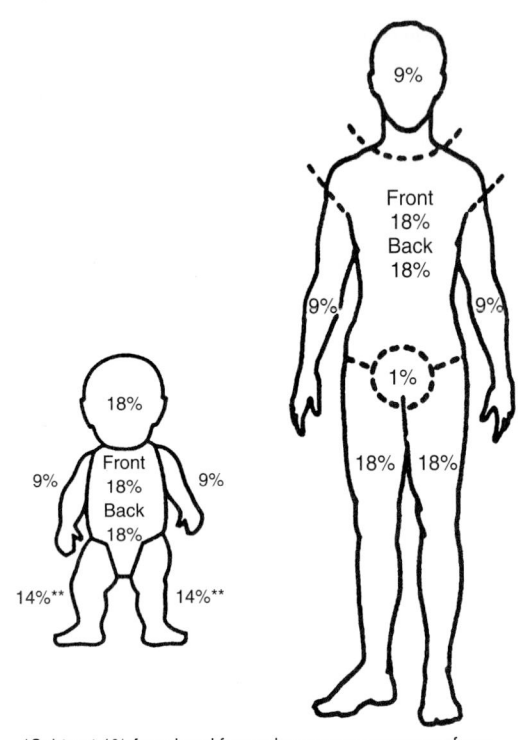

*Subtract 1% from head for each year over one year of age.
**Add 1/2% to each leg for each year over one year of age.

FIG. 14-1 Rule of 9's (for calculating percentage of body burned).

BURN SHOCK

Burn shock is initially hypovolemic in nature, characterized by decreased cardiac output, increased systemic vascular resistance (SVR), decreased perfusion, and hypotension. Histamine release induces capillary leak, edema formation, and arterial vasodilation. Prostaglandins and bradykinins also increase microvascular permeability. These reactions decrease in interstitial hydrostatic pressure and increase interstitial osmotic pressure and intravascular hydrostatic pressure, which further exacerbates the fluid flux. The combination of these factors lead to a dramatic increase in the tissue water content of the burned area that can double within 1 h. Thromboxane may lessen edema formation because it decreases blood flow to the injured area. Unfortunately, this response can lead to poor perfusion of the damaged skin and worsen the injury.

The extravasation of protein-enriched fluid from the intravascular to interstitial space leads to hypovolemia. Hypovolemia leads to tachycardia, hypotension, increased SVR, and decreased organ perfusion, if not corrected rapidly. The body's stress response to the burn and inflammatory process

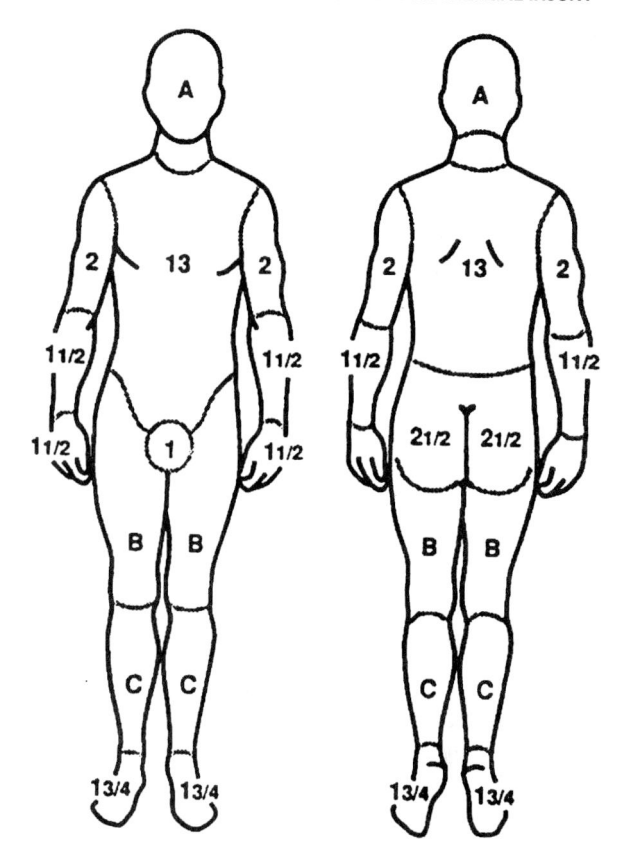

Area	0	1	5	10	15	Adult
A: half of head	9–1/2	8-1/2	6–1/2	5–1/2	4–1/2	3–1/2
B: half of thigh	2–3/4	3–1/4	4	4–1/4	4–1/2	4–3/4
C: half of leg	2–1/2	2–1/2	2÷3/4	3	3–1/4	3–1/2

FIG. 14-2 Lund and Browder Pediatric Burn Surface Area. Relative percentages of areas affected by growth (age in years).

leads to the release of catecholamines, angiotensin II, and vasopressin. These increase cardiac output and vasoconstriction, which help to decrease the microvascular extravasation. In patients with extensive burns (>40%), contractile dysfunction of the heart can occur despite adequate fluid resuscitation. Data suggest that oxygen free radicals, tumor necrosis factor, and interleukins act as direct cardiac depressants. The heart's response to endogenous and exogenous catecholamine is attenuated, which further blunts the cardiac response to the thermal injury.

INHALATIONAL INJURY

Concomitant with thermal injury to the skin, a patient may have an inhalational injury from the smoke created by the fire. Inhalational injury is caused by the carbonaceous material produced by the fire and the toxins released from the burning substances. The carbonaceous material enters the airway, irritating the mucosa and stimulating an inflammatory reaction. This reaction leads to a release of cytokines, free radical production, and complement activation. The epithelium of the tracheobronchial tree is destroyed, thereby eliminating the cilia responsible for clearing foreign material from the airway. Airway edema occurs, surfactant is deactivated, and mucous production increases as macrophages and leukocytes infiltrate the airways. Within 12 to 24 h, the tracheobronchial tree epithelium begins to slough, creating casts that obstruct the airway. In addition, the inflammation leads to acute lung injury characterized by decreased compliance and atelectasis, which make oxygenation and ventilation difficult. Inhalational injury complicates the management of any size burn and doubles the mortality rates in this population.

Carbon Monoxide

Although fires in enclosed spaces release many toxins, carbon monoxide and cyanide are the most prevalent and lethal. Incomplete combustion of carbon-containing substances, such as wood, coal, and gasoline, produces carbon monoxide. Carbon monoxide binds to hemoglobin with an affinity 200 to 250 times that of oxygen, thereby impairing hemoglobin's oxygen-carrying capacity. The oxygen disassociation curve shifts to the left, thus decreasing the ability to unload oxygen at the cellular level. Carbon monoxide also competitively inhibits cytochrome oxidative systems, thus decreasing the effectiveness of oxygen use.

In severe cases of carbon monoxide poisoning, a patient has changes in neurologic status and cardiac arrhythmias. Neurologic symptoms range from tinnitus and dizziness to coma and seizures depending on the levels of carbon monoxide in tissue. The readings on the pulse oximeter will be falsely elevated because it measures the binding of hemoglobin but does not differentiate between binding of oxygen or carbon monoxide to the hemoglobin molecules. A co-oximeter can accurately determine oxygen saturation in the blood and measure the carbon monoxide level. Toxicity occurs with levels above 10%; levels above 55% are considered lethal. The mainstay of therapy for carbon monoxide is 100% oxygen, which decreases the half-life of carbon monoxide from 250 min to less than 60 min. Because of this relationship, some physicians favor hyperbaric oxygen therapy to further decrease the half-life of carbon monoxide. Unfortunately, the data do not demonstrate long-term benefit from this therapy.[2]

Cyanide

Plastics with high nitrogen content such as polyurethane and acrocyanate glue found in laminates produce hydrogen cyanide when burned. Cyanide inhibits the cytochrome oxidative system by reversible inhibition of cytochrome oxidase (Fe^{3+}), which inhibits mitochondrial oxygen consumption. Cells then must use anaerobic metabolism to produce energy, which creates lactic acidosis and cell anoxia. Clinically, the patient experiences headache, dizziness, tachycardia, and tachypnea that can progress to death, if not reversed. Cyanide levels are not readily measured at institutions so one must look for metabolic acidosis out of proportion to hypovolemic shock and elevated lactate levels to make this diagnosis quickly.

Therapy for cyanide poisoning is administration of a cyanide antidote kit consisting of sodium thiosulphate and sodium nitrite. Sodium thiosulphate is a substrate used by the liver to metabolize the cyanide, which is a slow process. Sodium nitrite forms methemoglobin that will neutralize cyanide to cyanomethemoglobin. Unfortunately, methemoglobin also decreases oxygen-carrying capacity and oxygen delivery, potentially increasing a patient's existing hypoxia from the inhalational injury. It is prudent to add sodium thiosulphate quickly to the regimen of an inhalational injury victim with lactic acidosis but caution should be used with nitrite administration.[3]

MANAGEMENT ISSUES

Airway and Ventilation

In the initial stabilization phase, a child's airway must be evaluated for evidence of burns, inhalational injury, or other trauma. Evidence that the airway may be burned includes blistering or eschar on the lips or nasal area, singeing of the nasal hairs, and erythema or swelling of the airway. The patient also may have a brassy cough, stridor, or a hoarse voice. If a child has evidence of airway injury or has difficulty breathing, with tachypnea, stridor, wheezing, and retractions, he has an inhalational injury. Respiratory compromise also may lead to a depressed neurologic status. If there is a history of trauma in addition to the burn, a child should be examined for facial injury such as broken bones, significant lacerations, and airway fractures.

If a child has had thermal injury to the airway, edema in the first several hours after injury will obstruct the airway. A child's airway is narrower than an adult's airway, and mild swelling can produce significant distress. Although an awake intubation may be ideal in this type of patient, it can be very difficult in a child and usually one needs to examine other options. Many times a child can be intubated in the initial period with direct laryngoscopy after adequate sedation. However, some children may need to be taken to the operating room for a deep inhalational anesthetic and intubation, as for a patient with epiglottitis. In this situation, use of a fiber-optic scope, Bullard laryngoscopes, or a laryngeal mask airway to guide fiber-optic intubation may be beneficial. After successful intubation, a bronchoscopy is completed to further evaluate the damage to the proximal and distal airways.

When evaluating for inhalational injury by bronchoscopy, the more distal the evidence of airway injury, the greater the likelihood of acute lung injury. Acute lung injury causes difficulty with oxygenation, ventilation, and increased secretions. Therapies for acute lung injury include a ventilation strategy of adequate positive end expiratory pressure (PEEP) (10 to 15), minimal fraction of inspired oxygen (<0.60), low tidal volumes (5 to 8 mL/kg), and bronchodilators. Patients also will develop thick secretions and casts, which place them at high risk for an obstructed endotracheal tube and major bronchi. Aggressive pulmonary toilet with frequent suctioning is necessary to decrease this risk. If traditional methods of ventilation do not provide adequate oxygenation or ventilation, other therapies such as high-frequency oscillation, surfactant, nitric oxide, and even extracorporeal membrane oxygenation (ECMO) might be beneficial. None of these therapies is better than conventional ventilation strategies for improvement after acute lung injury.

Cardiovascular

A burned child may be tachycardic, with deceased pulses and capillary refill. She also may be hypotensive and hypothermic. The inflammatory response of the burn rapidly creates hypovolemia in a child, which can lead to end-organ damage without immediate attention. Venous access is challenging in this population. Ideally, two large-bore intravenous lines can be placed in the upper extremities through unburned skin. If unburned skin is not available, one may access the burned area. If attempts at peripheral access are unsuccessful, alternative access sites must be used. Interosseous lines, cut-down venous lines, and central venous catheters, preferably short lines with wide diameters, can be attempted, depending on the supplies and expertise immediately available.

Fluid resuscitation in this population begins with isotonic crystalloid fluids such as lactated Ringer's or normal saline. Initially, a child does not require glucose-containing products because catecholamine release causes hyperglycemia. As volume resuscitation begins, fluid is distributed in the interstitial and intravascular spaces. Only one-third of the volume will remain intravascular, so the patient will become edematous during resuscitation. Hypertonic saline in the first 24 h can be used to decrease the total fluid requirement by increasing osmotic pressure and pulling fluid from the interstitial space. Care must be taken not to exceed a sodium level of 160 mEq/L. Colloids do not decrease capillary leak and are expensive, so they are usually avoided during the first 8 to 12 h of fluid resuscitation.

There are many variations of the appropriate formula to use to estimate the fluid requirements of a burn patient. The Parkland formula recommends calculating 4 mL × kilograms × %TBSA, giving half of this fluid in the first 8 h after the burn and the rest during the next 16 h. Children have higher relative evaporative losses than adults because of their relatively large surface area, so many burn centers add maintenance fluids to this formula at the rate of 1500 to 2000 mL by body surface area (m^2). The only way to ensure that fluid resuscitation is adequate is to resuscitate to physiologic end-points and evaluate capillary refill, heart rate, blood pressure, urine output, and neurologic status. One should maintain urine output between 1 and 2 mL/(kg · h) in a small child and between 0.5 and 1 mL/(kg · h) an older patient. If urine output exceeds this rate, fluids should be decreased to prevent excess edema in the lungs and nonburned areas. If there is inadequate urine output, fluid rate should be increased.

If the patient has adequate urine output and still appears hypotensive, she may be exhibiting cardiac depression from the direct cardiac depressants released during the inflammatory response. A patient also may have entered the second phase of the burn inflammatory response with a high cardiac output (15 to 20 L/min) and a very low SVR (<300) because of ongoing inflammatory mediators. These conditions may require inotropic or vasopressor support or both. If a patient appears to have an adequate cardiac output but no SVR, then a pure α-agonist such as neosynephrine is a good choice for therapy. If the patient is not adequately resuscitated, this medication will increase ischemia to the skin beds and the kidneys, so it should be used cautiously. If the cardiac function appears depressed, such as relative bradycardia in the face of hypotension or echocardiogram (ECHO) evidence of diminished function, medication with α and β properties will work best. Examples are dopamine, epinephrine, and norepinephrine. Some experts advocate use of a Swan–Ganz catheter, if medication appears necessary. At the very least, one should closely observe central venous pressure (CVP), urine output, and perfusion.

Fluids, Electrolytes, and Nutrition

Electrolyte abnormalities are common in the first few days after a large burn because of the massive fluid shifts and the loss of protein-enriched fluid through the skin. Hypocalcemia and hypomagnesemia occur early in the course of the resuscitation, which can lead to tetany and cardiac contractility problems, if not corrected. In addition, during the first 24 h one may see hyperkalemia if the patient has rhabdomyolysis, particularly if there is an electrical injury. Hypernatremia occurs on the second or third day because of changes in the sodium pump at the skin site and the massive sodium replacement in the first 24 h. Fluids may be changed to include less sodium in the second 24 h. Glucose may be added if a patient's glucose is within normal limits or low. Hypophosphatemia can weaken the respiratory muscles if phosphate is not replaced. Hypoalbuminemia results from the protein loss from the wounds. Although albumin replacement does not change the absolute amount of albumin measured in the blood, it may decrease the total fluid requirement for the second 24-h period and throughout the later stages of therapy.

Although fluid requirements are highest in the first 24 h, a patient will require fluids until the burns have been adequately re-epithelialized, through healing, grafting, or coverage with artificial skin. Most fluid should be delivered in the form of enteral nutrition, but a patient is likely to continue to require some intravenous fluids of a crystalloid or a colloid nature. Blood products will be required for large burns.

Good nutrition is essential for burn patients to heal. Burns cause an individual to be catabolic and can double the calorie requirements for children. For these reasons, enteral nutrition is started immediately on a child's arrival to the burn center through nasogastric or nasojejunal tubes. Nasojejunal tubes are preferable because the patient can be fed despite the gastric ileus from a burn injury, narcotics, or subsequent sepsis. Because of their nutritional needs, intubated patients who tolerate their feedings should be fed until they go to the operating room, rather than observing the restriction against solids for 6 to 8 h before surgery. If the patient has a nasojejunal tube, enteral feedings can be continued during the operation.

Infection

Although febrile in the first several days after their injury, burn patients are rarely infected. Sepsis develops later from line infections or infections originating from burned, decaying skin. Burn debridement within the first week after the injury and topical atibiotics have greatly decreased the risk of infection. Central venous lines changed at regular intervals decrease the risk of infection. Intubation and ventilation increase the risk of tracheitis, pneumonia, and sinusitis. Foley catheters increase the risk of urinary tract infections. For these reasons, close attention is given to the need for each device. If a patient has burn wound sepsis, therapy must include debridement in the operating room. The need for debridement may require taking a hemodynamically unstable patient to the operating room.

The use of prophylactic antibiotics should be avoided because they do not improve survival and increase bacterial resistance. Parenteral antibiotics should be reserved for evidence of invasive disease, i.e., positive blood, cerebrospinal fluid, or urine culture or generalized sepsis. The risk of invasive candidal infection is high in burn patients and increases their mortality, so it should be considered during any septic episode.

Hematologic Concerns

Initially the burn patient will have a normal complete blood cell count, and the hematocrit may rise in the first 24 h because of hemoconcentration. Over the next several days, however, anemia will result from the reabsorption of interstitial fluid, hemolysis from the initial injury, blood loss, and decreased red blood cell production. Anemia will be compounded by operations in which large blood volumes will be lost during the debridement process. Iron replacement should start as soon as the patient tolerates enteral feeds, but children with large burns will require red blood cell (RBC) replacement during their initial hospitalization. In children with smaller burns, the hematocrit can decrease to 20, usually without hemodynamic instability, and the risks of transfusion can be avoided.

In children with large burns, significant blood loss can lead to dilutional coagulopathy from loss of clotting factors and platelets. Replacement with fresh frozen plasma (FFP), cryoprecipitate, and platelets may be necessary. If thrombocytopenia persists despite hemostasis and platelet replacement, alternative causes must be considered including alloantibodies and heparin-induced antibodies to platelets.

Renal Issues

Rhabdomyolysis occurs from deep burns that involve muscle, electrical injury, and compartment syndrome. Serum creatinine kinase levels and urine myoglobin levels should be checked, as should an urinalysis for the presence of blood without RBCs on the microscopic examination. If the patient has significant rhabdomyolysis, urine output must be increased to avoid direct renal injury from myoglobin. Sodium bicarbonate should be added to the fluids to alkalinize the urine and mannitol, 0.25 g/kg every 6 h, should be given to facilitate elimination of the toxin.

In addition to rhabdomyolysis, renal failure may develop in the burn patient from acute tubular necrosis from hypovolemia, uncompensated volume loss in the operating room, and nephrotoxic medications. Some patients will require continuous venous hemodialysis or limited dialysis because of renal failure. Adequate intravascular volume must be assured at all times to minimize renal failure.

Neurologic Trauma

The patient who has suffered a significant inhalational injury may have neurologic injury as a result of anoxia from inadequate oxygenation or toxic gases, such as cyanide and carbon monoxide. In these patients, careful evaluation of neurologic status at frequent intervals is necessary to monitor for seizure activity and further depression of mental status. Anoxia, regardless of the origin, may cause significant brain edema and cellular death. In severe cases, these changes can lead to coma and brain death. No specific therapy decreases the edema associated with anoxia. Therapy is supportive. Significant carbon monoxide exposure has caused a variety of neuropsychiatric syndromes, which develop 2 to 300 days after exposure. Again, therapy is supportive.

Pain Management

Thermal injury itself and the resultant therapies, including dressing changes and hydrotherapy, are very painful. This pain is best relieved by use of opioids. For the extubated and alert patient, a patient-controlled anesthesia (PCA) pump is appropriate. A pump will allow the child to control medication and safely increase the dose during painful procedures. Fentanyl lollipops have been used effectively for hydrotherapy in children without the side effect of nausea. Intermittent morphine dosing and Tylenol with codeine also are effective for relief of pain during simple dressing changes and hydrotherapy.

For some patients, the use of an opioid alone is not satisfactory to reduce the anxiety and pain experienced with a particular procedure. The addition of a benzodiazepine, such as midazolam, to morphine or fentanyl is effective. However, this combination increases the incidence of respiratory depression. Ketamine also may be useful. It has the advantage of providing amnesia and an anesthetic with one medication. Unfortunately, a child may experience dysphoria that is attenuated with benzodiazepines. Propofol can be used but it does not provide analgesia and can cause apnea and hypotension. Narcotics are required to supplement propofol use, further increasing side effect risk. The key issue is to be certain sufficient analgesics have been administered.

OPERATING ROOM MANAGEMENT

Surgical Procedures

Surgery for burn patients may begin on presentation to the burn unit. If a patient has circumferential burns of the extremities, he is at risk for compartment syndrome and loss of a limb. Burned extremities require prompt escharotomies or fasciotomies. The chest with circumferential burns can severely restrict the chest wall, decreasing pulmonary compliance and severely limiting a patient's ability to ventilate and oxygenate his lungs. The patient should have all pulses evaluated. If perfusion is compromised, compartment pressure must be reduced quickly with an escharotomy or fasciotomy. In escharatomy, the surgeon makes a mid-axial incision through the eschar with an electrocautery, being careful to avoid the subcutaneous tissue. This therapy should relieve the pressure, allow return of the pulses, or improve chest wall movement. Fasciotomies are also done with an electrocautery but the area is opened into the fascial plane. Bleeding can be excessive during or after a fasciotomy.

Surgeons begin to excise the burned skin early in a large burn to decrease colonization with bacteria and subsequent sepsis. This is a bloody procedure performed in the operating room. A dermatome or knife is used to excise the burned skin in a tangential fashion. The goal is to have a viable bed that may be fat or fascia. If dissection is to the fat layer, blood loss will be increased because of its rich capillary beds. The fascial plane has less bleeding but may not produce an equal cosmetic result.

With either procedure, hemostasis must be achieved after debridement. For extremities, the surgeon may use tourniquets to decrease the amount of bleeding. For all areas, the surgeon uses a topical diluted epinephrine solution or topical thrombin and ace wraps.

After hemostasis, the surgeon covers the excised area with a skin graft from the patient, donor skin, or artificial skin. The surgeon obtains a donor skin graft from the patient by using the dermatome to cut a thin piece of skin from a nonburned area. In children, the surgeon prefers the buttocks or upper thighs, if available, for cuts because these areas are hidden under clothing. Any area of skin may be used. The surgeon may inject the skin subcutaneously with a mixture of diluted epinephrine to stretch the skin and make it smoother for excision.

In electrical burns or very deep thermal burns, an extremity may have extensive injury, and significant portions may be necrotic. In these cases, amputation of the extremity may be necessary to prevent infection and promote healing.

Children with extensive burns will continue to have operations for years to come for reconstructive procedures and elimination of scar tissue. The head and neck may require extensive reconstruction to alleviate airway obstruction and recreate the face. Extremities require multiple additional surgeries to regain better function. Burn scars can be disfiguring and create medical problems such as immobile necks and scoliosis. Thus airway management may continue to be a challenge.

Preparation for the Operating Room

The anesthetic for a burn patient requires substantial preplanning. The anesthesiologist should carefully evaluate any burn patient preoperatively. Current medication and allergies should be reviewed. One should ask about any medical comorbidity or concomitant injuries with the burn that might complicate the anesthetic management such as inhalational injury or neurologic injury. Examination of the patient's airway and the intubation history are crucial in the preoperative preparation because burns or previous surgeries and intubations may have made the neck immobile, the landmarks distorted, or the airway narrow. An adequate number of blood products must be prepared. Temperature in the operating room must be adjusted to prevent hypothermia in the patient, especially the small child. The anesthesiologist may place a child under warming lights, a forced air blanket, or on a warming blanket for the procedure. One should know the position a child will be placed for surgery. The child may need to be on his side or prone for part or all of the case.

Induction and Maintenance

The choice of an anesthetic for the burn patient depends on the anesthesiologist and the patient. Inhalational and intravenous medications may be used effectively. The choice will depend on the hemodynamic stability of the patient, her tolerance level to medications, especially opioids; and the mode of ventilation.

One drug that is absolutely contraindicated is succinylcholine. From as little as 24 h after injury to 1 year after the injury, succinylcholine is life threatening. Thermal injury to the skin causes denervation and immobilization of the skin and muscle membrane in the area. Denervation and immobilization lead to a proliferation of acetylcholine receptors. Cholinergic agonists activate the membrane receptors. The receptors depolarize, releasing a large amount of intracellular potassium, which causes life-threatening hyperkalemia.

The burn patient's intravascular status changes rapidly with volume shifts between plasma and interstitial fluid. Increases in volume and changes in hepatic and renal elimination may alter the volume of distribution for many medications. For these reasons, it is not unusual to increase doses of medications, such as nondepolarizing muscle relaxants, to achieve the same plasma levels and clinical response.

Monitoring

The patient undergoing burn surgery with greater than 20% of the body affected will lose substantial quantities of blood. Therefore, one must have monitoring devices in place to help estimate volume resuscitation. Ideally, one should have an arterial line for continuous blood pressure monitoring and to facilitate blood sampling for hematocrit and arterial blood gases. Two large-bore intravenous lines or one single lumen central catheter and one peripheral intravenous line for volume resuscitation are required. A Foley catheter also allows continuous monitoring of urine output, which should remain at 1 to 2 mL/(kg · h) in the child. An esophageal or rectal temperature probe should be used to continuously monitor the temperature. Children will become hypothermic quickly. At a body temperature below 35°C, coagulopathy will be problematic. Surgery should be discontinued well in advance of this occurrence.

Airway and Ventilation Issues

It cannot be emphasized enough that careful evaluation of the airway of the burn patient is crucial. If the patient has had burns to the mouth or face, he may not be able to open his mouth for direct laryngoscopy. If there are burns to the neck, he may not be able to flex or extend his neck. The subglottic region may be narrow from inhalational injury and scarring or previous intubations. The evaluation should include direct visual examination and a review of previous intubation history.

An intubated patient still poses challenges to an anesthesiologist. Care should be taken that the tube is secure and properly placed before beginning the case. The patient may be placed in the prone position and a loose tube can easily become dislodged during the turning process. One also needs to be aware of the reason for the initial intubation and what the critical care team believes are the current conditions of the airway, i.e., edematous upper airway or acute lung injury. Patency of the endotracheal tube or tracheostomy tube is important and often threatened. Burn patients often have thick secretions that can easily occlude the airway. Suctioning may be required frequently throughout the surgery to prevent occlusion.

If a patient's lungs have been mechanically ventilated because of acute lung injury, mechanical ventilation with an intensive care unit ventilator may be necessary to ensure adequate oxygenation and ventilation. Anesthesia machines cannot easily generate the high minute ventilation required for a burn patient. If the patient requires greater than 5 of PEEP, more than 50% fraction of inspired oxygen, or greater than 50 peak inspiratory pressure (PIP) on volume control ventilation, then the intensive care unit ventilator should be available.

Fluid Management

After the airway has been managed, the next anesthetic challenge in a burn patient is fluid management. The patient has rapid fluid shifts during bleeding for harvesting and debridement. Bleeding can be brisk and difficult to quantify because of its diffuse nature. Transfusing packed RBCs and FFP (fresh frozen plasma) may be prudent before the first incision in a large burn case Red blood cells and FFP may be given together to simulate whole blood. If large blood loss is anticipated (one blood volume or greater), then giving platelets during the case will help with hemostasis of the vascular beds after debridement. For large burns (>25%) in a child weighing less than 20 kg, 5 U of packed RBCs (PRBCs), 5 U of FFP, and 5 single units of platelets should be available. For children weighing more than 20 kg, these numbers should be doubled. If the anesthesiologist notes hemodynamic instability that does not quickly correct, he should have the surgeons stop cutting and apply hemostasis techniques until the patient has been adequately resuscitated with fluid. A reasonable rule of thumb is that, for every 1% of TBSA grafted, there is a 2% blood volume loss, e.g., 20% excision equals a 40% blood volume loss.

Other Issues

The patient may absorb large amounts of the diluted (1:10,000 or less) epinephrine infusion during the case and become hypertensive. Hypertension can create a false sense of security about fluid status and cause the anesthesiologist to underestimate fluid requirements. As the epinephrine effect is lost, the patient becomes hypotensive. However, if this response is sustained, the anesthesiologist may have to temporarily block it with a short-acting antihypertensive or increased inhalation anesthesia.

Hypothermia is a substantial problem in the burn operating room. Coagulation is impaired. Hemodynamics are challenged. Blood warmers should be used for fluids and blood products. A forced air warmer should cover unoperated sites. If the intensive care unit ventilator is used, a humidifier can also reduce heat loss. Should the body temperature fall below 36°C, the operative procedure should be shortened.

The management of the burn patient challenges the anesthesiologist in many ways. Initial airway management includes many difficult airways and maintenance of the airway can be difficult because of secretions and multiple operating positions. Fluid resuscitation is critical in the initial burn surgeries and requires close attention to the surgical field. Coagulopathy and temperature instability further complicate these anesthetics. In the end, for an injured child, the cosmetic and functional improvements provided by these extensive surgeries demand our care and vigilance.

REFERENCES

1. MacLennan N, Heimbach DM, Clullen BF: Anesthesia for major thermal injury. *Anesthesiology* 89:749, 1998.
2. Tibbles PM, Edelsberg JS: Medical progress: hyperbaric-oxygen therapy. *N Engl J Med* 334:1642, 1996.
3. Breen PH, Isserles SA, Westley J, et al: Combined carbon monoxide and cyanide poisoning: a place for treatment? *Anesth Analg* 80:671, 1995.

15 | The Child With Cancer
Joseph Rossi, MD

Although the incidence is increasing, cancer in the pediatric population remains relatively rare (7500 new cases annually vs. 1.1 million cases/year in adults).[1] According to the National Cancer Institute's Surveillance, Epidemiology and End Result program, new disease occurs at a rate of 133.3 per 1,000,000 children each year[2] (Table 15-1). However, with improved therapy modalities, mortality from pediatric cancer and its treatment is decreasing. By some estimates, 80% of children treated for cancer are expected to be long-term survivors.[1] In 1991, 1 in 1000 adults had been treated for childhood cancer and 180,000 to 220,000 childhood cancer survivors were living in the United States.[3] Those numbers have certainly increased in the past decade. Others estimate that by 2010 1 in 250 adults, ages 20 to 45 years, will be a survivor of a childhood cancer.[4] Thus, the likelihood is increasing that anesthesia will be indicated for a patient with cancer or a cancer survivor.

Providing care for the pediatric cancer patient may take place in the operating room for primary or metastatic tumor resection, diagnostic staging, or central line placement. Conversely, care outside the operating room includes diagnostic procedures (e.g., lumbar punctures, bone marrow biopsies, imaging studies) and therapeutic interventions (e.g., radiation therapy). The anesthesiologist also may be involved in the treatment of cancer pain. Care is frequently provided for potential cancer victims (e.g., cervical node biopsies) who may present with little more than vague complaints (Table 15-2).

ONCOLOGIC EMERGENCIES

Acute emergencies in the pediatric oncology patient may require immediate care (Table 15-3).[5] These situations often involve the anesthesiologist in the operating room, radiology suite, or the emergency department. Some of these issues are described elsewhere in this text (e.g., increased intracranial pressure and imminent herniation from tumors in the central nervous system [CNS]) or are inherently obvious in the care of any child (e.g., massive organomegaly with respiratory compromise and aspiration risks), but other emergencies merit further discussion.

Masses of the Mediastinum

The anesthesia and surgical literatures are replete with case reports of unanticipated cardiorespiratory arrest in patients with anterior mediastinal masses. One or more factors contribute to this occurrence: obstruction of the major airways with the inability to ventilate, superior vena cava syndrome, and cardiac or great vessel (specifically the main pulmonary artery) compression with hypoxemia despite the ability to ventilate. Whereas some children have an established diagnosis, others for seemingly unrelated procedures might be at risk for a mediastinal mass. For example, malignant neoplastic disease is but one possible diagnosis in the child for excisional biopsy of a neck mass (Table 15-4).[6]

Cancerous and noncancerous masses occur within all compartments of the mediastinum (Table 15-5).[7] Although intraoperative catastrophes have been

TABLE 15–1 Annual U.S. Cancer Incidence Rates Among Children Younger Than 15 Years*

Type	All ages Rate	All ages %	<1 Rate	<1 %	1–4 Rate	1–4 %	5–9 Rate	5–9 %	10–14 Rate	10–14 %
All histologic types	133.3		218.4		174.9		106.8		111.0	
Acute lymphoblastic leukemia	30.9	23.2	20.0	9.2	60.8	34.8	27.3	25.6	15.6	14.0
All primary central nervous system tumors	27.6	20.7	32.8	15.0	32.3	18.5	29.4	27.5	21.8	19.7
Neuroblastoma	9.7	7.3	55.2	25.3	17.6	10.1	3.0	2.8	0.7	0.6
Non-Hodgkin's lymphoma	8.4	6.3	1.9	0.9	6.9	3.9	9.0	8.4	10.4	9.4
Wilm's tumor	8.1	6.1	21.7	9.9	16.7	9.5	5.8	5.4	1.1	1.0
Hodgkin's lymphoma	6.6	5.0	0.2	0.1	0.6	0.4	4.9	4.6	13.5	12.2
Acute myelogenous leukemia	5.6	4.2	10.6	4.9	6.2	3.5	4.4	4.1	5.8	5.2
Rhabdomyosarcoma	4.5	3.4	6.4	2.9	5.8	3.3	5.0	4.7	2.6	2.3
Retinoblastoma	3.9	2.9	24.7	11.3	7.6	4.3	0.3	0.6	0.0	0.0
Osteosarcoma	3.4	2.6	0.0	0.0	0.4	0.2	1.9	1.8	7.5	6.7
Ewing's sarcoma	2.8	2.1	0.6	0.3	0.8	0.5	2.4	2.3	436.0	4.1
All other histologic types	21.8	16.4	44.3	20.2	19.2	11.0	13.1	12.2	27.4	24.7

*Rates are standardized to the 1980 SEER population and reported per million children per year.
Source: Modified from Gurney JG, Severson RK, Davis S, et al: Incidence of cancer in children in the United States. *Cancer* 15:2186, 1995.

TABLE 15–2 Presenting Symptoms of Childhood Cancer

Fever	Lymphadenopathy (especially supraclavicular)
Pallor	
Bone or joint pain	Headache (especially on rising)
Gait disturbance (limp)	Diplopia
Gingival hyperplasia	Proptosis
Petechiae, ecchymoses or purpura	Nausea/vomiting (especially on rising)
Hepatomegaly and/or splenomegaly	
Mood/personality alterations	Lethargy
Papilledema	Fatigue
New onset seizures	Hypertension
Orthopnea	Cranial nerve palsy
Night sweats	Persistent cough
Torticollis	Abdominal mass
Sinusitis	Weight loss
Hoarseness	Dysphagia
	Ataxia
	Epistaxis

reported with *anterior* mediastinal masses, significant cardiorespiratory compromise has occurred with lesions in other compartments. Moreover, noncancerous lesions of the mediastinum may result in pulmonary and cardiac decompensation.[8] Lymphomas account for 87% of the malignant masses of the anterior mediastinum.[6] Conversely, 16% to 36% and 54% to 81% of children with non-Hodgkin's and Hodgkin's lymphomas, respectively,[9] and 8% of children with leukemias have anterior mediastinal masses on presentation.[5] Because lymphomas can double in size in days, anesthetic evaluation of these patients should include a recent chest x-ray.[6]

Several signs and symptoms suggest the presence of an anterior mediastinal mass (Table 15-6).[10] However, only 40% to 60% of patients have respiratory symptoms,[6,11] and only orthopnea has been shown to correlate with risk of respiratory collapse on induction of anesthesia (Figure 15-1).[12] Presenting symptoms are often nonspecific and include fever, malaise, mild cough, lymphadenopathy, or neck mass (Table 15-4). Cyanosis and stridor are late and ominous signs. Similarly, a new onset murmur may be the only sign of compression of the heart and pulmonary vessels. In seeking a mediastinal mass, the anesthesiologist must be vigilant in determining the need for a chest x-ray.

Children with anterior mediastinal masses often present for general anesthesia to secure tissue for diagnosis. When possible, diagnoses should be made in other ways—bone marrow biopsy, thoracentesis of pleural effusions, or biopsy of extrathoracic masses under local anesthesia. Because of the risks, it has historically been proposed that, if a diagnosis could not be made from tissue obtained without general anesthesia, a symptomatic patient should receive empiric radiation therapy to reduce the mass effect. However, because this has often yielded equivocal results that have led to suboptimal treatment, this approach has been questioned.[9,11] Thus, at some point general anesthesia may be sought to help provide a diagnosis.

Given the need for general anesthesia for children with intrathoracic masses and the dubious reliability of the history and physical examination, evaluative tests have been proposed. Two tests, used in conjunction, may best predict respiratory compromise under general anesthesia.[13] Cross-sectional area of the trachea, measured at its narrowest portion by computed

TABLE 15–3 Pediatric Oncologic Emergencies

Emergency	Signs and symptoms	Laboratory/radiology	Oncologic conditions
Superior vena cava syndrome	Shortness of breath, facial swelling, syncope	Anterior mediastinal mass	Non-Hodgkin's lymphoma, T-cell leukemia, teratoma, thyroid cancer, thymoma, Hodgkin's disease, sarcoma neuroblastoma
Spinal cord compression	Back pain, radicular pain, leg weakness or paralysis, extremity weakness, neck pain	MRI: epidural mass Radiograph: lytic lesion	Neuroblastoma, sarcoma, lymphoma, leukemia, astrocytoma, ependymoma, metastases
Increased intracranial pressure	Headache	CT/MRI:mass	Brain tumor
Brain herniation	Morning vomiting, diplopia, ataxia, Cushing's triad, increase in head size, cerebrovascular accident	Hydrocephalus, hemorrhage, thrombus	Brain metastasis, CNS; leukemia, abscess
Massive hepatomegaly	Huge liver, cardio-respiratory failure	Coagulation studies	Neonatal stage IV-S neuroblastoma
Hyperleukocytosis	Headache, altered consciousness, respiratory distress, priapism, none	WBC >200,000/mL; tumor lysis syndrome acidosis	Leukemia

(continued)

Leukopenia	Fever, infection, opportunistic infections	WBC <1500/mL ANC <500/mL ALC <1000/mL	Leukemia, post-chemotherapy
Coagulopathy	Bruising, petechiae, epistaxis, hemorrhagic diathesis	Thrombocytopenia increased PT, PTT	Leukemia, post-chemotherapy, acute promyelocytic leukemia, sepsis, vitamin K deficiency
Cerebrovascular accident	Headache, altered consciousness, local neurologic deficit	CT/MRI: hemorrhage, thrombus	Asparaginase, coagulopathy, methotrexate, vasculopathy, radiation vasculitis
Anemia	Pallor, heart failure	Hb <2-5 g/dL	Leukemia, hemorrhage
Tumor lysis syndrome	Abdominal mass, symptoms of leukemia	Hyperuricemia, hyperphosphatemia, hypocalcemia, hyperkalemia, increased blood urea nitrogen, creatinine	Acute lymphoblastic leukemia, Burkit's lymphoma, other lymphoma or leukemia, other tumors
Hypercalcemia	Vomiting, lethargy, decreased urine output	Increased calcium	Non-Hodgkin's lymphoma, alveolar rhabdomyosarcoma, leukemia

ALC, absolute lymphocyte count; ANC, absolute neutrophil count; CNS, central nervous system; CT, computed tomography; Hb, hemoglobin; MRI, magnetic resonance imaging; PT, prothrombin time; PTT, partial thromboplastin time; WBC, leukocyte.
Source: Modified from Kelly KM, Lange B: Oncologic emergencies. *Pediatr Clin North Am* 44:809, 1997.

TABLE 15–4 Common Causes of Neck Masses in Children

Inflammatory
- Ludwig's angina
- Parapharyngeal abscess
- Inflammatory node abscess
  - Viral
  - Bacterial
    - *Streptococcus* or *Staphylococcus*
    - Tuberculosis (scrofula) or atypical mycobacteria
  - Toxoplasmosis

Superficial benign mass
- Epidural inclusions
- Lipoma
- Fibroma

Congenital
- Hemangioma
- Cystic hygroma
- Brachial cleft cyst
- Thyroglossal duct cyst
- Goiter
- Ranula
- Dermoid–epidermoid

Neoplastic
- Benign
  - Neurogenic tumors
    - Neurilemona
    - Neurofibroma
- Malignant (has a benign component)
  - Cancer of thyroglossal duct remnants
  - Fibrosarcoma
  - Lymphoma (Hodgkin's or non-Hodgkin's)
  - Rhabdomyosarcoma
  - Leukemia
  - Thyroid malignancy
  - Salivary gland malignancy
  - Metastatic neoplasm
    - Tongue
    - Floor of the mouth
    - Lip
    - Mediastinum
    - Sinus/nasopharynx
    - Larynx
- Miscellaneous
  - Salivary gland disease
  - Thyroid/parathyroid disease
  - Esophageal diverticulum
  - Torticollis

Source: Modified from Viswanathan S, Campbell CE, Cork RC: Asymptomatic undetected mediastinal mass: a death during ambulatory anesthesia. *J Clin Anesth* 7:151, 1995.

TABLE 15–5 Tumors of the Mediastinum

Location	Presentation
Anterior division	
Lymphomas	Tracheal and lung compression
Lymphangiomas (cystic hygroma)	Cardiac tamponade
Teratomas	Superior venacaval syndrome
Thymomas and thymic cysts	
Middle division	
Bronchogenic cysts	Airway obstruction
Granulomas	Stridor
Lymphomas	Obstructive emphysema
Posterior division	
Enteric cysts, duplications	Airway obstruction
Neuroblastoma	Recurrent pneumonias
Ganglioneuroma, neurofibroma	Dysphagia

Source: Modified from Davis PJ, Hall S, Deshpande JK, et al: Anesthesia for general, urologic, and plastic surgery. In *Smith's Anesthesia for Infants and Children,* 6th ed. Motoyama EK, Davis PJ, eds. St. Louis, Mosby, 1996, p 588.

TABLE 15–6 Evaluation of Patients With Anterior Mediastinal Masses

	History	Physical	Laboratory
Airway	Cough Cyanosis Dyspnea Orthopnea	Decreased breath sounds Wheezing Stridor Cyanosis	Chest roentgram (x-ray), anteroposterior and lateral Chest computed tomography: tracheal cross sectional area versus predicted values Pulmonary function tests, peak expiratory flow rates versus predicted values
Cardiovascular system	Dizziness or fainting Change in color, pallor Orthopnea Headacne Facial swelling Exacerbation of symptoms with Valsalva maneuver	Neck or facial edema Jugular venous distention Papilledema New onset murmur Blood pressure changes or pallor with postural changes Increased pulsus paradoxus	Echocardiogram or radionuclide scan: impediment of cardiovascular system Electrocardiogram

Source: Modified from Halpern S, Chatten J, Meadows AT, et al: Anterior mediastinal mass: anesthesia hazards and other problems. *J Pediatr* 102:407, 1983.

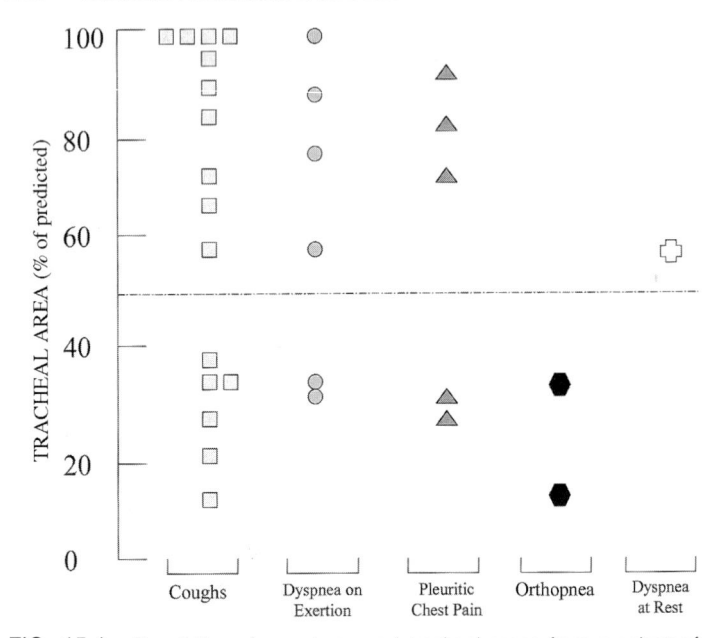

FIG. 15-1 Correlation of symptoms and tracheal areas from a cohort of 42 children with anterior mediastinal masses. *(Modified from Shamberger RC, Holzman RS, Griscom NT, et al: CT quantitation of tracheal cross-sectional area as a guide to the surgical and anesthetic management of children with anterior mediastinal masses.* J Pediatr Surg *26:138, 1991.)*

tomography (CT) and expressed as a percentage of predicted value, has been shown to correlate with the risk of respiratory collapse during general anesthesia.[12] Retrospective studies have cautioned that patients with tracheal sizes of less than 50% to 66% predicted may represent a high-risk group.[12] Further, in a study of the benefit of pulmonary function tests, general anesthesia was conducted safely in all patients who had peak expiratory flow rates (PEFRs) of greater than 50% predicted.[13] As PEFRs are affected by position (Figure 15-2),[13] measurements should be completed with the patient supine. Interestingly, not all children with less than 50% predicted PEFR were shown to have evidence of tracheal narrowing on CT (Figure 15-3).[13] Decreases in PEFRs were attributed either to *bronchial* compression limiting expiratory flow or to significant decrease in total lung capacity caused by the mass. Although all patients with both tracheal areas and PEFRs of greater than 50% predicted safely underwent general anesthesia, no conclusions regarding risks could be made in children with PEFRs of less than 50%. Quite possibly these patients would have done well. Thus, the two tests used in conjunction select patients at *low* risk. An electrocardiogram and an echocardiogram provide information on cardiac impingement by masses and should be completed in patients with signs of superior vena cava compression (Table 15-6) or in the presence of new heart murmurs.

Planning a course for safe general anesthesia requires an understanding of the pathophysiology of respiratory failure in patients with anterior mediasti-

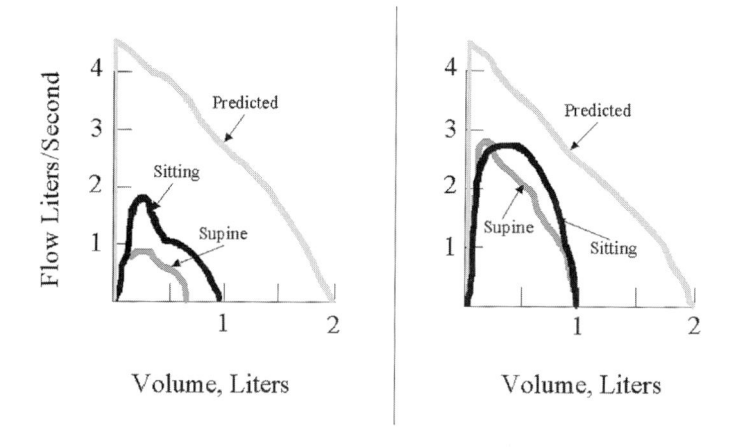

Presentation | Post Chemotherapy

FIG. 15-2 Pulmonary function flow testing in patients with anterior mediastinal masses at presentation and post chemotherapy. *(Modified from Shamberger RC, Holzman RS, Griscom NT, et al: Prospective evaluation by computed tomography and pulmonary function tests of children with mediastinal masses.* Surgery *118:468, 1995.)*

nal masses. With induction of general anesthesia, lung compliance decreases and lung retractive forces increase. These effects, along with cephalad displacement of the diaphragm while in the supine position, combine to significantly decrease functional residual capacity. Negative intrathoracic pressure, normally transmitted to the trachea during spontaneous ventilation, is lost with muscle relaxation and the use of positive pressure ventilation. As this negative pressure works to expand intrathoracic airways on inspiration, narrowing of the airways may become critical with the loss of spontaneous ventilation. Further, gas exchange decreases as laminar airflow through a compressed trachea becomes turbulent at high flow rates seen with positive pressure ventilation. Likewise, turbulent airflow may occur with spontaneous ventilation in patients with tachypnea, coughing, or increased work of breathing for any reason (e.g., hypoxemia, hypercarbia, pain).

When prior evaluation suggests a patient is at high risk for intraoperative complications, plans for general anesthesia prepare for the worst outcome. A sensitive but complete discussion of concerns, risks, and goals should take place with the family and patient as appropriate for age and ability to understand. Capability for rigid bronchoscopy by an experienced practitioner should be readily available. Although rarely needed, cardiopulmonary bypass must be anticipated for certain patients. Standard monitoring and intravenous access are secured before induction of anesthesia. Judicious use of preoperative sedation under close observation and EMLA cream may aid in patient preparation. Children with signs of superior vena cava syndrome should have intravenous access placed in a lower extremity. Direct intraarterial blood pressure monitoring before induction is occasionally indicated.

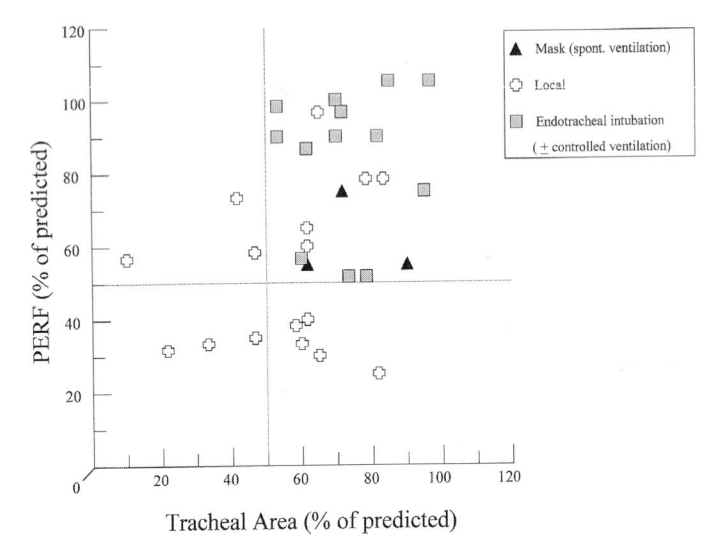

FIG. 15-3 The correlation between peak expiratory flow rate (PEFR) and tracheal area in a cohort of 31 children with anterior mediastinal masses evaluated prospectively. Children with PEFRs and tracheal areas less than 50% predicted are to the left and below the lines; all received local anesthesia and did well. Children with PEFRs and tracheal areas greater than 50% predicted received general anesthesia and did well. Although this study could not demonstrate that these children would have had anesthetic problems, it did confirm that these parameters (>50% PEFR and tracheal area) were safe for the administration of general anesthesia. *(Modified from Shamberger RC, Holzman RS, Griscom NT, et al: Prospective evaluation by computed tomography and pulmonary function tests of children with mediastinal masses.* Surgery 118:468, 1995.)

Gradual inhalation induction proceeds with the patient in the semi-Fowler or sitting position. Sevoflurane, with its rapid onset and offset properties, may be the ideal potent agent. One hundred percent oxygen is used and the patient allowed to breathe spontaneously as long as possible. If intubation is deemed necessary, it should be accomplished with topical anesthesia of the airway. The use of positive pressure ventilation and neuromuscular relaxants should be avoided.

Ideally the procedure should be completed without alteration in patient position because any change may be associated with the sudden loss of patent airways. Because cardiac or respiratory decompensation can occur at any time, constant vigilance is mandatory. Wheezing or increased peak inspiratory pressure may portend inadequate ventilation and needs to be investigated promptly. Although other reasons for increased peak inspiratory pressures (such as light anesthesia) exist, one must assume that extratracheal compression of the airways is responsible. Change in positioning, especially if the patient was altered from the original position, may resolve the obstruction. At times, a prone position may be needed. Although flexible fiber-optic bronchoscopy may confirm the diagnosis of tracheal compression and aid in directing the endotracheal tube beyond the obstruction, time should not be wasted because rigid bronchoscopy may be necessary to maintain a patent airway. Profound hypoxemia despite adequate tidal volumes also can occur at any time and suggests compression of the great vessels. Maintaining adequate preload will help, but relief of compression may be possible only with the lateral or prone position. Failure of this maneuver will mean the necessity of cardiopulmonary bypass.

Emergence and extubation can be as troublesome as induction and intubation. Upon emergence, anxiety and pain may cause coughing and tachypnea, leading to less effective, turbulent airflow and cyanosis. If reintubation becomes necessary, the same anesthetic concerns exist as before the surgical procedure. Therefore, a period of observation after extubation in the operating room may be beneficial. However, as long as the patient is stable, continued intubation with initiation of therapy may be considered. With an adequate tissue sample for definitive diagnosis, rapid tumor diminution may occur with prompt administration of radiation or chemotherapy (Figure 15-2). A safe, successful extubation can be accomplished days later.

In summary, all patients with newly diagnosed leukemia or lymphoma need a current chest x-ray despite previous negative studies,[6] as should any patient with dyspnea or positional intolerance. Even though a careful history and physical examination will suffice for the vast majority of asymptomatic children with neck masses, chest x-rays may be indicated in those having a biopsy of supraclavicular or low cervical masses. When in doubt, a chest x-ray is needed. If a mass is found, a chest CT is mandatory and pulmonary function tests with flow volume loops should be considered. General anesthesia for high-risk patients is best avoided. But when tissue biopsy is deemed imperative, judicious well-conducted anesthesia will depend on one's vigilance, preparation, and skill.

Spinal Cord Compression

Acute compression of the spinal cord occurs in 4% of children at time of diagnosis of cancer.[5] Most cases are due to epidural compression from extension of a paravertebral tumor through the intervertebral foramina. Direct extension of tumor from the vertebral column and internal growth of CNS malignancies are less common. Causative tumors include neuroblastoma, Ewing's sarcoma, non-Hodgkin's lymphoma, Hodgkin's disease, osteosarcoma, rhabdomyosarcoma, and astrocytoma. Eighty percent of patients present with localized pain anywhere along the vertebral column, which may or may not radiate. Back pain is usually the first symptom and often present for weeks before diagnosis. Later symptoms include sensory or motor deficits and bladder and bowel dysfunction. Without prompt relief of spinal cord compression, deficits become permanent. Magnetic resonance imaging identifies the tumor and degree of compression. Should the tissue diagnosis be in doubt, surgical decompression with biopsy is indicated. When the tumor is known to be sensitive to treatment, radiation or chemotherapy may be preferable.

Tumor Lysis Syndrome

Tumor lysis syndrome is a constellation of major metabolic perturbations due to spontaneous or therapy-induced necrosis of a large tumor load.[5] Although most often associated with hematopoietic malignancies (such as Burkitt's lymphoma or acute lymphoblastic leukemia [ALL]), it has been described with solid tumors as well (stage IV-S neuroblastoma, hepatoblastoma). Massive cell lysis leads to hyperkalemia, hyperphosphatemia with secondary hypocalcemia, and hyperuricemia from cellular nucleic acids. Hypocalcemia may result in mental status changes, seizures, and cardiac arrest. Cardiac arrest also may result from hyperkalemia. High uric acid concentrations crystallize in the acidic environment of the urine collecting system, causing an obstructive nephropathy and acute renal failure. Renal failure also may be aggravated by deposition of renal calcium phosphate precipitates, dehydration, and tumor infiltration of the kidney or compression of the ureters. The acute renal failure contributes to hyperkalemia, hyperphosphatemia, and hyperuricemia. Encephalopathy from cerebral edema, multisystem organ failure, and death may soon ensue. Therapy (Table 15-7) is directed toward preventing renal failure and correcting the electrolyte abnormalities.

Coagulopathies

Coagulopathies in cancer patients have varied etiologies. Thrombocytopenia may be secondary to decreased platelet production (as seen with tumor infiltration of the bone marrow or after chemotherapy) or increased platelet consumption (as seen with sepsis or with some forms of acute myeloid leukemia [AML]). Qualitative platelet dysfunction occurs in uremia, and an acquired von Willebrand's disease with platelet dysfunction may occur with Wilms' tumor. Consumption of coagulation factors and disseminated intravascular coagulation may be associated with massive hepatomegaly or hemorrhage secondary to tumor necrosis or cerebrovascular accidents. Rarely, children may present with hypercoagulable states. Patients with platelet counts below 20,000/µL commonly receive platelet transfusions to reduce the risk of spontaneous intracerebral hemorrhage. Transfusions also should be completed in patients with platelet counts below 50,000/µL and about to undergo invasive procedures. However, after multiple exposures to random donor platelets, development of alloimmunization may cause persistent thrombocytopenia despite transfusions. Although a single-donor platelet transfusion may help, it

TABLE 15–7 Management of Tumor Lysis Syndrome

Hydration	D5 ¼ NS + 50–100 NaHCO$_2$ mEq/L, without potassium, 3–6 L/(m^2/d)
	Maintain urine specific gravity < 1.010
Alkalinization	Maintain urine pH at 7.0–7.5
	Reduce NaHCO$_3$ if serum bicarbonate >30 mEq/L or urine pH >7.5
	Acetazolamide, 5 mg/kg/d orally
Uric acid reduction	Allopurinol, 100 mg/m^2, every 8 h orally
	Urate oxidase, 100 U/kg, IV or IM daily (investigational)
Diuretics	Avoid if hypovolemic
	Furosemide, 1 mg/kg, IV every 6 h
	Mannitol, 0.5 g/kg IV every 6 h
Phosphate reduction	Aluminum hydroxide, 50 mg/kg, orally every 8 h

D5 ¼ NS, 5% dextrose with 0.25% normal saline; IM, intramuscularly; IV, intravenously; NaHCO$_3$, sodium bicarbonate.
Source: Modified from Kelly KM, Lange B: Oncologic emergencies. *Pediatr Clin North Am* 44:809, 1997.

may be necessary to accept a lower platelet count. Under these circumstances, intraoperative transfusions of platelets may be indicated depending on the planned procedure. When transfusing platelets into an immunocompromised host, care should be given to ensure that the platelets have been irradiated and filtered for white blood cells (WBCs). The former will reduce risk of graft-versus-host disease (GVHD). The latter will decrease the risk of platelet resistance with future transfusions, cytomegalovirus infections, and WBC-mediated febrile transfusion reactions. Similar considerations should be given when transfusing erythrocytes.

Hyperleukocytosis

By definition, hyperleukocytosis is a WBC count greater than 100,000/µL.[5] However, WBCs between 200,000 and 300,000/µL are not uncommon in acute leukemias and values in excess of 600,000/µL can occur in children with chronic myelogenous leukemia. Such numbers represent a massive tumor load and place the patient at risk for tumor lysis syndrome. In addition, high numbers of circulating leukemic blast cells greatly increase the blood viscosity, leading to complications from leukostasis in the pulmonary, renal, and cerebral vasculatures. Neurologic symptoms include headaches, mental status changes, and seizures, whereas pulmonary symptoms present as dyspnea and hypoxemia. Damage to lungs, kidney, and brain result from ischemic infarctions secondary to hyperviscosity. Thrombocytopenia associated with leukemia compounds the danger of CNS hemorrhage. Hematocrits greater than 30 and dehydration result in increased viscosity of the blood. As myeloblasts are less pliant than lymphoblasts, patients with acute myelogenous leukemia also are at greater risk for stroke. Tumor lysis syndrome is more common in acute lymphoblastic leukemia. Therapy is to reduce WBC count by leukophoresis or exchanging transfusions. This should be accomplished before the induction of anesthesia, when possible.

DIAGNOSES

Caring for the pediatric oncology patient requires a basic understanding of the child's diagnosis.

Acute Lymphoblastic Leukemia[14,15]

Acute lymphoblastic leukemia is the most common pediatric malignancy, accounting for roughly 25% of all childhood cancers and 75% of all leukemias. Peak incidence occurs at age 2 to 3 years.[2] Despite a steady increase in the incidence, most cases lack plausible causal explanation. Conclusive data linking ALL to environmental factors such as viruses, low dose radiation, and electromagnetic fields remains elusive. Although associated with some pre-existing disorders such as trisomy 21, Fanconi's anemia, DiGeorge's syndrome, and other congenital immunodeficiency states, the vast majority of cases arise sporadically. However, specific genetic alterations can be shown in more than 90% of cases.

Phenotypically, ALL is divided into T-cell and B-cell types, with the latter commonly subclassified into "B-cell precursors" and mature (or simply) "B-cell." Presenting symptoms are vague and nonspecific and include fever, pallor, bruising, bone or joint pain, anorexia, fatigue, and abdominal pain. Seventy-three percent of children have no or only mild lymphadenopathy. As many as 14 % have significant hepatosplenomegaly, 8% have a mediastinal mass on presentation, and 4% have CNS symptoms. Forty-six percent present with a hemoglobin of less than 7.5 g/dL, 21% with a WBC count in excess of 50,000/µL, and 20% with a platelet count below 20,000/µL. Another 50% have a platelet count below 100,000/µL.[14] Diagnosis is by bone marrow biopsy.

Of the many variables that have been linked to ALL prognosis, response to treatment is the most predictive. The patient's age at diagnosis and initial leukocyte count are the two most reliable indicators of the response to therapy. Favorable prognostic factors include age 1 to 10 and initial WBC counts less than 50,000/µL. Combination chemotherapy is tailored so that the most aggressive therapy is reserved for unfavorable prognostic factors. Therapy for B-cell leukemia is of short duration (<6 months) but very intensive, consisting of high-dose cyclophosphamide, vincristine, doxorubicin, methotrexate, and cytarabine. T-cell and precursor B-cell leukemias typically require 2 to 3 years of therapy. Although current protocols vary, all contain four stages: remission induction, intensification-consolidation, prevention of CNS disease, and continuation of remission. Remission induction, the elimination of as many leukemic cells as biologically possible, usually includes vincristine, prednisone, and L-asparaginase, with or without doxorubicin or daunorubicin. Intensification-consolidation uses multiple agents to eradicate residual cells and minimize the development of resistant cells. More intensive systemic therapy and intrathecal agents (methotrexate, cytarabine, prednisone) have largely replaced CNS radiation in all but the highest-risk patients and those with known CNS disease. Allogeneic bone marrow transplantation (BMT) is the treatment of choice for relapse. Annually, 1500 children become long-term survivors. Sequelae include second malignancies (CNS tumors and AML) and side effects of chemotherapy and radiation therapy.

Acute Myelogenous Leukemias[16]

With only 350 to 500 new cases annually, AML occur with one-fifth to one-sixth the frequency of ALL. The incidence of AML is fairly consistent throughout childhood and adolescence.[2] Acute myeloid leukemia is associated with conditions of chromosomal or genetic abnormalities, most notably Down's syndrome, radiation exposure, and previous chemotherapy. Like ALL, AML presents with symptoms of bone marrow infiltration and failure: bone pain, fever, bruising, and pallor. Hepatosplenomegaly occurs in one-half of cases, but lymphadenopathy is surprisingly rare. Ten percent of patients have CNS involvement on presentation. White blood cell counts can be substantial, with 20% of patients having counts greater than 100,000/µL. Tumor lysis syndrome is rare, whereas symptoms and complications of hyperleukocytosis are more common. Patients with promyelocytic leukemia may present with thromboses and a consumptive coagulopathy.

Compared with ALL, therapeutic regimens for AML are less well established. There are several reasons for this. Because AML is divided into eight subtypes differentiated by morphology and histochemical criteria, there are few patients of any one subtype to enroll into protocols to determine the most efficacious treatment. Further, all subtypes of AML are more resistant to treatment than ALL. Induction regimens necessary for marrow aplasia result in greater toxicities. Five percent to 15% of patients succumb early to their disease or its treatment. Chemotherapy consists of anthracyclines, cytarabine, etoposide, and 6-thioguanine. Overall, 70% to 85% will succeed with induction, but only half will remain in remission. Subsequent therapy depends on the morphologic category and the patient's response to initial treatment. Although some children will continue with consolidation chemotherapy, most will proceed to allogeneic BMT once remission is accomplished. Future chemotherapeutic regimens may provide greater long-term survival without the need for BMT.

Central Nervous System Tumors[17]

Primary malignant tumors of the brain are the most common solid neoplasm and the second most common cancer of childhood and adolescence.[2] One in five children age 14 years or younger with newly diagnosed cancer has a malignant brain tumor. The incidence is highest in children younger than 6 years and steadily declines with age. Children 4 to 11 years of age tend to have infratentorial tumors, whereas younger and older children more often have supratentorial lesions. Across all age groups, 45% of neoplasms arise in the cerebellum, 20% to 27% in the cerebrum, 9% to 15% in the brainstem, 3% to 14% within the fourth ventricle, and 10% are midline (e.g., pituitary adenomas, craniopharyngiomas, optic gliomas). Neurologic symptoms, initially subtle and nonspecific, localize with tumor progression. These can include headache, morning nausea and vomiting, somnolence, irritability, increased head circumference, lost of developmental milestones, ataxia, gait disturbance, torticollis, cranial nerve palsies, seizures, hemiparesis, and diabetes insipidus. With larger masses or tumors causing obstructive hydrocephalus, increased intracranial pressure is observed.

Astrocytomas (40%) comprise the largest histologic type of all primary intracranial tumors. Of these, 58% are supratentorial and 42% are infratentorial. The other histologic types are medulloblastomas and other primitive neuroectodermal tumors (24%), gliomas (14%), ependymomas (8%), craniopharyngiomas (6%), and other (8%). In addition, other malignancies may metastasize to the brain. These include leukemias, lymphomas, neuroblastomas, Wilms' tumor, retinoblastoma, and rhabdomyosarcomas of the head and neck.

Therapy is mostly by surgical excision. Postoperative adjunctive care includes radiation therapy in children older than 3 years. Because of neurodevelopmental consequences of CNS radiation, chemotherapy is favored in children younger than 3 years. The principles of providing anesthetic care for intracranial surgical procedures and for children with increased intracranial pressure are described elsewhere in this text.

Non-Hodgkin's Lymphoma[18,19]

Hodgkin's and non-Hodgkin's lymphomas (NHL) comprise the third most common group of malignancies in children and adolescents and account for 12% of newly diagnosed pediatric cancers. In the United States, NHL shows a male predominance (75%) and a peak incidence at age 14 years. Females do not exhibit a single peak age of incidence.[2] However, frequency and incidence vary markedly throughout the world. Although there is a strong correlation between Ebstein–Barr virus and NHL in equatorial Africa, no such relation has been observed in industrialized countries. In addition, congenital and acquired immunodeficiencies (including solid organ transplants) are associated with NHL.

Non-Hodgkin's lymphomas comprise three histologic subtypes. Of the 30% to 35% of NHL patients with *lymphoblastic lymphomas*, 50% to 80% present with lymphadenopathy that is most often supradiaphragmatic. Anterior mediastinal masses (50% to 70% of patients with lymphoblastic lymphoma), massive pulmonary effusions, or rare pharyngeal masses may cause respiratory compromise. Potential cardiovascular symptoms are due to superior vena cava syndrome, pericardial effusions, or tamponade. Moderate hepatosplenomegaly, retroperitoneal lymphadenopathy, and renal masses are not uncommon, but CNS involvement is rare. Bone marrow infiltration by the cancerous lymphoblast is common. Because the lymphoblast of lymphoblastic NHL is indistinguishable from that of ALL, the diagnosis is determined by the percentage of marrow cells consisting of lymphoblasts.

Burkitt's lymphoma accounts for 40% to 50% of NHLs. Abdominal masses originating from the bowel, kidney, or gonads and often accompanied by ascites is the presenting symptom in 80% of patients. Symptoms range from a change in bowel habits to acute perforation of the bowel. Extraperitoneal sites include the anterior mediastinum (with or without pleural effusions), bone marrow, CNS, tonsillar bed, and thyroid. Lymphomatous masses may cause intussusception or mimic acute appendicitis or tonsillitis. Children with endemic (African) Burkitt's lymphoma may present with a jaw mass large enough to compromise the airway. *Large cell lymphomas* make up the remaining 15% to 30% of NHLs and present as masses occurring virtually anywhere. Extensive pulmonary lesions and anterior mediastinal masses may be clinically significant. However, tumors are rare in the CNS and bone marrow.

All childhood lymphomas have very high growth fractions and potential doubling times ranging from 12 h to a few days. Consequently, these children often present with large tumor loads that leave them at risk for quickly evolving complications (Table 15-8).[19] At the same time, because these tumors are very sensitive to antineoplastic therapy, a definitive tissue diagnosis may be lost subsequent to initiation of therapy. Hence, diagnostic procedures need to be expeditious yet safe. When tissue sampling under general anesthesia is considered prohibitively dangerous, the diagnosis may need to be made with tissue obtained in other ways. Such alternatives include obtaining cells from blood, bone marrow, or pleural effusions and by fine needle aspiration or superficial nodal biopsies without general anesthesia.

Due in part to their high growth fraction, all childhood NHLs respond to a wide range of chemotherapeutic agents. Specific agents are chosen to maximize cell death and minimize systemic toxicity, and the duration of chemotherapy differs markedly according to the stage and histology. Radiation has little role in treatment with the possible exception of extensive intracranial disease and those with symptomatic anterior mediastinal masses. Likewise, because these tumors are so responsive to chemotherapy, surgery has limited applications. Patients who relapse are candidates for allogeneic BMT.

Hodgkin's Disease[20,21]

Hodgkin's lymphoma is rare in children younger than 5 years and has peak occurrences at age 25 years and in the elderly. Some divide the earlier peak into a pediatric form in children younger than 14 years and a young adult form in those 15 to 34 years old. Although Ebstein–Barr virus (as well as her-

TABLE 15–8 Complications Associated With Non-Hodgkin's Lymphomas at the Time of Presentation

Complications related to space-occupying lesions
  Superior vena cava syndrome and superior mediastinal syndrome
  Spinal cord compression and other neurological emergencies
  Pleural and pericardial effusions
  Pulmonary embolism secondary to a large intraabdominal mass
  Obstructive uropathy
  Pharyngeal obstruction
Metabolic complications
  Tumor lysis syndrome
  Hypercalcemia
  Syndrome of inappropriate antidiuretic hormone secretion
  Hypoglycemia/hyperglycemia
Gastrointestinal complications
  Gastrointestinal bleeding, fistulae, intestinal obstruction
Complications associated with massive mediastinal disease
  Anesthetic problems, cardiac arrest
  Central line placement problems
Cytokine-mediated complications
  Cancer cachexia
  Fever, malaise
Hematological complications
  Bone marrow infiltration
  Pancytopenias

Source: Modified from Shad A, Magrath I: Non-Hodgkin's lymphoma. *Pediatr Clin North Am* 44:863, 1997.

pes virus 6 and cytomegalovirus) have been implicated, data supporting an infectious etiology of Hodgkin's disease are controversial. However, Hodgkin's lymphoma is associated with congenital or acquired immunodeficiency states.

In children Hodgkin's disease presents as painless lymphadenopathy that is most often cervical or supraclavicular but occasionally axillary or inguinal. Although two-thirds of patients will have mediastinal *lymphadenopathy* at presentation, a mediastinal *mass* is seen on chest x-ray in 17% to 40% of children. Mediastinal masses are more common in children older than 12 years and are almost always found when supraclavicular nodes or low cervical lymph nodes are enlarged. Whereas most masses are small and clinically insignificant in the non-anesthetized patient, one-third are larger than 30% of the diameter of the chest. The triad of fevers, night sweats, and weight loss, commonly associated with Hodgkin's disease in adults, occurs in only 20% to 30% of children. Likewise, hepatosplenomegaly is rare.

A discussion of the proper diagnostic evaluation of Hodgkin's lymphoma, including the implications of staging, is beyond the scope of this text. However, a chest CT should always be completed before any staging laparoscopy. Preferred therapy is tailored to maximize success and minimize long-term sequelae. Physically mature individuals are more likely to have high-dose radiation therapy, whereas younger patients receive low-dose radiation therapy and chemotherapy. Common regimens include nitrogen mustard, oncovin (vincristine), procarbazine, and prednisone (MOPP); adriamycin (doxorubicin), bleomycin, vinblastine, and dacarbazine (ABVD); or alternating courses of the two. Bone marrow transplantation is an alternative for those who relapse.

Neuroblastoma[22,23]

The neuroblastoma family of tumors consists of neuroblastomas, ganglioneuroblastomas, and gangliomas. As embryonic neoplasms of neural crest tissue, neuroblastomas are malignancies of infancy and early childhood. Because they constitute 25% of all tumors, neuroblastomas are the most common malignancy in the first year of life.[2] They are also the most common extracranial solid tumor throughout childhood. The most common presentation is an abdominal mass (67%) with or without pain; other common symptoms are relatively nonspecific (e.g., fever, irritability, failure to thrive). However, the capacity of neuroblastomas to arise anywhere in the sympathetic nervous system and metastasize early produces a full range of unique, sometimes critical, presenting symptoms. Very young infants may have significant cardiorespiratory symptoms due to massive hepatomegaly with inferior vena cava compression. Likewise, respiratory compromise or superior vena cava syndrome may be seen with posterior mediastinal masses. Spinal cord compression, secondary to paraspinal tumors extending through neural foramina, may present as pain, paresis, or paralysis. A medical emergency, these symptoms become irreversible if not promptly treated. Rarely tumor necrosis and hemorrhage leads to anemia and shock, and tumor lysis syndrome has been described. Marrow infiltration may cause myelosuppression and an immunocompromised state with its risk of overwhelming sepsis. Although 90% of neuroblastomas secrete catecholamines and the diagnosis often is made by identifying urinary metabolites, rarely does a child present with symptoms of catecholamine excess (e.g., hypertension, tachycardia, diaphoresis). When hypertension is seen, it usually is in response to hyperreninemia due to renal artery compression by tumor. Proptosis and periorbital ecchymoses ("raccoon eyes") may be seen with metastases to the head, and Horner's syndrome may denote thoracic disease. Paraneoplastic syndromes of secretory watery diarrhea or opsoclonus/myoclonus with ataxia and developmental delay may also be seen. Skin metastases appear as bluish nodules. Bone metastases may cause pain and gait disturbances.

Based on age and tumor biology, patients are categorized into low, intermediate, and high risk for treatment failure. Therapy is dictated so that poorer risks receive more aggressive therapy. Infants younger than 365 days at presentation are most often, but not always, considered low risk. Surgery, with complete or partial tumor debulkment, is the mainstay of therapy. Because of long-term sequelae in the young, external beam radiation therapy is used less frequently in favor of multiple agent chemotherapy. However, intraoperative radiation therapy may have important applications in the future.[24] Chemotherapy usually consists of cisplatin or carboplatin with an epipodophyllotoxin (etoposide or tenoposide) or doxorubicin with cyclophosphamide. Bone marrow transplantation is used for high-risk patients and those who relapse.

Wilms' Tumor (Nephroblastoma)[25–27]

Like neuroblastomas, Wilms' tumors are of embryonic origin and predominantly a disease of early childhood years. Eighty percent and 98% of cases present by ages 5 and 7 years, respectively. Wilms' tumor represents 6.7% of all childhood neoplasms (Table 15-1)[2]. Although most cases arise sporadically, a number of congenital anomalies (cryptochidism, hypospadias and other genitourinary malformations, aniridia, isolated hemihypertrophy, syndromes associated with gigantism such as Beckwith–Wiedemann and Sotos' syndromes) confer an increased risk for developing Wilms' tumor.

The usual presentation is as a silent mass found serendipitously by family or physician. Abdominal pain (33%), hypertension (25%), and hematuria (10-25%) may also be seen. Necrosis and intratumoral hemorrhage may lead to a rapidly expanding mass, fever, anemia, and hypotension. Rarely polycythemia, acquired von Willebrand's disease, or hypercalcemia may occur. Metastases are to lung, liver, and, infrequently, brain. Diagnostic evaluation determines intravascular extension into the inferior vena cava or right atrium (4% of cases) or the presence of bilateral disease (6%).

With unilateral disease, en bloc total nephroureterectomy, with staging and inspection of appropriate nodes, is accomplished with care to avoid tumor spillage. Partial nephrectomy is reserved solely for patients with bilateral disease or anticipated inadequate postoperative renal function. The need for bilateral nephrectomies is rare. Care of the patient is complicated by intravascular tumor thrombosis of the inferior vena cava and right atrium. Proper preparation and monitoring are dictated by the possibility of massive hemorrhage (>50 mL/kg) and the necessity of cardiopulmonary bypass. Intraoperative deaths from tumor emboli have been reported. When indicated, surgical excision is supplemented by local radiation therapy and chemotherapy (doxorubicin, actinomycin D, vincristine, cyclophosphamide).

Other Malignancies

The seven diagnoses presented thus far account for 75% of all malignancies of childhood and adolescence. Most of the remaining 25% include rhabdomyosarcoma, retinoblastoma, Ewing's sarcomas, osteogenic sarcoma, hepatic tumors, and germ cell tumors. The reader is referred to a pediatric text for further information of these and other malignancies. However, some points pertinent to the practice of anesthesiology can be made. Surgical excision of these solid masses is rarely the sole therapy. Thus, many patients will have received chemotherapy or radiotherapy before presenting to the operating room.

Although they arise anywhere, roughly 40% of *rhabdomyosarcomas* occur in the head and neck. *Retinoblastomas* are tumors of infancy and early childhood and present with leukocoria or strabismus. Therapy focuses on preservation of vision, so patients require anesthesia on a regular basis for evaluation or surgical treatment. As a family of highly malignant small cell tumors, *Ewing's sarcomas* include extracranial primitive neuroectodermal tumors and spread early to lung and bone. Forty-one percent occur in femur and pelvis. *Hepatic blastomas* and *hepatocellular carcinomas* are the most common gastrointestinal tumors. Although chemotherapy may reduce tumor size or eradicate metastases, complete resection is necessary for cure. Major bleeding should be anticipated. *Germ cell tumors* represent 1% of all childhood cancers and occur most often in testes and ovaries; extragonadal sites include the sacrococcygeal area, anterior mediastinum, brain, and retroperitoneum. *Sacrococcygeal teratomas* are a subset of germ cell tumors. Presenting in infancy, most often in the neonatal period, sacrococcygeal teratomas are usually small, benign, and easily resected. However, they can be massive and highly vascular and may cause high-output congestive heart failure. Surgical resection of these tumors is associated with extremely high perioperative morbidity and mortality.[28]

Langerhan's Cell Histiocytosis[29]

Previously known as histiocytosis X, Langerhan's cell histiocytosis also includes the former diagnoses of Letterer–Siwe disease, Hand–Schuller–Christian syndrome, and eosinophilic granuloma. As a disease of abnormally proliferating but normal functioning histiocytes, Langerhan's cell histiocytosis is not a malignancy per se. Rather, it is considered an immunologic dysfunction. However, because of its similarities with pediatric cancers, including the need for chemotherapy, it is included in this chapter.

Langerhan's cell histiocytosis has two basic presentations. *Solitary lesions* occur as single or multiple well-circumscribed tumors in bone. Most common in the skull, they also occur in femurs, vertebrae, and mandible. *Disseminated disease* involves one or more organ systems with the following frequencies: bone 100%, skin 88%, liver 71%, lung 54%, lymph nodes 42%, spleen 25%, pituitary 25%, bone marrow 18%, and CNS 16%. Disease progression can be clinically significant. Pulmonary disease may result in cough, tachypnea, dyspnea, cyanosis, pneumothorax, and pleural effusions. Other complications are hepatic failure with hepatosplenomegaly, hematologic dysfunction with marrow failure, diabetes insipidus, growth failure, panhypopituitarism, and hyperosmolar syndrome. Thyroid and pancreatic infiltrations lead to deficiencies of these organs. Treatment of solitary lesions is by surgical curettage and radiotherapy. Disseminated disease requires chemotherapy: prednisone, vinblastine, etoposide, mercaptopurine, and cyclosporine.

THERAPIES

Chemotherapy

Although surgical resection remains the primary therapeutic option for most pediatric tumors, almost all malignancies require chemotherapy or radiation therapy as a component of treatment.[30–31] Caring for the pediatric oncology patient requires an understanding of the clinical consequences of these therapeutic options. As chemotherapeutic agents are limited by their clinical toxicities, combination chemotherapy with multiple agents minimizes side effects. Table 15-9 lists systemic effects of many chemotherapeutic agents commonly used in pediatric oncology. Further discussion of two therapies, the anthracyclines and bleomycin, follow several general observations.

Bone marrow suppression causes varying degrees of pancytopenia, although not all cell lines may be affected equally. Nadir counts of granulocytes, platelets, and red cells occur most frequently at 7 to 14 days after administration of chemotherapy. However, some agents induce a late myelosuppression weeks after administration. Further, recovery to normal values is highly variable across agents and from child to child. Further, as patients approach their nadir blood counts, values may drop precipitously. Because of these factors, when indicated, a complete blood and platelet count should be obtained no more than 24 h before induction of anesthesia.

In addition to the malignancy, chemotherapy-induced myelosuppression causes an immunocompromised state. The risk for overwhelming sepsis is particularly critical with WBC counts below 1500/µL and absolute neutrophil counts below 500/µL. Scrupulous hand washing by staff and reverse isolation techniques (mask, gown, and gloves) should be practiced vigilantly. Additional patient safety is provided by protective isolation in preoperative holding areas and the postanesthetic care unit. New intravenous or intraarterial lines may be considered when in situ lines are older than a few days.[30] If

TABLE 15-9 Classification and Side Effects of Selected Chemotherapeutic Agents*

Classification	Drug	Toxicity	Notes
Alkylating agents			
Nitrogen mustards	Cyclophosphamide (Cytoxan)	Myelosuppression Cardiomyopathy Pulmonary infiltrates/fibrosis SIADH Hepatitis/VOD Hemorrhagic cystitis Inhibition of plasma cholinesterase Mucosal ulceration/stomatitis	High doses only, acute effect 10–15 d after administration High doses only, hyponatremia may lead to seizures
	Ifosfamide	Myelosuppression Hepatitis/VOD Nephrotoxicity Hemorrhagic cystitis	
	Mechlorethamine	Myelosuppression Hepatitis/VOD	
	Melphalan	Myelosuppression Hepatitis/VOD	
	Chlorambucil	Myelosuppression Hepatitis/VOD	
Alkyl sulfonates	Busulfan	Delayed myelosuppression Pulmonary fibrosis Hepatitis/VOD Inhibition of plasma cholinesterase Secondary leukemias	
Nitrosoureas	Carmustine (BCNU) and Lomustine (CCNU)	Delayed myelosuppression Pulmonary infiltrates/fibrosis Hepatitis/VOD	

(continued)

TABLE 15-9 Classification and Side Effects of Selected Chemotherapeutic Agents* (continued)

Classification	Drug	Toxicity	Notes
Antimetabolites			
Folic acid analog	Methotrexate	Acute renal failure	
		Secondary leukemias	
		Myelosuppression	
		Pulmonary infiltrates/fibrosis	
		"CVA-like" syndrome, seizure, lethargy/coma	Intrathecal or high-dose intravenous administration, usually transient
		Hepatic fibrosis/cirrhosis	With chronic administration
		Nephrotoxicity	
		Mucosal ulceration/stomatitis	
Pyrimidine analogs	5-Fluorouracil (5-FU)	Myelosuppression	
		Cardiac ischemia	Chest pain with ECG changes
		Acute cerebellar syndrome	
		Mucosal ulceration/stomatitis	
	Cytarabine (ARA-C, cytosine arabinoside)	Myelosuppression	
		Pulmonary infiltrates/fibrosis	
		Seizures, acute cerebellar syndrome	Intrathecal or high-dose intravenous administration
		Pancreatic dysfunction	
		Hepatic dysfunction	
		Mucosal ulceration/stomatitis	
Purine analogs	Azathioprine	Delayed myelosuppression	
	6-Mercaptopurine	Delayed myelosuppression	
		Pancreatitis	
Natural products			
Antimitotic drugs	Vinblastine	Myelosuppression	
		Peripheral neuropathy	Parasthesias, decreased DTRs, weakness of distal limbs musculature, vocal cord paralysis

(*continued*)

	Vincristine	Myelosuppression	
		Cardiac ischemia	Chest pain with ECG changes
		SIADH	Hyponatremia may lead to seizures
		Peripheral neuropathy	Parasthesias, decreased DTRs, weakness of distal limbs musculature, vocal cord paralysis
Epipodophyllotoxins	Etoposide (VP-16) and Teniposide (VM-26)	Myelosuppression	
Antibiotics	Dactinomycin (Actinomycin D)	Myelosuppression	
	Doxorubicin (Adriamycin) (*anthracycline*)	Myelosuppression	
		Arrhythmias	
		Cardiomyopathy	
	Daunorubicin (Cerubidine) (*anthracycline*)	Myelosuppression	
		Cardiomyopathy	Early onset complication, see text
	Idarubicin (Idamycin) (*synthetic anthracycline*)	Myelosuppression	
		Cardiomyopathy	Late onset complication, see text
	Bleomycin	Pulmonary infiltrates/fibrosis	See text
		Thrombotic or hemorrhagic cerebrovascular accident	Presents with focal neurologic symptoms, seizures, or lethargy/coma
	L-Asparaginase	Coagulopathy	Decreased production of clotting factors
			Decreased production of protein SC and/or III leading to spontaneous thrombosis
		Pancreatitis	Hyperglycemia due to insulin deficiency
		Anaphylaxis	
Miscellaneous agents	Cisplatin	Myelosuppression	
		Cardiomyopathy	
		Cerebrovascular accident	Ischemic (hypomagnesemic arterial spasm) or thrombotic (direct endothelial injury)

(*continued*)

TABLE 15–9 Classification and Side Effects of Selected Chemotherapeutic Agents* (*continued*)

Classification	Drug	Toxicity	Notes
		Seizures	Multifactorial
		Lethargy/coma	Multifactorial
		Peripheral neuropathy	Optic/sensory neuritis
		Elecytrolyte disturbances	Hypokalemia, hypocalcemia, hypomagnesemia, hypophosphatemia
	Carboplatin	Nephrotoxicity	
		Ototoxicity	
		Peripheral neuropathy	Optic/sensory neuritis
		Ototoxicity	
	Procarbazine	Pulmonary infiltrates/fibrosis	
		Acute cerebellar syndrome	
Hormones and related	Adrenocorticosteroids	Multiple systemic side effects including immunosuppression, hypertension and adrenal suppression	

CVA, cerebrovascular accident; DTR, deep tendon reflexes; ECG, electrocardiogram; SIADH, syndrome of inappropriate antidiuretic hormone (ADH) secretion; VOD, venoocclusive disease: hepatomegaly, increased serum transaminases, hyperbilirubinemia, and ascites.
*Compiled from Chabner et al.,[31], Eskeni et al.,[30] and Kelly and Lange.[5]

done at all, central lines should be accessed with aseptic technique. Special considerations for transfusing blood products in immunocompromised patients have been mentioned.

Stomatitis is painful swelling and ulceration of the oral mucosa secondary to chemotherapy. As patients are unable or unwilling to open their mouths, evaluation of airway may be difficult. Although opening the mouth is less painful with induction of anesthesia, intubation may be complicated by friable tissue and further trauma to the oral cavity. As most chemotherapeutic agents induce nausea and vomiting, occasional dehydration and electrolyte disturbances may be encountered. Electrolyte perturbations also can be seen with renal insufficiency (secondary to chemotherapy or tumor). Stomatitis may compound dehydration.

The anthracycline class of antineoplastic agents includes doxorubicin (Adriamycin), daunomycin, and several synthetic analogs (idarubicin, epirubicin, and mitoxanthrone).[31] Although the other drugs have been used primarily for the leukemias, doxorubicin is one of the most widely used antineoplastic agents in pediatric oncology. Doxorubicin also has extensive applications in adult neoplastic disease. Unfortunately, the use of anthracyclines is limited by early and late onset cardiotoxicities (Figure 15-4).[4]

Early and late cardiotoxicities are differentiated from each other by the interval of time from completion of anthracycline therapy to onset of symptoms. *Acute toxicity* (Figure 15-4, group 2) presents as electrocardiographic

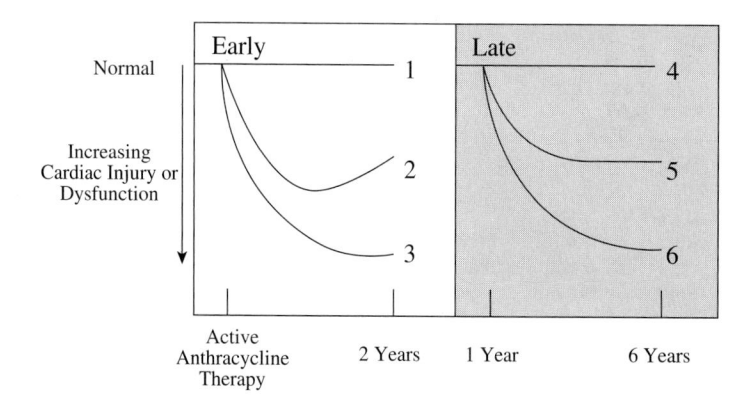

Years Since Completion of Anthracycline Therapy

FIG. 15-4 Theoretic patterns of cardiac injury or ventricular dysfunction during anthracycline therapy and after completion of therapy. Group 1 had no abnormalities, group 2 had transient injuries, and group 3 had persistent injuries. For group 3 patients, these changes may remain stable or progress. Most reversible cardiac dysfunction occurs during the first 2 years after treatment. Group 4 had no cardiac dysfunction, group 5 had stable dysfunction 6 years after treatment, and group 6 had progressive cardiac dysfunction during the same time period. It is unclear whether the dysfunction in group 6 eventually becomes stable. *(Modified from Grenier MA, Lipschultz SE: Epidemiology of anthracycline cardiotoxicity in children and adults. Semin Oncol 25[suppl 10]:72, 1998.)*

(ECG) changes during or shortly after infusion of doxorubicin and usually subsides within 1 to 2 weeks. Associated with catecholamine release, these effects are transient but may be clinically significant. The most common finding is sinus tachycardia; other ECG changes include ST depression, T-wave flattening, prolongation of QT interval, ventricular and supraventricular tachycardias, and different degrees of heart block.[32]

Subacute toxicity (also group 2) manifests as a pericarditis–myocarditis syndrome with ECG changes and acute but reversible left ventricular failure. Acute decrease in ejection fraction has been seen after a single dose of doxorubicin.[31] Pericardial effusions occur rarely and there have been reports of sudden death, presumably due to malignant arrhythmias. Although most patients improve with cessation of therapy, the onset of congestive heart failure within 4 weeks of anthracycline administration carries an especially grave prognosis.[33] Fortunately, alterations in dosing regimen have decreased the incidence of these subacute effects.

The remaining cardiotoxicities are irreversible, often progressive, and poorly responsive to therapy. By definition, *early onset chronic cardiomyopathy* (group 3) presents within 1 year of completion of therapy. Symptoms include electrophysiologic changes, diminished exercise capacity and left ventricular function, and overt congestive heart failure. Clinically significant early onset cardiotoxicity is rare in children, occurring less than 1% of the time.[34] However, damage to the heart is permanent and may progress even after the cessation of therapy. Early congestive heart failure carries a poor prognosis.[35]

Clinically significant late onset cardiomyopathy presents after a latency period of 1 or more years, during which the patient may be outwardly healthy. With onset of symptoms, cardiac function may stabilize (Figure 15-4, group 5) or continue to deteriorate (group 6). More concerning is *late onset asymptomatic cardiomyopathy* (group 4), which remains quiescent unless the patient is stressed. In these patients deterioration of cardiac function has been precipitated by sepsis, volume overload, tumor infiltration, and severely anemic states. One investigation has suggested that an event as innocuous as a viral illness may trigger the onset of significant deterioration.[33] It is a distinct possibility that these two groups denote one continuum, with dysfunction eventually developing in all asymptomatic patients. Acute decompensation with ensuing death in a previously asymptomatic patient has been reported as late as 10 years after cessation of therapy.[36]

Predisposing risk factors increase the incidence of cardiomyopathy. Foremost among these is the patient's cumulative dose of anthracycline. In 1979 Von Hoff et al. reported that the risk of congestive heart failure increases logarithmically with the administration of doxorubicin beyond a threshold dose of 550 mg/m^2.[35] Although many subsequently considered this a "safe" dose, such a concept is misleading. In reporting on adults and children in congestive heart failure with a mortality of 60%, Von Hoff et al. failed to recognize significant symptoms of toxicity at lower doses. Further, patients exhibited a wide variation in response. Some patients suffered from congestive heart failure at doses of 40 mg/m^2, whereas others had no such symptoms at doses in excess of 1000 mg/m^2. Subsequent work examining left ventricular function with echocardiograms determined that "nearly all children who had received a cumulative dose of ≥400 mg/m^2 were at increased risk of late-onset cardiotoxicity."[4] In another study, 65% of patients who had received 280 to 550 mg/m^2 of doxorubicin showed decreased ventricular function at 6.4 years after the final dose.[37]

Seventy-one percent of those patients developed progressive disease (i.e., Figure 15-4, group 6). Thus, individual patients may have lower thresholds and develop toxicity at significantly lower doses.

Additional risk factors include extremes of age at diagnosis, interval since completion of therapy, certain dosing regimens, female sex, thoracic radiation exposure, and possibly trisomy 21.[4] Although pre-existing heart disease and hypertension also increase the risk, these factors are likely of greater significance in adult patients.[38] Concomitant risk factors may account for patient variability. Thus, in determining a "safe dose" of doxorubicin, each patient must be considered individually. The effect of risk factors on cardiac function is summarized in Figure 15-5.[4]

Guidelines for assessing cardiac function have been proposed to monitor asymptomatic patients at risk for the development of significant disease (Figure 15-6).[36] The Cardiology Committee of the Children's Cancer Study Group recommended continued regular monitoring regardless of the presence or absence of immediate deterioration. Corrected QT interval on ECG may prove to be a useful screening test,[39,40] but its reliability has yet to be validated. Serial radionuclide angiocardiography dependably shows preclinical deterioration of cardiac function in adult patients. However, its sensitivity, specificity, and predictive accuracy have not been established in children. In its place, serial echocardiography is used to monitor reductions in systolic function. Although there are limitations even with this familiar study,[4,36,38] sensitivity can be increased by linking echocardiography with exercise or low-dose dobutamine infusions.[38] Interestingly, the 1992 recommendations of the Cardiology Committee of the Children's Cancer Study Group for increased surveillance at the 300-mg/m^2 threshold have recently been supported in a clinical study.

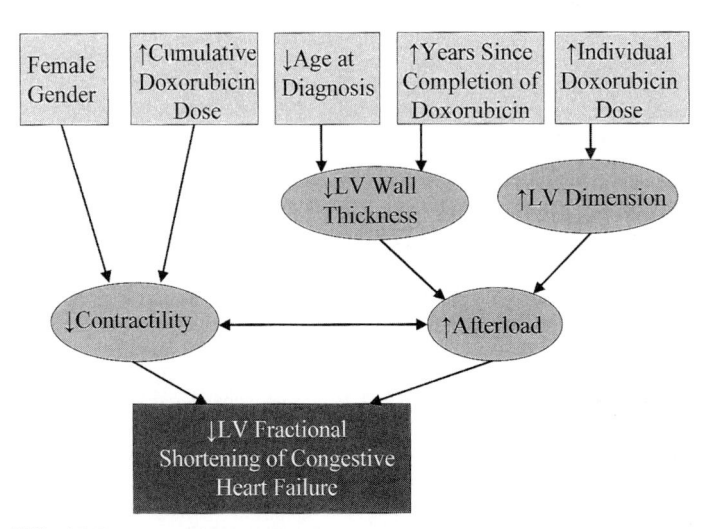

FIG. 15-5 The relation between cardiac and noncardiac findings in long-term survivors of childhood malignancy treated with anthracycline therapy. *(Modified from Grenier MA, Lipschultz SE: Epidemiology of anthracycline cardiotoxicity in children and adults. Semin Oncol 25[suppl 10]:72, 1998.)*

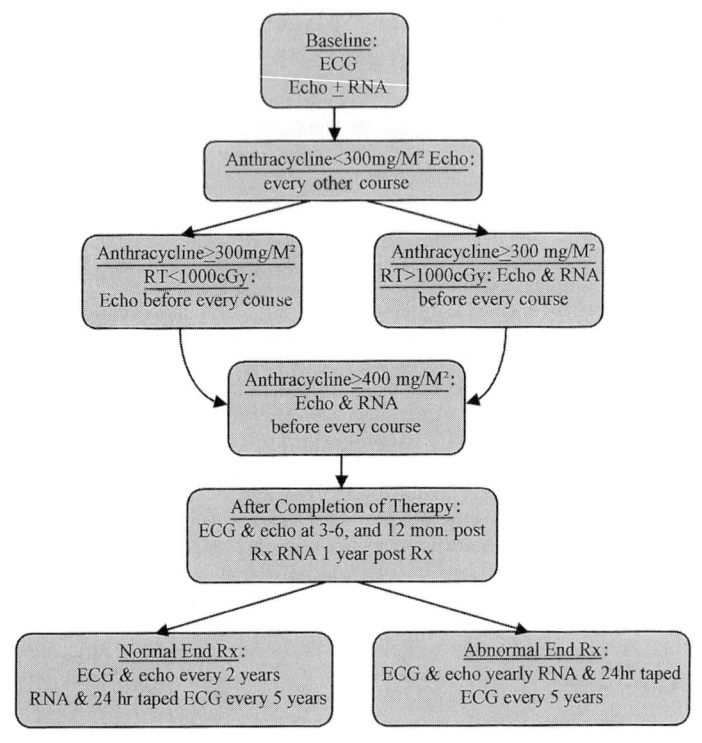

```
Baseline:
ECG
Echo ± RNA
  │
  ▼
Anthracycline<300mg/M² Echo:
every other course
  │
  ├──────────────────────┐
  ▼                      ▼
Anthracycline≥300mg/M²   Anthracycline≥300 mg/M²
RT<1000cGy:              RT>1000cGy: Echo & RNA
Echo before every course before every course
  │                      │
  └──────────┬───────────┘
             ▼
Anthracycline≥400 mg/M²:
Echo & RNA
before every course
             │
             ▼
After Completion of Therapy:
ECG & echo at 3-6, and 12 mon. post
Rx RNA 1 year post Rx
             │
  ┌──────────┴──────────┐
  ▼                     ▼
Normal End Rx:          Abnormal End Rx:
ECG & echo every 2 years  ECG & echo yearly RNA & 24hr taped
RNA & 24 hr taped ECG every 5 years  ECG every 5 years
```

FIG. 15-6 Frequency of monitoring patients receiving anthracyclines. ECG, electrocardiogram; ECHO, echocardiogram; Rx, therapy; RT, radiation therapy; RUA, radionuclide angiocardiogram. *(Modified from Steinherz LJ, Graham T, Hurwitz R, et al: Guidelines for cardiac monitoring of children during and after anthracycline therapy: report of the cardiology committee of the children's cancer study group.* Pediatrics *89:942, 1992.)*

Nysom et al. studied low-risk children 8 years after therapy and found few echocardiographic abnormalities in patients having received less than 300 mg/m² of doxorubicin.[34] Further, on endocardial biopsies, few anatomic changes of doxorubicin were noted at doses no larger than 240 mg/m².[34] However, Nysom et al. excluded patients suffering early onset toxicity and those having received mediastinal radiotherapy. Once again, even with doxorubicin doses lower than 300 mg/m², few broad generalizations can be supported and it is recommended that each patient be considered individually.

In summary, some patients who have received anthracyclines will be at higher risk for cardiotoxicity. Because of acute and subacute toxicities, patients who have received anthracyclines less than 4 weeks before anesthesia evaluation may be at higher risk for adverse intraoperative events. The risk may similarly be increased in those with risk factors for chronic cardiomyopathy. Because serial monitoring has shown transient improvement only to have cardiomyopathy with congestive heart failure occur years later, recent echocardiographic and a preanesthetic evaluations by a cardiologist may be prudent for anyone who has received anthracyclines regardless of the interval since chemotherapy or the patient's clinical status in the interim. Further, in recognition of the limitations of echocardiograms, one needs to limit intraoperative situations that may increase cardiac work (e.g., hypovolemia, severe anemia). Moreover, one should anticipate that at times inotropic support of cardiac output may be necessary regardless of cumulative dose of anthracycline or echocardiographic results.

Bleomycin (BLM) toxicities differ from other chemotherapeutic drugs, because BLM is used extensively for its activity against lymphomas, testicular tumors, and carcinomas of the head and neck.[31] Although BLM is favored because of minimal myelosuppression, 2% to 40% of recipients develop pulmonary toxicity. A dry cough, fine rales, and diffuse basilar infiltrates on chest x-ray are the most common findings. Roughly 5% to 10% of patients develop clinically significant pulmonary fibrosis and 1% of all patients will succumb to the pulmonary effects of BLM. Certain traits are thought to increase the incidence of fibrosis. These include advanced age, pre-existing pulmonary disease, prior thoracic radiation therapy, and a cumulative dose larger than 250 to 450 mg.[41]

Since the publication of Goldiner et al.'s landmark paper in 1978,[42] fractional inspired oxygen has been considered to potentiate BLM-induced pulmonary toxicity. Their original paper described five adult patients who had received BLM and developed fatal pulmonary disease consistent with acute respiratory distress syndrome 3 to 10 days after general anesthesia. A retrospective review of these patients found that all had been given fractional inspired oxygen concentrations of at least 0.35 and "excessive crystalloids." Twelve subsequent patients with comparable BLM doses underwent general anesthesia during which oxygen concentration was limited to no more than 0.25, and the fluid management was tightly controlled with more invasive monitoring and the use of colloids in favor of crystalloids. None of these patients developed acute respiratory distress syndrome. Goldiner et al.'s conclusions purported the importance of minimal fractional inspired oxygen concentration and fluid balance during anesthesia.

Numerous case reports and a multitude of animal models support Goldiner et al.'s original contention. However, the issue has always been controversial and other investigators have argued against those conclusions. In a recent review of the literature, Mathes[41] identified several factors that might contribute to the increased toxicity seen with supplemental oxygen:

1. Pre-existing pulmonary injury from BLM is a major risk factor for the development of significant oxygen-induced pulmonary injury.
2. Recent exposure to BLM (i.e., less than 1 to 2 months before supplemental oxygen) may be a major risk factor. The rationale is that there may be inadequate time for BLM levels to decrease in lung tissue.
3. Secondary risk factors that may contribute to BLM-induced pulmonary injury include renal insufficiency (thereby allowing delayed clearance of BLM) and a total dose in excess of 450 mg (roughly 240 mg/m^2).

Those patients with one or more risk factors may be susceptible to further injury by oxygen and therefore should have their intraoperative and postoperative oxygen concentrations limited. In those without risk factors, fractional inspired oxygen likely has little effect. Unfortunately, the best way to identify "pre-existing pulmonary injury" is not apparent. Whereas some investigators insist that the earliest symptoms are detected with serial pulmonary function tests, others contend that PFTs are not predictive of postoperative problems and that evidence of injury is better supported by a history and physical examination positive for tachypnea, dyspnea, dry cough, and rales. All agree that routine preoperative chest x-rays are not particularly useful because radiologic changes are a late sign of disease.

A more recent retrospective study of these same patients concluded that intraoperative fractional inspired oxygen during prolonged surgeries was not a risk for the development of postoperative "oxygen saturation problems."[43] Surmising that BLM-induced fibrosis compromises the lungs' ability to handle large volumes of fluids, the investigators concluded that "intravenous fluid management, including transfusion" was the most significant variable affecting postoperative pulmonary morbidity. Ironically, this is one of the conclusions (in addition to limiting inspired oxygen concentrations) reached by Goldiner et al. 20 years before.

In summary, excessive use of oxygen may or may not be detrimental to the pediatric patient who has previously received BLM. Each patient needs to be considered individually for the presence of BLM-induced lung disease, renal insufficiency, and the total dose and duration since last BLM. Further, anesthesia caregivers must be thorough in searching for clinical effects of pulmonary toxicity. However, regardless of the potential for oxygen-induced toxicities, this debate may be moot. Limiting excessive fractional inspired oxygen and intravenous crystalloids is sound clinical practice that should be applied to all patients and not just those having received BLM. If, during the course of anesthesia, a child requires additional support, alternative measures such as the use of positive end-expiratory pressure and colloids should be used.

Radiation Therapy[44,47]

Because 80% of pediatric cancer patients are now expected to survive to adulthood,[1] greater emphasis has been placed on the long-term toxicities of care, especially radiation therapy. Although its role is diminishing, external beam radiation therapy (EBRT) continues to have applications in adjunctive care of childhood neoplasms. Further, use of intraoperative radiation therapy (IORT) has become more common. Thus, anesthesiologists will be asked to provide care during EBRT and IORT and to patients with sequelae of radiation therapy.

Established treatment protocols for all primary CNS tumors include EBRT of the cranium and spine. Children younger than 3 years with CNS tumors usually are excluded because of significant neuropsychological sequelae. External beam radiation therapy is used for CNS metastases of other tumors (notably leukemias) and is still considered for CNS prophylaxis in leukemic patients without evidence of CNS disease. Further, EBRT has applications in testicular ALL relapse, Hodgkin's lymphomas, neuroblastomas, Wilm's tumors, Ewing's sarcomas, retinoblastomas, and rhabdomyosarcomas.[45] Total body irradiation is used in preparation for BMT. Enthusiasm for EBRT is mitigated by its significant long-term complications to irradiated fields (Table 15-10). Although dose-dependent toxicity affects every organ system to different degrees, cardiac, pulmonary, and airway effects are especially important to anesthesia care providers. The cardiac effects are especially pervasive.[46]

TABLE 15–10 Sequelae of Radiation Therapy*

Site	Effects
Central nervous system	Neurocognitive deficits
	Leukoencephalopathy
	Ischemic cerebrovascular accident
	Ototoxicity
Neuroendocrine	Hypothalamus—growth hormone deficiency
	Pituitary—thyroid, prolactin, gonadal and adrenal deficiency
Eye	Lens—cataract
	Lacrimal gland—decreased tear production
	Retinopathy
	Optic neuropathy
Maxillofacial abnormalities	Xerostomia
	Trismus
	Fibrosis of tissue with facial deformities
	Osteoradionecrosis
Teeth	Agenesis, root shortening enamel hypoplasia, microdontia
Thyroid	Clinical/subclinical hypothyroidism
Cardiovascular	Acute and delayed pericarditis
	Pericardial fibrosis
	Asymptomatic chronic pericardial effusion with rare tamponade
	Valvular defects
	Coronary artery disease
	Conduction defects
	Restrictive cardiomyopathy with rare severe heart failure
Pulmonary	Pneumonitis
	Restrictive lung disease from pulmonary fibrosis
	Decreased diffusion capacity
	Decreased chest wall compliance in younger children
Gastrointestinal/hepatic	Esophageal strictures
	Enteritis/duodenal ulcers
	Radiation injury to bowel with fistulae and perforations
	Hepatitis
	Hepatic venoocclusive disease
Genitourinary	Glomerular dysfunction and chronic renal insufficiency
	Secondary hypertension—may be benign, malignant, or hyperreninemic
	Renal growth arrest
	Hemorrhagic cystitis
Ovary	Ovarian failure, sterility
	Delayed pubertal development
Testes	Oligo/azoospermia
	Delayed pubertal development/testosterone deficiency due to Leydig cell failure
Musculoskeletal	Retarded long bone growth/growth failure
	Pathological fractures from radiation osteitis
	Avascular necrosis femoral head
	Kyphoscoliosis
Surgical	Postoperative wound dehiscence
Secondary malignancies	Leukemia (latency 7 y)
	Solid tumors of bone, brain, and breast and malignant melanoma (latency 10–15 y)

*Compiled from Kalapurakal and Thomas,[44] Grossi,[3] Hancock et al.,[46] Kelly and Lange.[5]

Because sequelae are the result of the dose of radiation per session and the total exposure, toxicities are best minimized by increasing the number of treatments. *Fractionated* therapy involves daily sessions that allow smaller doses and time for healing of surrounding healthy tissue. *Hyperfractionated* therapy, multiple sessions each day, allows for greater total dose with comparable toxicity.[47] General anesthesia or sedation provides a reliably motionless patient to optimize delivery of radiation with minimal damage to surrounding tissue. Usually short and painless procedures, the challenge of providing anesthesia for EBRT lies in having intermittent access to patients during the procedure. Caregivers are required to be in an adjacent room. A simulation or planning session, where fields to be irradiated are plotted and marked, tend to be longer and may require general anesthesia. Preanesthetic evaluation includes full assessment of a child's diagnosis, significance of coexisting conditions, and complications of prior therapy. Because no one anesthetic method has been shown to be superior, anesthesiologists should practice to their comfort level given the remote nature of the practice and the occasional need for a prone position.

To optimize care and limit damage to healthy tissue by EBRT, many centers use IORT.[24,48] Intraoperative radiation therapy involves surgical resection of a tumor with intracavitary application of radiation therapy. Fewer long-term complications result from limited doses of radiation and the ability to exclude healthy tissue through operative mobilization and shielding. Used mostly in adults, IORT recently has been used in pediatric patients with neuroblastoma, rhabdomyosarcoma, Wilm's tumor, extraosseous Ewing's sarcoma, osteosarcomas, and others. Early work suggests greater cure rates and decreased need for EBRT.[24,48] Although anesthesia for IORT may require interdepartmental transport during surgery, the entire procedure may be accomplished in dedicated operating suites with linear accelerators. Care during IORT entails the same principles as those during EBRT, including being physically removed from the patient.

Bone Marrow Transplant and Graft Versus Host Disease

"Bone marrow transplantation is the process of replacing an individual's diseased, defective, or damaged marrow elements with healthy donor marrow cells."[49] Donor cells may be supplied by one's own (*autologous*) or someone else's (*allogeneic*) bone marrow, peripheral blood stem cells, or umbilical blood. Applications extend beyond oncology: possible candidates include any one of numerous hematologic, immunologic, or metabolic diseases.[49,50]

As applied to oncology patients, BMT permits aggressive antineoplastic regimens without regard for hematopoietic toxicity. Suitable candidates are determined by the patient's type of cancer, its course and extent, and the availability of suitable donor cells. Although a full discussion of candidate suitability is beyond the scope of this text, applications of BMT have been applied to the following neoplastic diagnoses: acute myelogenous leukemia in first remission, chronic myelogenous leukemia, high-risk ALL, recurrent leukemia of any type, and certain stages of lymphomas, neuroblastomas, Wilms' tumors, Ewing's sarcomas, and intracranial CNS tumors. Patients with solid tumors generally receive autologous transplants, whereas patients with hematologic tumors receive matched allogeneic transplants.

When allogeneic transplants are used, preparative regimens also must provide adequate immunosuppression to allow engraftment. Agents used include chemotherapy (high-dose cyclophosphamide, cytosine arabinoside, etoposide, thiotepa, melphalan, and busulfan) with or without total body irradiation. Toxicities of these agents and total body irradiation have been discussed, but it should be emphasized that the profound myelosuppression and prolonged immunosuppression lasts weeks after preparative regimen and BMT. Until full grafting takes place, risk of infection does not decrease for up to 100 days posttransplant.

Complications of BMT include the toxicities of preparative regimen (total body irradiation and chemotherapy), fatal infection (especially in those with GVHD), failure to engraft, recurrent neoplastic disease, secondary malignancies, and acute and chronic GVHD. All patients having received allogeneic stem cells are at risk to develop acute or chronic GVHD. Further, any immunocompromised patient who receives nonirradiated WBCs through transfusions of blood products may get GVHD. Because it is mediated by immunocompetent donor T lymphocytes, GVHD can occur even when the donor and recipient have identical human leukocyte antigens due to the presence of untypable, minor antigens. Among siblings with identical human leukocyte antigens, the risk of developing acute GVHD is as high as 20%.[50] Prophylactic regimens include cyclosporine, methotrexate, tacrolimus, and prednisone.

Acute GVHD presents with symptoms in one or more of its target organs: skin, liver, and gastrointestinal tract. Cutaneous symptoms manifest as a maculopapular rash, whereas gastrointestinal symptoms include cholestatic jaundice, anorexia, dyspepsia, and a mucoid, watery diarrhea. Skin biopsy, endoscopy, and colonoscopy with biopsies confirm the diagnosis. Coagulopathies secondary to liver disease and post-BMT thrombocytopenia usually preclude liver biopsies. Treatment includes prednisone, tacrolimus, and psoralin with ultraviolet light.

Chronic GVHD may follow acute GVHD (with or without resolution of the latter) or may occur de novo without prior acute GVHD. However, by definition, it does not occur until 80 days post-BMT. Manifestations range from mild, consisting mostly of oral lesions, to severe, with several organ systems involved. Cutaneous involvement consists of epidermal atrophy and focal dermal fibrosis. Generalized scleroderma results in joint contractures and debility. Alopecia and hair loss also may occur. Ocular symptoms of keratoconjunctivitis sicca include burning, pain, and photophobia. Gastrointestinal symptoms include oral lesions, atrophy, and dryness. Cholestatic jaundice, restrictive pulmonary disease, gastrointestinal system, and neuromuscular system involvement also may occur. Therapy, consisting of more aggressive regimens of the same agents used to treat acute disease, lasts for months.

Cancer Pain

Pain relief is one of the foremost concerns of families and children with cancer. Studies of children with cancer report that 50% of inpatients and 25% of outpatients experience pain regularly.[51,52] However, many have the perception that pain is underappreciated or undertreated by caregivers. Meg Durbin, a pediatrician whose child had cancer, placed "prompt and adequate pain relief" foremost on her parents' wish list for interactions with their children's doctors.[53] The reasons for insufficient treatment range from inability to adequately assess a child's pain to caregiver's fears of addiction, respiratory depression, and "giving up." Further, failure to fully comprehend a family's needs and desires, especially during the terminal stages of disease, may lead to parental dissatisfaction with their child's care.[51,52]

Ironically, pain in the pediatric oncology patient is due mostly to the toxicities of therapy (Table 15-11).[52] In one report, treatment-related pain accounted for 67% and 80% of the pain experienced by hospitalized patients and outpatients, respectively.[51] This is because tumor-related pain dissipates with effective antineoplastic therapy. Only in the terminal stages of disease does pain related to the advancement of cancer become difficult to alleviate. Of the causes of tumor-related pain (Table 15-12), pain from invasion of tumor into bone and bone marrow is most common. Neuropathic pain, whether due to effects of tumor or treatment, is especially difficult to treat. In addition to the treatment-related pain outlined in Table 15-11, a child may experience pain secondary to the diagnosis of cancer (e.g., lumbar punctures and bone marrow biopsies) and pain from secondary infections due to immunosuppression.

As full volumes have been written on the subject, it would be foolish to conclude that any reasonably complete discussion of this topic could be accomplished within one chapter of one text. For an excellent, concise discus-

TABLE 15–11 Pain Syndromes Associated With Therapy in Patients With Cancer

Cause	Characteristics	Treatment
After surgery		
Acute postoperative	Wound or referred pain	Epidural catheters, opioids, NSAIDs
Limb amputation	Stump or phantom pain	Prophylaxis with preemptive regional anesthesia; antiepileptics or TCAs or mexiletine, calcitonin, topical agents, intrathecal catheters
Nerve trauma	Burning, lancinating pain, dysesthesia, hyperalgesia	Injection with local anesthesia and steroid; neurolysis, antiepileptics/TCAs/mexiletine
After chemotherapy or radiation therapy		
Vincristine	Symmetric polyneuropathy or glove and stocking burning	Antiepileptics/TCAs/mexiletine, capsaicin
Mucositis	Intense pain with swallowing or defecation	Opioids, topical agents

NSAID, nonsteroidal anti-inflammatory drug; TCA, tricyclic antidepressant.
Source: Modified from Galloway KS, Yaster M: Pain and symptom control in terminally ill children. *Pediatr Clin North Am* 47:711, 2000.

TABLE 15-12 Tumor-Related Pain Syndromes in Patients With Cancer

Cause	Characteristics	Treatment
Infiltration of bone by tumor	Constant aching ± muscle pain	Palliative radiation, steroids, fracture stabilization, calcitonin/etidronate, opioids, nonsteroidal anti-inflammatory drugs, baclofen, benzodiazepines, neurolysis
Metastatic fractures close to nerves	Acute pain ± muscle spasm	
Vertebral body fractures	Back or coccygeal pain ± neurologic defect	
Infiltration or compression of nerves by Tumor		Palliative radiation, steroids, surgical decompression, adjuvant drugs (tricyclics, antiepileptics), neurolytic nerve blocks, epidural or intrathecal techniques, opioids notoriously ineffective; cord compression is an oncologic emergency
Peripheral nerve	Burning, dysesthesia, lancinating pain	
Plexus or nerve root	Radicular pain	
Meningeal carcinomatosis	Headache, neck stiffness, cranial nerve deficits	
Spinal cord compression	Severe neck and back pain with upper motor neuron neurologic deficits	
Gastrointestinal or genitourinary obstruction of hollow viscus	Poorly localized, dull, "sickening" pain with superimposed cramping	Decompress (nasogastric, bladder catheter) anticholinergics, actreotide
Visceromegaly, tumor invasion of abdominal/pelvic/thoracic organs	Poorly localized, dull, often referred to as *somatic dermatomes*	Neurolytic nerve blockade (e.g., celiac plexus, hypogastric plexus intercostals), epidural/intrathecal catheters, opiods
Stretching of periosteum or fascia	Severe, localized pain	Palliative radiation, surgical debulking, steriods, opioids, potential neurolysis, epidural or intrathecal catheter
Inflammation	Severe, localized pain	Steroids, NSAIDs, surgical drainage where appropriate, opioids, potential neurolysis, epidural or intrathecal catheter
Elevated intracranial pressure	Headache, nausea or vomiting, behavioral changes	Surgical decompression, steroids

NSAID, nonsteroidal anti-inflammatory drug.
Source: Modified from Galloway KS, Yaster M: Pain and symptom control in terminally ill children. *Pediatr Clin North Am* 47:711, 2000.

sion on the subject, the reader is directed to recent reviews by Miser[51] and Galloway.[52] However, some salient points can be made in this chapter.

Like any chronic or unrelenting pain syndrome, cancer "pain" is a constellation of physical, psychological, and emotional discomforts. (Figure 15-7).[52] Because of this, effective therapy needs to address more than the physical component. Further, other symptoms related to cancer and its therapy contribute to patient discomfort. Symptoms such as nausea and vomiting, pruritus, agitation, and dyspnea can make patients even more miserable and tax overburdened coping mechanisms. Treating the patient's "pain" often requires relief of these additional symptoms. Caregivers also need to address the family unit. Understanding the family's "pain" and needs will help the anesthesiologist to more effectively treat the child's discomfort (see The Emotional Stress of Disease).

With these caveats, treatment of the chronic or unrelenting pain is approached in a stepwise fashion modeled after the World Health Organization paradigm (Figure 15-8).[52] Nonsteroidal anti-inflammatory drugs and opioids can be supplemented by tricyclic antidepressants, antiepileptic agents, mexiletine, and clonidine. These latter agents are especially useful for neuropathic pain where nonsteroidal anti-inflammatory drugs and opioids often

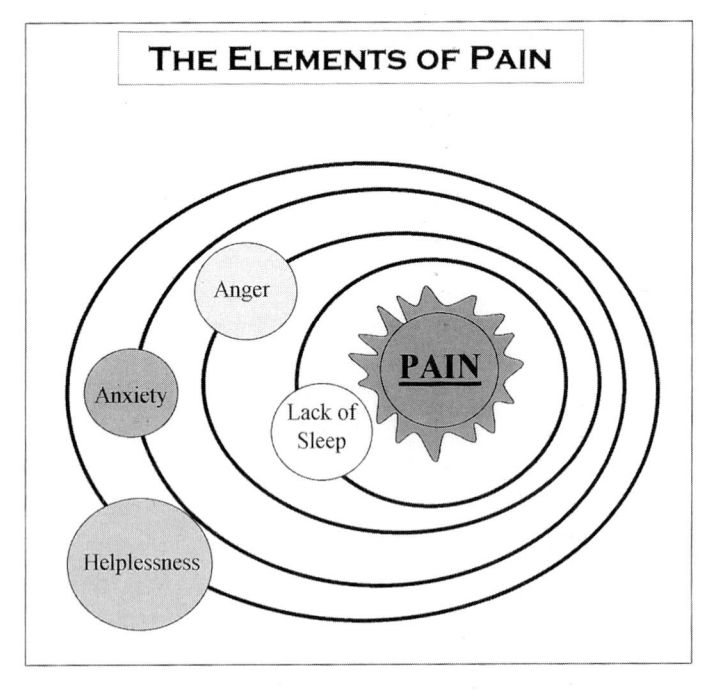

FIG. 15-7 The interactions between pain, lack of sleep, anxiety, anger, and helplessness. *(Modified from Galloway KS, Yaster M: Pain and symptom control in terminally ill children.* Pediatr Clin North Am *47:711, 2000.)*

Step Four
Invasive Therapy

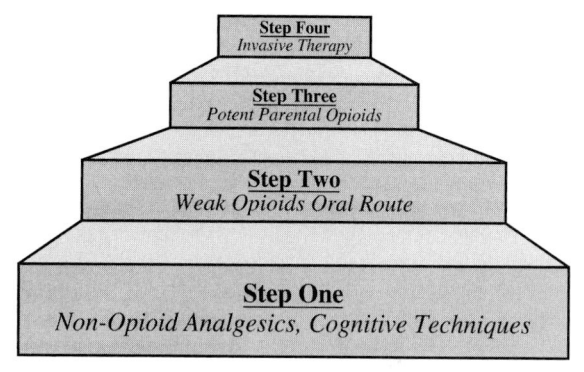

Step Three
Potent Parental Opioids

Step Two
Weak Opioids Oral Route

Step One
Non-Opioid Analgesics, Cognitive Techniques

FIG. 15-8 The World Health Organization pain management stepwise approach. *(Modified from Galloway KS, Yaster M: Pain and symptom control in terminally ill children.* Pediatr Clin North Am *47:711, 2000.)*

fail. For acute exacerbations of pain related to surgery, patient-controlled analgesia with opioids or regional anesthesia may prove useful. However, because of prior long-term use, these patients often require larger doses of opioids than would normally be expected for a given procedure. For certain patients with unrelenting pain, invasive therapy with neuraxial or neurolytic agents may be appropriate.[52,54] Because the pain of pediatric cancer is more often diffuse than localized, these modalities often are not used. However, especially with neuropathic pain and in the later stages of disease progression, these mechanisms may provide profound pain relief and allow for less sedation. Properly placed epidural and intrathecal catheters may be maintained for several weeks. The reader is directed to Galloway[52] and Collins[54] for a more complete discussion of these more invasive techniques.

The Emotional Stress of Disease

Few events can be more emotionally traumatic to parents than being told that their child has cancer. Likewise in children, the diagnosis of cancer generates concerns ranging from fears of separation to anxiety over body image and acceptance among peers. Long-term psychological effects are not uncommon, especially for the older child who has attained more sophisticated developmental milestones. For health care professionals to best treat the child, they need to better appreciate these emotional consequences.

Although most studies agree that there are long-term effects of having one's child treated for cancer, reports of the effects on parents of childhood cancer survivors yield inconsistent results. Some investigators contend that parents cope well with the extreme stress. Other researchers find that mothers of pediatric cancer survivors are at risk for a variety of psychological difficulties, including depression, anxiety, and marital discord. This is consistent with the long-held notion that parents, especially mothers, of seriously ill children are at risk for psychological maladjustment. In one study, severe posttraumatic stress symptoms were found in 39.7% of the mothers and 33.3% of the fathers.[55] Although those with stress symptoms may not meet criteria for posttraumatic stress disorder, the presence of symptoms indicates significant psychological disturbance. Further, symptoms have been noted to persist.[55,56] Years after completion of therapy, parents of childhood cancer survivors exhibited an 84% prevalence of loneliness and uncertainty of the well-being of their children.[56] Other symptoms such as sleep disturbances, anxiety, depression, and disease-related fear were less frequent but still present.[57] Stuber et al. reported posttraumatic stress symptoms more than 2 years after end of therapy.[55] The health care provider should anticipate the emotional impact of childhood cancer on parents to persist over time.

The level of parental anxiety and distress correlates with the likelihood that the child will develop posttraumatic stress disorder; similar results were found in the cancer survivors. The level of posttraumatic stress symptoms observed in 12.5% of children correlated with a clinical diagnosis of posttraumatic stress disorder.[55] Although less pervasive than in their parents, this prevalence is between that of survivors of severe childhood burns (6.7%) and child victims of sexual abuse (20.7%).[55] For patients and their parents, the origin of traumatic events included the life threat of the diagnosis, the repeated intrusive procedures, and the threat to body integrity. In the study by Stuber et al., medical procedures were frequently recalled as traumatic events.[55] This suggests that psychological effects associated with invasive procedures persist well past the end of treatment for children and their parents.

The potential of posttraumatic stress symptoms in children many years after treatment has important implications. Children and adults exposed to traumatic events can have difficulties with academic performance and learning problems. Personality development also can be influenced by trauma. Such a combination of effects on cognition and personality could compound the learning difficulties identified in pediatric cancer patients treated with cranial irradiation or intrathecal chemotherapy.

"Parents perceive themselves as providers for their children, whom they are supposed to protect from fear, hurt and pain. The diagnosis of cancer represents an assault on a parent's identity and sense of adequacy as guardian."[58] Many parents of children with cancer feel that they are unable to help their children. As the diagnosis is accepted, guilt becomes significant and anger may be directed at the health care personnel caring for their children. The stress of illness and hospitalization can cause psychological regression in patients and their parents. Sleep disturbances and fatigue common during treatment may exacerbate this problem. Even after the end of therapy, for the patient or parents with posttrauma symptoms, hospitals and health care providers can be reminders of their cancer experience.

In the process of sorting through these emotions, parents develop unique ways of coping and interacting with health care professionals. Whereas some families seem easier to work with and take less of the doctor's time, other parents expect to participate in treatment decisions. Such parents typically ask endless questions, require detailed explanations, and monitor the expertise of medical personnel. All parents quickly learn to shield their child from unnecessarily painful procedures performed without adequate anesthesia or by inexperienced individuals. Doctors may label as "difficult" these parents who make requests and take more of their time.[53]

Despite these challenges, doctors who cannot eliminate physical ailments can help to heal by showing compassion and empathy to children and their families. Although showing patience and offering latitude may seem difficult at times, in the end the patient and family benefit.

CONCLUSION

Provision of care for the pediatric oncology patient requires an appreciation for the medical, surgical, and psychological principles described within this chapter. Each child must be evaluated individually with a thorough understanding of the diagnosis, course of therapy, and psychological needs. Care can be facilitated with preprinted forms generated with the aid of the oncology department. Ideally, forms include medication therapy (agents, last dose, cumulative dosage), radiation therapy (site, last dose, cumulative dose), complications of treatment, and recent laboratory data and imaging results (e.g., chest x-rays, echocardiograms) with dates of completion. Many institutions have dedicated oncology pharmacists who might provide some of this data on short notice.

Prepared with this information, the anesthesiologist is ready to approach the patient and family with sensitivity and patience. As with any child, but especially with one who is chronically and potentially terminally ill, the patient includes the whole family. In my opinion, *every* cancer patient is a candidate for preoperative sedation. Oncology patients must regularly tolerate unpleasant experiences. As many children will return often, they will come to dread trips to the operating room that include an unpleasant induction. If the child has previously received sedation for procedures, families are knowledgeable about the benefits of sedation for that child.

Families may be suspicious of new medical personnel and will be keenly aware of routine. Because they understand the risks of infection, parents may be vocally protective of central lines. If indwelling central lines are accessed at all, sterile technique should be practiced diligently.[46] When appropriate, these patients may make good candidates for parental presence on induction of general anesthesia. Children with cancer often have an unexpectedly greater need for pain therapy. This should be anticipated to avoid a painful emergence.

Caring for the pediatric oncology patient or cancer survivor is as rewarding as it is challenging. Given the child's exposure to the medical system and the likelihood of the child's return, the anesthesia care provider has a strong opportunity to influence the child and family's experience that may last a lifetime.

REFERENCES

1. Donaldson SS: Lessons from our children. *Intl J Radiat Oncol Biol Phys* 26:739, 1993.
2. Gurney JG, Severson RK, Davis S, et al: Incidence of cancer in children in the United States. *Cancer* 75:2186, 1995.
3. Grossi M: Management and long term complications of pediatric cancer. *Pediatr Clin North Am* 45:1637, 1998.
4. Grenier MA, Lipschultz SE: Epidemiology of anthracycline cardiotoxicity in children and adults. *Semin Oncol* 25(suppl 10):72, 1998.
5. Kelly KM, Lange B: Oncologic Emergencies. *Pediatr Clin North Am* 44:809, 1997.
6. Viswanathan S, Campbell CE, Cork RC: Asymptomatic undetected mediastinal mass: a death during ambulatory anesthesia. *J Clin Anesth* 7:151, 1995.

7. Davis PJ, Hall S, Deshpande JK, et al: Anesthesia for general, urologic, and plastic surgery. In *Smith's Anesthesia for Infants and Children,* 6th ed. Motoyama EK, Davis PJ, eds. St. Louis, Mosby, 1996, p 588.
8. Furst SR, Burrows PE, Holzman RS: General anesthesia in a child with a dynamic, vascular anterior mediastinal mass. *Anesthesiology* 84:976, 1996.
9. Ferrari LR, Bedford RF: General anesthesia prior to treatment of anterior mediastinal masses in pediatric cancer patients. *Anesthesiology* 72:991, 1990.
10. Halpern S, Chatten J, Meadows AT, et al: Anterior mediastinal masses: anesthesia hazards and other problems. *J Pediatr* 102:407, 1983.
11. Shamberger RC: Preanesthetic evaluation of children with anterior mediastinal masses. *Semin Pediatr Surg* 8:61, 1999.
12. Shamberger RC, Holzman RS, Griscom NT, et al: CT quantitation of tracheal cross-sectional area as a guide to the surgical and anesthetic management of children with anterior mediastinal masses. *J Pediatr Surg* 26:138, 1991.
13. Shamberger RC, Holzman RS, Griscom NT, et al: Prospective evaluation by computed tomography and pulmonary function tests of children with mediastinal masses. *Surgery* 118:468, 1995.
14. Mahoney DH: Acute lymphoblastic leukemia. In *Oski's Pediatrics: Principles and Practice,* 3rd ed. McMillan JA, DeAngelis CD, Feigan RD, et al, eds. Philadelphia, Lippincott Williams & Wilkins, 1999, p 1493.
15. Pui C-H: Acute lymphoblastic leukemias. *Pediatr Clin North Am* 44:831, 1997.
16. Steuber CP: Acute myeloid leukemia. In *Oski's Pediatrics: Principles and Practice,* 3rd ed. McMillan JA, DeAngelis CD, Feigan RD, et al, eds. Philadelphia, Lippincott Williams & Wilkins, 1999, p 1501.
17. Chintagumpala MM, Mahoney DH: Malignant brain tumors. In *Oski's Pediatrics: Principles and Practice,* 3rd ed. McMillan JA, DeAngelis CD, Feigan RD, et al, eds. Philadelphia, Lippincott Williams & Wilkins, 1999, p 1511.
18. McClain KL: Non-Hodgkin's lymphoma. In *Oski's Pediatrics: Principles and Practice,* 3rd ed. McMillan JA, DeAngelis CD, Feigan RD, et al, eds. Philadelphia, Lippincott Williams & Wilkins, 1999, p 1509.
19. Shad A, Magrath I: Non-Hodgkin's lymphoma. *Pediatr Clin North Am* 44:863, 1997.
20. McClain KL: Hodgkin's disease. In *Oski's Pediatrics: Principles and Practice,* 3rd ed. McMillan JA, DeAngelis CD, Feigan RD, et al, eds. Philadelphia, Lippincott Williams & Wilkins, 1999, p 1507.
21. Hudson MM, Donaldson SS: Hodgkin's disease. *Pediatr Clin North Am* 44:891, 1997.
22. Castleberry RP: Biology and treatment of neuroblastoma. *Pediatr Clin North Am* 44:919, 1997.
23. Strother DR, Dreyer ZE: Neuroblastoma. In *Oski's Pediatrics: Principles and Practice,* 3rd ed. McMillan JA, DeAngelis CD, Feigan RD, et al, eds. Philadelphia, Lippincott Williams & Wilkins, 1999, p 1517.
24. Haas-Kogan DA, Fisch BM, Wara WM, et al: Intraoperative radiation therapy for high-risk pediatric neuroblastoma. *Int J Radiat Oncol Biol Phys* 47:985, 2000.
25. Chintagumpala MM, Steuber CP: Wilms' tumor. In *Oski's Pediatrics: Principles and Practice,* 3rd ed. McMillan JA, DeAngelis CD, Feigan RD, et al, eds. Philadelphia, Lippincott Williams & Wilkins, 1999, p 1515.
26. Petruzzi MJ, Green DM: Wilms' tumor. *Pediatr Clin North Am* 44:939, 1997.
27. King DR, Groner JI: Renal neoplasms. In *Pediatric Surgery,* 3rd ed. Ashcraft KW, ed. Philadelphia, WB Saunders, 1997.
28. Teitelbaum D, Teich S, Cassidy S, et al: Highly vascularized sacrococcygeal teratoma: description of this atypical variant and its operative management. *J Pediatr Surg* 29:98, 1994, p 1535.
29. McClain KL: Langerhan's cell histiocytosis. In *Oski's Pediatrics: Principles and Practice,* 3rd ed. McMillan JA, DeAngelis CD, Feigan RD, et al, eds. Philadelphia, Lippincott Williams & Wilkins, 1999.
30. Eskeni AE, Mogul MJ, Yeager AM, et al: Management of the child with malignant disease in the pediatric intensive care unit. In *Textbook of Pediatric Intensive Care,* 3rd ed. Roger MC, ed. Baltimore, Williams and Wilkins, 1996, p 1433.

31. Chabner BA, Allegra CJ, Curt GA, et al: Antineoplastic agents. In *Goodman's and Gilman's the Pharmacological Basis of Therapeutics,* 9th ed. Hardman JG, Limbird LE, eds. New York, McGraw-Hill, 1996, p 1233.
32. McQuillan PJ, Morgan GA, Ramwell J: Adriamycin cardiomyopathy. *Anaesthesia* 43:301, 1988.
33. Ali MK, Ewer MS, Gibbs HR, et al: Late doxorubicin-associated cardiotoxicity in children: the possible role of intercurrent viral infection. *Cancer* 74:182, 1994.
34. Nysom K, Holm K, Lipsitz SR, et al: Relationship between cumulative anthracycline dose and late cardiotoxicity in childhood acute lymphoblastic leukemia. *J Clin Oncol* 16: 545, 1998.
35. Von Hoff DD, Layard MW, Basa P, et al: Risk factors for doxorubicin-induced congestive heart failure. *Ann Intern Med* 91:710, 1979.
36. Steinherz LJ, Graham T, Hurwitz R, et al: Guidelines for cardiac monitoring of children during and after anthracycline therapy: report of the Cardiology Committee of the Children's Cancer Study Group. *Pediatrics* 89:942, 1992.
37. Sorensen K, Levitt G, Bull C, et al: Anthracycline dose in childhood acute lymphoblastic leukemia: issues of early survival versus late cardiotoxicity. *J Clin Oncol* 15:61, 1997.
38. Hale JP, Lewis IJ: Anthracyclines: cardiotoxicity and its prevention. *Arch Dis Child* 71:457, 1994.
39. Nousiainen T, Vanninen E, Rantal A, et al: QT dispersion and late potentials during doxorubicin therapy for non-Hodgkin's lymphoma. *J Intern Med* 245:359, 1999.
40. Schwartz CS, Hobbie WL, Truesdell S, et al: Corrected QT interval prolongation in anthracycline-treated survivors of childhood cancer. *J Clin Oncol* 11:1906, 1993.
41. Mathes DD: Bleomycin and hyperoxia exposure in the operating room. *Anesth Analg* 81:624, 1995.
42. Goldliner PL, Carlon GC, Cvitkovic E, et al: Factors influencing postoperative morbidity and mortality in patients treated with bleomycin. *BMJ* 1:1664, 1978.
43. Donat SM, Levy DA: Bleomycin associated pulmonary toxicity: is perioperative oxygen restriction necessary? *J Urol* 160:1347, 1998.
44. Kalapurakal JA, Thomas PRM: Pediatric radiotherapy: an overview. *Radiol Clin North Am* 35:1265, 1997.
45. Fortney JT, Halperin EC, Hertz CM, et al: Anesthesia for pediatric external beam radiation therapy. *Int J Radiat Oncol Biol Phys* 44:587, 1999.
46. Hancock SL, Donaldson SS, Hoppe RT: Cardiac disease following treatment of Hodgkin's disease in children and adolescents. *J Clin Oncol* 11:1208, 1993.
47. Holzman RS: Anesthesia and sedation for procedures outside the operating room. In *Smith's Anesthesia for Infants and Children,* 6th ed. Motoyama EK, Davis PJ, eds. St Louis, Mosby, 1996, p 703.
48. Gunderson LL, Willett CG, Harrison LB, et al: Intraoperative irradiation: current and future status. *Semin Oncol* 24:715.731, 1997.
49. Ogden AK, Steuber CP: Bone marrow transplantation for childhood leukemia. In *Oski's Pediatrics: Principles and Practice,* 3rd ed. McMillan JA, DeAngelis CD, Feigan RD, et al, eds. Philadelphia, Lippincott Williams & Wilkins, 1999, p 1505.
50. Sanders JE: Bone marrow transplantation for pediatric malignancies. *Pediatr Clin North Am* 44:1005, 1997.
51. Miser AW, Miser JS: The treatment of cancer pain in children. *Pediatr Clin North Am* 36:979, 1989.
52. Galloway KS, Yaster M: Pain and symptom control in terminally ill children. *Pediatr Clin North Am* 47:711, 2000.
53. Durbin M: From both sides now: a parent-physician's view of parent–doctor relationships during pediatric cancer treatment. *Pediatrics* 100:263, 1997.
54. Collins JJ, Grier HE, Sethna NF, et al: Regional anesthesia for pain associated with terminal pediatric malignancy. *Pain* 65:63, 1996.
55. Stuber ML, Christakis DA, Houskamp B, et al: Posttrauma symptoms in childhood leukemia survivors and their parents. *Psychosomatics* 37:254, 1996.
56. Van Dongen-Melman JE, Pruyn JF, De Groot A, et al: Late psychosocial consequences for parents of children who survived cancer. *J Pediatr Psychol* 20:567, 1995.

57. Pelcovitz D, Goldenberg B, Kaplan S, et al: Postraumatic stress disorder in mothers of pediatric cancer survivors. *Psychosomatics* 37:116, 1996.
58. Hersh SP, Wiener LS, Figueroa V, et al: Psychiatric and psychosocial support for the child and family. In *Principles and Practice of Pediatric Oncology,* 3rd ed. Pizzo PA, Poplack DG, eds. Philadelphia, Lippincott-Raven, 2000, p 1241.

16 | The Child With Neurological Problems

Frank Mazzeo, MD
Bruno Bissonnette, MD

In perhaps no other area of anesthesiology does the anesthetic technique have as significant an impact on morbidity and outcome as it does in pediatric anesthesiology. The manipulation of physiologic and anatomic factors can profoundly attenuate morbidity and improve long-term outcome. Because central nervous system development is not complete until the end of the child's first year, important pathophysiologic differences exist between adults and children. In this chapter we explore some common clinical scenarios in pediatric neuroanesthesia and incorporate the relevant neurophysiology.

THE CHILD WITH INCREASED INTRACRANIAL PRESSURE (ICP)

History and Physical

The clinical presentation of the child with increased ICP will depend on the age of the patient, the degree of increased ICP, and the duration of increased ICP.[1] Neonates and infants with increased ICP may present with irritability, lethargy, poor feeding, and a bulging anterior fontanelle. Patients with more severe increases in ICP are more likely to be lethargic and moribund than irritable. As ICP increases to more critical levels, vomiting, decreasing level of consciousness, gait disturbances, and oculomotor palsies may develop. With severe increases, cranial nerves may be affected and compromise the child's ability to protect the airway. Causes of increased ICP include tumors, trauma, obstruction of cerebrospinal fluid (CSF) drainage, subarachnoid hemorrhage, and cranial deformities.

Physiology

The cranium has a fixed volume and is comprised of 70% brain tissue, 10% CSF, 10% extracellular fluid, and 10% blood, so any increase in one compartment will lead to decreases in one or more of the other volumes, an increase in ICP, or both.

A decrease in CSF volume is usually the first compensatory response to an increase in volume in one of the other compartments. When decreases in CSF volume can no longer compensate for an increase in volume of one of the other compartments, or when increased CSF volume itself is increased, ICP will increase. An additional compensatory mechanism present in the pediatric patient is the presence of open fontanelles and suture lines that can expand and, hence, compensate for slow, progressive increases in intracranial volume. Normal ICPs are 8 to 18 cmH$_2$O in adults and 2 to 4 cmH$_2$O in children and may be subatmospheric in newborns.[2] In general, the ICP increases more rapidly in children and infants than in adults. Therefore, cerebral blood flow (CBF) also is compromised sooner. As a result, children are much more likely to have sudden neurologic deterioration. Cerebral blood flow depends on the cerebral perfusion pressure (CPP), which is derived from the mean arterial pressure (MAP) minus the ICP or central venous pressure (CVP), whichever is greater. Thus, patients with increased ICP may need a higher MAP to maintain adequate CBF. Cerebral blood flow is autoregulated in the normal brain. Cerebral blood flow in children is autoregulated at values higher than in adults. The autoreulation curve for infants and neonates is lower and to the left.

Cerebral blood flow also depends on arterial partial pressure levels of carbon dioxide ($Paco_2$) and alveolar oxygen. Hypercarbia and hypoxia will cause cerebral vasodilitation and an increase in CBF and cerebral blood volume (CBV). Although an increase in CBF may be beneficial in the setting of increased ICP, the increase in CBV is not and may exacerbate the increase in ICP. In addition to hypercarbia and hypoxia, all of the volatile anesthetic agents increase CBV and ICP as a result of cerebral vasodilitation. Some of this volatile anesthetic effect can be attenuated by concurrent gentle hyperventilation. For these reasons, it is probably best to maintain patients slightly hypocapneic and always well oxygenated.

Preoperative Assessment of the Neurosurgical Patient

In recent years there has been dramatic progress in the assessment of the neurosurgical patient because of improved diagnostic imaging techniques and an increased understanding of cerebral metabolism and physiopathology. In parallel to that progress, biochemical investigations have produced information on neurotransmission and molecular mechanisms underlying brain function. This opens up the field of therapies related to neurotransmission.

Despite advancing technologies, the most important aspect of the preoperative assessment remains the clinical history and physical examination. The anesthetic workup of the neurosurgical child must be done in step by step.[3] Central to the neuroanesthetic is the assessment of intracranial hypertension. The history and physical findings of intracranial hypertension differ somewhat according to age group. The clinical presentation of the patient with intracranial hypertension differs according to the underlying disease and the age group. As in subarachnoid hemorrhage, sudden massive increases in ICP may cause coma. Double vision due to vertical oculomotor palsies (sunset sign) and absent venous pulsation of the retinal vessels may be present on fundoscopy. Dysphonia, dysphagia, or gait disturbances also may be noted. Injury to the third cranial nerve may result in ptosis. Injury to the sixth cranial nerve produces a strabismus from a loss of abduction. Nausea and vomiting are common and older children will complain of morning headaches. Papilledema may be noted on fundoscopy. As ICP reaches threshold levels, a decreased level of consciousness and signs of brain herniation may develop.[3]

Four imaging modalities that aid in the assessment of intracranial hypertension are skull x-rays, ultrasonography, computed tomography (CT), and magnetic resonance imaging (MRI). Skull x-rays might show the "beaten copper sign," universal suture stenosis, or splitting of the sagittal sutures caused by chronically increased ICP. In infants and young children, the cranial sutures should be narrower than 2 mm and should not have bridges or closures.[4] Ultrasonography of the brain is useful in premature infants and neonates. It is relatively inexpensive, it does not require sedation, and it can be performed at the bedside anterior to the fontanel. The real-time sector scanner can visualize virtually all parts of the brain.[5]

In the past two decades, the development of CT and MRI has revolutionized the investigation of brain disease. It is essential to anesthesiologists to become familiar with these modalities of preoperative assessment and review them before proceeding with the anesthetic management. The preoperative evaluation of these images, among others, will facilitate the identification of the neuroanesthetic considerations and help plan the anesthetic technique most appropriate to use for a given surgical procedure. The identification of highly vascularized tumors on MRI, the assessment of brain structure shifts, decisions pertaining to the use of mannitol are examples of how these tests can aid in the anesthetic preparation.

Neurosurgical patients may be receiving anticonvulsant medication. Recognition of the child's seizure history and any potential drug interaction is important. Patients with a suprasellar tumor such as craniopharyngioma frequently have pituitary dysfunction and therefore should have a complete endocrine evaluation including thyroid and adrenal function studies.

Premedication

Preoperative sedation in pediatric neurosurgical patients should not be administered on a routine basis. Due to the negative consequences of hypoventilation and hypoxemia on cerebral circulation, sedatives and narcotics should not be given to unmonitored children. Two scenarios are outlined: the child with intracranial hypertension and the child with a hypervascularized lesion.

In the first case, hypotension and hypercarbia may lead to cerebral vasodilatation and increased ICP. The loss of airway protection may compromise oxygenation. For these reasons, sedatives and narcotics should be avoided in the preoperative period.

In the second scenario, if the child has a large hypervascularized lesion and normal ICP, one should avoid sustained pressure variations and in particular hypertensive episodes. These children may benefit from some degree of sedation to avoid precipitating a preoperative hemorrhage. Several agents and routes can be used. Rectal pentobarbital (4 mg/kg) or orol or rectal chloral hydrate (50 mg/kg) can be administered to small children 1 h before surgery. Nasal midazolam is a rapid premedicant but sometimes painful during administration.[6-8] Ketamine by any route is not recommended in pediatric neuroanesthesia. Cardiovascular and respiratory monitoring is recommended. The emotional preparation of the child is essential and can be accomplished by the anesthesiologist and the parents working in concert. Accurate, honest information for the child and parents forms the cornerstone of emotional preparation. In older children, a simple explanation of what may be expected, before the induction of anesthesia, will reduce any element of surprise and the incidence of hemodynamic responses in a hostile environment.

Clonidine premedication has been used in adult neuroanesthesia with disparate results. In a recent study, clonidine blunted the blood pressure response to pin holder application.[9] Other research found that addition of clonidine at the same dosage (150 g) did not change the blood pressure response to pin insertion.[10] Its use as premedication in 3- to 12-year-old children with American Society of Anesthetists Physical Status 1 and 2 has been reported with good results,[11,12] but its use in infants and pediatric neurosurgical procedures has not been well studied. Therefore, according to experience presently available, clonidine should not be used in pediatric neuroanesthesia.

Laboratory Data

Electrolyte disturbances and volume depletion may result from persistent vomiting that is common in the setting of increased ICP.

Patient Positioning

Prevention of position-related injuries is important. Patient positioning and theater organization should be planned before the procedure and in concert with the neurosurgeon. Specific material for patient positioning should be prepared before the induction. Ventilation may be compromised by incorrect positioning. It is mandatory to ensure that chest excursion remains adequate, especially if the patient is prone. The use of suitable bolsters or a frame will allow the abdomen to be pendulous and aid respiratory movement. A 10° head-up position often is used to improve cerebral venous return and reduce brain venous congestion. However, the most recent data have indicated that there is no reduction in CBV in an anesthetized patient when the table is lifted in a progressive head-up position.[13] In addition to information obtained by the usual monitoring devices, it is desirable to visually observe a body part, such as a hand or foot, during the procedure to assess peripheral perfusion and adequacy of gas exchange. All lines, endotracheal tube connectors, and the neck (access to compress carotid arteries or jugular veins) should be visible and accessible.

Induction

Rapid control of the airway is essential in the child with increased ICP. This is best achieved with a rapid sequence induction using pentothal, atropine, and succinylcholine followed by manual hyperventilation and intubation. Fasiculations, seen in adults who have received succinylcholine, seem to be less of a problem in children. The potential for increasing ICP with succinylcholine is attenuated by its ability to facilitate rapid control of the airway. It should be avoided in patients with pre-existing conditions that predispose them to hyperkalemia. These include closed head injury, subarachnoid hemorrhage, myopathies, and other neurologic conditions that result in loss of motor neuron function. If succinylcholine is contraindicated, a 1-mg/kg dose of rocuronium will allow for excellent intubating conditions within a period only slightly longer than that of succinylcholine.

Another pharmacologic way to decrease the increase in ICP associated with laryngoscopy is the use of intravenous lidocaine. In a dose of 1 to 2 mg/kg, lidocaine will attenuate the systemic hypertension and concomitant increase in ICP that occurs with laryngoscopy, if given 60 to 90 s before intubation. A single dose of fentanyl (3 to 5 µg/kg) also will attenuate the increase in systemic blood pressure and ICP associated with laryngoscopy. There is little risk of residual respiratory effect unless the patient is obtunded preoperatively or the procedure is very short.

Rarely does a child with increased ICP present to the anesthesiologist without an intravenous line. In this situation, the potential increase in ICP that may result from the stimulation associated with intravenous placement must be weighed against the potential problems associated with a mask induction. This is especially problematic in the patient with a full stomach. Essentially, the fastest way to obtain airway control, with the least amount of stimulation, is probably the safest. One method is to let the child breathe nitrous oxide during intravenous placement and then follow with an intravenous induction. An alternative method is to induce anesthesia through a

25-gauge butterfly needle that can be placed with minimal sympathetic stimulation. If intravenous access is difficult, it must be kept in mind that a smooth inhalational induction, with assisted ventilation to avoid hypercapnia, may be less injurious to the child with high ICP than multiple failed attempts at gaining intravenous access. In this case, sevoflurane may have an advantage over halothane because induction is faster and control of the airway is achieved with less coughing.

Monitoring

The patient with elevated ICP may already have an ICP monitor in place. An arterial blood pressure line also may be justified if the CPP is marginal or dramatic hemodynamic changes are anticipated.

Maintenance

Anesthesia can be maintained with N_2O, isoflurane, and an appropriate muscle relaxant. Local anesthetic can be administered by the surgeon at the sight of surgical incision to minimize the amount of sympathetic stimulation associated with skin incision. A single 3- to 5-μg/kg dose of fentanyl will provide intraoperative analgesia with little risk of postoperative respiratory or neurologic depression.

Gentle hyperventilation, with Pa_{CO_2} levels in the range of 28 to 32 reduce ICP. Intraoperatively, other measures may be needed to reduce ICP. An easy nonpharmacologic method of decreasing the ICP is to position the head appropriately. Raising the head 15° to 20° and keeping the neck unflexed or turned to the side improves venous drainage and thus may decrease ICP. Other methods to decrease ICP involve the use of diuretics or steroids.

Furosemide, a loop diuretic, can be given to induce a systemic diuresis, decrease CSF production and cerebral edema, and thereby reduce ICP. It should be given in a dose of 0.5 to 1 mg/kg intravenously. If given with mannitol, the dose should be reduced to 0.2 to 0.4 mg/kg. Mannitol is an osmotic diuretic, given in a dose of 0.25 to 0.5 g/kg, to increase osmolality and reduce cerebral edema and ICP. If given too quickly, it can transiently increase CBV and ICP and cause hemodynamic instability. Therefore, we recommend that a 0.5-g/kg dose be given over 20 to 30 min. It also may cause electrolyte disturbances. The use of diuretics mandates the use of a Foley catheter to document urine output and prevent bladder distention. In additon to diuretics, dexamethasone, a corticosteroid, can be given in the dose of 0.1 mg/kg (up to 10 mg) during induction and every 6 h thereafter to reduce cerebral edema in the penumbral area surrounding a tumor. Unfortunately, this effect on ICP is delayed and may take several hours, or days, for a clinically apparent effect.

Fluid administration to neurosurgical patients depends on the pathology being treated. A frequent problem in pediatric brain injury is the development of cerebral edema, with a resultant increase in ICP. There is no perfect protocol for fluid replacement in neurosurgical patients with increased ICP. However, the maintenance of cerebral perfusion should represent the optimal goal of fluid therapy. The intravenous solution should maintain an isovolemic, iso-osmolar, and relatively iso-oncotic intravascular volumes. For example, a patient with increased ICP and/or a brain mass requires a fluid regimen that adequately balances the intravascular volume with efforts to dehydrate the brain mass. In a patient undergoing insertion of a ventricular shunt or repair of myelomeningocele, fluid management should replace third-space losses.

Emergence

Before extubation the patient should be awake with intact airway reflexes. Unfortunately, many of these patients are neurologically impaired and have poor airway reflexes at baseline. These patients certainly have a greater risk for aspiration and perhaps should have their stomachs suctioned before extubation or be nursed in a lateral decubitus position.

HYDROCEPHALUS

Hydrocephalus results from an increase in CSF volume within the ventricular system. The causes include excessive CSF production, obstruction of the CSF pathway, or decreased reabsorbtion of CSF.[14] These patients often present to the operating room for revision of a pre-existing malfunctioning shunt. Hydrocephalus also may result from a subarachniod hemorrhage, particularly in the neonate or premature infant.

Preoperative Assessment

In any patient with hydrocephalus, it is essential to evaluate the ICP by assessing the patient's level of consciousness and symptomatology.[15] Other important aspects of the preoperative assessment for patients with hydrocephalus are nil per os (NPO; nothing by mouth) status (realizing that patients with increased ICP have delayed gastric emptying); fluid and electrolyte disturbances (that may have resulted from persistent vomiting); diabetes insipidus or syndrome of inappropriate secretion of antidiuretic hormone (SIADH); coexisting pathology such as neoplasm; and age-dependent phenomena (postoperative apneas in the premature patient).

Induction and Maintenance

The method of induction will depend on the patient's NPO status and whether the patient has increased ICP. The principles for securing the airway in both instances were discussed in the preceding section. Maintenance of the anesthetic also will depend on whether ICP has increased. If so, the patient should be hyperventilated to a $Paco_2$ level of 25 to 30 mmHg. The anesthetic can be maintained with N_2O and sevoflurane, isoflurane, or halothane. The judicious use of local anesthesia at the surgical site will reduce the need for opiod medications intraoperatively and postoperatively.

Emergence

As with the patient with increased ICP, the patient with hydrocephalus should have intact airway reflexes before extubation. The child's preoperative neurologic status also may affect the decision to extubate immediately postoperatively. Some children may be neurologically impaired at baseline with poor airway protection and impaired gag reflexes. As a precautionary measure, it is prudent to extubate these patients while they are in the lateral decubitus position and carefully observe them until they have fully recovered.

INTRACRANIAL TUMORS

In children, brain tumors are the second most common type of neoplasm, after leukemia.[16] Posterior fossa tumors account for half of the tumors, with the remainder being supratentorial in origin. Expanding space-occupying lesions are associated with increased ICP, decreased CPP, and potential ischemia. Tumors also are associated with hydrocephalus, so many of the anesthetic considerations that are valid for the patient with increased ICP and hydrocephalus are valid for the patient with a brain tumor.

SUPRATENTORIAL CRANIOTOMY

Anesthetic considerations for a supratentorial craniotomy are (1) management of increased ICP, (2) a full stomach and delayed gastric emptying secondary to increased ICP, (3) electrolyte disturbances, (4) the presence of SIADH or diabetes insipidus (DI), and (5) appropriate positioning of the patient with the head slightly elevated to promote venous drainage.

Preoperative Assessment

The preoperative assessment for these children should include an assessment of the ICP. On the one hand, these children also may show signs of hypervolemia, low osmolarity, and cerebral edema if they suffer from SIADH. On the other hand, these children may have undergone aggressive brain dehydration and subsequent hypovolemia.

Induction and Maintenance

Induction should be aimed at preventing any increases in ICP. At the Hospital for Sick Children, a standard induction for this type of patient consists of thiopental, lidocaine (1.0 mg/kg), fentanyl (2 to 3 µg/kg), and a nondepolarizing muscle relaxant. The thiopental dose should be reduced if hypovolemia is suspected. Gentle manual hyperventilation with isoflorane titrated to the patient's blood pressure can be done before intubation. After intubation the patient should be hyperventilated to reduce ICP. Maintenance for most of these patients includes the use of isoflorane, nitrous oxide, and fentanyl. For neuroprotective purposes, we also allow our patients to cool passively to 34.5°C to 35°C.

Placement of an arterial blood pressure line after induction will allow close blood pressure monitoring and easy blood sampling. Patients with increased ICP are hyperventilated to a $Paco_2$ of 25 to 30 mmHg. Excessive hyperventilation may lead to profound vasoconstriction and ischemia. For patients with impaired oxygenation, positive end-expiratory pressure (PEEP) may be introduced gradually. However, the overaggressive use of PEEP may lead to decreased cerebral venous drainage, causing the ICP to increase and a concomitant decrease in MAP. Together, they may lead to a decrease in CPP and greater potential for ischemia. Because PEEP also increases dead space ventilation, the gradient from $Paco_2$ to end-tidal partial pressure of carbon dioxide ($EtCO_2$) gradient may be increased and the $Etco_2$ level may no longer accurately reflect the $Paco_2$ level. Hence, after PEEP is introduced, a blood gas should be checked, not only to determine whether oxygenation has improved but also to determine whether the relation of $Paco_2$ to $Etco_2$ has changed.

Emergence

The decision for immediate postoperative extubation will depend on the smoothness of the intraoperative course, the presence of neurologic deficits, and the success of surgical intervention. In the absence of complications, the trachea can be extubated when the patient is fully awake and has an intact gag reflex. Neuromuscular blockade should be reversed and normothermia obtained.

Postoperative problems may include abnormal temperature homeostasis, analgesia and neurologic assessments, hypertension, seizures, and fluid or electrolyte disturbances. These patients may develop neurogenic hyperthermia postoperatively, which can be detrimental to long-term outcome. Cooling measures need to be taken if this condition develops.

The overaggressive use of opioid analgesics may interfere with postoperative neurologic assessment. Use of local anesthesia for a field block or superficial cervical plexus block will reduce the need for postoperative opioid use. Nonopioid analgesics such as acetaminophen or ketorolac also can be used to reduce the postoperative opioid requirements, although the ketorolas should be avoided if postoperative bleeding is a concern. Because inadequate control of pain can lead to hypertension and subsequent increased ICP, it needs to be treated aggressively, yet judiciously. After adequate analgesia is obtained, hypertension can be treated with an antihypertensive such as labetalol or hydralizine. These vasodilators also may cause cerebral vasodilatation and increased ICP, something that may not be desirable postoperatively. However, after the resection of a large supratentorial tumor, increased ICP generally is not a problem.

Postoperatively, patients are also at risk of developing a seizure disorder. For this reason, many neurosurgeons will choose to give anticonvulsants prophylactically. Dilantin can be given in a dose of 20 mg/kg but must be given over 20 to 30 min to avoid arrhythmias and hypotension.

Diabetes insipidus also may develop postoperatively, especially after pituitary surgery. The diagnosis is confirmed by an inappropriately low urine osmolarity in association with a rising serum osmolarity. Treatment includes fluid replacement and administration of vasopressin or 1-3-desamino-8-D-arginine vasopressin (DDAVP). DDAVP can be given intranasally in a dose of 0.025 to 0.15 mL twice a day or intravenously in a dose of 0.3 µg/kg, up to a maximum dose of 20 µg.

POSTERIOR FOSSA CRANIOTOMY

There are four types of tumors that commonly occur in the posterior fossa. Medulloblastoma, cerebellar astrocytoma, and brainstem glioma occur in near equal proportions and account for 90% of all posterior fossa tumors.[17] The remainder consist of ependyomas (7%), acoustic neuromas (3%), meningioma, ganglioma, and so forth. Children with Arnold–Chiari malformations also will undergo posterior fossa craniotomy for decompression. In addition to the presence of increased ICP and a potentially full stomach, other anesthetic considerations are air embolism secondary to unusual positioning and brainstem compression that may result in hypertension, arrythmias, and upper airway dysfunction.

Preoperative Assessment

The preoperative considerations are similar to those for supratentorial craniotomy. A review of the radiologic study (MRI, CT, etc.) before surgery may alert the anesthesiologist to potential intraoperative problems. Reviewing these with the neurosurgeon or neuroradiologist is especially helpful for anesthesiologists not well versed in neuroanatomy.

Positioning

The prone position is the one most used for patients undergoing posterior fossa craniotomy, with the sitting position accounting for 30% of all posterior fossa craniotomies, although this figure will differ widely from institution to institution. Special concerns for patients in the prone position are ensuring that flexion of the head does not interfere with ventilation of the patient or jugular venous drainage. Special attention should be paid to the eyes by making sure that they are adequately protected from any pressure.

If the surgery is to take place in the sitting position, the patient is at greater risk for venous air embolism, and special monitoring, such as a precordial Doppler, should be used. A sudden decrease in blood pressure and a decrease in $EtCO_2$ level may be the first physiologic signs of venous air embolism. If a venous air embolism does occur, one must inform the surgeon to flood the surgical field, ventilate with 100% oxygen (and turn off the nitrous gas), attempt to withdraw air through CVP, if one is present, and treat hemodynamic compromise with vasopressors and fluids. Jugular venous compression may prevent further air entrainment. Cardiac compressions may be necessary to break the air lock in the right ventricular outflow tract. The routine use of PEEP in sitting patients may reduce air embolism, but this is controversial.

Monitoring

In addition to standard monitors, a precordial Doppler is often used when the patient is in the sitting position. Somatosensory evoked potentials also may be monitored during removal of intramedullar or brainstem tumors.

Induction

In addition to the concerns of maintaining CPP and avoiding exacerbations and intracranial hypertension, patient positioning may lead to kinking or obstruction of the endotracheal tube. For that reason, many neuroanesthesiologists prefer a reinforced endotracheal tube or a nasotracheal tube. Another option is an orotracheal tube with a soft bite block. Oral airways have been associated with severe oropharyngeal edema in patients undergoing posterior fossa surgery.

Maintenance

No single anesthetic technique has been shown to be superior, so we recommend tailoring the anesthetic to the individual needs of the patient and surgeon. Local anesthetic infiltration along the skin incision may reduce intraoperative and postoperative narcotic requirements. Maintenance with a combination of fentanyl, isoflurane, and a nondepolarizing muscle relaxant is a reasonable choice. Decreasing the ICP will reduce the amount of retractor pressure necessary and allow for adequate cerebral perfusion. This can be accomplished with a combination of mannitol, furosemide, and hyperventilation. Dexamethasone also may be helpful in this regard. After the tumor is removed, the $PaCO_2$ can be returned to normal.

Emergence

The site of surgery will play an extremely important role in determining whether the child should be extubated immediately postoperatively or remain sedated and intubated until surgical swelling has decreased. For instance, a patient with an intrabulbar tumor or a high intramedullary spinal tumor may have adequate respiratory efforts immediately postoperatively but may quickly deteriorate as postsurgical edema worsens. If the patient is to be extubated immediately postoperatively, the use of narcotics in combination with intravenous lidocaine (1.0 mg/kg) may improve emergence by decreasing coughing and straining on the endotracheal tube. Another alternative is to extubate the child while using a deep insoluble inhalational agent such as sevoflurane, which may allow for neurologic assessment sooner than a more soluble agent such as halothane. Postoperative analgesia can be obtained with morphine, codeine, and/or acetaminophen (40 mg/kg rectally or 15 to 20 mg/kg orally).

MYELODYSPLASIA

Seventy percent of babies with hydrocephalus have some abnormality in their spinal cords or columns. Myelodysplasia occurs when the neural tube fails to fully close. A herniation of the meninges is called a *meningocele*, and a herniation containing neural elements is referred to as a *myelomeningocele*. Most children with myelomeningocele also have Arnold–Chiari type 1 malformation and therefore will be prone to hydrocephalus. Timely closure of the defect is essential in preventing infection. If the defect is closed within the first 48 h, the rate of ventriculitis is less than 7%. Delaying closure more than 48 h increases the infection rate to 37%.[18] Further, the likelihood of progressive neural damage and decreased motor function is increased with any delay in closure.

Preoperative Assessment

In addition to associated pathology (e.g., Arnold–Chiari malformation) and age-related pathophysiology, these patients may present unique positioning and airway management problems. The neuroplaque should be protected, so the patient should be positioned on the side or, with proper padding, can be carefully placed on the back for the induction. A lateral decubitus position, with the head rotated, usually provides an adequate intubating position. These patients are also subject to large third-space losses and hypothermia.

Monitoring

Blood transfusion may be necessary, especially for patients with large defects, and skin grafting is common. Encephaloceles require a craniotomy for repair. An arterial line should be placed for repeat hemoglobin measurements and continuous blood pressure monitoring in these children. Nasal encephaloceles may require the semisitting position for their repair, so a central venous line and a precordial Doppler may be justified.

Induction

Positioning for induction can be problematic for this patient population and will require induction in a lateral decubitus position or supine with padding and a cushioned ring to protect the neural sac. Induction can be accomplished with atropine, thiopental, and a muscle relaxant. We prefer to use succinylcholine in these cases because of the awkward positioning resulting in difficult mask ventilation. Alternatives include awake intubation in the premature infant after intravenous atropine, or the intubation may be done without muscle relaxants under deep inhalational anesthesia. Patients with nasal encephaloceles may present a problem in that face mask fit is often less than optimal and, hence, does not allow adequate control of the airway.

SPINAL CORD SURGERY

Common diseases of the spinal cord requiring surgery include herniated discs, spondylosis, syringomyelia, primary or metastatic tumors, hematomas or abscesses, and trauma. In all cases, compression of the spinal cord may produce ischemia,[19] interstitial edema and venous congestion[20] and may interfere with nerve transmission.[21,22] Maintaining spinal cord perfusion pressure and reducing spinal cord compression are crucial. Intraoperative monitoring of spinal cord function includes (1) the wake-up test, (2) somatosensory evoked potentials, and (3) motor evoked potentials. The wake-up test remains the traditional method to assess anterior spinal cord (i.e., motor) function. Evoked potential monitors (e.g., somatosensory evoked potentials) measure only the response of the sensory nervous system. This limitation can be overcome by use of motor evoked potentials.[23,24]

HEAD INJURY

Unintentional injury is the leading cause of death among children in the United States.[25] It is a major cause of morbidity and mortality and the most frequent cause of pediatric trauma hospitalization.[26,27] Skull fractures are present in more than 25% of all children with head injuries[28] and in more than 50% of fatal cases of childhood head trauma.[29] The incidence of posttraumatic intracranial hematomas varies considerably, but some children with head injuries require surgical treatment.[30] Failure to recognize the presence of a hematoma may transform an otherwise mild head injury into a fatal or permanently disabling one. Adults suffer more hematomas than children, but children have diffuse cerebral edema more frequently.[31]

Epidural hematomas most often are the result of a laceration of the middle meningeal artery during a deceleration injury. Children do not necessarily have an overlying skull fracture. It represents 25% of all intracranial hematomas in the pediatric population and a true neurosurgical emergency. Children often do not have the initial alteration in the state of consciousness commonly observed in adults. Children old enough to talk complain of an increasing headache and then become confused or lethargic. Rapid development of hemiparesis, posturing, and pupillary dilation occurs frequently and may confuse the diagnosis. Rapid expansion of the hematoma causes herniation of the temporal lobe downward through the tentoria incisura. Anisocoria is an early sign. Herniation is associated with bradycardia, slowed and irregular breathing, and widened pulse pressure (Cushing's triad).

Subdural hematomas are associated with parenchymal contusion, blood vessel laceration, and cortical damage. The mass effect of the contused and edematous brain may prompt surgical removal of the hematoma if the brain region involved is not functionally important. Severe edema and elevated ICP often lead to persistent neurologic deficits.

Intracerebral hematomas are rare but carry a poor prognosis. Surgery usually is avoided for fear of damaging viable brain tissue.

Anesthetic Considerations

Resuscitation and Stabilization

Airway, breathing, and circulation are essential components of the initial clinical assessment. Traumatized patients may present acid–base and electrolyte imbalances and abnormalities of glucose homeostasis and body temperature control.

Neurologic Status

The Glasgow Coma Scale provides a means of detecting changes in the patient's condition. Symptoms of raised ICP must be evaluated.

Associated Injuries

Pediatric trauma often occurs from high-velocity energy transfer, which leads to injuries to the neck, chest, and abdominal organs.

Full Stomach

Vomiting leads to pulmonary aspiration and respiratory complications.

Age-Related Pathophysiology

Monitoring

Arterial catheter and central venous line placements are indicated. A urinary catheter should be inserted unless contraindicated by an associated bladder neck injury. Central body temperature should be monitored at all times. Computed tomography is the procedure of choice for evaluation of head injury during the first 72 h after the accident.

Induction and Maintenance

The association of head injury and neck injury occurs so often in infants and children that tracheal intubation must be accomplished with axial traction. The presence of a neck collar will serve only as a reminder of a cervical spine fracture rather than a proper means of cervical spine stabilization. Patients should be hemodynamically stable before anesthesia is induced. In a hemodynamically stable patient, anesthesia can be induced rapidly with atropine, thiopentone or propofol, lidocaine, and succinylcholine or a nondepolarizing muscle relaxant such as rocuronium. The use of ketamine with propofol may reduce ICP[32] and thus may be useful in clinical circumstances where immediate evacuation of the hematoma requires that hemodynamic stability cannot be reached before induction.

Maintenance of Anesthesia

Evacuation of an intracranial hematoma usually requires a craniotomy, which may suddenly decrease ICP and allow upward movement of the brainstem through the tentoria incisura. This may result in transient hemodynamic instability and cardiac arrhythmias.

Emergence and Postoperative Management

Patients with severe head injury remain intubated after surgery to provide ventilatory support and control elevated ICP. Transfer to an intensive care unit is indicated for continued care.

REFERENCES

1. Welch K: The intracranial pressure in infants. *J Neurosurg* 52:693, 1980.
2. Lang EW, Chestnut RM: Intracranial pressure. Monitoring and management. *Neurosurg Clin North Am* 5:573, 1994.
3. Brown K: Preoperative assessment of neurologic function in the neurosurgical patient. In *Cerebral Protection, Resuscitation and Monitoring: A Look Into the Future of Neuro Anesthesia.* Bissonnette B, ed. Philadelphia, WB Saunders, 1992, p 645.

4. Hodges FI: Pathology of the skull. In *Radiology Diagnosis—Imaging—Intervention: Neuroradiology and Radiology of the Head and Neck.* Tavaras J, ed. Philadelphia, JB Lippincott, 1989, p 123.
5. Grant E, Richardson J: Infant and neonatal neurosonography technique and normal anatomy. In *Radiology Diagnosis—Imaging—Intervention: Neuroradiology and Radiology of the Head and Neck.* Tavaras J, ed. Philadelphia, JB Lippincott, 1989, p 453.
6. Lejus MC, Renaudin M, Testa S, et al: Midazolam for premedication in children: nasal vs. rectal administration. *Eur J Anaesthesiol* 14:244, 1997.
7. Geldner G, Hubmann M, Knoll R, et al: Comparison between three transmucosal routes of administration of midazolam in children. *Paediatr Anaesth* 7:103, 1997.
8. Malinovsky JM, Populaire C, Cozian A, et al: Premedication with midazolam in children. Effect of intranasal, rectal and oral routes on plasma midazolam concentrations. *Anaesthesia* 50:351, 1995.
9. Costello TG, Cormack JR: Clonidine premedication decreases hemodynamic response to pin-holder application during craniotomy. *Anesth Analg* 86:1001, 1998.
10. Favre JB, Gardaz JP, Ravussin P: Effect of clonidine on ICP and on the hemodynamic responses on nociceptive stimuli in patients with brain tumors. *J Neurosurg Anesthesiol* 7:159, 1995.
11. Reimer EJ, Dunn GS, Montgomery CJ, et al: The effectiveness of clonidine as an analgesic in paediatric adenotonsillectomy. *Can J Anaesth* 45:1162, 1998.
12. Nishina K, Mikawa K, Shiga M, et al: Oral clonidine premedication reduces minimum alveolar concentration of sevoflurane for tracheal intubation in children. *Anesthesiology* 87:1324, 1997.
13. Lovell AT, Marshall AC, Elwell CE, et al: Changes in cerebral blood volume with changes in position in awake and anesthetized subjects. *Anesth Analg* 90:372, 2000.
14. Gascon G, Leech R: Medical evaluation. In *Hydrocephalus: Current Clinical Concepts.* Leech R, Brunback R, eds. St Louis, CV Mosby, 1991, p 105.
15. Bissonnette B: Anesthetic management of a child with hydrocephaly or with a ventricular shunt. *Ann Fr Anesth Reanim* 16:122, 1997.
16. Duffner PK, Cohen ME, Freeman AI: Pediatric brain tumors: an overview. *CA Cancer J Clin* 35:287, 1985.
17. Bruno L, Schut L: Survey of pediatric brain tumors. In *Pediatric Neurosurgery: Surgery of the developing nervous system.* McLaurin RL, ed. New York, Grune & Stratton, 1992, p 361.
18. Charney EB, Weller SC, Sutton LN, et al: Management of the newborn with myelomeningocele: time for a decision-making process. *Pediatrics* 75:58, 1985.
19. Sandler AN, Tator CH: Effect of acute spinal cord compression injury on regional spinal cord blood flow in primates. *J Neurosurg* 45:660, 1976.
20. Kato A, Ushio Y, Hayakawa T, et al: Circulatory disturbance of the spinal cord with epidural neoplasm in rats. *J Neurosurg* 63:260, 1985.
21. Kobrine AI, Evans DE, Rizzoli HV: Correlation of spinal cord blood flow, sensory evoked response, and spinal cord function in subacute experimental spinal cord compression. *Adv Neurol* 20:389, 1978.
22. Griffiths IR, Trench JG, Crawford RA: Spinal cord blood flow and conduction during experimental cord compression in normotensive and hypotensive dogs. *J Neurosurg* 50:353, 1979.
23. Lam A: Do evoked potentials have any value in anesthesia? In *Cerebral Protection, Resuscitation and Monitoring: A Look Into the Future of Neuro Anesthesia.* Bissonnette B, ed. Philadelphia, WB Saunders, 1992, p 657.
24. Grundy BL: Intraoperative monitoring of sensory-evoked potentials. *Anesthesiology* 58:72, 1983.
25. Guyer B, MacDorman MF, Martin JA, et al: Annual summary of vital statistics—1997. *Pediatrics* 102:1333, 1998.
26. Bruce DA, Schut L, Bruno LA, et al: Outcome following severe head injuries in children. *J Neurosurg* 48:679, 1978.

27. Lavelle JM, Shaw KN: Evaluation of head injury in a pediatric emergency department: pretrauma and posttrauma system. *Arch Pediatr Adolesc Med* 152:1220, 1998.
28. Harwood-Nash D: Fractures of the petrous and tympanic parts of the temporal bone in children: a tomographic study of 35 cases. *AJR* 110:598, 1970.
29. Freytag E: Autopsy findings in head injuries from blunt forces. Statistical evaluation of 1,367 cases. *Arch Pathol* 75:402, 1963.
30. Hendrick E, Harwood-Nash D, Hudson A: Head injuries in children: a survey of 4465 consecutive cases at the Hospital for Sick Children, Toronto, Ontario, Canada. *Clin Neurosurg* 11:46, 1964.
31. Bruce DA, Alavi A, Bilaniuk L, et al: Diffuse cerebral swelling following head injuries in children: the syndrome of "malignant brain edema." *J Neurosurg* 54:170, 1981.
32. Albanese J, Arnaud S, Rey M, et al: Ketamine decreases intracranial pressure and electroencephalographic activity in traumatic brain injury patients during propofol sedation. *Anesthesiology* 87:1328, 1997.

17 | Systemic Disorders Commonly Seen in Pediatric Anesthesia

Terrance A. Yemen, MD, FRCP(C)
James Michael Jaeger, MD, PhD, FCCP

Fortunately, the most common scenario in pediatric anesthesia is that of an otherwise healthy child in need of a straightforward surgical procedure; the preschool child with recurrent ear infections scheduled for myringotomy and pressure equalization (PE) tube placement comes to mind. Unfortunately, for some of us, life has become more complicated. We now commonly see children with significant, life-threatening disorders scheduled for simple and complex surgeries. The fact that many of these children are scheduled for outpatient surgery or, at best, seen the morning of surgery adds to the complexity of their anesthetic care. This chapter highlights several, relatively common systemic disorders encountered in pediatric anesthesia and not covered in detail elsewhere in this text. Although volumes can be written about each of these disorders, it is the purpose of this chapter to discuss those aspects of the disease process and anesthetic management most pertinent to the practicing anesthesiologist. A basic understanding of these diseases and their perioperative management is essential to any physician dealing with children on a day-to-day basis.

SICKLE CELL DISEASE

Etiology

The prevalence of sickle cell disease (SCD) in North America and the United Kingdom depends on the ethnic distribution in a given area. The gene responsible for SCD is thought to be present in 10% to 15% of the African-American population. The highest incidence appears to be among those of African-Caribbean decent. The high incidence of sickle cell trait (SCT) carriers in these populations has led to the suggestion that all patients be screened whenever the population at risk exceeds 15% of a demographic region. Sickle cell disease also is found in populations of the Middle East, the Mediterranean, India, and parts of South America. Young children who are heterozygous for the SCT gene are believed to have a relative resistance to falciparum malaria. This may account for the high incidence of the gene in those populations who live in malaria-endemic areas, although this has not been well documented.

Pathophysiology

The structure of hemoglobin is composed of two paired subunits. These subunits contain protoheme and globin. The globin molecule is responsible for many of the spatial characteristics of hemoglobin, not the least of which is its affinity for oxygen. The relationship of the various subunits also determines the physical properties of solubility and polymerization. In general, polymerization is enhanced by acidosis and deoxygenation. There are a variety of globin chains, which are characterized by the number and the sequence of amino acids. Commonly these variations are designated by the symbols α, β, γ, δ, ε, ζ, and θ. Normally, adult hemoglobin (Hb) consists primarily of HbA (95%), designated as α_2 or β_2. The hemoglobinopathies are a result of the production of abnormal hemoglobin molecules, as in SCD, or a given subunit, as in the thalassemias.

The molecular basis for SCD disease was discovered in 1957 and shown to be the result of the substitution of a single amino acid, valine for glutamic acid, at position 6 of the β-chain. Polymerization is increased as a result and the subsequent alignment of multiple polymers results in "sickling." A portion of the sickling process is reversible. Those sickled cells that do not reverse produce viscous, rigid cell bodies that have a tendency to adhere to the vascular endothelium. The result is the hemolysis of red blood cells, and capillary and/or arteriolar vaso-occlusion. It is this pathophysiology that is the basis for the acute crisis and chronic effects of SCD. In addition, there is an increase in serum coagulability and a decrease in splenic function. The defect in splenic function results in defective immune opsonization and ineffective phagocytosis. Susceptibility to infection by encapsulated organisms subsequently occurs. Interestingly, the presence of fetal hemoglobin (HbF) decreases polymerization and offers some protection against sickling, resulting in milder forms of SCD.

Patients who are heterozygous, SCT, or HbC (S-C disease) are at lesser risk of vaso-occlusive episodes. The various sickle cell states and their significance are presented in Table 17-1.

The natural history or progression of SCD is the result of chronic hemolysis punctuated by several acute crises. Chronic intermittent vaso-occlusion results in damage to all vascular beds. Reticulocytosis, hyperbilirubinemia, decreased growth, vision and hearing losses, cardiac failure, pulmonary insufficiency, renal failure, splenic infarction, destruction of joints and bones, skin ulcerations, and infection can occur.

An acute SCD crisis is characterized by an acute vaso-occlusive event. Severe pain, infarction of organs, priapism, acute splenic sequestration, and acute chest syndrome may occur. Acute splenic sequestration is generally seen in children younger than 2 to 3 years and results in profound shock and anemia. Aplastic crisis is the result of an acute drop in red cell production, usually secondary to a viral infection (paravirus B19).

Acute chest syndrome results from pulmonary vaso-occlusion. Signs and symptoms are similar to those of pneumonia and may make the diagnosis confusing for the unsuspecting. Chest radiographs show patchy or complete opacification of the lungs. Respiratory failure is common with acute chest syndrome. Acute chest syndrome is a common indication for hospitalization and accounts for up to 25% of deaths of patients with SCD. The complications of SCD are summarized in Table 17-2.

Anesthetic Management

The first issue in the anesthetic management of patients with SCD is that of screening. Screening of patients for SCD is controversial, like all screening programs. The issues of cost effectiveness are always at the forefront of such discussions. In simple terms, the identification of those patient groups at risk and the taking of a careful history are the first steps in the screening process. The screening of high-risk demographic groups is common in most centers, although studies on this particular issue are surprisingly scarce. Screening programs may be preconceptual, antenatal, neonatal, or during the later years of life. Hemoglobin electrophoresis provides an accurate diagnosis in all age

TABLE 17–1 Characteristics of the Various Sickle Cell States

Syndrome	Genotype	Clinical severity			Neonatal screening	Electrophoresis					Solubility test
		Hemolysis	Vasoocclusion			% HbA	% HbS	% HbF	% HbA$_2$	% HbC	
Sickle cell anemia	S-S	++++	++++	FS	0	80–95	2–20	<3.5	0	Positive
Sickle β^0 thalassemia	S-S^0	+++	+++	FS	0	80–92	2–15	3.5–7	0	Positive
Sickle HbC disease (HbSC)	S-C	+	++	FSC	0	45–50	1–5	N/A	45–50	Positive
Sickle β$^+$ thalassemia	S-B$^−$	+	+	FSA or FS	5–30	0	2–10	3.5–6	0	Positive
Sickle trait	A-S	0	0	FAS	50–60	35–45	<2	<3–5	0	Positive
Normal	A-A	0	0	FA	95–98	0	<2	<3–5	0	Negative

F, fetal hemoglobin; S, sickle hemoglobin; C, hemoglobin C; A, hemoglobin A; Hb, hemoglobin; N/A, not available.
Source: Adapted from Lane PA: Sickle cell disease. *Pediatr Clin North Am* 43:639, 1996.

TABLE 17–2 Complications in Patients With Sickle Cell Disease

Crisis	Complication
Hemolytic of painful crisis	Precipitated by cold, dehydration, hypoxia, infection, acidosis, stress, fatigue, and menstruation Unpredictable onset and variable duration Less frequent in those patients with higher HbF levels Aggressive analgesia needed; narcotics and NSAIDs are useful
Overwhelming infection	High risk of infection with encapsulated organisms such as *Streptococcus pneumoniae* and *Haemophilus influenzae*
Aplastic crises	Often the result of infection with paravirus B19 Usually in the preschool child or infant Requires transfusion Usually self-limiting
Acute chest syndrome	Leading cause of death in patients with SCD Multifactorial pathophysiology; atypical pneumonia, pulmonary sequestration, infarction, and fat embolism
Stroke	Present in 15–20% of SCD patients
Acute splenic sequestration	Sudden enlargement with acute cardiovascular collapse Often associated with infection Major cause of mortality in children <2 y
Bone and skin involvement	Dactylitis (hand and foot syndrome) Femoral head necrosis Leg ulceration *Salmonella* osteomyelitis
Hypersplenism	
Priapism	Up to 12% of children
Retinopathy	Vitreous hemorrhage, retinal detachment
Biliary disease	Cholelithiasis and cholecystitis
Uropathy	Glomerulopathy and tubular dysfunction

HbF, fetal hemoglobin; NSAID, nonsteroidal anti-inflammatory drug; SCD, sickle cell disease.
Source: Adapted from: Development and disease in childhood. In *Paediatric Anaesthesia*. Sumner E, Hatch DJ, eds. New York, Oxford University Press, 1999, p 1.

groups. It defines the exact nature of the defect allowing appropriate management of high-risk patients with SCD (S-S), without unduly treating low-risk patients such as those with SCT or SCD (S-A, S-C). Many centers use a sodium metabisulfite test (Sickledex) to screen children at high risk of SCD. Although often very useful, it has a number of significant limitations. First, false-negative tests do occur. Second, the test is not useful in the neonatal age group. Third, Sickledex does not distinguish between children with SCD from those with only SCT. An electrophoresis must be done to determine the exact disorder in any child who has a positive result. This is important given that SCT patients rarely ever have disease-related anesthetic complications and SCD patients most certainly do.

The second issue, relating to the management of SCD, is an understanding of the anesthetic morbidity and mortality. For a number of years the care of patients with SCD has varied greatly from one institute to another. Until the past decade very little information was available to determine appropriate guidelines. Early reviews demonstrated an increased surgical morbidity and mortality in SCD patients. Some reported mortality rates as high as 10%.[1] A more recent study from 1994 reported a perioperative mortality rate of 1.1%.[2] Although this is much lower than originally thought, it was still much higher than the risk for the average healthy patient. In fact, 7% of all deaths in that study were surgically related, with the mean age of death at only 42 years. Fully one-third of patients died from an acute event, even though none had diagnosed organ failure before death.

Given these humbling statistics, patients with SCD have been traditionally managed perioperatively with blood transfusionss. Typically, SCD patients were transfused to raise their Hb values to greater than 10 g/dL and lower their levels of HbSS to less than 30%. Although clearly done in the patient's best interests, the transfusion of blood products is not benign and there are few data to support or refute such a therapeutic approach.

At this same time another report appeared in the literature.[3] That report examined SCD-affected children who had not been transfused perioperatively. Although there no deaths were reported, more than 25% of the patients experienced postoperative complications. The investigators suggested that transfusion is unnecessary for children undergoing minor surgical procedures. The data were interesting but not compelling. The Cooperative Study of Sickle Cell Disease Group also published data from almost 4000 patients having surgery. The mortality rate was 1.1% and, unfortunately, offered no new insights into SCD management.[4]

In 1995 a study examining the benefit of perioperative transfusion therapy was released.[5] Thirty-six centers participated in that study involving more than 600 cases. Patients were randomized into aggressive therapy (transfusion up to 10 g/dL and HbS values of less than 30%) and simple therapy (nontransfusion). Despite the differences in Hb levels, both groups had the same complication rates postoperatively, including mortality. The rate was in excess of 30%. Interestingly, 14% of the complications were related to the transfusions in the aggressive-therapy group. The aggressive-therapy group received twice as much blood as the simple-treatment group and had a longer average hospital stay (4 vs. 2.5 days, respectively).

In a 1997 follow-up study, the results of 364 patients with SCD having cholecytectomy were published.[6] That study was conducted with aggressive and simple treatment protocols. Although the complication rate was the same for both groups, serious SCD-related complications, such as acute chest syndrome, were twice as common in the simple-treatment group (19%).

In 1999 another follow-up study reported that 8 of 29 patients who had simple myringotomies had serious perioperative complications.[7] That study highlighted the significant anesthetic risk these patients incur with even minor surgery.

Although those recent studies have suggested that complication rates are the same in transfused and nontransfused patients, a few important caveats should be noted. A significant collaboration occurred among the surgeons, hematologists, and anesthesiologists in these studies. All patients were carefully monitored and followed for any and all complications. Patients were also aggressively hydrated preoperatively 8 h or more before the surgery. Patients were actively warmed and all hypoxic events were treated aggressively. The single most important lesson learned from those studies may be the value of coordinated active management of patients with SCD.

The value of aggressive transfusion therapy in the perioperative management of SCD is in doubt. Perhaps it should be reserved for those patients having extensive surgery, in particular procedures such as thoracotomy and cardiopulmonary bypass. However, if one is to obtain results comparable to, or better, than those in the studies cited, then attention to routine care and detail is paramount.

Perioperatively, careful attention should be paid to a complete systems review. The medical condition of the child, especially those issues affecting hydration and oxygenation, should be optimized. A preoperative Hb level is required, in addition to any other blood deemed relevant by review of the history and physical examination. The choice of anesthetic matters less than its careful management. Children should not be allowed be become dehydrated from extensive fasts. An intravenous line is recommended for all children with SCD, if only for the purpose of hydration. Fluids should be warmed and measures should be taken to prevent hypothermia in the operating and recovery rooms. Monitoring and treatment for hypoxia should be aggressive because of its effect on the polymerization of abnormal Hb.

The use of regional anesthesia has been questioned in adults, especially obstetric patients, but there are no data to refute its use in providing postoperative pain relief in other patient subgroups. In fact, the use of local analgesics may prevent episodes of hypoxia that occur with narcotic analgesia and sedation.

Patients should have postoperative nausea and vomiting carefully monitored and treated to avoid the possibility of dehydration, especially in the outpatient. The management of these patients should involve a multidisciplinary approach. All relevant subspecialties should be involved in all phases of care.

Summary

Sickle cell disease is a common hemoglobinopathy encountered in pediatric anesthesia. Although there is a variety of subtypes, SCD (S-S) is associated with significant morbidity and mortality. Sickle cell disease is a multisytemic disease affecting all organ systems and should be approached as such. Careful preoperative preparation, including consultation with hematology, is invaluable. Attention to the basics of anesthesia appear to be as or more important than transfusion therapy for most patients. Further studies should identify those patients who specifically might benefit from aggressive transfusion management.

DIABETES MELLITUS

Etiology

Diabetes mellitus has been recognized as a disease entity for centuries, with scrolls describing its clinical features as long ago as 1550 B.C. Although most young patients with diabetes lead happy and productive lives in these prosperous times, it was only 80 years ago that children and adults with diabetes died within 2 years of the diagnosis.[8]

Diabetes is classified as two main types: insulin-dependent disease (type 1) and non–insulin-dependent disease (type 2; Table 17-3). Diabetes mellitus is certainly one of the most common endocrine disorders seen by anesthesiologists. It eventually affects 3% to 10% of the population in Western developed countries, with rates as high as 20% in Scandinavia.[9] Interestingly, it is strikingly less common in the underdeveloped countries of Latin America and Asia. For the purposes of this chapter, the discussion of diabetes concentrates on type 1 disease, previously called juvenile onset diabetes.

The etiology of diabetes is unclear but environmental, genetic, infectious, and immune factors have been implicated. The etiology is strongly associ-

TABLE 17–3 Classification of Diabetes Mellitus

Diabetes
  Insulin dependent (IDDM), or type 1
  Non-insulin dependent (NIDDM), or type 2
    Nonobese
    Obese
  Malnutrition-related diabetes mellitus
  Diabetes associated with disease states
    Pancreatic
    Hormonal
    Drug or chemical induced
    Genetic
    Miscellaneous
Impaired glucose tolerance
  Nonobese
  Obese
  Associated with certain diseases such as pancreatic
  Gestational diabetes mellitus

Source: World Health Organization.

ated with class 2 human leukocyte antigens. Viruses such as Coxsackie B and toxins are suspected agents in some patients. Children of a parent with type 1 disease have an increased risk of disease, with a cumulative risk up to 10% by age 30 years.

Pathophysiology

The pathophysiology of diabetes mellitus is complex and fascinating but clearly beyond the scope and purpose of this text. However, the basic concepts should be highlighted.

The diagnosis of diabetes is made by finding an abnormal glucose level, most commonly fasting blood sugar. Insulin deficiency and resistance are the basic defects responsible for the disease. Insulin is a low-molecular-weight protein and a significant anabolic hormone. It is secreted and stored in the β-islet cells of the pancreas. It is released in response to a rise in serum glucose and amino acids, usually as a result of eating. Approximately 95% of the insulin is released into the portal circulation, with half of that insulin being cleared by the liver on first-pass metabolism. The kidneys clear the remainder of the insulin. Basal insulin secretion is approximately 1 U/h, with a plasma half-life of 5 min and a biologic half-life of 20 min.

The effects of insulin are anabolic and stimulate the movement of glucose into muscle and adipose tissue. Glucose is converted into glycogen and triglycerides. Insulin inhibits the breakdown of muscle and fat. In addition, hepatic glycogen synthesis is stimulated.

The deficiency of insulin in diabetes mellitus leads to a catabolic state. Glucose and potassium uptake by cells is limited. This leads to hyperglycemia. Gluconeogenesis is activated with a resultant breakdown of muscle and adipose tissues. The free fatty acids are oxidized in the liver and ketone bodies are produced. Those bodies add to the metabolic acidosis and electrolyte disturbance. Patients develop polydypsia, polyuria, hyperglycemia, and ultimately ketoacidosis. Those affects are treatable with exogenous insulin therapy.

Surgery and anesthesia increase secretion of catecholamines, corticotropin, cortisol, growth hormone, and glucagon. Obviously these responses are directly proportional to the site, extent, and duration of the surgery and the anesthetic technique. In general, surgery is a catabolic event. In the diabetic patient, the surgical response is superimposed on a patient whose ability to produce and respond to insulin is already impaired, and the catabolic results are exaggerated.

Anesthetic Management

The goal of the pediatric anesthesiologist in managing the child with diabetes mellitus is straightforward. Fortunately, diabetic children rarely have the vascular, neurologic, and renal complications commonly associated with adult diabetics, especially type 2 disease. As such, the management of these children is focused on glucose homeostasis.[9–13] The fundamentals of their care can be summarized as follows:

1. Identify related or coexisting diseases
2. Correct any acid–base, fluid, and electrolyte disorders before surgery
3. Achieve a satisfactory control of blood glucose
4. Avoid hypoglycemia
5. Provide insulin to inhibit catabolic proteolysis, lipolysis, and ketogenesis

The safest, simplest, and, we believe, most effective method of managing these issues is by the use of an infusion of glucose and insulin. There are many methods of achieving an effective solution and infusion. We do not believe there is only one successful protocol. Some physicians prefer to have a single infusion of dextrose mixed with regular insulin. An example is the use of 50 g/L of dextrose with 20 U of regular insulin at a rate of 1.5 mL/(kg · h). We often use this method by putting the 20 U of regular insulin into a bag of 5% dextrose in lactated Ringer's solution at the rate of 1.5 mL/(kg · h). This provides enough substrate to ensure that glucose is metabolized and avoids hyper- and hypoglycemia. It also avoids giving insulin without giving dextrose. Both glucose and insulin should be given to avoid hypoglycemia and promote an anabolic state (or at least minimize the catabolic one).

Other physicians prefer to have a concentrated infusion of insulin and run a separate infusion of dextrose. For example, they would make a solution consisting of 50 U of regular insulin in 50 mL of saline. The starting rate of insulin delivery is 0.05 µg(kg · h). A separate infusion of dextrose is also administered. The techniques differ from each other but, in our experience, the results are the same.

Some physicians prefer to have patients continue administering their own insulin at home on the morning of surgery but only one-half to one-third of their intermediate insulin levels. Although this technique has the advantage of simplicity, it is associated with a greater incidence of hypoglycemia, especially if there is a delay in admitting the patient and starting a dextrose infusion. We also have found that control of hyperglycemia is erratic with this technique.

Regardless of the method chosen, blood sugars must be monitored carefully with the use of "point of care testing" such as Acutest.™ We prefer to have the baseline value taken at the time of admission and check values every 2 h for stability. If the values are not, then we check blood glucose levels at least every hour. In our experience, excluding those patients on steroids, control of blood sugars with an insulin infusion is very simple and blood glucose levels are surprisingly stable. Although there is some debate on this topic, we try to keep the blood sugars between 5 and 10 mmol/L ($\cong$90 to 180 mg/dL). We pay careful attention to sudden changes in glucose levels to avoid any surprising peaks or troughs in blood glucose. In the event that the infusion needs changing, we increase or decrease the infusion in increments of 10%.

A few other points should be made. Although it would seem self-evident, it is surprising that diabetic children are commonly placed at the end of a surgical list. A clear effort must be made to ensure that these children are scheduled at the beginning of the day or at least in the early morning. This is especially true now that patients are outpatients or admitted on the day of surgery. These patients usually have been fasting since the night before and will not have had intravenous access until they are admitted to the hospital. Failure to address this issue increases the incidence of erratic blood glucose control. Some of these young children are very brittle diabetics!

Dehydration is the enemy of all diabetics. The liberal use of a balanced salt solution is very important in the management of young diabetics. An intravenous solution should be started at the first opportunity and continued until the child is drinking. Control of nausea and vomiting is very important, especially in the outpatient setting. Diabetic patients do not tolerate fasting for extended periods. Arrangements should be made for an appropriate discharge. The decision to discharge the diabetic patient should consider extending the recovery period necessary for an otherwise healthy patient for a given surgery and must ensure adequate hydration and glucose control postoperatively. These children cannot be hurried out the door, in a manner of speaking!

The overall care of these children is enhanced by consultations with their pediatricians.[14] This allows a coordinated effort in their perioperative management and avoids unnecessary alterations in insulin dosing, which often is due to mixed and confused messages between care providers. Many good pediatric hospitals have multidisciplinary protocols to aid in the management of the diabetic child having surgery.

Summary

Diabetes mellitus is the most common hormonal and metabolic disturbance that anesthesiologists see. Children are fortunately usually spared the ravages of this disease until late in life but very brittle with regard to their glucose homeostasis, with a strong propencity toward ketoacidosis. Careful management of blood glucose and hydration is the hallmark of good care for these children. The early use of insulin and dextrose infusions allows the tight control of glucose levels perioperatively and avoids ketosis. These children are not routine outpatients and adjustment to discharge criteria and times should be made to avoid postoperative complications.

CEREBRAL PALSY

Etiology

Cerebral palsy (CP) traditionally is defined as a nonprogressive disorder of motion and posture. It is the end result of damage to the central nervous system that can occur during the antenatal, perinatal, or portnatal period. It is the leading cause of motor disability in childhood, with an incidence of 1 to 2 per 1000 births in Western countries. Interestingly, this incidence has not changed significantly over the past decade or two, despite a greater understanding of the role of perinatal medicine in indentifying and preventing this disorder. It is reasonable to assume that two factors are responsible for this fact. First, the incidence of hypoxia perinatally was overestimated, as was its effect on the incidence of CP. Second, the survival rate of very-low-birth-weight infants during that period increased. It is these children who have such a high incidence of motor disabilities.[15]

Cerebral palsy in the premature infant is commonly the result of a periventricular hemorrhage producing a spastic diplegia. Antenatal causes, to a lesser degree, include antenatal infection, thyroid disease, and neuronal migration disorders. Postnatal causes include meningitis, encephalitis, hydrocephalus, trauma, neurosurgical lesions, and their treatment.[16]

Pathophysiology

The central neurologic lesion is static and does not change over time. However, its clinical presentation and associated complications do change over time. Almost all CP children have associated findings or system complexes such as cognitive impairment, seizures, hearing or visual defects, and communicative and behavioral problems. In addition, many of these children develop systemic problems secondary to the original disorder such as gastrointestinal, respiratory, and orthopedic complications. In general terms, the likelihood of developing these complications is increased by the degree of spasticity associated with CP.

Spasticity is the result of abnormalities of the cerebral cortex. Athetosis results from the involvment of the basal ganglia and ataxia from defects in the cerebellum.

Many methods have been used to classify CP with the use of etiologic, neurologic, and clinical criteria.[16] The Swedish classification has been widely accepted as the most useful by addressing the movement disorder and its location (Table 17-4).

Spastic CP is the most commonly seen variation and is associated with the formation of contractures, especially those of the limbs. Spastic diplegia and hemiplegia are associated with the most favorable prognosis. In spastic quadraparesis, all four limbs are involved and intellectual impairment and seizures are common accompaniments. Bulbar muscles are also commonly involved with CP quadraparesis, affecting breathing and swallowing. The end result is malnutrition, aspiration pneumonias, obstructive and central sleep apnea, and respiratory failure. The prognosis is least favorable in

TABLE 17–4 Swedish Classification of Cerebral Palsy*

Spastic (70%)	Dyskinetic (10%)	Ataxic (10%)	Mixed (10%)
Quadriplegia (27%)	Distonia, twisting of torso and extremities	Intention tremor and head tremor	Spastic athetoid, etc.
Diplegia (21%)	Athetosis, slow, distal purposeless movements		
Hemiplegia (21%)	Chorea, proximal, jerky movements		

*All percentages are expressed as portions of the total population of children with cerebral palsy.
Source: Mutch L, Alberman E, Hagberg B, et al: Cerebral palsy epidemiology: where are we now and where are we going? *Dev Med Child Neurol* 34:547, 1992.

that group.[17] Dyskinetic CP is commonly associated with deafness and dysarthria. Intelligence levels in that group are generally below normal. Ataxic CP results in impaired balance and speech. Intellectual disorders and seizures are common in such children. The prognosis for functional improvement in that group is also poor.

Anesthetic Management

The anesthetic management of CP children depends on a preanesthetic evaluation of seven basic problems[18] and their subsequent management:

1. Behavior and communication problems
2. Visual and hearing defects
3. Epilepsy
4. Respiratory problems
5. Gastrointestinal problems
6. Medications
7. Pain management

Intellectual impairment is common in CP patients, especially those with quadraparesis. Its overall incidence is 50% in children with CP. In addition, there are hearing, visual, and speech deficits. Speech deficits also occur in CP children with normal or high intelligence. Therefore, the anesthesiologist must become familiar with the abilities and problems of individual patients to find an effective method of communication. A common mistake is to assume that these children do not understand us or cannot express their concerns and wishes. Each child must be assessed individually.[19] Communication with the principal care providers is the best approach to sorting out these potentials and limitations. The CP children with hearing and visual impairments can be particularly challenging in this regard. Special arrangements should be made to take advantage of communication devices and methods that are effective for these children. Depression and emotional labilities are not uncommon in older adolescents and should be addressed.

Epilepsy occurs in one-third of CP children. It is most common in those with spastic CP and least so with ataxic forms of CP. Tonic–clonic seizures are the most common expression. Antiseizure medications should be continued up to and including the morning of surgery. Most of these medications are not available in intravenous preparations. Fortunately, most have long therapeutic half-lives (24 to 36 h), so that dosing usually can restart the night of surgery or the next day, if need be. Medications also can be given through the gastrointestinal tube, if present, unless the surgery involves the bowel. The role of anesthetic medications is controversial in patients with epilepsy, but most of our medications are anticonvulsant (sodium pentathol) or have little to no effect (propofol and inhalational agents excluding ethrane). Some medications, e.g., methohexital, are only proconvulsant in particular forms of epilepsy. Children with temporal lobe epilepsy should not received methohexital.

Unfortunately, respiratory failure is a common cause of death in CP patients. Most respiratory complications are the result of three problems: chronic aspiration of oropharyngeal secretions and food, spinal deformities that often include severe chest wall malformations, and sleep apnea. These patients typically develop restrictive lung disease. In addition, in those children with spastic quadraparesis and histories of prematurity, the restrictive lung disease is compromised further by tracheomalacia. These children often have a significant collapse of the trachea and main stem bronchi requiring constant intervention, including the placement of airway stents. Thus, preoperative assessment is directed at defining respiratory function and reserve for a given patient.

Drooling and excessive secretions are common throughout the perioperative period and often difficult for the child to manage without risk of aspiration. This is especially true for those children who are sedated postoperatively with pain medications. These patients often benefit greatly from continued use of antisialogues such as 10 to 20 µg/kg glycopyrulate given intravenously or orally.

Malocclusion is very common in CP children and clearly accentuated with growth during the adolescence period. In addition, gingival hypertrophy occurs with some of the antiseizure medications, especially phenytoin (Dilantin). Loose teeth and dental caries are common in CP. In our experience, these children are usually easy to ventilate by mask, and intubation is usually simple to moderate in difficulty.

A thorough and complete evaluation is best accomplished through the coordinated efforts of the anesthesiologist, surgeon, and pediatric pulmonologist. Usually these children require frequent surgeries and hospitalizations. As a result, they are closely followed by a variety of physicians who can provide invaluable information about children with CP that is not otherwise possible with a 10-min preassessment on the morning of surgery. Pulmonary function tests and blood gases are necessary, or useful, only for extensive surgeries such as scoliosis instrumentation, in our experience.

Gastrointestinal problems increase in severity and are concordant with the degree of spasticity. Almost all CP children with some spasticity have motility problems and gastroesophageal reflux. Commonly, these children are recommended for, or have had, a fundoplication procedure. Such procedures reduce the incidence of gastric reflux and aspiration but do little to prevent the aspiration of oropharyngeal secretions. In fact, such procedures often worsen the degree of aspiration secondary to preventing the children from swallowing their secretions and worsening feeding problems. Placement of a gastric feeding tube is invariable after antireflux surgery in CP patients. All of these factors aggravate the chronic nutritional problems of CP. As a result, many CP children are cachectic. The institution of aggressive feeding and the use of total parenteral nutrition are beneficial in selected cases preoperatively. It should be considered especially in those children who appear catabolic even before surgery and will be nil per os (NPO; nothing by mouth) for several days postoperatively.

Like most children with a multisystemic disease, CP patients receive many different and sometimes uncommon drugs. Phenytoin, in addition to causing gingival hyperplasia, upregulates nicotinic receptors on skeletal muscle. The end result is a resistance to nondepolarizing muscle relaxants. In addition, phenytoin and pentobarbital increase cytochrome P450 activity in the liver and, hence, increase the rate of metabolism for some medications. Both drugs appear to affect the mean alveolar concentration (MAC) of intravenous agents by producing unpredictable results at times for intravenous induction agents and lipid soluble narcotics. This effect is most noticeable when trying to sedate these children for minor procedures or radiologic examinations. Increasing the usual recommended dosage by 25% or more is often necessary.

Although frequently mentioned and questioned, succinylcholine is not contraindicated in CP patients. Its pharmacodynamics are inconsistent in many acquired upper motor neuron lesions. Its administration is not associated with hyperkalemia.

Sedative premedications should be used with caution because their effects are often unpredictable and the presence of a mixed sleep apnea syndrome aggravates the potential for obstruction, apnea, and hypoxia. The dose and type of sedative premedication should be chosen carefully and administered on a strictly individual basis. These same factors affect the use of sedatives, especially narcotics, at the end of surgery and during the postoperative period. They should be carefully titrated to effect with the use of small doses at more frequent intervals, thereby avoiding overtreatment.

Either intravenous or inhalational induction techniques are appropriate. The choice depends on the situation. Many of these children have easy venous access, but others do not. The ability to communicate safety and parental and patient choice should be the determinants.

These children may receive two unique drugs,[18] baclofen and botoxin. Baclofen, a γ-aminobutyric acid b agonist, is given to children with CP who have severe spasticity. It inhibits spasticity and allows increased muscle activity for ambulation. It is poorly absorbed orally. Given intrathecally, it produces a greater positive effect at lower doses and with fewer complications. Usually an implantable intrathecal infusion pump is used to administer the drug. Side effects include apathy, muscle weakness, and urinary retention. These side effects are reversible and treatable with flumazenil and physostigmine. Serious side effects, usually a result of an overdosage, include loss of consciousness, respiratory arrest, and severe hypotonia. Cessation of the baclofen infusion and supportive care must be emergently instituted in such a circumstance. This critical situation is usually the result of pump failure or improper programming of the baclofen infusion pump.

Botulinum neurotoxin is used to treat localized spasticity. It causes a dose-dependent reversible inhibition of acetylcholine release from skeletal muscle. The effect occurs only at the injection site and systemic absorption is low. Side effects usually are limited to tenderness or pain at the site of injection. Occasionally fatigue and generalized muscle weakness are observed. Because these injections are painful, anesthesia is requested at times. However, in our experience, moderate sedation using oral midazolam is all that is required for the vast majority of children.

Postoperative pain management is discussed in detail in Chapter 23, but a few points deserve attention here. Postoperative pain management is affected by three problems: (1) inability for many children to communicate their discomfort, (2) unpredictable response to sedative analgesics, and (3) muscle spasms. Othropedic procedures make up the majority of surgical procedures these children undergo. Pain management is most effective if it is administered before emergence from anesthesia. These children benefit from regional anesthetic blocks more than any other group of children. Regional blocks minimize the amount of sedative analgesic required and decrease the time until oral feeds can start again. They also reduce the degree of muscle spasm that is so common after bone and tendon work. Intermittent or continuous infusions of local anesthetics, given caudally or epidurally, work well. We prefer to use only local anesthetics in our infusions and avoid adding sedative drugs that might potentiate loss of adequate airway reflexes or sleep apnea so common in these children. In addition, children with CP are quite prone to nausea and vomiting, and local anesthesia negates or reduces the need for narcotics, which are commonly emetic in potential. The use of nonsteroidal analgesics also is highly recommended. Parents are commonly relied upon to assess the degree of discomfort. It is often hard to judge the behavior of these children in response to pain when meeting them the day of surgery. Parents are often good judges of their child's behavior (e.g., excitement vs. panic).[19]

Two miscellaneous points should be made. First, many of these children are very thin and often malnourished. Careful attention is necessary, even during short procedures, to avoid hypothermia. The admission temperature should be carefully recorded. Children with CP, especially those with spastic quadraparesis, commonly have baseline hypothermia, with oral temperatures between 35.5°C and 36.5°C. The aggressive use of warmed fluids, overhead heaters, and heating blankets, especially during prepping, is strongly recommended and beneficial in our experience. Second, although latex allergy has been reported in this group of patients, it is not common.[20] The likelihood of latex allergy in this group may correlate with the number of latex exposures, especially during their numerous surgical exposures. It does not occur with the frequency that has been reported with children with meningomylocoeles, and CP children do not have the same propensity for the allergic reaction.

Summary

Cerebral palsy is the most common neuromuscular disorder encountered in pediatric anesthesia. Most medical problems associated with CP, with the exception of cerebral and cerebellar functions, are related to the degree of spasticity. Most surgical procedures are also related to the treatment of spasticity. A detailed history and physical examination are required preoperatively because these children often have a diverse assortment of medical problems as they mature. These children generally do well with anesthesia. The achievement of success is related to an understanding of the disease process, the selection and use of appropriate anesthetic drugs, and the postoperative attention given to sedation and pain management.

MUSCULAR DYSTROPHY

Etiology

Duchenne's muscular dystrophy (DMD) is the most severe of the dystrophies and represents a significant challenge in pediatric anesthesia. For these reasons, this particular variant is the focus of this section.

Duchenne's muscular dystrophy is believed to be inherited and transmitted as an X-linked recessive trait. It reportedly occurs with an incidence of 13 to 33 per 100,000 male births, depending on the country. The rare occurrence of DMD in females is the result of karyotype abnormalities such as Turner's syndrome or partial defects of dystrophin in female carriers. It usually manifests before children reach school age but occasionally presents as late as the second decade of life in very few individuals.

Pathophysiology

Duchenne's muscular dystrophy usually presents as a combination of hypotonia and muscular weakness.[21,22] Walking often is delayed in these children, with early weakening of the hip extensors and gluteal musculature. Gower's maneuver, where the hands "climb up" the legs to stand upright, is commonly noted. Enlargement of the distal muscles, pseudohypertrophy, often is present from birth and usually involves the muscle of the calf but can also involve the tongue. Proximal muscle weakness is characteristic, but cranial nerves, muscles, and sphincters are always spared.

The phenotypic expression differs across individuals, but by the second decade of life most of those affected have lost the ability to walk. Eventually these people become wheelchair or bed bound. Kyphoscoliosis and a multitude of contractures are common. The function of the diaphragm remains surprisingly intact, but weakness of the other inspiratory and expiratory muscles results in restrictive lung disease and recurrent pneumonias. Lung disease remains the single most common cause of death, with an average life expectancy of 20 years or younger.

Clinical cardiomyopathy becomes apparent in the second decade of life but is subclinically present from the earliest manifestations. Typically these patients have an increased algebraic sum of R and S waves, with tall precordial R waves. Sinus tachycardia is present in most patients. A dilated cardiomyopathy develops in many DMD patients and has been cited as the most common cause of death in DMD patients younger than 10 years.[23] These patients typically present with unresolving pulmonary edema.

Mental impairment also occurs. The degree of mental impairment is not related to the degree of muscle impairment. It is not progressive and not accounted for by the physical handicaps these children have. Emotional problems, especially depression, are not uncommon during later years.

The principal defect in DMD involves the production of the protein dystrophin. Dystrophin is a cytoskeletal protein found in low concentrations localized at the sarcolemma. It is also present in different concentrations in the brain, heart, and smooth muscle. Although it is not entirely clear, dystrophin may be involved in the linking of the cytoskeleton of the muscle to the extracellular matrix, but more research is necessary to elicit its true importance.

Originally, the diagnosis was based on the history and physical examination, creatine kinase levels, muscle biopsy, and electromyography. As a result of gene mapping, evidence of gene dysfunction is now also required. Demonstration of a mutation in the dystrophin gene can be done by DNA analysis and will detect about two-thirds of affected patients. More accurately, electrophoretic analysis of the dystrophin protein allows detection of all DMD patients.

The treatment of DMD patients currently is nonspecific. Gene therapies are expected to be available in the next decade, their approval for general use notwithstanding. Because these children develop contractures and kyphoscoliosis, we as pediatric anesthesiologists most commonly see DMD patients when they present for corrective orthopedic procedures, especially spinal fusion.

Anesthetic Considerations

Children with DMD comprise only a small group of the patients that present for surgery, but they are a significant anesthetic challenge and definitely a high-risk population for perianesthetic complications. The two most important aspects in treating DMD patients in the operating room relate to their respiratory and cardiac functions.[23]

Several articles have appeared over the years detailing the anesthetic management of DMD patients. Most of these have focused on the respiratory impairment so commonly present. Given that respiratory failure is the primary cause of death for DMD patients in the second decade of life, this is not surprising. What is surprising is the lack of attention paid to the cardiac status of these patients. In our experience, the most common unexpected complications are the result of cardiac decompensation.

Most DMD patients are wheelchair- or bed-ridden when they present for surgery and, hence, have very low activity levels. Thus, it is unrealistic that these children would be symptomatic for heart disease until the final stages of cardiac failure. Therefore, many of these children will have significant cardiac disease that is clinically expressed only when they are physically stressed. Unfortunately, it is not possible to physically stress these children preoperatively. The challenge is to assess their cardiac functions to predict their cardiac responses to surgical stress. This stress results from a variety of factors: hypothermia, acute blood loss and rapid fluid shifts, the endocrine response to surgery, and the productions of stress hormones and mediators, just to mention a few.

Cardiac performance in DMD patients usually is assessed noninvasively while they are at rest.[23] Most commonly, we request echocardiograms to assess the ventricular wall size and motion and look for evidence of dilated myopathy. Ejection fractions also can be measured within reason. Unfortunately, no assessment has been truly indicative of perioperative cardiac morbidity. It is not uncommon to have a relatively normal cardiac appearance and function on echocardiography only to have the child develop hypotension and pulmonary edema postoperatively. In addition, some centers advocate a "stress" echocardiogram using an infusion of dopamine or other vasoactive drugs to pharmacologically stress the heart during the examination. The shortening fraction also can be measured. Measurements of less than 30% shortening are thought by some to be indicative of significant cardiac compromise. Further studies will be necessary to determine the validity of such tests in DMD children undergoing major surgery.

Until more accurate and reliable information is available, the anesthesiologist is advised to order a preoperative cardiac assessment of the child knowing that false-negative examinations do occur but that at least most of those with dilated asymptomatic cardiac disease will be identified. Accordingly, the choice of anesthetic drugs and technique should be determined by the fragile and unpredictable cardiac status of DMD patients. We suspect that this problem will become greater in the next few years as pulmonary care continues to improve and more children live longer, thereby exposing their cardiac problems.

Respiratory concerns are the same as those for any patient with restrictive lung disease and limited respiratory reserve. A pediatric pulmonologist should be consulted preoperatively to assess baseline function and optimize pulmonary mechanics before the planned surgery. Pulmonary hygiene is very important in these patients and anesthetic plans should include active pulmonary toilet and support. In addition, these patients often have a borderline nutrition. The respiratory muscle weakness inherent in the disease process is aggravated by their poor nutrition status and compounded by an increased work of breathing. Some degree of postoperative respiratory support is required for all but the simplest of surgeries or healthiest of DMD children.

There is some controversy regarding the relation between DMD and malignant hyperthermia (MH). Although there is no conclusive evidence to suggest a direct correlation between the two, many medical centers and patient societies consider DMD patients at risk for MH and avoid all triggering agents. Other centers consider these children at risk of rhabdomyolysis but not necessarily of MH. Rhabdomyolysis has been reported with halothane, isoflurane, and sevoflurane.[24] These patients develop an acute breakdown of skeletal muscle with myoglobinuria. Many of the other dignostic features of MH are absent, suggesting that these patients have a truly unique problem. The rhabdomyolysis can be halted by the administration of dantrolene. Hyperkalemia, secondary to the rhabdomyolysis, has been reported as a cause of death in such patients. Consequently, the use of inhalational agents remains controversial, with some centers continuing to use them with DMD patients and others strongly advocating against their use. Unfortunately, the incidence of rhabdomyolysis secondary to the use of inhalational agents is not known but is undoubtedly rare. The question then remains: Do the benefits of inhalational agents in anesthesia outweigh the risks?

In these days of convenient and effective intravenous anesthetic drugs, we suggest that total intravenous anesthesia is a safe and viable alternative. Certainly, succinylcholine should never be used in a child with a myopathy. In fact, the U.S. Federal Drug Administration investigated several reports of rhabdomyolysis, hyperkalemia, and death in young male children in whom the diagnosis of DMD was made postmortem and condemned the routine use of succinylcholine in pediatric patients.

Summary

Like all systemic disorders, a consultation with the primary pediatric caregivers is important to maximize the patient's health before surgery and anesthesia. This is especially true when assessing the child with DMD. Consultation with a pediatric pulmonologist and cardiologist is very helpful in determining anesthetic management and risk. The significance of cardiopulmonary status cannot be overstated when providing anesthetic care for these patients. Caution should be exercised when choosing anesthetic drugs and techniques to avoid rare but life-threatening complications.

TABLE 17–5 Etiology of Chronic Renal Failure in Children

Glomerular diseases
   Glomerulonephritis
   Focal glomerulosclerosis
   Membranoproliferative glomerulonephritis
Developmental anomalies
   Posterior urethral valves
   Urinary reflux with pyelonephritis
Hereditary
   Alport's disease
   Polycystic renal disease
   Cystinosis
   Oxalosis
   Nephrolithiasis
Others
   Hemolytic uremic syndrome
   Vascular
   Iatrogenic

RENAL FAILURE

Etiology

Fortunately, renal failure is less common in children than in adults. The causes of renal failure in the pediatric population in part depend on age. Basically, the etiology of renal failure falls into four categories (Table 17-5). The largest category, representing approximately 40% of cases, is aquired glomerular disease. In this category, glomerulonephritis is the most common disease. Typically this disease presents in school-age children and is rare in infants. Developmental anomalies comprise the second category. For the most part, posterior urethral valves and ureteral reflux are the two common entities. Ureteral reflux results in a condition of chronic pyelonephritis, if left untreated, and renal failure is the end result. This condition is two to three times as common in females as in males. Most of these diseases present by age 5 years. Hereditary conditions constitute the third category and includes a diverse and relatively uncommon group of diseases such as Alport's disease, cystinosis, and polycystic kidney disease. This group also presents by age 5 years. Many miscellaneous entities constitute the last category: vascular problems, renal injury secondary to hypoxia, hemolytic uremic syndrome, and iatrogenic disease. The clinical presentation of this group covers all age groups, but many occur in the neonate and young infant.

Pathophysiology

The definition of renal failure in children differs from that in adults and depends on the age of presentation. In neonates glomerular filtration rates below 15 mL/min are commonly used to define renal failure. In infants 3 months to 1 year of age, rates between 20 and 25 mL/min determine the diagnosis. For older children, the adult rate, below 30 mL/min, is used.[25,26]

The pathophysiology of renal failure initially depends on the etiology and extent of disease. In the early phases of renal failure, the type of fluid derangement depends on which portion of the renal system is most affected. For example, if the medullary portion of the kidney is impaired, the ability to concentrate urine will be lost and these children are prone to polyuria, with salt and water wasting. Clearly, these children are at risk of dehydration, especially during a prolonged fast. Replacement fluids consist of electrolytes and free water. When glomerular function is impaired but the medullary function is intact, then salt and water retention occur and these children are prone to overhydration, with edema and hypertension. Some children may have only a portion of the tubular apparatus affected. In these conditions, such as pyelonephritis, the kidney may have lost the ability to preferentially reabsorb sodium. The end result is hyponatremia, which is aggravated by salt restriction and the administration of free water. Seizures and death are the end results.

Once renal failure becomes chronic, many systemic abnormalities occur. The loss of glomerular filtration results in fluid and salt retention. Eventually the child becomes hypertensive, with secondary cardiac conditions such as cardiac failure and pulmonary edema. Potassium balance is also affected and puts the child at risk for hyperkalemia, particularly when the patient is catabolic or acidotic.

Acidosis occurs because the kidney can no longer adequately excrete hydrogen ions, primarily in the form of ammonium. The presence of acidosis affects appetite, growth, and bone formation.

Calcium and phosphate metabolisms are affected, resulting in a loss of bone density. Hypocalcemia occurs and results in an ineffective secondary hyperparathyroidism.

Several other hormones are affected. The clearance of gastrin is reduced and the incidence of hypergasrtic ulcers is greatly increased in 60% to 70% of patients with end-stage renal failure. Secretin and cholecystokinin also are affected. Nutrition status is another issue. Patients are in a constant state of catabolism, which is compounded by a decreased appetite.

Renal failure decreases red cell survival and iron use and eventually anemia develops. Platelet factor III conversion and platelet adhesion also are impaired. This defect is partly improved with dialysis.

The treatment for chronic renal failure in children is similar to that in adults. The first step is the replacement and balancing of electrolytes, water, and acid balance. Salt and water restriction with bicarbonate administration is a basic measure. Vitamin D analogs are given to reduce parathyroid hormone levels and improve calcium balance. Erythropoietin and iron supplements can be given to improve anemia. Growth hormone also can be given to improve anabolism and growth. Dietary supplements are always necessary.[27,28]

Dialysis and renal transplantation are the final steps in pediatric chronic renal failure.[25,29] Peritoneal dialysis and hemodialysis are used. Peritoneal dialysis is associated with a high incidence of peritoneal infection, about once per year per dialysis patient. Peritoneal dialysis is considerably more convenient for the child and parents because it can be done in the home, thereby minimizing loss of school time and decreasing hospital stay. Hemodialysis has the disadvantage of frequent visits to a hospital, infection, and risk of damage to, or disconnection from, the arterial–venous fistula. Renal transplantation is the preferred definitive method of treatment because it offers overall improvement compared with dialysis.[30] Problems associated with renal transplantation are immunosuppression and its attendant risks of infection, Cushing's syndrome, and the increased risk of malignancy.

Anesthetic Considerations

The basic anesthetic considerations for the child with end-stage renal disease revolve around fluid and electrolyte balance and secondary complications, especially anemia and hypertension.

NPO orders should take into account their effect on the child's preoperative fluid balance. Electrolytes should be measured preoperatively within a day of surgery. In addition, the aggressive treatment of hypertension results in children who are relatively hypovolemic secondary to fluid restriction and antihypertensive medication. Therefore, once anesthesia is induced, it is hypotension that is commonly encountered and not necessarily hypertension. The clinician should be careful not to treat anesthesia-induced hypotension with aggressive fluid administration. Instead, the use vasopressors may be more appropriate. The aggressive administration of intravenous fluids exacerbates the pre-existing condition of hypertension in the recovery room. With regard to fluid administration and hypertension, many of these children are receiving β-blockers and are prone to hypoglycemia if they fast for extended periods. The serum glucose should be monitored during prolonged surgical procedures.

Anesthetic inductions should consider the high incidence of gastric disease and nausea in end-stage renal patients. A rapid sequence induction is a reasonable consideration for most children with an intravenous line in place.

Certainly, those children with acute peritonitis secondary to peritoneal dialysis are at risk for gastric aspiration and should be considered as having "full stomachs."

The loss of renal function partly dictates the choice of anesthetic drug. Many nondepolarizing muscle relaxants depend wholly or partly on renal excretion. Their use and dosing should be modified accordingly. The use of a neuromuscular monitor is very advantageous in these children. The use of succinylcholine is not contraindicated in renal failure, but it should be used cautiously in any child whose pre-existing potassium levels are elevated. A rise of 0.5 to 1.0 meq/dL of potassium can be expected in all patients. Some clinicians question the use of morphine in patients with renal failure. Although morphine pharmacokinetics are altered in renal failure, our experience shows that it can be used safely if titrated carefully with appropriate monitoring for respiratory depression postoperatively.

The disorders of coagulation are improved with dialysis. As such, it is recommended that, when surgery is elective, the timing of the procedure be coordinated with nephrologists to allow dialysis of the patient within 24 h of surgery. This is especially important when the surgery involves extensive dissections or surgeries associated with postoperative bleeding such as tonsillectomies.

Children who have had renal transplantation are immunosuppressed. The anesthesiologist should be wary of infections and the risks of cross-contamination. Steroid supplementation may be necessary during the surgery and postoperatively. Many children return to the operating room secondary to transplant complications. An assessment of renal function is warranted each time because posttransplant renal physiology is not static.

Conclusion

End-stage renal disease in children usually is the result of etiologies different from those in adults. However, the end result is similar. Management of fluid and electrolytes, hypertension, the avoidance and treatment of infection, and altered drug metabolism are the cornerstones of anesthetic management. When possible, the child should be dialyzed just before surgery. Like most children with major metabolic illnesses, the margin for error is minimal. Attention to the details is paramount.

HEPATIC FAILURE

Etiology

It is clearly beyond the scope of this chapter to cover the many diverse and complex issues of pediatric hepatic disease and failure. Rather, the purpose of this section is to emphasize, for the reader, the concept that hepatic disease in children covers a broad range of entities. Each disease has its own prognosis and treatment, but end-stage hepatic failure, like renal failure, has a common pathophysiologic pathway regardless of the cause.

The etiology of hepatic failure in children is broad and diverse. Acute hepatic failure is usually the result of an insult from one of four broad categories: infection, toxic, metabolic, or ischemia. However, hepatic failure is not always fulminant and may be the result of a more insidious disease that is marginally dysfunctional but stable at the beginning and then progresses to complete hepatic failure over months or years. The more common causes of hepatic disease encompassing all age groups are outlined in Table 17-6.[31–33]

TABLE 17–6 The Causes of Liver Disease in Infants and Children

Type	Etiology	Anesthetic considerations
Neonatal hepatitis	Idiopathic	Avoid anesthesia during acute inflammatory phase
Hepatitis of the newborn (TORCH)	Toxoplasmosis, syphilis, rubella, cytomegalo and herpes viruses	As above
Postnatal	Hepatitis A, B, or C	As above, complications uncommon compared to adults
Biliary atresia	Embryonic and perinatal causes unknown	10% have associated anomalies Coagulopathy, malnutrition and infection
Tumors	Unknown	
Benign		When resected, bleeding can be massive and the surgical procedure commonly interferes with venous return and cardiac filling
Cavernous hemangioma		
Hemangioendothelioma		
Focal nodular hyperplasia		
Hepatic adenoma		
Malignant		Heart failure is not an uncommon associated finding secondary to hepatic function and failure
Hepatoblastoma		
Hepatocellular carcinoma		
Mesenchymoma		Chemotherapeutic agents commonly used. Side effects are common and unique for each (see Chapter 15, The Child with Cancer)
Cystic disease		
Choledochal cyst	Unknown	Bleeding, portal hypertension and cholangitis commonly found
Caroli's disease		
Congenital hepatic fibrosis		
Solitary cysts		
Polycystic disease		Renal failure common
Metabolic	Multiple (see appropriate reference text)	Multiple (see appropriate reference text); most involve the monitoring of electrolytes and glucose metabolism

This is by no means a complete list, but it covers 98% of the hepatic diseases seen by most clinicians.

Pathophysiology

The pathophysiology depends on the age of the child affected and the etiologic agent involved. Only the basic concepts are covered in this section. The pathophysiologic and resultant anesthetic considerations are summarized in Table 17-7.

TABLE 17–7 Hepatic Dysfunction and Anesthetic Considerations

Cardiopulmonary dysfunction
  Ascites
  Intrapulmonary shunting
  Edema
  Intravascular
    Repletion: hypoalbuminemia and/or hyperaldosteronism
    Depletion: diuretics and/or blood loss (varices, etc.)
  Increased risk of aspiration due to increased abdominal girth and pressure
Nutrition status
  Malnutrition with generalized wasting
  Magnesium, zinc, and potassium depletion
  Hypoalbuminemia
Renal status
  Heart failure
  Hypovolemia
  Infection
  Cholestatic jaundice
  Hepatorenal syndrome
Immune status
  Increased risk of bacterial and viral infections
Coagulation problems
  Decreased synthesis of coagulation factors
  Decreased clearance of coagulation inhibitors
  Decreased platelet number and function
  Disseminated intravascular coagulopathy
Metabolic
  Decreased first-pass metabolism of drugs
  Decreased hepatic clearance of drugs and toxins, oxidative pathways especially, glucoronidation minimally affected
  Decreased drug binding by albumin and α_1 acid glycoprotein

As with all systemic diseases, the initial lesion primarily affects one organ (the liver in this case), but eventually most of the body's systems are involved. The pathophysiologic derangements encountered with end-stage liver disease include the decompensation of other organ systems as they respond and adjust to the primary insult.[34]

The liver is responsible for three broad functions: synthesis, metabolism, and excretion. In end-stage liver disease, all three functions are impaired. However, early in hepatic disease the impairment may be related primarily to only one function. Therefore, the pathophysiologic processes depend on the etiologic agent involved and the stage of disease development.

A defect in synthesis may alter the production of albumin and α_1-acid glycoprotein. Because both proteins are involved in drug binding, the free fractions of a number of drugs might increase when administered, although this usually is significant in end-stage disease.

The liver is also the production source for the coagulation factors I, II, V, VII, IX, and X; factors II, V, IX, and X are vitamin K dependent. The absorption of vitamin K is codependant on liver function. A decrease in these factors leads to defects in coagulation that may or may not respond to vitamin K administration. The liver produces bile acids, cholesterol, various globulins and lipoproteins, and glucose. All of these are important in the processes of digestion, nutrition, and immunology.

One of the principal metabolic functions of the liver is the conversion of ammonia to urea. The failure of the liver to adequately carry out this function strongly correlates with hepatic failure. The inability to convert ammonia to urea is aggravated further by portosystemic shunting. Urea is hard to measure and quantify for clinical use. As such, ammonia levels are followed and correlate, within reason, with hepatic function.

Portal hypertension is a common accompanying feature resulting in esophageal varices. Bleeding from these varices can be significant and life threatening. In addition, portal hypertension results in hypersplenism. Sequestration of platelets is increased, further aggravating the defects in coagulation.

End-stage hepatic disease eventually leads to ascites and generalized edema formation and is accompanied by secondary hyperaldosteronism. Intrapulmonary shunting is increased, with a heightened potential for hypoxia and respiratory infections. The presence of significant ascites further aggravates those problems by displacing the diaphragm and decreasing residual lung volume and functional residual capacity. Fluid overload eventually occurs and, with cardiac demands already increased by shunting, cardiac failure ensues.

The kidneys also may be affected. The combination of heart failure, hypo- or hypervolemia, and cholestasis increases the risk of renal failure. For reasons not well understood, hepatorenal syndrome also may occur.

Hepatic encephalopathy may occur. This problem is well described but poorly understood. It is not caused directly by, but is associated with, cerebral edema. Children may show an altered level of consciousness with mood swings, motor dysfunction, and altered brainstem responses. The presence of hepatic encephalopathy is associated with a significantly increased anesthetic risk.

Anesthetic Considerations

The conduct of anesthesia depends on the degree of hepatic failure (see Table 17-7). The general condition of the child should be assessed. Nutritional, neurologic, cardiorespiratory, renal, and coagulation status should be thoroughly reviewed and addressed.

The selection of anesthetic drugs should be determined by alterations in first-pass effects, metabolism, and drug binding that occurs with hepatic failure. The vast majority of anesthetic drugs can be used safely in these patients as long as appropriate alterations in drug dosing occur and patients are carefully monitored.

The induction of children with hepatic failure should be determined by patients' cardiorespiratory reserves and the presence of ascites. The presence of ascites significantly reduces the safe period of apnea after induction and may increase the likelihood of gastric reflux and aspiration.

Caution should be exercised in the decision to place a nasogastric tube. The presence of esophagel varices may make the placement difficult and persistent attempts can result in disruption of the varices and massive bleeding. Substantial venous access, with large-bore catheters, is recommended in all children with hepatic failure, especially those with portal hypertension.

The emergence and extubation of children with hepatic failure should be tempered by the pre-existing presence of ascites and the patients' neurologic status. Prominent ascites will increase the risk of hypoxia and aspiration, especially in a child who is neurologically impaired. Patients with hepatic encephalopathy should be monitored in an intensive care setting.

As in the case of renal failure, children with hepatic failure may be the recipients of organ transplants.[35] With successful transplantation, many of the issues we have discussed are rectified. However, it is not uncommon for these children to reappear in the operating room to resolve a surgical complication from the original transplantation surgery. On these occasions, hepatic function may be only partly improved. In addition, these children have the same considerations posttransplant as children with renal transplantation. Immunosuppression is fundamental to the care of the posttransplant child. Care should be exercised in avoiding cross-contamination of infectious materials. Steroid coverage during the perioperative period should be organized. Cyclosporin therapy, a mainstay of immunosuppression for organ transplants, may potentiate the effects of some anesthetic drugs, especially fentanyl and the barbiturates.

CONCLUSION

Hepatic failure in children is the result of different etiologic agents. As in their adult counterparts, end-stage hepatic failure has a common pathophysiologic pathway. Hepatic failure is a multisystemic entity. A complete review of all systems will identify associated complications and provide the necessary information to administer an appropriate anesthetic.

REFERENCES

1. Holxmann L, Finn H, Licthtman HC, et al: Anesthesia in patients with sickle cell disease: a review of 112 cases. *Anesth Analg* 48:566, 1969.
2. Platt OS, Brambiller DJ, Rosse WF, et al: Mortality in sickle cell disease: life expectancy and risk factors for early death. *N Engl J Med* 303:1639, 1994.
3. Griffin TX, Buchanan GR: Elective surgery in children with sickle cell disease without preoperative blood transfusion. *J Pediatr Surg* 28:681, 1993.
4. Koshy M, Weiner J, Miller S, et al, and The Cooperative Study of Sickle Cell Disease: Surgery and anesthesia in sickle cell disease. *Blood* 86:3676, 1995.
5. Vichinsky EP, Haberkern CM, Neumayr L, et al, and The Preoperative Transfusion in Sickle Cell Disease Study Group: A comparison of conservative and aggressive transfusion regimens in the perioperative management of sickle cell disease. *N Engl J Med* 333:206, 1995.
6. Haberkern CM, Neunayr L, Orringer EP, et al: Cholecystectomy in sickle cell anemia patients: perioerative outcome of 364 cases from the National Preoperative Transfusion Study. *Blood* 89:1533, 1997.
7. Waldron P, Pegelow C, Neumayr L et al: Tonsillectomy, adenoidectomy and myringotomy in sickle cell disease: perioperative morbidity. Preoperative Transfusion in Sickle Cell Disease Study Group. *J Pediatr Hematol Oncol* 21:129, 1999.
8. Kelnar CJH: The historic background. In *Childhood and Adolescent Diabetes.* Kelnar CJH, ed. London, Chapman and Hall, 1995, p 123.
9. McAnulty GR, Robertshaw HJ, Hall GM: Anaesthetic management of patients with diabetes mellitus. *Br J Anaesth* 85:80, 2000.
10. Eldridge AJ, Sear JW: Peri-operative management of diabetic patients. Any changes for the better since 1985? *Anaesthesia* 51:45, 1996.
11. Peters A, Kerner W: Perioperative management of the diabetic patient. *Exp Clin Endocrinol Diabetes* 103:213, 1995.
12. Anonymous: American Diabetes Association: clinical practice recommendations 2000. *Diabetes Care* 23(suppl 1):S1, 2000.
13. Silverstein JH, Rosenbloom AL: New developments in type 1 (insulin-dependent) diabetes. *Clin Pediatr* 39:257, 2000.

14. Houston EC, Cunningham CC, Metcalfe E, Newton R: The information needs and understanding of 5–10-year-old children with epilepsy, asthma or diabetes. *Seizure* 9:340, 2000.
15. Eicher PS, Batshaw ML: Cerebral palsy. *Pediatr Clin North Am* 40:537, 1993.
16. Mutch L, Alberman E, Hagberg B, et al: Cerebral palsy epidemiology: where are we now and where are we going? *Dev Med Child Neurol* 34:547, 1992.
17. DeLuca PA: The musculoskeletal management of children with cerebral palsy. *Pediatr Clin North Am* 43:1135, 1996.
18. Nolan J, Chalkiadis GA, Low J, et al: Anesthesia and pain management in cerebral palsy. *Anaesthesia* 55:32, 2000.
19. Biersdorff KK: Incidence of significantly altered pain experience among individuals with developmental disabilities. *Am J Mental Retard* 98:619, 1994.
20. Delfico AJ, Dormans JP, Craythorne CB, Templeton JJ: Intraoperative anaphylaxis due to allergy to latex in children who have cerebral palsy: a report of six cases. *Dev Med Child Neurol* 39:194, 1996.
21. Roland EH: Muscular dystrophy. *Pediatr Rev* 21:233, 2000.
22. Urtizberea JA: Therapies in muscular dystrophy: current concepts and future prospects. *Eur Neurol* 43:127, 2000.
23. Shapiro F, Sethna N, Colan S, et al: Spinal fusion in Duchenne muscular dystrophy: a multidisciplinary approach. *Muscle Nerve* 15:604, 1992.
24. Obata R, Yasumi Y, Suzuki A, et al: Rhabdomyolysis in association with Duchenne's muscular dystrophy. *Can J Anaesth* 46:564, 1999.
25. Moudgil A, Bagga A: Evaluation and treatment of chronic renal failure. *Indian J Pediatr* 66:241, 1999.
26. Bagga A: Management of acute renal failure. *Indian J Pediatr* 66:225, 1999.
27. Kari JA, Gonzalez C, Ledermann SE, et al: Outcome and growth of infants with severe chronic renal failure. *Kidney Int* 57:1681, 2000.
28. Lowrie LH: Renal replacement therapies in pediatric multiorgan dysfunction syndrome. *Pediatr Nephrol* 14:6, 2000.
29. Van Dyck M, Bilem N, Proesmans W: Conservative treatment for chronic renal failure from birth: a 3-year follow-up study. *Pediatr Nephrol* 13:865, 1999.
30. Platt JL: Xenotransplantation of the kidney: a pediatric perspective. *Pediatr Nephrol* 13:966, 1999.
31. Bernard O: Cholestatic childhood liver diseases. *Acta Gastroenterol Belg* 62:295, 1999.
32. Sokal EM, Bortolotti F: Update on prevention and treatment of viral hepatitis in children. *Curr Opin Pediatr* 11:384, 1999.
33. Reynolds M: Pediatric liver tumors. *Semin Surg Oncol* 16:159, 1999.
34. D'Agata ID, Balistreri WF: Evaluation of liver disease in the pediatric patient. *Pediatr Rev* 20:376, 1999.
35. Mazariegos GV, Reyes J: What's new in pediatric organ transplantation. *Pediatr Rev* 20:363, 1999.

18 | The Child With Allergies
Robert S. Holzman, MD, FAAP

Pediatricians have long been concerned about the immaturity of the immune system in the first years of life and the development of allergic disease. T-cell function, especially the capacity to produce cytokines, is diminished in early childhood and the production of interferon-γ and interleukin-4 is reduced. Even lower interferon-γ levels have been found in the cord blood of newborns with family histories of atopy. Differences in other immune cell types (natural killer cells, antigen-presenting cells, and B cells) and irregularities in immunoglobulin (Ig) E synthesis may play a role in the development of allergy in childhood.

Epidemiologic data have shown an increased prevalence and severity of atopic diseases (asthma, eczema, and allergic rhinitis) during the past 15 to 20 years.[1,2] Gastrointestinal allergy to food at an early age may be an etiology of more generalized allergies in older patients. The symptoms of allergic gastroenteropathy may be those of classic allergic reactions or may include gastrointestinal dysfunction such as diarrhea, malabsorption, and protein-losing enteropathy.[3] Immediate allergy to food is believed to be a type I hypersensitivity reaction involving mast cells and food-specific IgE antibodies. Fatal and near-fatal anaphylactic reactions to food in children and adolescents have been reported.[4] Frequent intestinal infections and reduced secretory IgA, which are associated with malnutrition, alter intestinal permeability and result in an increased uptake of food antigens. The increased antigenic load combined with factors such as an atopic predisposition may initiate an abnormal mucosal immune response, resulting in chronic enteropathy during the more vulnerable childhood period.[5,6]

Family history also plays an important role in the development of allergy.[1,7] Forty-four percent of allergic children have at least one atopic relative, with 19.5% having an atopic brother or sister. Odds ratio calculations favor an association between family history and development of allergy in children, especially with an increasing number of affected family members.[8]

Anesthesiologists frequently treat children who have allergies. Atopic disease, rhinitis, conjunctivitis, and upper respiratory infections seem to be associated phenomena, although the biology of the association is poorly understood.[9] Recognizing and understanding the importance of clinical allergy and basic immunochemistry are important because provocative factors may be avoided in high-risk patients.[10,11] Exaggerated side effects of routinely administered medications (e.g., anticholinesterases, histamine releasers) or procedures (intubation of the trachea) that affect airway responsiveness may be appropriately anticipated. In addition, children with frequent infections may have primary or secondary immunodeficiency diseases.

Anaphylaxis in hospitalized children (including but not limited to the operating room) was caused by exposure to latex in 27%, food in 25%, drugs in 16%, and venoms in 15%; 58% occurred outside the hospital. Only 35% had histories of prior allergy to the causative agent. Respiratory (93%) and skin (93%) symptoms were by far the most common. A few patients with known past anaphylaxis had epinephrine self-administration devices available; fewer still used them![4,12] The incidence of anaphylaxis during anesthesia ranges from 0.5 to 16.3 per 10,000.[13–15] Cardiovascular collapse has consistently been reported as the most common sign. Whereas a history of drug allergy is found in more than one-third of patients, the majority do not have such a history. Moreover, the majority of patients with such a history do not react.[16]

Anaphylaxis during anesthesia has been attributed to induction agents, in particular muscle relaxants. A review of 826 patients referred to an Anesthetic Allergy Clinic in Australia over a 17-year period revealed severe immediate anaphylactic reactions in 54%; in 59% a muscle relaxant was involved.[13] Of 452 patients evaluated in an allergy and anesthesia clinic in Nice, France, 62 patients experienced anaphylaxis, 57 due to muscle relaxants, 4 to latex, and 1 to gelatin. By avoiding drug re-exposure and offering alternate methods of anesthesia (e.g., regional block), subsequent allergic reactions were avoided.[17] In a 20-year (1964 to 1984) review of the French and English literature, 975 cases of life-threatening anaphylactoid reactions due to parenterally administered anesthetic drugs were found. The greatest number of cases was due to muscle relaxants (51%) and hypnotic drugs (42.3%). In another recent series, the allergens involved were muscle relaxants (70%), latex (12.6%), hypnotics (3.6%), benzodiazepines (2.0%), opioids (1.7%), colloids (4.7%), and antibiotics (2.6%).[18] Although neuromuscular blocking drugs accounted for most of the cases of anaphylactoid reactions (59% to 70%), the incidence of latex-related reactions is increasing.[15] There were 57 reports of possible allergic reactions in the perioperative period cited in the Australian Incident Monitoring Study, representing about 3% of the first 2000 incidents; 19 of the 59 were judged as "very likely allergic responses," which represented nearly 1% of the first 2000 incidents.[16] Although an anaphylactic reaction is a rare event during anesthesia, the high incidence of morbidity and mortality makes these reactions a major concern.

CLINICAL MANIFESTATIONS OF ALLERGIC REACTIONS

All four types of immunopathologic reactions described by Gell and Coombs can be seen during anesthesia (Table 18-1). The primary target organs of anaphylaxis in humans are the cutaneous, gastrointestinal, respiratory, and cardiovascular systems (Table 18-2). In a large series of fatal anaphylactic reactions occurring *outside* the operating room, 70% of patients died from respiratory complications and 24% from cardiovascular complications. Evaluation and treatment of patients who develop anaphylaxis *inside* the operating room is challenging even for the experienced physician (Table 18-3). In addition to multiple medications having been given virtually simultaneously, patients are also unconscious and draped, potentially obscuring early signs and symptoms of anaphylaxis. During general and regional anesthesia and even during deep sedation, cardiovascular signs predominate.[13,19] Further, anesthetics alter mediator release, possibly delaying early recognition. Conscious patients often describe a sense of impending doom in addition to other signs and symptoms of allergic reactions.

TREATMENT OF ANAPHYLAXIS

Anaphylactic reactions must be recognized early because death can occur within minutes. Morbidity and mortality are associated primarily with compromised cardiovascular and respiratory functions. Therefore, close monitoring of vital signs, airway patency, and ventilation is most important in

TABLE 18–1 Classification of Immunopathologic Reactions According to the Scheme of Gell and Coombs

Reaction type	Description	Antibody	Cells	Other	Clinical reactions
I	Anaphylactic (reagenic), immediate hypersensitivity	IgE	Basophils, mast cells		Anaphylaxis, urticaria
II	Cytotoxic or cytolytic	IgG, IgM	Any cell with isoantigen	C', RES	Coombs + hemolytic anemia; drug-induced nephritis; transfusion reaction; Rh disease
III	Immune complex disease	Soluble immune complexes (Ag–Ab)	None directly	C'	Serum sickness; drug fever; glomerulonephritis
IV	"Delayed" or cell-mediated hypersensitivity	None known	Sensitized T lymphocytes		Contact dermatitis

Ag–Ab, antigen–antibody; C', complement; Ig, immunoglobulin; RES, reticuloendothelial system.
Source: Gell P, Coombs R: Classification of allergic reactions responsible for clinical hypersensitivity and disease. In Gell P, Coombs R, Hachman P, eds. *Clinical Aspects of Immunology*, Oxford, Blackwell Scientific Publications, 1975; and Weiss ME, Adkinson NF: Immediate hypersensitivity reactions to penicillin and related antibiotics. *Clin Allergy* 18:515, 1988.

TABLE 18–2 Clinical Manifestations of Anaphylaxis

System	Signs and symptoms
Cutaneous	Pruritis
	Flushing*
	Erythema*
	Urticaria/angioedema*
Gastrointestinal	Nausea
	Abdominal pain
	Diarrhea
	Vomiting
Respiratory	Laryngeal edema
	Hoarseness
	Dysphonia
	"Lump" in throat
	Chest tightness
	Dyspnea
	Cough
	Wheezing*
	Cyanosis*
	Increase in peak airway pressure*
Cardiovascular	Light-headedness
	Faintness
	Syncopy
	Tachycardia*
	Hypotension*
	Dysrhythmias*

*Signs and symptoms most likely to occur during anesthesia.

assessing the severity of the reaction and response to therapy. Treatment of anaphylactic reactions can be divided into initial and secondary therapies (Table 18-4).

DETERMINING THE CAUSE OF ALLERGIC REACTIONS

In contrast to a patient electively seeking consultation from an allergist, patients who have had allergic reactions in the operating room require diligent postoperative evaluation to identify the cause and to guide selection and use

TABLE 18–3 Differential Diagnosis of Anaphylaxis

Vasovagal reaction
Dysrhythmia
Myocardial infarction
Overdose of medication or illicit drugs
Pulmonary embolism
Seizure disorder
Cerebral vascular accident
Aspiration
Globus hystericus
Fictitious asthma
Hereditary angioedema
Physical or idiopathic urticaria
Serum sickness
Carcinoid tumors
Systemic mastocytosis

TABLE 18–4 Management of Anaphylaxis

Initial therapy	Secondary therapy
1. *Stop administration or reduce absorption of offending agent* *If antigen given subcutaneously* Venous tourniquet proximal to site Epinephrine (1:1000) into antigen site *If latex is suspected* Consider potential routes of administration, including mucosal contact and inhalation Remove all latex from surgical field Change to non-latex gloves 2. *Maintain airway and administer 100% oxygen* Aerosolized epinephrine if not already intubated Intubation, cricothyrotomy, or tracheostomy 3. *Rapid intravascular volume expansion* 25–50 mL/kg (2–4 L in adult) of crystalloid or colloid for hypotension 4. *Administer epinephrine* 0.01-mL increments of 1:1000 IV; titrate as needed 10 mL of 1:10,000; endotracheal administration in adults 5. *Discontinue all anesthetic agents* 6. *Consider use of MAST*	1. *Administer antihistamine* Diphenhydramine: 1 mg/kg IV or IM (maximum dose 50 mg) Ranitidine: 1 mg/kg IV (maximum dose 50 mg) 2. *Administer glucocorticoids* Hydrocortisone: 5 mg/kg initially and then 2.5 mg/kg q 4–6 h Methylprednisolone: 1 mg/kg initially and 0.8 mg/kg q 4–6 h 3. *Adminster aminophylline (may be ineffective during inhalational anesthesia)* Loading dose: 5–6 mg/kg Continuous infusion: 0.4–0.9 mg/(kg/h) (check blood level) 4. *Administer inhaled β_2 adrenergic agonists* 5. *Continuous catecholamine infusion* Epinephrine: 0.02–0.05 μg/(kg/min) (2–4 μg/kg min in adults) Norepinephrine: 0.05 μg/(kg/min) (2–4 μg/min in adults) Dopamine: 5–20 μg/(kg/min) 6. *Administer sodium bicarbonate* 0.5–1 mg/kg initially; titrate using arterial blood gas analysis

IM, intramuscularly; IV, intravenously; MAST, military anti-shock trousers.

of future medications. The evaluation starts with a detailed history including concurrent illnesses and earlier allergic and anesthetic episodes. It is helpful for the anesthesiologist to prepare a flow diagram of the allergic reaction, temporally identifying the clinical manifestations of the reaction and the medications received, including indications, when initiated, doses, and duration of therapy. Equally important information includes previous exposure to the same or structurally related medications, the effect of drug discontinuation, the response to treatment, and any previous diagnostic testing or rechallenge. Medications should be considered with regard to their known propensity for causing anaphylaxis. In general, agents that have been used for long, continuous periods before the onset of an acute reaction are less likely to be implicated than agents recently introduced or reintroduced. However, in the perioperative period, patients commonly receive many medications in quick succession, making a diagnosis by history alone difficult.

In Vivo Immunodiagnostic Tests

Skin testing for immediate hypersensitivity reactions has an established role in the evaluation of IgE-mediated penicillin allergy and is also useful in the evaluation of allergy to muscle relaxants, barbiturates, chymopapain, streptokinase, insulin, latex, and miscellaneous drugs. Epicutaneous (scratch) testing should be performed before the more definitive intradermal test. Skin testing must be done in the absence of medications that will affect the skin test response (especially H_1 antihistamines, tricyclic antidepressants, and sympathomimetic agents). Appropriate positive (histamine) and negative (diluent) controls should be used.

Delayed (tuberculinlike) skin tests have little, if any, place in the evaluation of drug allergy. Patch tests may be of value in cases of contact dermatitis.

In Vitro Immunodiagnostic Tests

Although elevations of total serum IgE have been reported after allergic reactions, the level of IgE is rarely, if ever, helpful in establishing the diagnosis of an allergic drug reaction. Assessment of complement activation includes assaying for decreases in complement components (C4, C3, or total hemolytic complement C_H50) and the generation of products of complement activation (C3a, C4a, C5a, etc.). If positive, these assays may implicate complement activation in specific reactions. Washed leukocytes containing basophils with IgE antibody on their cell surfaces will release histamine and other mediators when incubated with relevant antigens. This test has been used to demonstrate sensitivity to thiopental, muscle relaxants, and penicillins. Recent assays that measure serum tryptase, a protease released specifically from mast cells, appear promising in the confirmation of mast cell–mediated allergic reactions. Serum tryptase may remain elevated for hours after release from mast cells.[20–22]

Radioallergosorbent testing (RAST) measures circulating allergen-specific IgE antibody. When appropriately done, the RAST correlates well with skin test end-point titration, basophil–histamine release, and provocation tests. Radioallergosorbent tests have been developed to measure IgE antibody to insulin, chymopapain, muscle relaxants, thiopental, trimethoprim, protamine, and latex.

REQUIREMENT FOR DRUG USE IN THE FUTURE

If a patient has had an allergic reaction to a medication in the past but requires its use again, the risks and benefits of readministration must be evaluated carefully. When equally effective and non–cross-reacting alternative drugs are available, they should be used. If these choices fail, induce unacceptable side effects, or are clearly less effective, then cautious administration of the drug with the use of a premedication regimen or a desensitization protocol may be considered.

Premedication regimens have been tested, validated, and used most often in patients who have had previous reactions to radiocontrast media and require the administration of radiocontrast again. These reactions are not IgE mediated. There is little evidence supporting the use of premedication with antihistamines or steroids to prevent IgE-mediated anaphylaxis; therefore, the use of these drugs is not recommended for reactions mediated by IgE antibodies.

SPECIFIC ALLERGIC REACTIONS OFTEN SEEN BY THE ANESTHESIOLOGIST

Penicillin Antibiotics

Penicillin antibiotics are the most common medications that cause allergic drug reactions. Available data do not permit exact conclusions about the true frequency of allergic reactions to penicillin, but they are reported to occur in 0.7% to 8% of treatment cases in different studies,[23] with anaphylactic reactions occurring in 0.004% to 0.015%. Fatality from penicillin anaphylaxis occurs about once in every 50,000 to 100,000 treatment cases, resulting in 400 to 800 deaths per year. The β-lactam ring in penicillin opens spontaneously under physiologic conditions and forms the penicilloyl group, also known as the *major determinant*. Benzylpenicillin also can be degraded by other metabolic pathways to form additional antigenic determinants. These derivatives are formed in small quantities and stimulate a variable immune response; hence, they have been termed the *minor determinants*.

Individuals with a history of previous penicillin reactions have a four- to six-fold increased risk for subsequent reactions to penicillin compared with those without previous histories. However, most serious and fatal allergic reactions to penicillin and β-lactam antibiotics occur in those who have never had a previous allergic reaction. Sensitization of these individuals may have occurred from their last therapeutic course of penicillin or (less likely) by occult environmental exposures. Penicillin anaphylaxis has not been reported in patients with negative skin tests; therefore, negative skin tests indicate that penicillin antibiotics may be safely given. A limited number of patients with positive skin tests has been treated with therapeutic doses of penicillin. The risk of an anaphylactic or accelerated allergic reaction ranges from 50% to 70% in such patients. Therefore, if skin tests are positive, equally effective non–cross-reacting antibiotics should be substituted when available.

Cephalosporins

Like penicillins, cephalosporins possess a β-lactam ring but the six-membered dihydrothiazine ring replaces the five-membered thiazolidine ring. Allergic reactions were reported shortly after cephalosporins came into clinical use and cross-reactivity between cephalosporins and penicillins was observed. Primary cephalosporin allergy in non–penicillin-allergic patients also has been reported. Although the incidence of clinically relevant cross-reactivity between penicillin and the cephalosporins is unknown and probably small, it cannot be discounted on statistical grounds because life-threatening anaphylactic cross-reactivity has occurred. Therefore, patients with positive skin tests to any penicillin reagent probably should not receive cephalosporin antibiotics unless alternative drugs are clearly less desirable. If cephalosporin drugs are used, they should be administered cautiously, possibly with the use of a modified desensitization protocol.

Vancomycin

Hypotension is the most serious immediate adverse effect associated with the use of vancomycin. Direct myocardial depression and nonimmunologically mediated histamine release (not true anaphylaxis) have been reported as mechanisms of vancomycin-induced hypotension. In humans, hypotension occurs most commonly when the drug is rapidly infused or when it is administered in a concentrated solution. In addition to hypotension, vancomycin can produce "red man's syndrome," an intense erythematous discoloration of the upper trunk, arms, and neck. To minimize the risk of reactions, vancomycin should be infused over a period of at least 60 min and in a dilute solution (500 mg/dL).

Muscle Relaxants

Evidence supporting an IgE-mediated mechanism of allergic reactions after the administration of muscle relaxants includes positive Prausnitz–Kustner tests, basophil–histamine release studies, inhibition of basophil–histamine release after desensitization to anti-IgE, and the demonstration of drug-specific IgE antibodies in sera from patients who had adverse reactions to muscle relaxants. It appears that IgE antibodies are directed against the quaternary or tertiary ammonium ions in muscle relaxants.

Extensive in vitro cross-reactivity has been reported between the muscle relaxants and other compounds that contain quaternary and tertiary ammonium ions. Insofar as these compounds occur widely in many drugs, foods, cosmetics, disinfectants, and industrial materials, patients may become cross-sensitized to muscle relaxants through environmental contact. Sensitization to ammonium ion epitopes in cosmetics has been postulated to explain the predominance of reactions in women. Muscle relaxants with a rigid backbone between the two ammonium ions such as pancuronium and vecuronium appear to be less likely than flexible molecules to initiate anaphylaxis.

Barbiturates

Allergic reactions have been reported after the administration of thiobarbiturates, especially thiopental.[19] Proposed mechanisms for thiobarbiturate reactions include nonimmunologically induced mediator release and IgE-mediated reactions.[24] Positive immediate skin tests to thiopental have been reported in patients who had anaphylactic reactions after the induction of general anesthesia. The predictive value of the RAST to thiopental is uncertain and requires further study, but skin testing appears to be useful.[25]

Local Anesthetics

Despite widespread self-reporting of adverse reactions to local anesthetics, true allergic reactions to injected local anesthetics are exceedingly rare. Reactions to local anesthetics are often the result of vasovagal reactions, toxic reactions (probably caused by accidental intravascular injection), side effects from epinephrine, or psychomotor responses such as hyperventilation during stressful procedures. Toxic symptoms often involve the central nervous and cardiovascular systems and may result in slurred speech, euphoria, dizziness, excitement, nausea, emesis, disorientation, or convulsions. Sympathetic stimulation from coadministered epinephrine or anxiety may result in tremors, diaphoresis, tachycardia, and hypertension. Rarely, urticaria, bronchospasm, and anaphylactic shock follow the administration of local anesthetics, which is clinically consistent with an IgE-mediated reaction. Immunoglobulin E–mediated sensitivity has, on rare occasions, also been reported to paraben preservatives used in local anesthetics. In a patient with a history suggestive of an IgE-mediated reaction or possible methylparaben sensitivity, preparations without methylparaben should be used for testing, challenge, and treatment. Preparations without epinephrine should be used for skin testing because epinephrine may obscure a positive skin test or induce toxic effects.

Narcotics

Narcotics most commonly cause nonimmunologically mediated histamine release from skin mast cells. Studies in vitro have suggested that the skin mast cell is uniquely sensitive to narcotics, whereas the gastrointestinal and lung mast cells and the circulating basophils do not release histamine when exposed to narcotics. Most opiate-induced reactions are self-limiting and cutaneous, restricted to hives and pruritus, or mild hypotension easily treated by fluid administration. Because codeine, morphine, and meperidine routinely cause positive skin responses secondary to nonimmunologic skin mast cell histamine release, skin tests must be interpreted cautiously and accompanied by the skin testing of normal control subjects.

Radiocontrast Media (RCM)

Fatal reactions occur in about 1 per 50,000 intravenous radiocontrast administrations and result in as many as 500 deaths per year. The incidence of vasomotor reactions (nausea, vomiting, flushing, or warmth) caused by RCM injections is 5% to 8%. *Anaphylactoid* reactions (urticaria, angioedema, wheezing, dyspnea, hypotension, or death) occur in 2% to 3% of patients receiving intravenous or intraarterial infusions. Most reactions begin 1 to 3 min after intravascular administration. Patients with a previous reaction to RCM have approximately a 33% (range 17% to 60%) chance of a repeat reaction on re-exposure.

There is no evidence that IgE-mediated mechanisms play a role in RCM reactions. Histamine release is a prominent feature, although elevations in plasma histamine have occurred without hemodynamic changes or anaphylactic reactions. Activation of serum complement occurs after the intravascular injection of RCM by the classic or alternative pathway. Production of anaphylatoxins with subsequent mast cell and basophil mediator release may be the cause of RCM reactions. However, RCM are capable of inducing histamine release from mast cells and basophils in the absence of complement activation, possibly due to hypertonicity.

Pretreatment of high-risk patients with prednisone and diphenhydramine 1 h before RCM administration reduces the risk of reactions to 9%. The addition of ephedrine 1 h before RCM administration results in a further reduction in the reaction rate to 3.1%. Almost all reactions in pretreated patients are of no clinical importance.

Protamine

Intravenous protamine may provoke life-threatening allergic reactions after cardiopulmonary bypass, cardiac catheterization, hemodialysis, and pheresis. Diabetic adults receiving daily subcutaneous injections of insulins containing protamine have a 40- to 50-fold increased risk for life-threatening reactions when given protamine intravenously. Because protamine is produced from the matured testis of salmon or related species of fish belonging to the family Salmonidae or *Clupeidae*, individuals allergic to fish may have serum antibodies directed against protamine. However, evidence supporting this is limited to rare case reports. Previous exposure to intravenous protamine given for reversal of heparin anticoagulation may increase the risk for a reaction on subsequent protamine administration.

Some protamine reactions may be associated with complement activation through protamine–heparin complexes or the interaction of protamine and complement-fixing antiprotamine IgG antibody. Thus, it appears likely that more than one mechanism may be responsible for the adverse reactions associated with protamine.[26]

Natural Rubber Latex

Although natural rubber latex products have been used for many years, hives and life-threatening reactions to latex have been described only recently. It was shortly after embracing universal precautions that reports describing hives, swelling, upper and lower respiratory symptoms, and cardiovascular collapse or cardiac arrest appeared. The patients who have had severe reactions often have a history of hives, swelling, or respiratory distress with rubber products such as gloves or rubber balloons, or easy susceptibility to allergy.[27–32]

Certain populations are at increased risk for natural rubber latex allergy. These include health care workers who have increased occupational exposure to latex, usually in the form of gloves, and patients with prolonged or frequent exposure to latex products.[27] Those with spina bifida or congenital urinary tract abnormalities seem particularly susceptible.[33–42] Careful questioning appears to be effective as a guide to latex avoidance in susceptible individuals.[30] Multiple additional allergies often are found in patients with latex allergy. Cross-reactivity with tropical fruits is not uncommon and such a history may heighten suspicion for latex allergy.

Avoidance of latex products is the only effective prophylaxis. Because prophylactic drug protocols have proven ineffective, a latex-safe environment has been advocated.[42–45] It has also been suggested that patients in identified high-risk pediatric groups such as children with urologic birth defects and spina bifida be offered latex-free exposure in the operating room from birth.[46] The efficacy of latex precautions for the prevention of allergic reactions in children with spina bifida is well established.[43,47]

REFERENCES

1. Paty E, Paupe J, de Blic J, et al: Allergic children. *Rev Prat* 46:975, 1996.
2. Nevot S, Lleonart R, Casas R: Atopic dermatitis today. *Allerg Immunol (Paris)* 25:203, 1997.
3. Moon A, Kleinman RE: Allergic gastroenteropathy in children. *Ann Allerg Asthma Immunol* 74:5, 1995.
4. Sampson HA, Mendelson L, Rosen JP: Fatal and near-fatal anaphylactic reactions to food in children and adolescents. *N Engl J Med* 327:380, 1992.
5. Ahmed T, Fuchs GJ: Gastrointestinal allergy to food: a review. *J Diarr Dis Res* 15:211, 1997.
6. James JM, Burks AW: Food-associated gastrointestinal disease. *Curr Opin Pediatr* 8:471, 1996.
7. Aberg N, Sundell J, Eriksson B, et al: Prevalence of allergic diseases in schoolchildren in relation to family history, upper respiratory infections, and residential characteristics. *Eur J Allerg Clin Immunol* 51:232, 1996.
8. Mikawa H, Fukushima Y, Baba M: Survey of family history on allergy in 1-year-old and 6-year-old children. *Acta Paediatr Jpn* 38:601, 1996.
9. Schneider LC, Lester MR: Atopic disease, rhinitis and conjunctivitis, and upper respiratory infections. *Curr Opin Pediatr* 9:537, 1997.

10. Rothe MJ, Grant-Kels JM: Atopic dermatitis: an update. *J Am Acad Dermatol* 35:1, 1996.
11. Wood RA, Doran TF: Atopic disease, rhinitis and conjunctivitis, and upper respiratory infections. *Curr Opin Pediatr* 7:615, 1995.
12. Dibs SD, Baker MD: Anaphylaxis in children: a 5-year experience. *Pediatrics* 99:E7, 1997.
13. Fisher MM, Baldo BA: The incidence and clinical features of anaphylactic reactions during anesthesia in Australia. *Ann Fr Anesth Reanim* 12:97, 1993.
14. Middleton EJ, Reed C, Ellis E: *Allergy: Principles and Practice,* 4th ed. St Louis, Mosby, 1992.
15. Theissen JL, Zahn P, Theissen U, et al: Allergic and pseudo-allergic reactions in anesthesia. I: pathogenesis, risk factors, substances. *Anasth Intens Notfall Schmerz* 30:3, 1995.
16. Currie M, Webb RK, Williamson JA, et al: The Australian Incident Monitoring Study. Clinical anaphylaxis: an analysis of 2000 incident reports. *Anaesth Intens Care* 21:621, 1993.
17. Occelli G, Amedeo J, Raucoules M, et al: Evaluation of the activities and value of allergo-anesthetic consultation in Nice hospital since 1985 to 1991. *Therapie* 47:423, 1992.
18. Laxenaire MC: Drugs and other agents involved in anaphylactic shock occurring during anaesthesia. A French multicenter epidemiological inquiry. *Ann Fr Anesth Reanim* 12:91, 1993.
19. Levy J: *Anaphylactic Reactions in Anesthesia and Intensive Care.* Boston, Butterworth-Heinemann, 1992.
20. Fisher MM, Baldo BA: The diagnosis of fatal anaphylactic reactions during anaesthesia: employment of immunoassays for mast cell tryptase and drug-reactive IgE antibodies. *Anaesth Intens Care* 21:353, 1993.
21. Laroche D, Dubois F, Lefrancois C, et al: Early biological markers of anaphylactoid reactions occurring during anesthesia. *Ann Fr Anesth Reanim* 11:613, 1992.
22. Volcheck GW, Li JT: Elevated serum tryptase level in a case of intraoperative anaphylaxis caused by latex allergy. *Arch Intern Med* 154:2243, 1994.
23. Blanca M: Allergic reactions to penicillins. A changing world? *Eur J Allerg Clin Immunol* 50:777, 1995.
24. Binkley K, Cheema A, Sussman G, et al: Generalized allergic reactions during anesthesia. *J Allerg Clin Immunol* 89:768, 1992.
25. Moscicki RA, Sockin SM, Corsello BF, et al: Anaphylaxis during induction of general anesthesia: subsequent evaluation and management. *J Allerg Clin Immunol* 86:325, 1990.
26. Weiss M, Adkinson NJ: Allergy to protamine. In *Clinical Reviews in Allergy: Anesthesiology: Anesthesiology and Allergy.* Vervloet D, ed. New Brunswick, Humana Press, 1991.
27. Charpin D, Vervloet D: Epidemiology of immediate-type allergic reactions to latex. *Clin Rev Allerg* 11:385, 1993.
28. Moneret-Vautrin DA, Beaudouin E, Widmer S, et al: Prospective study of risk factors in natural rubber latex hypersensitivity. *J Allerg Clin Immunol* 92:668, 1993.
29. Pecquet C: Allergic contact dermatitis to rubber. Clinical aspects and main allergens. *Clin Rev Allerg* 11:413, 1993.
30. Rankin KV, Jones DL, Rees TD: Latex reactions in an adult dental population. *Am J Dent* 6:274, 1993.
31. Salkie ML: The prevalence of atopy and hypersensitivity to latex in medical laboratory technologists. *Arch Pathol Lab Med* 117:897, 1993.
32. Swartz J, Braude BM, Gilmour RF, et al: Intraoperative anaphylaxis to latex. *Can J Anaesth* 37:589, 1990.
33. Beaudouin E, Prestat F, Schmitt M, et al: High risk of sensitization to latex in children with spina bifida. *Eur J Pediatr Surg* 4:90, 1994.
34. Dormans JP, Templeton JJ, Edmonds C, et al: Intraoperative anaphylaxis due to exposure to latex (natural rubber) in children. *J Bone Joint Surg (Am)* 76:1688, 1994.

35. Emans JB: Allergy to latex in patients who have myelodysplasia. Relevance for the orthopaedic surgeon. *J Bone Joint Surg (Am)* 74:1103, 1992.
36. Kelly KJ, Pearson ML, Kurup VP, et al: A cluster of anaphylactic reactions in children with spina bifida during general anesthesia: epidemiologic features, risk factors, and latex hypersensitivity. *J Allerg Clin Immunol* 94:53, 1994.
37. Pearson ML, Cole JS, Jarvis WR: How common is latex allergy? A survey of children with myelodysplasia. *Dev Med Child Neurol* 36:64, 1994.
38. Slater JE, Mostello LA, Shaer C, et al: Type I hypersensitivity to rubber. *Ann Allerg* 65:411, 1990.
39. Swartz JS, Gold M, Braude BM, et al: Intraoperative anaphylaxis to latex: an identifiable population at risk. *Can J Anaesth* 37:589, 1990.
40. Yassin MS, Sanyurah S, Lierl MB, et al: Evaluation of latex allergy in patients with meningomyelocele. *Ann Allerg* 69:207, 1992.
41. Steiner DJ, Schwager RG: Epidemiology, diagnosis, precautions, and policies of intraoperative anaphylaxis to latex. *J Am Coll Surg* 180:754, 1995.
42. Holzman RS: Latex allergy: an emerging operating room problem. *Anesth Analg* 76:635, 1993.
43. Holzman R: Clinical management of latex-allergic children. *Anesth Analg* 85:529, 1997.
44. Ortiz JR, Garcia J, Archilla J, et al: Latex allergy in anesthesiology. *Rev Esp Anestesiol Reanim* 42:169, 1995.
45. Tosi LL, Slater JE, Shaer CM, et al: The surgical implications of latex sensitivity in children with spina bifida. *Eur J Pediatr Surg* 1:34, 1993.
46. Ellsworth PI, Merguerian PA, Klein RB, et al: Evaluation and risk factors of latex allergy in spina bifida patients: is it preventable? *J Urol* 150:691, 1993.
47. Birmingham P, Dsida R, Grayhack, et al.: Do latex precautions in children with myelodysplasia reduce intraoperative allergic reactions? *J Pediatr Orthop* 16:799, 1996.

19 | The Four Hs: Hypertension, Hypotension, Hypoxia, and Hypercarbia

Josée Lavoie, MD, FRCPC

This chapter provides the reader with a rapid overview and differential diagnosis of significant intraoperative events. It includes algorithms that provide not only a visual appraisal of different situations but also plans of action. The treatment of specific disease entities is not included because it is beyond the scope of this chapter.

HYPERTENSION

Hypertension in the pediatric population is defined as an increase in resting blood pressure above the 95th percentile of normal values according to the patient's age.[1] Figure 19–1 lists normal pediatric blood pressure values according to age.[1] The reader is referred to Figure 19–2, which shows common etiologies of intraoperative hypertension. Figure 19–3 shows a plan of action for the anesthesiologist confronted with intraoperative hypertension. Initially, steps should be taken to deepen the anesthetic because awareness is associated with altered vital signs. One also should ascertain that the patient has sufficient analgesia. The patient's volume status also should be evaluated because hypervolemia may be a cause of hypertension. Some medications may cause hypertension when used alone or in combination. Exogenous catecholamines for inotropic use or to provide local vasoconstriction are obvious culprits; however, steroids and cyclosporine also may cause hypertension. The discontinuation of sodium nitroprusside may lead to rebound hypertension. Topically administered vasoconstrictors such as phenylephrine eye drops sometimes will cause systemic hypertension.

In a study of neonatal hypertension by Singh et al., the incidence of hypertension in neonates admitted to a neonatal intensive care unit was 0.81%, 40% of which was renal in origin.[2] In a similar study by Skalina et al., the incidence of hypertension in neonates admitted to intensive and intermediate care nurseries was 2%, 85% of which was due to renal dysfunction.[3] In both studies, the presence of an indwelling umbilical arterial catheter was considered a risk factor. Thus, neonates with an indwelling umbilical arterial catheter may be at greater risk of developing hypertension, and the catheter position and any signs of renal dysfunction must be carefully evaluated preoperatively.

Various disease states also may be responsible for intraoperative hypertension, the most common of which are listed in Table 19–1. Although rare, pheochromocytomas can occur in the pediatric age group. Characteristically, there is a high recurrence rate in children.[4] A more common endocrine tumor is the neuroblastoma. Sickle cell disease may be associated with hypertension, especially if it is accompanied by renal dysfunction. Vascular etiologies of hypertension include coarctation of the aorta, which may present in the

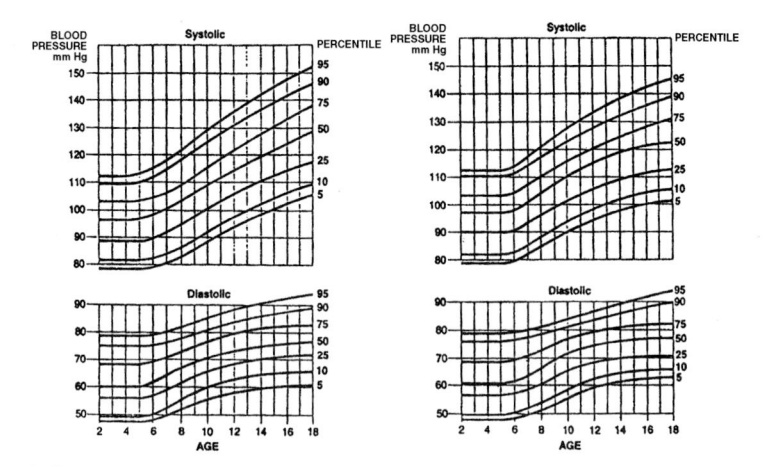

FIG. 19–1 Normal pediatric blood pressure values according to age. (*Reproduced with permission from Blumenthal S: Report of the task force on blood pressure control in children.* Pediatrics 59 (Suppl): 797, 1977.)

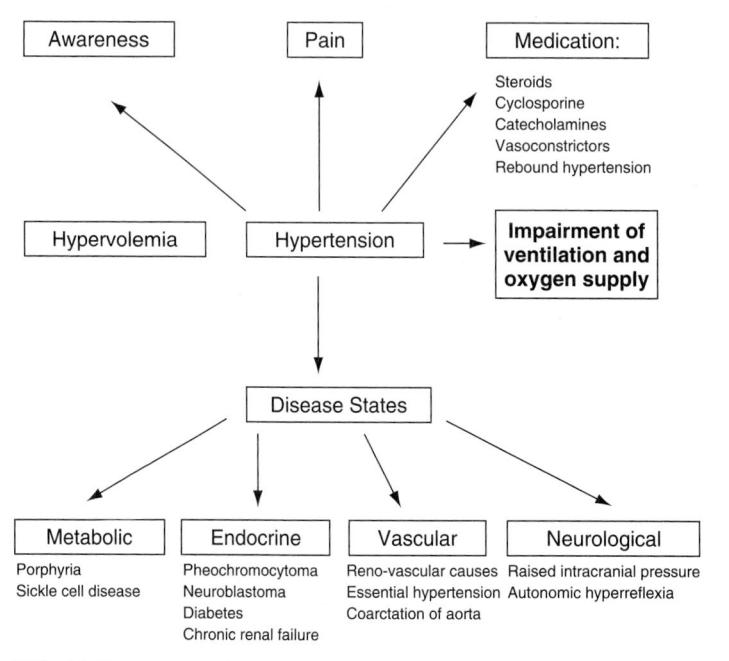

FIG. 19–2 Etiology of intraoperative hypertension.

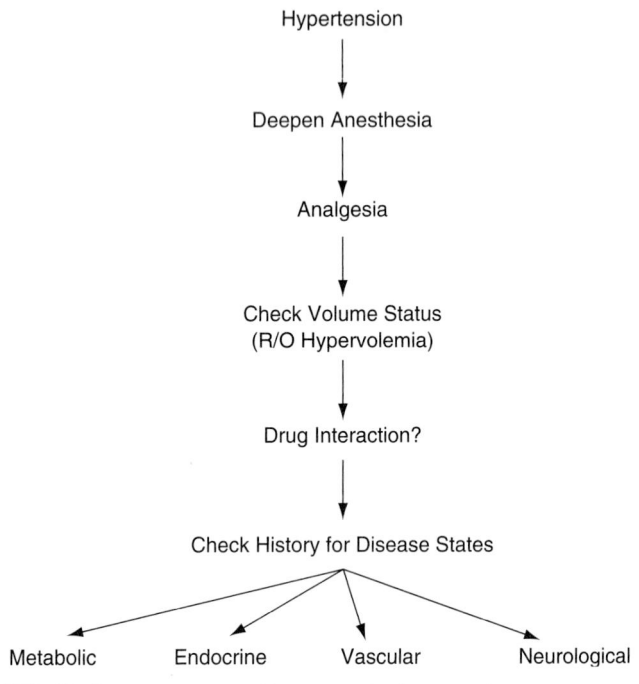

```
                    Hypertension
                         ↓
                  Deepen Anesthesia
                         ↓
                     Analgesia
                         ↓
                 Check Volume Status
                  (R/O Hypervolemia)
                         ↓
                  Drug Interaction?
                         ↓
             Check History for Disease States
              ↙        ↙        ↘        ↘
      Metabolic   Endocrine   Vascular   Neurological
```

FIG. 19–3 Management of intraoperative hypertension.

neonatal period (preductal) or later (postductal). Neurologic etiologies include raised intracranial pressure of any origin and autonomic hyperreflexia.

HYPOTENSION

The causes of intraoperative hypotension in children are outlined in Figure 19–4. Pediatric patients are at increased risk of incurring adverse events in the operating room, even more so in the neonatal period.[5] The most frequent causes of adverse events are of respiratory and/or cardiovascular origin.[5] A study of cardiac arrest due to anesthesia established that half of those arrests were due to failure to provide adequate ventilation and one-third resulted from an overdose of volatile anesthetic gases.[6] In infants, bradycardia may occur in 1.27% of patients undergoing anesthesia, whereas the incidence decreases to 0.65% in the third year of life.[7] The complication is hypotension in 30% of cases and the causes are overdose of inhalation agent in 35% and hypoxemia in 22% of patients.[7] The most recent study on anesthesia-related cardiac arrest in children found an incidence of 1.4 per 10,000 instances of anesthesia.[8] The mortality rate was 26%. The arrests were related mostly to medication (mostly cardiovascular depression from halothane) or were cardiovascular in origin. Infants younger than 1 year accounted for 55% of those arrests.

Hypotension may be associated with allergic reactions. Of interest in the pediatric population is the elevated incidence of latex sensitization that occurred in 59% of children with spina bifida versus 0% for the control group

TABLE 19–1 Disease Entities Associated With Hypertension

Renal
  Acute glomerulonephritis
  Hemolytic uremic syndrome
  Bilateral obstructive uropathy
  Congenital defects: polycystic kidneys, Ask–Upmark kidney, hypoplasic disorders
  Unilateral renal disorders
    Renal artery abnormalities, stenosis, neurofibromatosis, thrombosis, trauma, fistula, fibromuscular dysplasia, external compression
    Unilateral parenchymal disease, pyelonephritis, congenital defects, obstructive uropathy, radiation nephritis, infarction
    Perirenal masses
  Anaphylactoid purpura (Henoch–Schönlein) nephritis
  After renal transplantation (rejection, steroid-related)
  Acute renal failure
  After blood transfusions or volume expansion in patients with renal disease
  After genitourinary surgery
  After renal biopsy
  Tumors of the kidney (Wilms' tumor, juxtaglomerular cell tumors, tuberous sclerosis)
  Collagen disease (periarteritis, lupus erythematosus, dermatomyositis)
  Chronic glomerulonephritis and chronic pyelonephritis
  Heavy-metal poisoning
  Amyloidosis (familial form)
  Fabry's disease (angiokeratoma corporis diffusum)
  Familial nephritis (Alport's syndrome, medullary cystic disease)
  Renal tubular acidosis with nephrocalcinosis

Vascular
  Coarctation of the aorta
  Polycythemia
  Anemia (systolic only)
  Pseudoxanthoma elasticum
  Takayasu's arteritis
  Radiation aortitis
  Patent ductus arteriosus (systolic only)
  Arteriovenous fistula (systolic)
  Leukemia
  Subacute bacterial endocarditis
  Cardiac problems (heart block, aortic insufficiency)

Endocrine
  Pheochromocytoma
  Congenital adrenal hyperplasia
  Hyperthyroidism (systolic only)
  17-Hydroxylase deficiency
  Aldosteronism (primary)
  Neuroblastoma
  Cushing's disease
  Liddle's syndrome
  Hyperparathyroidism
  Ovarian tumors

Metabolic
  Diabetes mellitus (renal involvement)
  Gouty nephropathy
  Acute intermittent porphyria
  Hypercalcemia
  Hypernatremia

Neurologic
  Dysautonomia (Riley–Day syndrome)
  Neurofibromatosis
  Increased intracranial pressure (of any cause, especially tumors, infection, trauma)
  Guillain–Barré syndrome
  Poliomyelitis

Drug related
  Steroid administration (corticosteroids and desoxycorticosterone acetate)
  Heavy metals (mercury and lead)
  Reserpine overdose
  Amphetamine overdose
  Following intravenous α-methyldopa
  Following sympathomimetic drugs (nose drops, cough medicine, cold preparations)
  Excessive ingestion of licorice
  Use of birth control pills

Miscellaneous
  Burns
  Stevens–Johnson syndrome
  Cyclic vomiting with dehydration
  Hypertension related to stretching of the femoral nerve (leg traction)
  Renoprival hypertension

Source: Reprinted from Ingelfinger JR: Systemic arterial hypertension. In *Nadas' Pediatric Cardiology.* Fyler DC, ed. Philadelphia, Hanley & Belfus, 1992, p. 295.

```
                    ┌──────────────┐
                    │  Hypotension │
                    └──────────────┘
         ┌──────────────┼──────────────┐
         ▼              ▼              ▼
   ┌──────────┐   ┌──────────┐   ┌──────────┐
   │ Artifacts│   │ Pulmonary│   │   Shock  │
   └──────────┘   └──────────┘   └──────────┘
```

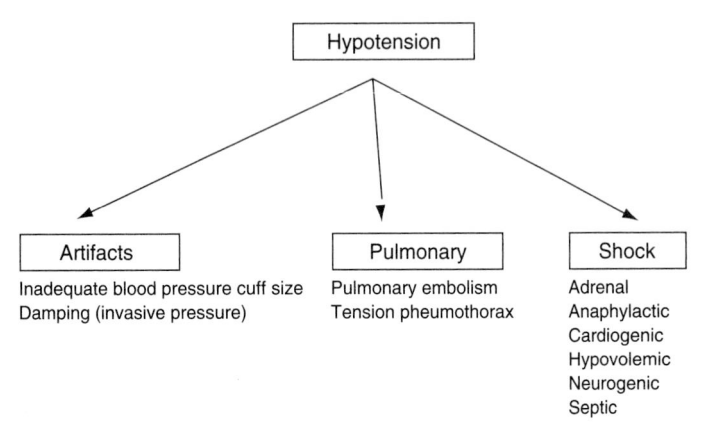

Inadequate blood pressure cuff size   Pulmonary embolism   Adrenal
Damping (invasive pressure)   Tension pheumothorax   Anaphylactic
                                                                                                        Cardiogenic
                                                                                                        Hypovolemic
                                                                                                        Neurogenic
                                                                                                         Septic

FIG. 19–4 Etiology of intraoperative hypotension.

according to Porri et al.[9] The mean number of previous anesthetics was also greater in the sensitized group (8.4 vs. 3.9). The following individuals are considered at risk: patients with myelodysplasia and/or genitourinary anomalies, sensitized health care workers, and patients with frequent exposure to latex. However, some patients who do not belong to any risk group may still be susceptible to latex allergy. Rueff et al. found a 27% incidence of latex sensitization in subjects not belonging to any risk group.[10] Primary prophylaxis by avoidance of latex exposure for patients at risk of latex sensitization has been successful in decreasing latex sensitization in those patients.[11]

Adrenal insufficiency may be iatrogenically induced as there are many subgroups of patients in the pediatric population who require steroid therapy: severe asthmatics, those with cystic fibrosis, those with Crohn's disease, those with junior rheumatoid arthritis, and some cancer patients. One should not neglect steroid supplementation should it be required for these patients.

A rapid evaluation of the airway and breathing should rule out a tension pneumothorax. Pulmonary embolism may occur suddenly intraoperatively in certain circumstances but is difficult to confirm. Hemorrhage and inadequate volume repletion, cardiac tamponade, and arrhythmias are possible cardiovascular causes of intraoperative hypotension. Hypocalcemia is not uncommon in pediatric patients receiving multiple transfusions and should be corrected promptly. Misuse of systemic vasodilators also may be responsible for intraoperative hypotension. Figure 19–5 suggests a plan of action for the management of intraoperative hypotension.

HYPOXIA

The intraoperative causes of hypoxia in the pediatric population are summarized in Figure 19–6. The neonate is at greater risk of developing hypoxia than an older infant because of its high oxygen consumption and low functional residual capacity. Another risk factor for intraoperative hypoxia is the presence of an upper respiratory tract infection (URI). Cohen et al. found that children with URI are two to seven times more likely to present respiratory-related adverse events perioperatively.[12] Further, if the child with a URI un-

```
                    ┌─────────────┐
                    │ Hypotension │
                    └──────┬──────┘
                           ↓
                    ┌─────────────┐
                    │   Confirm   │
                    │ Hypotension │
                    └──────┬──────┘
                           ↓
                    ┌─────────────┐
                    │ Discontinue │
                    │   Agents    │
                    │    with     │
                    │ Vasodilating│
                    │ Properties  │
                    └──────┬──────┘
                           ↓
                    ┌─────────────┐
                    │   Other     │
                    │  Probable   │
                    │   Cause?    │
                    └──┬────────┬─┘
                       ↓        ↓
                            Pulmonary
                           Auscultation
           ┌───────┐              ┌──────────────────────┐
           │ Shock │              │ Tension Pneumothorax │
           └───────┘              └──────────────────────┘
       Resuscitate                 Decompress
       according to
       probable cause
```

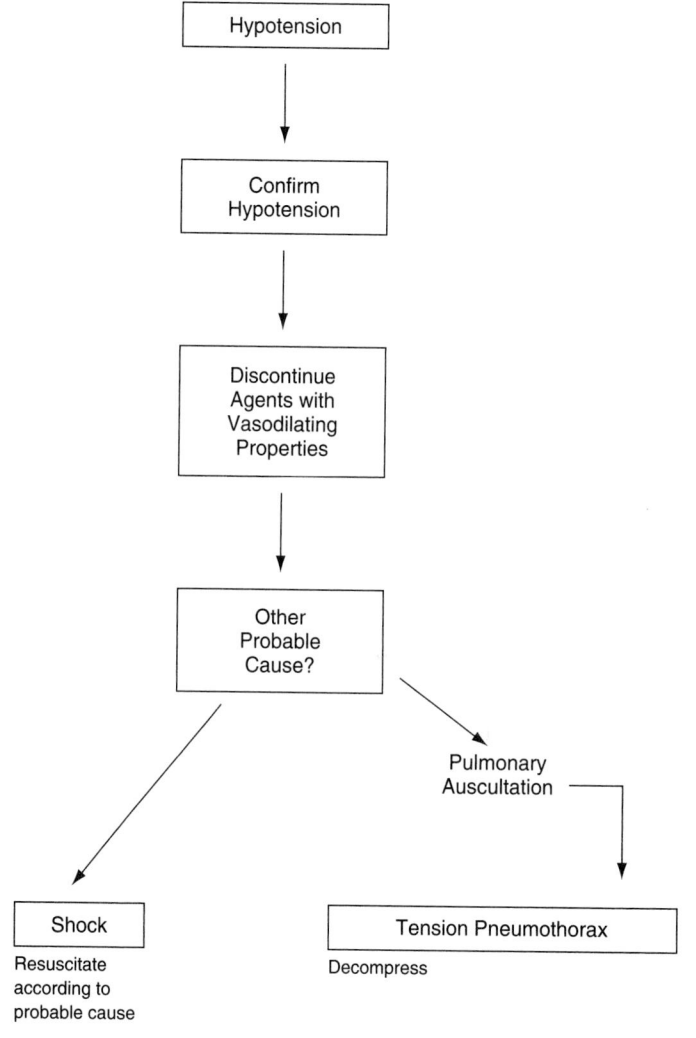

FIG. 19–5 Diagnosis and treatment of intraoperative hypotension.

derwent general anesthesia with endotracheal intubation, the risk of experiencing a respiratory-related complication increased 11-fold.[12] A study comparing the use of the laryngeal mask airway with the endotracheal tube in children with URI found that the intubated patients present with a significantly greater incidence of respiratory complications.[13] Bronchospasm may be responsible for hypoxia not only in patients with URI but also in patients with pulmonary pathologies such as asthma, cystic fibrosis, pulmonary embolism, aspiration pneumonitis, pneumonia, and pulmonary edema. Negative pressure pulmonary edema may occur after complete respiratory obstruction.

```
                                    ┌──────────────────────────┐
                                    │  Cyanotic Heart Disease  │
                                    └──────────────────────────┘
                                              ▲
                                 ┌──────────┐
                                 │  Hypoxia │
                                 └──────────┘
        ┌─────────────┐    ┌──────────┐   ┌────────────┐   ┌─────────────┐
        │  Physical   │    │ Toxicity │   │ O₂ Delivery│   │ Respiratory │
        │ Restriction │    └──────────┘   └────────────┘   └─────────────┘
        └─────────────┘
```

Physical Restriction	Toxicity	O$_2$ Delivery	Respiratory
CO$_2$ insufflation	CO poisoning	Circuit disconnection	Absorption atelectasis
Surgical position	Cyanide toxicity	Diffusion hypoxia	Endobronchial intubation
		Equipment malfunction	Esophageal intubation
		Hypoxic mixture	Pneumothorax
		Inadequate ventilation settings	Pulmonary edema
		Kinked circuit	Pulmonary embolism
			Respiratory depression

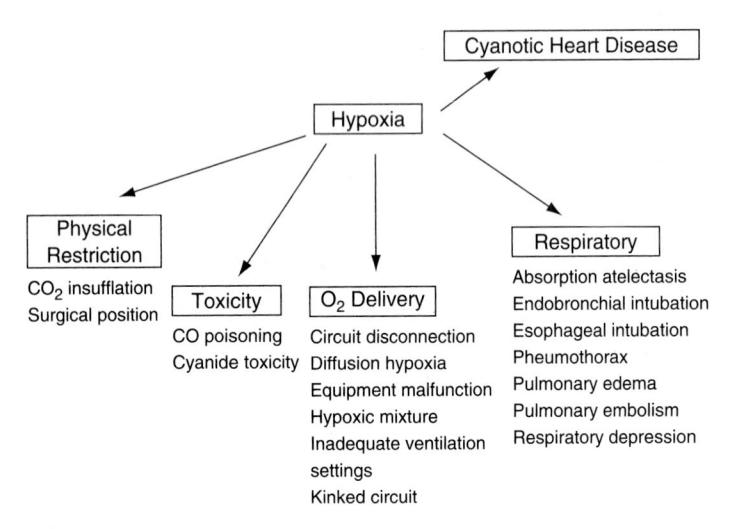

FIG. 19–6 Etiology of intraoperative hypoxia.

The incidence of congenital heart disease is 4 per 1000 live births, with a cyanotic ratio of 15%.[1] Patients with cyanotic lesions will present different degrees of chronic desaturation, which should be quantified preoperatively. Patients with acyanotic heart disease may become cyanotic should shunt reversal occur. Factors influencing reversal of shunt flow are increased pulmonary vascular resistances (positive end-expiratory pressure, hypoxia, high ventilating pressures), decreased systemic vascular resistances, and increased systemic venous pressures.

Intraoperatively, physical restriction on the diaphragm and lungs may occur secondary to carbon dioxide insufflation (pneumoperitoneum, pneumothorax), abdominal packing, surgical positioning, or pneumothorax.

Accidental administration of hypoxic mixtures can occur. Other intoxications such as cyanide poisoning secondary to sodium nitroprusside administration may present perioperatively. Carbon monoxide poisoning should be suspected in burn patients. Absorption atelectasis may occur in patients with severe pulmonary pathologies who are administered high inspired oxygen concentrations. Diffusion hypoxia is easily prevented by administration of 100% oxygen after discontinuation of nitrous oxide.

Disease entities characterized by extreme hypermetabolism may be responsible for the intraoperative occurrence of hypoxia. These should be sought and treated.

The anesthesia machine, breathing circuit, and central medical gas supply should be inspected to eliminate any obstruction, kinks, and disconnection and ascertain adequate ventilation settings. Further, the endotracheal tube position should be checked to rule out esophageal or endobronchial positioning of the tube. Figure 19–7 summarizes the management of intraoperative hypoxia.

CHAPTER 19 / THE FOUR Hs   319

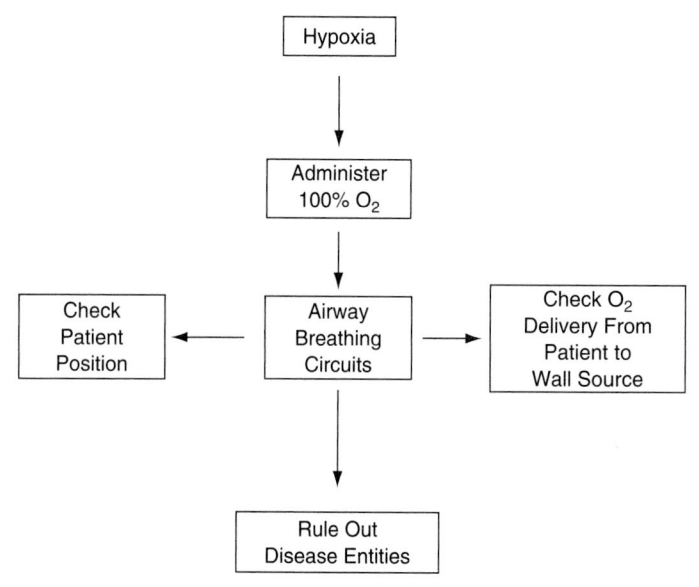

```
                    ┌─────────┐
                    │ Hypoxia │
                    └────┬────┘
                         │
                         ▼
                  ┌─────────────┐
                  │ Administer  │
                  │  100% O₂    │
                  └──────┬──────┘
                         │
   ┌──────────┐    ┌─────▼──────┐    ┌─────────────┐
   │  Check   │    │  Airway    │    │  Check O₂   │
   │ Patient  │◄───│ Breathing  │───►│ Delivery From│
   │ Position │    │  Circuits  │    │  Patient to │
   └──────────┘    └─────┬──────┘    │ Wall Source │
                         │           └─────────────┘
                         ▼
                  ┌─────────────┐
                  │   Rule Out  │
                  │Disease Entities│
                  └─────────────┘
```

FIG. 19–7   Management of intraoperative hypoxia.

HYPERCARBIA

There are multiple intraoperative events that can cause hypercarbia (Figure 19–8). The causes can be broken down into three categories: increased production, decreased elimination, and increased intake. By far the most common cause is hypoventilation.[14] Hypoventilation may be due to multiple factors: patient position, increased airway resistance, decreased compliance, inadequate ventilator settings, administration of respiratory depressants in a

```
                    ┌─────────────┐
                    │ Hypercarbia │
                    └──────┬──────┘
         ┌─────────────────┼─────────────────┐
         ▼                 ▼                 ▼
  ┌─────────────┐  ┌─────────────┐   ┌─────────────┐
  │ ↑Production │  │↓Elimination │   │   ↑Intake   │
  └─────────────┘  └─────────────┘   └─────────────┘
```

↑Production	↓Elimination	↑Intake
Sepsis	Tourniquet release	Sodium bicarbonate
Malignant hyperthermia	Hypoventilation	administration
Neuroleptic malignant	Equipment failure	Equipment failure
syndrome	↑Deadspace	
Thyroid storm	Pulmonary embolism	
Shivering		
Pheochromocytoma		

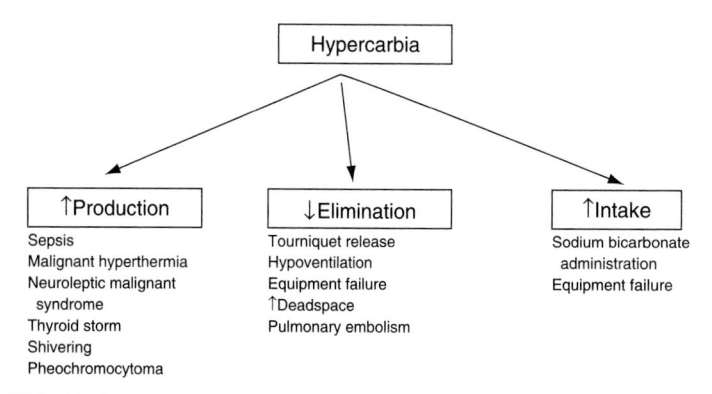

FIG. 19–8   Etiology of intraoperative hypercarbia.

```
┌─────────────────┐
│   Hypercarbia   │
└────────┬────────┘
         │
         ▼
┌─────────────────────┐      ┌──────────────────────────┐
│ ↑Minute Ventilation │─────▶│   Check Anesthesia       │
└────────┬────────────┘      │  Machine and Breathing   │
         │                   │  Circuit and Malfunction │
         ▼                   └──────────────────────────┘
┌──────────────────────────┐
│ Signs of Hypermetabolism?│
└──────────────────────────┘

R/O   Malignant hyperthermia
      Neuroleptic malignant syndrome
      Sepsis
      Shivering
      Thyroid storm
```

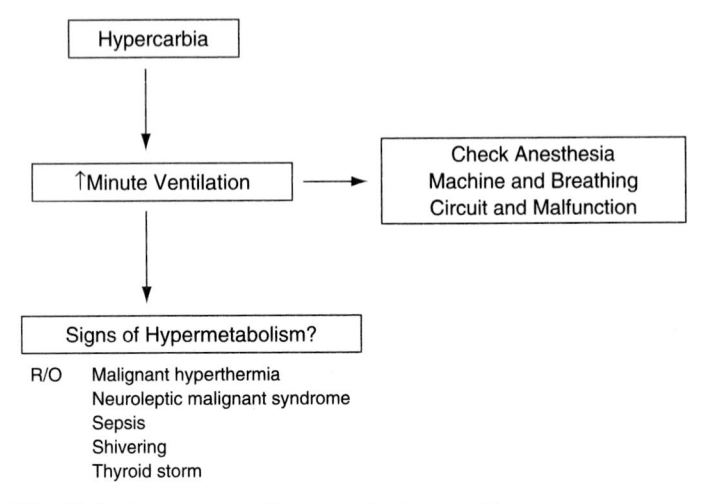

FIG. 19–9 Management of intraoperative hypercarbia.

spontaneously breathing patient, and disease entities involving the respiratory system such as obstructive tonsillar hypertrophy and asthma. Increased deadspace also may contribute to hypercarbia. Some factors responsible for increased deadspace are the carbon dioxide absorber, endobronchial intubation, hypovolemic shock with decreased pulmonary artery pressure, increasing positive end-expiratory pressure, and pulmonary embolism. Increased production, although rare, is usually the result of increased basal metabolism: sepsis, malignant hyperthermia, neuroleptic malignant syndrome, shivering, thyroid storm, and pheochromocytoma. The release of a tourniquet will cause acute hypercarbia. Increased intake may occur with inadequate fresh gas flows causing rebreathing or insufflation of carbon dioxide in a body cavity as an adjunct to surgical endoscopic techniques. Management of intraoperative hypercarbia first requires careful identification of its etiology. However, an increase in minute ventilation as an initial empiric step will correct most causes of hypercarbia due to hypoventilation, deadspace, and increased basal metabolism, but this may not treat the underlying problem. Figure 19–9 shows an algorithm for management of intraoperative hypercarbia.

REFERENCES

1. Fyler DC, ed: *Nadas' Pediatric Cardiology*. Philadelphia, Hanley & Belfus, 1992.
2. Singh HP, Hurley RM, Myers TF: Neonatal hypertension. Incidence and risk factors. *Am J Hypertens* 5:51, 1992.
3. Skalina ME, Kliegman RM, Fanaroff AA: Epidemiology and management of severe symptomatic neonatal hypertension. *Am J Perinatol* 3:235, 1986.
4. Ein SH, Pullerits J, Creighton R, et al: Pediatric pheochromocytoma. A 36-year review. *Pediatr Surg Int* 12:595, 1997.
5. Cohen MM, Cameron CB, Duncan PG: Pediatric anesthesia morbidity and mortality in the perioperative period. *Anesth Analg* 70:160, 1990.
6. Keenan RL, Boyan CP: Cardiac arrest due to anesthesia. A study of incidence and causes. *JAMA* 253:2373, 1985.

7. Keenan RL, Shapiro JH, Kane FR, et al: Bradycardia during anesthesia in infants. An epidemiologic study. *Anesthesiology* 80:976, 1994.
8. Morray JP, Geiduschek JM, Ramamoorthy C, et al: Anesthesia-related cardiac arrest in children. *Anesthesiology* 93:6, 2000.
9. Porri F, Pradal M, Lemiere C, et al: Association between latex sensitization and repeated latex exposure in children. *Anesthesiology* 86:599, 1997.
10. Rueff F, Thomas P, Reissig G, et al: Natural rubber-latex allergy in patients not intensely exposed. *Allergy* 53:445, 1998.
11. Cremer R, Kleine-Diepenbruck U, Hoppe A, et al: Latex allergy in spina bifida patients—prevention by primary prophylaxis. *Allergy* 53:709, 1998.
12. Cohen MM, Cameron CB: Should you cancel the operation when a child has an upper respiratory tract infection? *Anesth Analg* 72:282, 1991.
13. Tait AR, Pandit UA, Voepel-Lewis T, et al: Use of the laryngeal mask airway in children with upper respiratory tract infections: a comparison with endotracheal intubation. *Anesth Analg* 86:706, 1998.
14. Foltz BD, Benumof JL: Mechanisms of hypoxemia and hypercapnia in the perioperative period. *Crit Care Clin* 3:269, 1987.

20 | Blood Salvage and Conservation Techniques in Children

Josée Lavoie, MD

There has been growing concern over the safety of the blood supply since the identification of the human immunodeficiency virus (HIV) in the early 1980s. This discovery has increased public and medical awareness of other infectious risks from blood product transfusion such as hepatitis B and C transmission. Tremendous progress has been made to increase the safety of transfusions, and in the past 10 years the risk of transmitting infectious diseases has decreased significantly (Table 20-1). However, transmission of infectious diseases is not the only risk associated with transfusion of blood products; transfusion reactions are still quite common (Table 20-2). In fact, hemolytic transfusion reactions are more frequent than any other complication.[1] Clerical errors are not infrequent and may be responsible for most major ABO incompatibilities. Thus, heightened awareness that homologous blood transfusions may be associated with serious and potentially fatal side effects has increased interest in various modalities of blood conservation (Table 20-3). Many techniques have been developed in an effort to reduce perioperative bleeding and/or the incidence of homologous blood transfusions. In the pediatric group, application of blood conservation techniques may be even more crucial because of the small estimated blood volume. However, the added difficulty of the small estimated blood volume may make some techniques impossible to use. This chapter reviews the techniques of blood salvage and conservation that are applicable to children, with special emphasis on practical aspects.

AUTOLOGOUS BLOOD DONATIONS

Autologous blood donation programs have been widely instituted over the past 15 years and recently have been extended to include children and even infants as young as 9 months.[2] Most blood banks will accept children with a minimum weight of 20 kg; blood donations of 9 mL/kg are drawn every week and should cease 1 week before the planned surgical procedure. A recent study has shown that, in adolescents, blood donations with volumes up to double the standard per deposit are well tolerated.[3] Further, the increase in erythropoietin was greater and occurred earlier in the group of patients undergoing larger phlebotomies. This may increase compliance to autologous blood donation programs in adolescents by reducing the number of appointments. A minimum hemoglobin level of 110 g/L is generally required before the first donation and 105 g/L before subsequent donations. Four donations are usual, although some patients have donated up to 6 U sometimes at a rate of 2 U/week. All patients receive oral iron supplements daily from their enrollment in the autologous donation program until the day of surgery. In addition, some hospitals have set up their own autologous donation programs to include those patients weighing less than 20 kg to benefit a greater number of patients. Of course, the cost of predeposited autologous donations exceeds that of blood from the national blood supply. Unfortunately there is a ten-

TABLE 20–1 Risk of Transmitting Infectious Diseases During Transfusion of Blood Products

Risk factor	Estimated frequency Per million units	Per actual unit
Infection		
Viral		
Hepatitis A	1	1/1,000,000
Hepatitis B	7–32	1/30,000–1/250,000
Hepatitis C	4–36	1/30,000–1/150,000
HIV	0.4–5	1/200,000–1/2,000,000
HTLV types I and II	0.5–4	1/250,000–1/2,000,000
Parvovirus B19	100	1/10,000
Bacterial contamination		
Red blood cells	2	1/500,000
Platelets	83	1/12,000

HIV, human immunodeficiency virus; HTLV, human T-lymphotropic virus.

dency to overcollect, and it is estimated that up to 40% of autologous blood collected is never transfused, adding to the already higher administrative costs of autologous blood. A controversy also exists as to what should become of used autologous units. In most centers, these are discarded after the patient is discharged from the hospital.

Advantages of autologous transfusions include decreased rate of postoperative bacterial infection[4] compared with patients who had received homologous transfusions without the complications listed in Table 20-2. However, a recent study showed that transfusion of buffy coat–depleted red cells does not cause immediate suppression of immune function in the host.[5] Also, patients with rare blood types or antibodies that make routine cross-matching difficult may benefit from an autologous donation program. Risks include vasovagal reactions that seem to be more common in the pediatric population[6] and in the autologous donors,[7] thrombophlebitis, hematoma formation,

TABLE 20–2 Side Effects Associated With Transfusion of Homologous Blood and Blood Products

Immunosupression
  Postoperative infectious complications
  Cancer recurrence
Transmission of infectious diseases
  Virus
    Hepatitis
    Cytomegalovirus
    HIV
    HTLV
  Bacteria
  Parasites
Transfusion reactions
  Hemolytic
  Nonhemolytic
  Alloimmunization
  Transfusion-related acute lung injury

HIV, human immunodeficiency virus; HTLV, human T-lymphotropic virus.

TABLE 20–3 Blood Salvage and Conservation Techniques Used in Children

Autologous blood donations
Intraoperative blood salvage
Acute normovolemic hemodilution
Controlled hypotension
Antifibrinolytics and other pharmacologic means
Altered surgical technique
Preoperative embolization
Ultrafiltration of the extracorporeal circuit volume after cardiopulmonary bypass

---

arterial puncture, and misidentification of units collected with the potential for ABO incompatible transfusion. Contraindications for autologous donations include anemia, bacteremia, and significant hemoglobinopathies.

The introduction of autologous blood donation programs has allowed a significant decrease in the transfusion of homologous blood and blood products. In a study of 116 adolescents undergoing spinal surgery, the use of an autologous blood donation program preoperatively decreased the rate of homologous transfusion from 60% to 11%.[8] Eighty-nine percent of patients required only autologous blood during their surgical procedures.

The routine use of human recombinant erythropoietin to improve the number of autologous units collected is still being investigated, although there is an ever-increasing body of literature supporting its efficacy.[9,10] Human recombinant erythropoietin causes a dose-dependent increase of red blood cell production when administered in conjunction with iron supplementation. A recent study adressed the issue of using erythropoietin supplementation during a program of pediatric autologous blood collection and found that pediatric patients have a good endogenous erythropoietin response to mild anemia.[11] This response enabled patients to donate the required units of blood preoperatively without exceeding their iron stores. Iron supplementation alone was sufficient for red cell synthesis. In pediatric patients who are not anemic at the initiation of an autologous donation program, the addition of erythropoietin and its elevated cost does not seem to be justified.[11] However, in patients who were anemic before entering an autologous blood donation program, the use of erythropoietin allowed these patients to donate the required number of units preoperatively and thus justified the added costs.[12] Another clinical strategy consists of enhancing erythropoiesis by administering erythropoietin without preoperative autologous blood donations. This should provide a greater stimulus for increasing the patients' rate of erythropoiesis. Studies have demonstrated the effectiveness of this strategy in pediatric and adult patients.[13–15]

Cryopreservation

Currently there is growing interest in the use of cryopreservation as a means of conserving autologous blood.[16,17] This blood is drawn and then stored at −85°C with glycerol or hydroxyethyl starch used as a cryoprotective agent. Before transfusing the blood, it is thawed and the glycerol is removed by washing. Although the equipment needed for cryopreservation is expensive and not universally available, the technique presents several advantages. Most importantly, because the blood can be preserved for a longer period, the collection period can be extended and, hence, more blood can be collected. This allows the patient to recover completely, hematologically and hemodynamically, before the surgical procedure. The frozen washed erythrocytes have an in vivo survival that is similar to that of fresh erythrocytes.

Should the Same Criteria Be Used for Transfusion of Autologous and Allogeneic Red Cells?

A controversy exists as to whether the same criteria should be used to guide autologous and allogeneic blood transfusions. It is argued that, because the risks associated with the use of autologous blood transfusion are less than those associated with allogeneic blood, less stringent triggers for transfusion should be used to allow for a certain cardiac reserve in the face of impending needs. A higher hemoglobin concentration also might allow earlier ambulation and thus prevent postoperative complications.[18] Proponents of using the same guidelines claim that, although the risk associated with autologous transfusions may be lower, the literature has not provided adequate data in support of transfusion to higher hemoglobin levels, so the same criteria should be used to guide all blood product transfusions.[19]

Infected Patients and Autologous Blood Donations: Ethical Issues

It has been argued that allowing infected blood to be collected, stored, and transfused poses an increased risk to health care workers and other patients.[20,21] In an attempt to quantify the risk–benefit ratio of autologous transfusions in infected patients, Vanston et al. calculated days of life saved with the use of autologous blood transfusions.[22] Patients infected with hepatitis B would gain 70 days of life, those with HIV would gain 5.69 days, and those with hepatitis C would gain 0.95 days. However, with the current lower risks of infection, these numbers decrease dramatically, whereas the risk to the health care worker handling infected blood does not change. Vanston et al. concluded that the benefit to infected patients is negated by the increased cost and risks to the health care worker and other patients. However, it is also argued that patients should not be discriminated against on the basis of their infective status. Patients who are HIV positive may benefit greatly from autologous transfusions by avoidance of secondary viral infections, which may be more severe in this subset of patients and may enhance HIV viral replication and accelerate the clinical course of the disease.

Directed Donations

Directed donations for children have been advocated, although there is no evidence that such donations are safer. Indeed, a relative who has infection risk factors and who has been asked to donate for a child might find it difficult to avoid doing so. Starkey et al. found that, of 699,000 donors, directed donors tested positive more often than nondirected donors for infectious diseases such as human T-lymphotropic virus and hepatitis B virus.[23] However, directed donations serve another purpose: it provides fresh whole blood. Fresh whole blood less than 48 h old has been shown to significantly decrease bleeding after cardiopulmonary bypass in children.[24]

INTRAOPERATIVE BLOOD SALVAGE

This technique is seldom used in small children because of the relatively small volumes of blood lost, but a recent study has reported on the feasibility of intraoperative blood salvage in pediatric patients.[25] The in vitro study was performed using three different autotransfusion devices: the classic autotransfusion device with a 125-mL bowl, a device with a smaller 55-mL bowl, and a device based on the technology of cell separators. This study simulated clinical pediatric conditions where 100, 200, 300, and 400 mL of blood were processed. The cell separator device was the fastest, most efficient device and presented consistent hematocrits over 60%. The classic device was inefficient at levels of blood losses below 400 mL. The cell separator device seems to be the preferable option for use in pediatric surgery.

The salvage machines were designed for adults and the small volumes of blood lost by children are wasted in the dead spaces of the machines. For older children, there are 125-mL capacity (250 mL for adults) centrifugation bowls available. To collect blood, smaller reservoirs are available, which require a minimum of 400 to 700 mL of blood before processing can be initiated. The adult reservoirs require a minimum of 600 to 900 mL of blood.

Spain et al. assessed the quality of intraoperatively salvaged blood.[26] There was a low concentration of free hemoglobin especially in the pediatric patients, the heparin activity was minimal even in patients undergoing full anticoagulation, and fibrinogen was undetectable in the majority of samples, indicating a low level of residual plasma. The hematocrit of processed blood can vary but is usually around 50% to 55%. Further, because the salvaged blood is not stored, its concentration of 2,3-diphosphoglycerate does not decrease. Thus, salvaged blood can deliver more oxygen to the tissues in comparison with homologous blood.

Blood salvage is also used postoperatively because significant blood loss often follows major orthopedic procedures. This technique reinfuses unwashed, uncentrifuged, albeit filtered blood. Blood collected in the receptacles is reinfused at least every 6 h and the receptacles are then changed. Studies using red blood cells traced with chromium 51 have found that up to 75.9% of initial activity remained 4 days after infusion of postoperative shed blood.[27]

Contamination of the shed blood with malignant cells or bowel content as well as bacteremia or infection of the surgical site contraindicate the use of perioperative blood salvage. Some potential problems with intraoperative blood salvage include contamination, air embolism, and coagulopathy. Murray et al. reported on two patients with severe neuromuscular disease undergoing spinal surgery who subsequently developed disseminated intravascular coagulation.[28] These patients often incur great operative blood losses due to the presence of osteopenic bones secondary to their neuromuscular disease. The proposed explanation for the development of disseminated intravascular coagulation in these patients may be increased bone and tissue debris that may have been aspirated during scavenging and greater coagulation factor activation and red blood cell damage intraoperatively. In a retrospective study by Horst et al., the use of intraoperative blood salvage in trauma patients and the incidence of coagulopathy were evaluated.[29] Moderate to severe abormalities of coagulation occurred in 31% of patients. Coagulopathy was more frequent in patients receiving more than 15 U of salvaged blood.

ACUTE NORMOVOLEMIC HEMODILUTION (ANH)

Hemodilution has been used in patients of all ages, from infants to adults. With this technique, part of a patient's blood volume is withdrawn and replaced with colloid or crystalloid solutions. Circulating volume is thus maintained and a stock of autologous blood is available for later reinfusion. It is a rare source of fresh whole autologous blood available for transfusion. Because this blood is kept at room temperature and is not stored, it has a greater concentration of platelets and clotting factors than banked homologous blood. The presence of infection at the surgical site or malignancy does not contraindicate the use of ANH in contrast to intraoperative blood salvage. Further, when ANH is used, the red cell loss is decreased because the lost blood has been hemodiluted. This technique is useful for patients with multiple antibodies who are difficult to cross-match.

Hemodilution decreases viscosity and leads to improved tissue perfusion by reducing the peripheral vascular resistance and allows improved cardiac output due mainly to an increase in stroke volume. The mechanisms that are responsible for an increased stroke volume are increased venous return and a reduction in afterload due to decreased blood viscosity and peripheral vascular resistance. In addition, increased myocardial contractility may be responsible for the increase in stroke volume. Habler et al. measured myocardial contractility in dogs undergoing progressive and severe acute normovolemic hemodilution to a hematocrit of 20%.[30] An increase in myocardial contractility was demonstrated by load-independent variables such as end-systolic elasticity and preload recruitable stroke work. Total organ blood flow, including cerebral, renal, and hepatic blood flows, increases in proportion to the increase in cardiac output. The reduced oxygen content of blood may decrease tissue oxygen supply–demand ratio, but this phenomenon is partly compensated for by improved tissue perfusion (secondary to decreased blood viscosity), increased dissolved oxygen, improved oxygen extraction, and a rightward shift of the oxyhemoglobin dissociation curve.[31]

The minimum acceptable hematocrit varies but levels as low as 15% have been used; a value of 20% to 25% is a common end-point in children. In a recent echocardiographic study, a reduction in hemoglobin to 8 g/dL during ANH did not compromise systolic or diastolic myocardial function in healthy volunteers.[32] The addition of hyperoxic ventilation may allow further hemodilution; a recent study evaluated the effects of hyperoxic ventilation in dogs undergoing acute normovolemic hemodilution initially at 7 g/dL and then at profound levels of 3 g/dL.[33] The addition of hyperoxic ventilation improved tissue oxygenation, allowed for an additional exchange of 19% of the blood volume (from a level of 7 g/dL) before losing its beneficial effects and allowed further hemodilution to a hemoglobin of 3 g/dL without jeopardizing tissue oxygenation and myocardial function. However, high arterial partial pressure of oxygen induces cerebral vasoconstriction. Therefore, cerebral tissue oxygenation may be compromised during profound hemodilution if hyperoxic ventilation is used. This requires further investigation. Another study on critical hematocrit in intestinal oxygenation during severe ANH in rats found a critical hematocrit value of 16% for organ oxygen consumption and microvascular oxygen partial pressure.[34]

To achieve acute normovolemic hemodilution, blood is withdrawn according to the following formula:

$$\text{volume of blood withdrawn} = \frac{\text{EBV} \times (\text{preoperative hematocrit} - \text{desired hematocrit})}{\text{preoperative hematocrit}}$$

and substituted by an equal volume of a colloid or three times the volume of a crystalloid solution. The estimated blood volume (EBV) depends on the patient's age: 80 mL/kg for infants and 70 to 75 mL/kg for children. The blood collected need not be refrigerated if reinfused within 4 h.

The benefits of ANH have been contested recently by two studies.[35,36] According to Brecher et al. who used mathematical and computer modeling, the theoretic savings in red cell volume with the use of acute normovolemic hemodilution is less than expected when taking into account the decreasing hematocrit of the patient due to hemodilution and operative blood losses.[35] Feldman et al. also used a mathematical model to calculate the net red cell mass savings when using ANH.[36] With a preoperative hematocrit of 40%, the packed red cell equivalents saved would be 1.1 U if the patient was hemodiluted to a hematocrit of 25%; the units saved would increase to 2 with a hematocrit of 20% and to 3.4 with a hematocrit of 15%. Thus, blood savings would become significant with greater levels of hemodilution. Weiskopf also used mathematical analysis to examine the efficacy of ANH[37] and found that a higher initial hematocrit, larger circulating blood volume, and a lower target hematocrit increased the efficacy of ANH. In a recent study on the use of ANH during repair of craniosynostosis, Hans et al. found no reduction in the amount of homologous blood transfused.[38] Conversely, Copley et al. found that ANH reduces transfusion requirements in children undergoing spine surgery.[39]

The advantage of using this technique in children is that their cardiovascular systems are usually normal and high levels of hemodilution can be used without compromising major organ systems. Healthy children can easily tolerate hemodilution to 20%. In a study of hemodynamics and oxygenation during hemodilution, children responded to hemodilution levels as low as 16% by increasing their cardiac indexes (associated with decreased systemic vascular resistance and increased stroke volume) and increasing oxygen extraction.[40]

The effects of acute normovolemic hemodilution on hemostasis has been measured in humans and in a porcine model by McLoughlin et al.[41] During profound acute normovolemic hemodilution (hemocrit < 20%), a combined deficiency of several coagulation factors was more likely than thrombocytopenia or hypofibrinogenemia to be responsible for coagulation abnormalities. Also, significant coagulopathy develops before tissue oxygenation is compromised. However, when ANH is limited to a hematocrit of 20% to 25%, patients do not experience excessive blood loss.

Contraindications to hemodilution include evidence of end-organ dysfunction, significant hemoglobinopathies (sickle cell disease, thalassemia), anemia, and clotting disorders.

The use of acute hypervolemic hemodilution has been advocated to replace acute normovolemic hemodilution.[42] This technique consists of hemodiluting patients without removing autologous blood. Isoflurane is also used to achieve vasodilation. Mielke et al. found that the use of hypervolemic hemodilution was less time consuming, required less equipment, and thus was less expensive to use and that the amount of homologous blood transfused was the same when compared with the amount of acute normovolemic hemodilution. Further, because no autologous blood is withdrawn, there is no risk of blood contamination or clerical errors.

CONTROLLED HYPOTENSION

Another, older technique often used in combination with acute normovolemic hemodilution is controlled hypotension. Some controversy exists as to the level of acceptable lowest mean arterial pressure because of the concern over end-organ blood flow and spinal cord blood flow. Controlled hypotension affects cerebral blood flow. Vasodilators and volatile anesthetics affect the ratio of cerebral blood flow to the metabolic rate of oxygen consumption of the brain. Because hypocapnia also decreases cerebral blood flow, it is best avoided in combination with controlled hypotension, although no studies have evaluated the effects of this combination in children. Coronary blood flow is rarely compromised in children. Thus, factors that increase myocardial oxygen demand should not precipitate myocardial ischemia. The arterial partial pressure of oxygen should be maintained above 300 mmHg at all times during hypotension. A commonly used end-point is a mean arterial pressure of 50 to 60 mmHg.

Various drugs have been used to facilitate the induction of controlled hypotension. These drugs include ganglionic blockers (trimetaphan), vasodilators (sodium nitroprusside, nitroglycerin), the combined α- and β-adrenergic antagonist labetalol,[43] the β_1-selective antagonist esmolol, the calcium channel blocking agent nicardipine, and potent inhalation anesthetics.[44] Short-acting drugs are preferable to long-acting agents so that blood pressure can be easily restored in case of hemodynamic instability with minimal rebound effects. Drugs most commonly used for controlled hypotension and their mechanisms of action, dosages, advantages, and disadvantages are listed in Table 20-4.

Nicardipine is a recent addition to the armamentarium of drugs used to achieve controlled hypotension. In a recent study comparing its use to nitroprusside for controlled hypotension, nicardipine significantly reduced blood loss: blood loss was 761 mL in the nicardipine group versus 1297.5 mL in the nitroprusside group.[45] There was a significantly higher incidence of reflex tachycardia in the nitroprusside group. The time to restoration of baseline blood pressure was significantly higher in the nicardipine group than in the nitroprusside group (26.8 vs. 7.3 min). In a similar study by Bernard et al., the hypotension induced by nicardipine was maintained for 40 min after its discontinuation.[46] The slow restoration of mean arterial pressure without the rebound hypertension often associated with nitroprusside may be clinically advantageous. It may allow enough time for a stable blood clot to be formed and prevent increased blood loss secondary to hypertension.

The use of esmolol for hypotensive anesthesia in patients undergoing Lefort osteotomies has been compared with the use of nitroprusside.[47] Esmolol provided greater stability of controlled hypotension and a significant reduction in blood loss compared with the nitroprusside group (436 vs. 895 mL). A more recent study compared esmolol with nitroprusside for controlled hypotension during functional endoscopic sinus surgery.[48] Esmolol provided better operating conditions during the procedure, even at mild levels of hypotension. It is speculated that the hypotension caused by the β-antagonist results in increased sympathetic tone of mucous membrane vasculature causing vasoconstriction, thereby providing a dry surgical field. The onset times of various effects caused by esmolol have been studied: the decrease in heart rate was most rapid, followed by the decrease in blood pressure and the decrease in plasma renin activity.[49] Further, esmolol has minimal effects on pulmonary resistance and compliance, which makes it an attractive choice in patients with increased airway reactivity.

Contraindications to controlled hypotension include decreased end-organ blood flow, elevated intracranial pressure, anemia, significant hemoglobinopathies, polycythemia, allergy to the hypotensive agent, and hypovolemia.

TABLE 20-4 Agents Used to Achieve Controlled Hypotension

Agent	Mechanism of action	Dosage	Advantages	Disadvantages
Esmolol	β_1-Adrenergic antagonist	Bolus: 0.5–1 mg·kg Infusion: 100–300 µg·kg·min	Rapid onset and offset no increase in ICP, no effects of HPV, decreased myocardial O_2 consumption	Decreased CO, heart block, bronchospasm
Isoflurane	Negative inotropy vasodilation	End tidal concentration 1–3%	Rapid onset/offset, cerebral protection	Decreased CO, cerebral vasodilation, interferes with SSEP monitoring
Labetalol	β_1, β_2, α_1 antagonists	Bolus: 0.25–0.5 mg·kg Infusion: 0.25 mg·kg·h	No increase in ICP, no effects on HPV, rapid onset	Heart block, slow offset, decreased CO, bronchospasm
Nicardipine	Calcium channel blocker	1–10 µg·kg·min	Rapid onset, increased CO, no effect on airway reactivity, increased GFR/urine output, limited increase in HR	Slow offset, increased ICP, inhibits HPV
Nitroglycerin	Direct vasodilator	1–10 µg·kg·min	Rapid onset/offset, no coronary steal, increase in HR	Increased ICP, inhibits HPV, methemoglobinemia, inhibits platelet aggregation
Nitroprusside	Direct vasodilator	0.5–5 µg·kg·min; maximum 8 µg·kg·min	Rapid onset/offset, increased CO	Cyanide toxicity, increased ICP, inhibits HPV, rebound hypertension, coronary steal, tachycardia, photosensibility
Trimetaphan	Ganglionic blockade	10–200 µg·kg·min	Rapid onset/offset, no increased ICP	Bronchospasm, tachyphylaxis, mydriasis, ileus, urinary retention, inhibits plasma cholinesterase

CO, cardiac output; GFR, glomerular filtration rate; HPV, hypoxix pulmonary vasoconstriction; HR, heart rate; ICP, intracranial pressure; SSEP, somatosensory evoked potentials.

COMBINED TECHNIQUES

Various combinations of these blood-saving techniques have been used. A study on the use of combined intraoperative blood salvage and hemodilution during reconstructive spine surgery found that the use of combined techniques resulted in fewer transfusions of blood and blood products than the use of intraoperative blood salvage alone.[50] The use of intraoperative blood salvage alone decreased the units of red blood cells transfused but not the transfusion of plasma and platelets compared with patients receiving conventional transfusion therapy alone. Haberkern et al. found a 75% decrease in homologous blood transfusions in pediatric patients, aged 3.4 to 19.9 years, undergoing spinal fusion with combined acute normovolemic hemodilution and intraoperative blood salvage.[51] Conversely, Simpson et al. found no added benefits when using intraoperative blood salvage in patients with predeposited autologous blood undergoing spinal surgery.[52] One hundred fifty-five patients were enrolled in an autologous blood donation program before undergoing scoliosis surgery by posterior and/or anterior spinal fusion. Seventy-four of those patients constituted the study group on intraoperative blood salvage and 81 constituted the control group. There were no differences in the incidence of homologous blood transfusions between groups. However, there was an advantage, albeit not statistically significant, in using intraoperative blood salvage in older patients (16 to 18 years), with intraoperative blood losses over 2000 mL.

Lisander et al. compared combined blood saving methods in patients undergoing scoliosis surgery.[53] Five groups were compared: a control group, a group undergoing hemodilution, a group undergoing intraoperative blood salvage, a group undergoing a combination of hemodilution and intraoperative blood salvage, and a group undergoing a combination of hemodilution, intraoperative blood salvage, and controlled hypotension. The use of homologous blood products was significantly less in the two groups using a combination of blood-saving methods. No complications were observed in the patients during the study period.

There is some controversy with regard to the safety of controlled hypotension when combined with acute normovolemic hemodilution. End-organ tissue oxygenation may be compromised when adding hypotension to decreased oxygen content. This is especially true in adult patients with vascular disease. It also may decrease hepatic blood flow and oxygen delivery. However, controlled hypotension has been used safely in the pediatric population in combination with acute normovolemic hemodilution.[39,54,55] Hur et al. used acute normovolemic hemodilution, controlled hypotension, preoperative autologous blood donations, and intraoperative blood salvage for patients undergoing spinal fusion surgery.[54] Only 3.4% of patients required homologous blood transfusions. No complications occurred. It should be emphasized that hypovolemia added to controlled hypotension or acute normovolemic hemodilution will have deleterious effects on perfusion and oxygen delivery. Hypovolemia should be treated promptly in every circumstance.

The reader is referred to Table 20-5, which lists autologous blood collection techniques in selected surgical procedures that may benefit patients. Table 20-6 shows the shelf lives of autologous red blood cells.

ANTIFIBRINOLYTICS AND OTHER PHARMACOLOGIC MEANS

Although many studies using antifibrinolytics have been performed in adults, few pediatric studies have been published. The pediatric studies usually are limited to cardiac surgical patients.

TABLE 20–5 Autologous Blood Collection Techniques in Selected Surgical Procedures

Surgical procedure	PABD	IBS	PBS	ANH
Coronary artery bypass graft	+	+	+	+
Major vascular surgery	+	+	−[†]	+
Primary hip replacement	+	+	+	+
Revision hip replacement	+	+	+	+
Total knee replacement	+	−	+	−
Major spine surgery with instrumentation	+	+	+	+
Selected neurologic procedure (e.g., resection of arteriovenous formation)	+	+	−	+
Hepatic resections	+	+[‡]	−	+
Radical prostatectomy	+	+[‡]	−	+
Cervical spine fusion	−	−	−	−
Intervertebral discectomy	−	−	−	−
Mastectomy	−	−	−	−
Hysterectomy	−	−	−	−
Reduction mammoplasty	−	−	−	−
Cholecystectomy	−	−	−	−
Tonsillectomy	−	−	−	−
Vaginal and cesarean deliveries	−	−	−	−
Transurethral resection of the prostate	−	−	−	−

ANH, acute normovolemic hemodilution; IBS, intraoperative blood salvage; PABD, preoperative autologous blood donation; PBS, postoperative blood salvage.
[†]Inappropriate.
[‡]See discussion on selection of cancer patients for IBS.
Source: Reprinted with permission from Transfusion alert: Use of autologous blood. National Heart, Lung, and Blood Institute expert panel on the use of autologous blood. *Transfusion* 35:703, 1995.

Aprotinin in children deserves special consideration. This drug has been used in pediatric cardiac surgery and liver transplant surgery. It has proved useful in decreasing perioperative blood loss[56] and the inflammatory response in pediatric cardiac surgery. It is most useful in redo cardiac procedures and complex malformations.[56] This drug can sensitize some patients, and anaphylaxis can develop with re-exposure in certain patients.[57,58] Acute respiratory distress syndrome in a young patient receiving aprotinin for the first time has been reported.[59] An anaphylactoid reaction is hypothesized. There is also an isolated report of thrombosis of the fenestration in patients undergoing a fenestrated Fontan procedure.[60]

TABLE 20–6 Shelf Life of Autologous Red Blood Cells

Source of red blood cells	Shelf life
Units collected during perioperative blood salvage	6 h
Units collected during hemodilution	8 h
Thawed, previously frozen autologous red blood cells	24 h
Liquid-stored PABD units	35–42 d

PABD, Preoperative autologous blood donation.
Source: Reprinted with permission from Transfusion alert: Use of autologous blood. National Heart, Lung, and Blood Institute expert panel on the use of autologous blood. *Transfusion* 35:703, 1995.

The use of 1-desamino-8-D-arginine vasopressin (DDAVP) is effective for limiting blood loss in patients with hemophilia and some forms of von Willebrand's disease. It has not been effective in reducing blood loss in scoliosis surgery for patients with idiopathic or neuromuscular scoliosis.[61,62] Theroux et al. found no decreases in estimated intra- and postoperative blood losses or in the amount of packed erythrocytes transfused.[62] They studied 21 patients with severe cerebral palsy undergoing spinal fusion for scoliosis repair. Based on clinical experience, patients with neuromuscular scoliosis are at increased risk of bleeding during surgery. Although desmopressin increased the levels of factor VIIIC and von Willebrand factor, it did not decrease perioperative blood loss. Two patients developed transient hypotension during infusion of DDAVP. Because of the drug's potent antidiuretic hormone activity, patients receiving this drug should be monitored closely for hyponatremia and oliguria intraoperatively and postoperatively. However, Letts et al. found that DDAVP can be effective in a subgroup of neuromuscular patients undergoing scoliosis surgery.[63]

ε-Aminocaproic acid (EACA) administration in cardiac surgical patients decreased perioperative blood loss but did not significantly decrease blood product transfusion.[64] However, in cyanotic patients, blood loss and blood product transfusion were decreased when EACA was used.[65] Horwitz et al. studied the use of EACA for the prevention of bleeding in infants on extracorporeal membrane oxygenation.[66] Twenty-nine neonates were studied in that multicenter trial. The incidence of hemorrhagic complications did not improve with the use of EACA.

Tranexamic acid is a promising agent. It produces an antifibrinolytic effect by competitively inhibiting the activation of plasminogen to plasmin. It is also a weak non-competitive inhibitor of plasmin. It has an action mechanism approximately 10 times more potent than EACA. It has been effective in decreasing blood loss in pediatric patients undergoing repeat cardiac procedures.[67] Its efficacy has also been demonstrated in patients with cyanotic congenital heart disease undergoing cardiac surgery.[68] It was also effective in reducing hemorrhagic complications in patients undergoing congenital diaphragmatic hernia repair while on extracorporeal membrane oxygenation.[69] However, it may have been responsible for thrombotic complications. Adverse reactions include gastrointestinal disturbances (nausea, vomiting) and hypotension with rapid administration. The recommended dose for noncardiac cases is a 10 mg·kg bolus followed by an infusion of 1 mg·kg · h for 12 h.[70]

Oxygen-carrying volume-expanding solutions have been developed.[71] They are divided into hemoglobin-based oxygen carriers and perfluorocarbon emulsions. Lamy et al. studied diaspirin cross-linked hemoglobin solution in cardiac surgical patients and ofund a significant decrease in intraoperative exposure to homologous blood.[72] The usefulness of perfluorocarbon emulsions is limited by its low oxygen-carrying capacity, short intravascular persistence, brief shelf-life, temperature instability, and side effects such as marked uptake by the reticuloendothelial system and disruption of normal pulmonary surfactant mechanisms. Concerns about efficacy of these products and side effects will have to be resolved before these products appear in the operating room.

CONCLUSION

Blood conservation and salvage techniques are extremely useful in the pediatric population and can be performed safely and efficiently. Further, pediatric patients can tolerate lower levels of hematocrit, which may be advantageous when using acute normovolemic hemodilution. Various combinations of the techniques can and have been used safely, and this should allow a significant reduction of homologous transfusions, if not their elimination. Thus, to achieve optimal blood conservation in the pediatric population, combined methods should be used.

REFERENCES

1. Practice guidelines for blood component therapy. *Anesthesiology* 84:732, 1996.
2. Kemmotsu H, Joe K, Nakamura H, et al: Predeposited autologous blood transfusion for surgery in infants and children. *J Pediatr Surg* 30:659, 1995.
3. Erb T, Moller R, Christen P, et al: Increased withdrawal volume per deposit for pre-operative autologous blood donation in adolescents. *Vox Sang* 78(4):231, 2000.
4. Mezrow CK, Bergstein I, Tartter PI: Postoperative infections following autologous and homologous blood transfusions. *Transfusion* 32:27, 1992.
5. Tietze M, Klüter H, Troch M, et al: Immune responsiveness in orthopedic surgery patients after transfusion of autologous or allogeneic blood. *Transfusion* 35:378, 1995.
6. McVay PA, Andrews A, Kaplan EB, et al: Donation reactions among autologous donors. *Transfusion* 30:249, 1990.
7. Popovsky MA, Whitaker B, Arnold NL: Severe outcomes of allogeneic and autologous blood donation: frequency and characterization. *Transfusion* 35:734, 1995.
8. Moran MM, Kroon D, Tredwell SJ, et al: The role of autologous blood transfusion in adolescents undergoing spinal surgery. *Spine* 20:532, 1995.
9. Goodnough LT, Price TH, Friedman KD, et al: A phase III trial of recombinant human erythropoietin therapy in nonanemic orthopedic patients subjected to aggressive removal of blood for autologous use: dose, response, toxicity, and efficacy. *Transfusion* 34:66, 1994.
10. Schmoeckel M, Nollert G, Mempel M, et al: Effects of recombinant human erythropoietin on autologous blood donation before open heart surgery. *Thorac Cardiovasc Surg* 41:364, 1993.
11. Han P, Stacy D: Response of the erythron and erythropoietin to autologous blood donations in paediatric subjects. Is erythropoietin supplement necessary? *Vox Sang* 73:24, 1997.
12. Mercuriali F, Zanella A, Barosi G, et al: Use of erythropoietin to increase the volume of autologous blood donated by orthopedic patients. *Transfusion* 33:55, 1993.
13. Canadian Orthopedic Perioperative Erythropoietin Study Group: Effectiveness of perioperative recombinant human erythropoietin in elective hip replacement. *Lancet* 341:1227, 1993.
14. Kyo S, Omoto R, Hirashima K, et al: Effect of human recombinant erythropoietin on reduction of homologous blood transfusion in open-heart surgery: a Japanese multicenter study. *Circulation* 86:II-413, 1992.
15. Shimpo H, Mizumoto T, Onoda K, et al: Erythropoietin in cardiac surgery clinical efficacy and effective dose. *Chest* 111:1565, 1997.
16. Oga M, Ikuta H, Sugioka Y: The use of autologous blood in the surgical treatment of spinal disorders. *Spine* 17:1381, 1992.
17. Horn EP, Sputtek A, Standl T, et al: Transfusion of autologous, hydroxyethyl starch-cryopreserved red blood cells. *Anesth Analg* 85:739, 1997.
18. Miller RD, von Ehrenburg W: Controversies in transfusion medicine: indications for autologous and allogeneic transfusion should be the same: con. *Transfusion* 35:450, 1995.
19. Gould SA, Forbes JM: Controversies in transfusion medicine: indications for autologous and allogeneic transfusion should be the same: pro. *Transfusion* 35:446, 1995.
20. Yomtovian R, Kelly C, Bracey AW, et al: Procurement and transfusion of human immunodeficiency virus-positive or untested autologous blood units: issues and

concerns: a report prepared by the autologous transfusion committee of the American association of blood banks. *Transfusion* 35:353, 1995.
21. Macpherson CR: Ethical issues in autologous transfusion. *Transfusion* 35:281, 1995.
22. Vanston V, Smith D, Eisenstaedt R: Should patients with human immunodeficiency virus infection or chronic hepatitis donate blood for autologous use? *Transfusion* 35:324, 1995.
23. Starkey JM, MacPherson JL, Bolgiano DC, et al: Markers for transfusion-transmitted disease in different groups of blood donors. *JAMA* 262:3452, 1989.
24. Manno CS, Hedberg KW, Kim HC, et al: Comparison of the hemostatic effects of fresh whole blood, stored whole blood, and components after open heart surgery in children. *Blood* 77:930, 1991.
25. Booke M, Hagemann O, Van Aken H, et al: Intraoperative autotransfusion in small children: an in vitro investigation to study its feasability. *Anesth Analg* 88:763, 1999.
26. Spain DA, Miller FB, Bergamini TM, et al: Quality assessment of intraoperative blood salvage and autotransfusion. *American Surgeon* 63:1059, 1997.
27. Davis RJ, Agnew K, Shealy CR, et al: Erythrocyte viability in postoperative autotransfusion. *J Pediatr Orthop* 13:781, 1993.
28. Murray DJ, Gress K, Weinstein SL: Coagulopathy after reinfusion of autologous scavenged red blood cells. *Anesth Analg* 75:125, 1992.
29. Horst HM, Dlugos S, Fath JJ, et al: Coagulopathy and intraoperative blood salvage (IBS). *J Trauma* 32:646, 1992.
30. Habler OP, Kleen MS, Podtschaske AH, et al: The effect of acute normovolemic hemodilution on myocardial contractility in anesthetised dog. *Anesth Analg* 83:451, 1996.
31. Spahn DR, Leone BJ, Reves JG, et al: Cardiovascular and coronary physiology of acute isovolemic hemodilution: a review of nonoxygen-carrying and oxygen-carrying solutions. *Anesth Analg* 78:1000, 1994.
32. Bak Z, Abildgard L, Lisander B, et al: Transesophageal echocardiographic hemodynamic monitoring during preoperative acute normovolemic hemodilution. *Anesthesiology* 92:1250, 2000.
33. Habler OP, Kleen MS, Hutter JW, et al: Effects of hyperoxic ventilation on hemodilution-induced changes in anesthetized dogs. *Transfusion* 38:135, 1998.
34. Van Bommel J, Siegemund M, Henny P, et al: Critical hematocrit in intestinal tissue oxygenation during severe normovolemic hemodilution. *Anesthesiology* 94:152, 2001.
35. Brecher ME, Rosenfeld M: Mathematical and computer modeling of acute normovolemic hemodilution. *Transfusion* 34:176, 1994.
36. Feldman JM, Roth JV, Bjoraker DG: Maximum blood savings by acute normovolemic hemodilution. *Anesth Analg* 80:108, 1995.
37. Weiskopf RB: Mathematical analysis of isovolemic hemodilution indicates that it can decrease the need for allogeneic blood transfusion. *Transfusion* 35:37, 1995.
38. Hans P, Collin V, Bonhomme V, et al: Evaluation of acute normovolemic hemodilution for surgical repair of craniosynostosis. *J Neurosurg Anesthesiol* 12:33, 2000.
39. Copley LAB, Stephens Richards B, Safavi F, et al: Hemodilution as a method to reduce transfusion requirements in adolescent spine fusion surgery. *Spine* 24:219, 1999.
40. van Iterson M, van der Waart FJM, Erdmann W, et al: Systemic haemodynamics and oxygenation during haemodilution in children. *Lancet* 346:1127, 1995.
41. McLoughlin TM, Fontana JL, Alving B, et al: Profound normovolemic hemodilution: hemostatic effects in patients and in a porcine model. *Anesth Analg* 83:459, 1996.
42. Mielke LL, Entholzner EK, Kling M, et al: Preoperative acute hypervolemic hemodilution with hydroxyethylstarch: an alternative to acute normovolemic hemodilution? *Anesth Analg* 84:26, 1997.
43. Sum DC, Chung PC, Chen WC: Deliberate hypotensive anesthesia with labetalol in reconstructive surgery for scoliosis. *Acta Anaesthesiol Sin* 34:203, 1996.

44. Tobias JD. Sevoflurane for controlled hypotension during spinal surgery: preliminary experience in five adolescents. *Paediatr Anaesth* 8:167, 1998.
45. Hersey SL, O'Dell NE, Lowe S, et al: Nicardipine versus nitroprusside for controlled hypotension during spinal surgery in adolescents. *Anesth Analg* 84:1239, 1997.
46. Bernard JM, Passuti N, Pinaud M: Long-term hypotensive technique with nicardipine and nitroprusside during isoflurane anesthesia for spinal surgery. *Anesth Analg* 75:179, 1992.
47. Blau WS, Kafer ER, Anderson JA: Esmolol is more effective than sodium nitroprusside in reducing blood loss during orthognathic surgery. *Anesth Analg* 75:172, 1992.
48. Boezaart AP, van der Merwe J, Coetzee A: Comparison of sodium nitroprusside and esmolol-induced controlled hypotension for functional endoscopic sinus surgery. *Can J Anaesth* 42:373, 1995.
49. Ornstein E, Young WL, Ostapkovich N, et al: Are all effects of esmolol equally rapid in onset. *Anesth Analg* 81:297, 1995.
50. Blais RE, Hadjipavlou AG, Shulman G: Efficacy of autotransfusion in spine surgery: comparison of autotransfusion alone and with hemodilution and apheresis. *Spine* 21:2795, 1996.
51. Haberkern M, Dangel P: Normovolaemic haemodilution and intraoperative autotransfusion in children: experience with 30 cases of spinal fusion. *Eur J Pediatr Surg* 1:30, 1991.
52. Simpson MB, Georgopoulos G, Eilert RE: Introperative blood salvage in children and young adults undergoing spinal surgery with predeposited autologous blood: efficacy and cost effectiveness. *J Pediatr Orthop* 13:777, 1993.
53. Lisander B, Jonsson R, Nordwall A: Combination of blood-saving methods decreases homologous blood requirements in scoliosis surgery. *Anaesth Intens Care* 24:555, 1996.
54. Hur S-R, Huizenga BA, Major M: Acute normovolemic hemodilution combined with hypotensive anesthesia and other techniques to avoid homologous transfusion in spinal fusion surgery. *Spine* 17:867, 1992.
55. Rohling RG, Haers PE, Zimmermann AP, et al: Multimodal strategy for reduction of homologous transfusions in cranio-maxillofacial surgery. *Int J Oral Maxillofac Surg* 28:137, 1999.
56. Carrel TP, Schwanda M, Vogt PR, et al: Aprotinin in pediatric cardiac operations: a benefit in complex malformations and with high-dose regimen only. *Ann Thorac Surg* 66:153, 1998.
57. Bohrer H, Bach A, Fleischer F, et al: Adverse haemodynamic effects of high-dose aprotinin in a paediatric cardiac surgical patient. *Anaesthesia* 45:853, 1990.
58. Yanagihara Y, Shida T: Immunological studies on patients who received aprotinin therapy. *Jpn J Allergol* 34:899, 1985.
59. Vucicevic Z, Suskovic T: Acute respiratory distress syndrome after aprotinin infusion. *Ann Pharmacother* 31:429, 1997.
60. Reid RW, Babik B, Burrows FA, et al: Are synthetic antifibrinolytics associated with an increased incidence of baffle fenestration occlusion following modified Fontan procedure. *Anesth Analg* 82:S375, 1996.
61. Guay J, Reinberg C, Poitras B, et al: A trial of desmopressin to reduce blood loss in patients undergoing spinal fusion for idiopathic scoliosis. *Anesth Analg* 75:404, 1992.
62. Theroux MC, Corddry DH, Tietz AE, et al: A study of desmopressin and blood loss during spinal fusion for neuromuscular scoliosis. *Anesthesiology* 87:260, 1997.
63. Letts M, Pang E, D'Astous J, et al: The influence of desmopressin on blood loss during spinal fusion surgery in neuromuscular patients. *Spine* 23:475, 1998.
64. Williams GD, Bratton SL, Riley EC, et al: Efficacy of epsilon-aminocaproic acid in children undergoing cardiac surgery. *J Cardiothorac Vasc Anesth* 13:304, 1999.
65. Rao BH, Saxena N, Chauhan S, et al: Epsilon aminocaproic acid in paediatric cardiac surgery to reduce postoperative blood loss. *Indian J Med Res* 111:57, 2000.

66. Horwitz JR, Cofer BR, Warner BW, et al: A multicenter trial of 6-aminocaproic acid (Amicar) in the prevention of bleeding in infants on ECMO. *J Pediatr Surg* 33:1610, 1998.
67. Reid RW, Zimmerman AA, Laussen PC, et al: The efficacy of tranexamic acid versus placebo in decreasing blood loss in pediatric patients undergoing repeat cardiac surgery. *Anesth Analg* 84:990, 1997.
68. Zonis Z, Seear M, Reichert C, et al: The effect of preoperative tranexamic acid on blood loss after cardiac operations in children. *J Thorac Cardiovasc Surg* 111:982, 1996.
69. Van der Staak FHJ, de Haan AFJ, Geven WB, et al: Surgical repair of congenital diaphragmatic hernia during extracorporeal membrane oxygenation: hemorrhagic complications and the effect of tranexamic acid. *J Pediatr Surg* 32:594, 1997.
70. Horrow JC, Van Riper DF, Strong MD, et al: The dose-response relationship of tranexamic acid. *Anesthesiology* 82:383, 1995.
71. Dietz NM, Joyner MJ, Warner MA: Blood substitutes: fluids, drugs, or miracle solutions? *Anesth Analg* 82:390, 1996.
72. Lamy ML, Daily EK, Brichant JF, et al: Randomized trial of diaspirin cross-linked hemoglobin solution as an alternative to blood transfusion after cardiac surgery. *Anesthesiology* 92:646, 2000.

21 | Malignant Hyperthermia in Pediatric Anesthesia

Barbara Brandom, MD

This chapter presents a view of malignant hyperthermia (MH) in the practice of pediatric anesthesia. Clinical problems that still exist in the practice of pediatric anesthesia are discussed and illustrated with cases from the MH Hotline. In addition, planning for the anesthetic management of a MH-susceptible family and the management of an acute episode of MH are reviewed.

GENETICS

Malignant hyperthermia is a pharmacogenetic disease. The genetic basis for MH susceptibility is not entirely known. It is known that intracellular calcium is excessive during an MH episode. Several of the systems that affect intracellular calcium control may be involved in the progression of an MH episode. The calcium release channel in the terminal cisternae of the muscle cell, the ryanodine receptor (Ry1), or a protein directly coupled to this channel, the dihydropyridine receptor, may be abnormal in MH-susceptible muscle. Indeed, the first genetic association with MH susceptibility was in the Ry1 gene on chromosome 19q12-13.[1,2] Twenty mutations[3–5] in the Ry1 gene have been identified but the association between these and MH susceptibility is not well understood. An identical mutation occurring in different families may be associated with different phenotypes. Other loci, on chromosomes 1, 3, 5, 7, and 17,[6–10] have been proposed as associated with MH susceptibility. For example, the skeletal muscle α_2/δ-subunits (CACNL2A) of the dihydropyridine-sensitive L-type voltage-dependent calcium channel are located on 7q.

It is thought that the severe metabolic abnormalities occurring in MH are due to abnormalities of intracellular calcium homeostasis in muscle. It is also believed that muscle is the primary organ that is dysfunctional during an MH episode. But there are suggestions that metabolic abnormalities also occur in other tissues. This subject is controversial. However, ryanodine receptors do exist in tissues other than muscle. No doubt there are various phenotypic expressions of the genetic material responsible for MH. In addition, there are poorly defined environmental factors that affect the expression of MH susceptibility.[11–13] Further research in these areas is ongoing.

HISTORY

During the 1960s MH was observed in children under anesthetics in which potent inhalation anesthetics including ether and/or halothane were administered. Succinylcholine also may have been given. Anesthesia could proceed without apparent problems until muscle stiffness impaired ventilation and/or tracheal intubation was difficult. Body temperature was rarely continuously documented and there was no capnographic monitoring. The only documentation of body temperature was after subjective palpation, "the forehead felt warm." Ventricular dysrhythmias might have been observed. Blood gases and plasma potassium concentrations likely were documented only during the treatment of the cardiac arrest. Resuscitation was futile once the rectal temperature was very high and the metabolic acidosis profound. Hence, the term *malignant hyperthermia* fit the syndrome well.

The benefits of early recognition and treatment of MH became part of the continuing education of anesthesia practitioners. Anesthesiologists and the families of patients who had experienced MH episodes were strongly motivated to avoid another MH event. The introduction of dantrolene in 1979[14] allowed more than just symptomatic treatment of the acute episode. Dantrolene often was given preoperatively to patients thought to be MH susceptible. The Malignant Hyperthermia Association of the United States (MHAUS), incorporated in 1981, began to provide educational support to families and health care providers.

As the 1980s progressed, pulse oximetry and capnographic monitoring became widely applied. Respiratory difficulties were recognized more quickly. Anesthetics were aborted at the earliest sign of MH. Masseter rigidity was known to be an early sign of MH, but stiffness of the jaw occurred with alarming frequency, as often as 1 per 100 administrations of succinylcholine.[15] The practice of pediatric anesthesia began to change. Previously the surgical list had been almost completely composed of inpatients who were admitted the day before surgery. These children were easily separated from their parents after receiving narcotic and/or barbiturate premedication in their hospital rooms before their transport to the operating theater. Now increasing numbers of children arrived at the outpatient clinic with less than the usual amount of sleep and no food or drink. They received no premedication before separation from their parents. Therefore, one might expect that endogenous catecholamines were elevated in such patients. Epinephrine had been shown to significantly increase resting tension of normal muscle exposed to succinylcholine in the presence of halothane.[16] Although the trend toward same-day admission for all types of surgery has continued, the epidemic of masseter spasm has decreased as premedication, with different forms of benzodiazepine, has become popular, and the administration of succinylcholine is less common.

The concern of anesthesiologists to avoid episodes of acute MH resulted in the identification of many families thought to be MH susceptible. Muscle biopsies and standardized contracture testing were part of the effort necessary to reach a more definite diagnosis.[17] In the 1980s there were several MH diagnostic centers functioning in North America. The MH diagnostic test involves the exposure of a fresh piece of muscle from the patient's thigh to incrementally increased concentrations of caffeine and halothane. If a contracture occurs at a below-normal threshold, the patient is judged to be MH susceptible. This process is best performed after review of the patient's anesthetic and family histories and in concert with evaluation by a neurologist for other muscular disease.[18]

In 1989 the North American Malignant Hyperthermia Registry (NAMHR) was founded by Dr. Marilyn Larach. Reports of the diagnostic contracture tests and Adverse Metabolic/Musculoskeletal Reaction to Anesthesia Reports (AMRAs) are cataloged with the registry. Of the more than 450 AMRAs for the NAMHR in 2000, more than 50% described adverse anesthetic events in patients younger than 18 years. The most frequent age of patients called into the MH Hotline, the voluntary telephone consulting service provided by anesthesiologists with the support of the MHAUS, consistently ranges from neonatal to 5 years. These facts suggest that anesthetic problems, suggestive of MH, occur relatively more frequently in pediatric than in adult patients.

During the 1970s and 1980s[19-22] there were a number of published case reports describing a syndrome of cardiac arrest accompanied by rhabdomyolysis, fever, and hypercarbia in children who received inhalation anesthetics and succinylcholine. Those cases often were diagnosed as MH on the basis of the clinical findings. In 1 year alone several such cases were reported to the MHAUS Hotline. This led to a review of NAMHR data and the conclusion that succinylcholine given to children, usually boys, with occult myopathy was responsible for those deaths. The mechanism of cardiovascular collapse was extreme hyperkalemia rather than classic MH.[23]

Many possible MH families never present for contracture testing. Their children still have histories supporting the tentative diagnosis of "possible MH susceptible." Now, at the beginning of the 21st century, our most frequent anesthetic problem related to MH is how to anesthetize these patients. In our highly efficient outpatient surgical clinic, all pediatric patients receive the potent inhalation anesthetic "du jour." Halothane, sevoflurane, and all the other potent vapors are triggers of MH. With the advent of short-acting benzodiazepines, propofol, synthetic narcotics, and nondepolarizing neuromuscular blockers, it is simple to administer a "nontriggering anesthetic." Unfortunately the problem of identifying the individuals who must have only this type of general anesthesia remains.

DIAGNOSIS OF AN ACUTE EPISODE OF MH

Because MH is rare and there are many other diseases that also produce increased metabolism and muscle injury, it is very difficult to diagnose MH based on clinical findings. Nevertheless, the anesthesiologist must be prepared to evaluate the patient for evidence of MH (Table 21-1).

In classic MH, the metabolic rate may increase suddenly or slowly over the course of hours. A slow increase in the metabolic rate may be masked by compensatory increases in controlled ventilation.[24] With an increase in metabolic rate, tachycardia is commonly observed, but dysrhythmias may not occur in pediatric patients until the serum potassium is significantly elevated. As energy stores in the muscle are depleted, rigidity can occur and the permeability of the muscle cell increases. This allows potassium, myoglobin, and creatine kinase (CK) to move from the muscle cell to the extracellular fluid. Potassium concentrations in the blood may not be elevated initially, if potassium uptake by the liver balances the release from the muscle. Myoglobin may be bound by proteins in the blood and not appear in the urine until later in the acute episode. Testing the urine with a chemstrip will produce a positive test for blood when myoglobin or hemoglobin is present in that urine sample. Renal failure may result as a complication of myoglobinuria. Crea-

TABLE 21–1 Clinical Evidence of Malignant Hyperthermia

Increasing carbon dioxide production beyond that expected considering body core temperature
Increasing metabolic acidosis
Tachycardia
Arrhythmias
Hyperkalemia
Rigidity
Myoglobin and creatine phosphokinase elevation
Disseminated intravascular coagulation

tine kinase is released continuously by the damaged muscle. Peak CK levels often are observed 8 to 36 h after the initial muscle injury, but CK levels may not be elevated greatly.[25] Disseminated intravascular coagulation is another complication of severe muscle injury, as is cerebral edema.

When MH is suspected, vital signs, including core temperature, fluid balance, minute ventilation, and end-tidal carbon dioxide concentrations, should be documented carefully. Blood gases, electrolytes, myoglobin, CK, and coagulation function should be measured. Mixed venous blood samples will show changes in acid–base status more quickly than arterial specimens. Other studies, such as chest x-ray, complete blood counts, and cultures, should be obtained as indicated by the clinical condition of the patient. The suspicion that MH may be occurring should not delay evaluation and treatment of other medical conditions that may produce similar signs. Sepsis,[26] endocrine disease,[27] and other adverse drug reactions[28,29] are common problems that can also produce metabolic changes and muscle injury.

MH CASES

The following cases were called into the MH Hotline and all occurred between 1997 and 2000 inclusive. Hotline cases are randomly selected, blinded, and then reviewed by a committee to determine diagnostic and therapeutic consensus. Details that identify the patient, or provider, are excluded in these reviews. The ages of the patients reported here are approximate. All were younger than 18 years.

The first three cases were thought to be examples of MH by the review committee. In clinical practice, confirmation of a MH diagnosis may depend on events that occur weeks to months after the initial presentation. Nevertheless, these cases were judged to be definitely or very likely to be MH.

Case 1

A 10-year-old male had a sudden increase in end-tidal carbon dioxide and minute ventilation after 20 min of anesthesia with propofol, isoflurane, and nitrous oxide during orthopedic surgery on his leg. The patient had coughed on the endotracheal tube after mivacurium had been used to facilitate intubation, but there was no generalized rigidity. The leg tourniquet had been up for less than 20 min. It was not possible to lower minute ventilation, although end-tidal carbon dioxide could be kept at 35 mmHg. There was no obvious myoglobinuria and cardiovascular function was stable. Because the anesthesia provider felt the patient was definitely experiencing an MH crisis, treatment was begun before blood samples were taken. The patient was cooled. After the administration of 2 mg/kg of dantrolene, end-tidal carbon dioxide returned to normal, with normal minute ventilation. Bicarbonate and fluids also were given. No elevation of serum potassium or metabolic acidosis was observed. No fault in the ventilating system could be identified. The postoperative CK was 46,000 IU. There was respiratory muscle weakness that eventually resolved. The patient made a complete recovery and was appropriately referred to MHAUS for information, followed by a biopsy and a contracture test.

In this case no laboratory data were obtained before initiating treatment. This may be the best course of action when very few individuals are available to help process specimens and mix the dantrolene. In such cases it is very important that the anesthesia provider communicate the events to the patient, the family, and the NAMHR in written form. Completion of an

AMRA as soon as possible will allow the anesthetic events to be recorded in a confidential manner within the NAMHR. When the patient undergoes a muscle biopsy and contracture test to assess MH susceptibility, the data in the AMRA can be linked to the biopsy report. Only when definite evidence of MH susceptibility is documented in families can less invasive tests of MH susceptibility be developed in the future.

Case 2

A 3-year-old male was anesthetized with propofol and rocuronium for repair of a minor trauma to his hand. A tourniquet was in place. Anesthesia was maintained with nitrous oxide, isoflurane, and morphine for more than 2 h when an end-tidal carbon dioxide tension of 79 mmHg was noted. The heart rate increased from 150 to 220 beats per minute over 20 min, and temperature increased 2°C. An arterial blood gas showed a pH of 7.07, Po_2 of 113 mmHg, Pco_2 of 67 mmHg, and base deficit of −11.5 meqv/L. Dantrolene, 5 mg/kg, was given and decreases in end-tidal CO_2, heart rate, and temperature followed. As the heart rate slowed, the electrocardiogram (EKG) showed a wide complex QRS without a pulse. Cardiac compressions were given for 90 s. Normal sinus rhythm then returned. Dantrolene was given again and the child was transported to the pediatric intensive care unit, with the endotracheal tube in place. He then received 1 mg/kg dantrolene every 6 h for 24 h.

One might ask for more data with regard to resting heart rate, preoperative laboratory data, tourniquet time, and the presence of local anesthetic in the injured hand. Perhaps the child has an underlying muscle disease such as Duchenne's muscular dystrophy (DMD). Resting tachycardia and abnormal R-wave progression may be observed in the EKG of a child with DMD.[30,31] Perhaps the prolonged tourniquet time and its subsequent release contributed to the changes in vital signs. Could local anesthetic have contributed to the cardiac arrest? Postoperatively, serial CK levels, coagulation function and renal function should be followed so that complications are rapidly identified and treated. If the child has an occult myopathy, CK levels may remain elevated and referral to a neurologist is then indicated. Whether or not an occult myopathy is present, MH cannot be ruled out on the day of surgery. Therefore, continued treatment with dantrolene is indicated until the vital signs are stable and the acidosis has resolved. Then, if weakness of skeletal muscle is present, dantrolene administration may be stopped.

Case 3

A 4-month-old infant was anesthetized for gastrostomy before fundoplication of a hemidiaphragm. The infant had spasticity preoperatively and recently had a respiratory infection. There was no evidence of an intracardiac shunt or tracheoesophageal fistula. The anesthesia included halothane, fentanyl, and a nondepolarizing neuromuscular blocker, given to facilitate intubation. Arterial blood gases were drawn about 1 h after induction of anesthesia to assess respiratory status. At that time the carbon dioxide tension was 45 mmHg and the serum potassium was 9.9 meqv/L. Shortly thereafter, the heart rate was greater than 190 beats per minute and rectal temperature was 39.5°C. MH was suspected and treatment begun. The surgery was terminated and the halothane was discontinued. The patient was given 2.5 mg/kg dantrolene, 15 meqv $NaHCO_3$, 3.5 U insulin, 1.5 g dextrose, and 3 mg furosemide. Urine myoglobin testing was negative. Prothrombin and partial thromboplastin times were sent. Two hours later, the potassium was 6.1 meqv/L, CK levels were 17,230 IU, core temperature was 37°C, heart rate was 165 beats per minute, pH was 7.4, and the P_{CO_2} was 29 mmHg. Dantrolene, 1 mg/kg, was continued every 6 h for 24 h. On the day after the scheduled surgery, the CK level was 155,000 IU and arterial blood gases showed a pH of 7.37, P_{CO_2} of 52 mmHg, and HCO_3 of 29 meqv/L. Coagulation and renal function were normal. One dose of dantrolene, 2 mg/kg, had produced flaccidity, and then the rigidity of the legs recurred, without metabolic abnormality. The CK level was between 20,000 and 30,000 IU after tapering the dantrolene dose.

After tracheal extubation, diagnostic procedures were performed. The infant's spine was reported to be normal on magnetic resonance imaging. There was no definitive diagnosis of muscular disease, although muscle biopsy and evaluation of mitochondrial function were performed.

Probably the most accurate diagnosis for this case is a neuromuscular disease complicated by an acute MH episode. Documentation of the minute ventilation may be difficult if a Mapleson circuit, rather than a circle system, is used. This is often the case for infants. There may be a large gradient between end-tidal and arterial carbon dioxide tensions in normal infants and more so in those with respiratory disease. Exogenous heat is supplied commonly and actively to an infant. Thus, many of the early findings of MH are difficult to document in the small infant and easy to attribute to underlying respiratory disease and the effects of the interventions by the anesthesia provider. Creatine kinase levels may not return to normal in a patient with underlying myopathy. Six months after this episode, a tentative diagnosis of King–Denborough syndrome was made. This syndrome was one of the first to be identified with MH-like episodes during anesthesia.[32]

These three cases present somewhat similar anesthetic problems; abnormal vital signs and/or laboratory data reverted to normal after administration of dantrolene. In one, or perhaps even all three cases, there may have been an underlying myopathy. For research purposes, classic MH excludes patients with myopathy. However, for clinical purposes, the initial evaluation and treatment of the patient with acute MH are the same, whether or not there is a myopathy present. The diagnosis of a myopathy has different implications for the patient and family than that of classic MH without a myopathy. For that reason and to improve our understanding of the pathophysiology of these anesthetic complications, the patient should be referred for a thorough diagnostic evaluation.

A CASE OF MASSETER MUSCLE RIGIDITY

Case 4

After refusing spinal anesthesia, a healthy 16-year-old male received an intravenous induction agent and succinylcholine in anticipation of surgery on his lower extremity. No inhalation agents were given. The degree of muscle tension in the masseter was not reported, but laryngoscopy was said to be difficult, "a class III airway." There was no generalized rigidity. Due to the failure to intubate after three attempts, the case was canceled. Five hours later, the patient complained of severe myalgia, especially in the thighs. Creatine kinase levels at that time were 56,000 IU and potassium was 4.4 meqv/L. No dantrolene was given. The urine was very dark red and contained a "large" amount of blood. Fluids, bicarbonate, and diuretics were given. The next morning, the CK level was 99,000 IU, the urine was clear, and the serum creatinine was normal. The heart rate, temperature, and other vital signs were normal throughout this episode.

There was evidence of rhabdomyolysis but not of increased metabolism in this case. The diagnosis of masseter muscle rigidity was supported by the available data, but the diagnosis of MH *was not* well supported by the same data. For that reason, there could be some disagreement regarding the diagnosis of MH in this case. Although it is important to test the patient for susceptibility to MH, the patient might have had an unrelated myotonia. Baseline CK levels should be documented and the patient referred to a neurologist and MH diagnostic biopsy center.

Increased epinephrine[16] and temperature levels[33] in the presence of a potent inhalation anesthetic can increase the resting tension of the normal masseter muscle, even more than is usually observed after succinylcholine.[34,35] Therefore, one may well wonder when a patient, whose masseter was not completely relaxed, should be referred for thorough diagnostic evaluation and when the patient should be considered at the upper end of the distribution of normal responses. Evaluation of the myalgia in this case showed evidence of a severe muscle injury. Myalgia may be noted on the day of surgery or the day after. Such a patient should be evaluated thoroughly so that the best recommendations can be made and complications such as renal failure after exposure to anesthetic drugs and adjuncts can be avoided in the future.

DISASTER IN THE RECOVERY ROOM

Case 5

A previously healthy, large, 13-year old male underwent 2 h of uncomplicated halothane anesthesia for elective surgery on his lower extremity. Postoperatively, he appeared to be recovering, as expected, when he reported "feeling sick." A cardiac arrest followed. Potassium was greater than 10 meq/L. He was resuscitated with bicarbonate, epinephrine, calcium chloride, dextrose, and insulin. He had a fever up to 40°C. He was actively cooled with ice packs and cold intravenous fluids. Acute oliguric renal failure occurred. Prothrombin and partial thromboplastin times were prolonged and the platelet count was less than 100,000/mL, but a clinical coagulopathy did not develop. Dantrolene was not given during the acute event and had no apparent effect when given more than 18 h after surgery. The patient became metabolically stable but died of hyperkalemia before institution of dialysis.

This patient may have had an occult myopathy such as Becker's muscular dystrophy. In Becker's dystrophy, dystrophin is less than normal but greater than in DMD. Thus, patients may not develop signs of skeletal muscle weakness until adolescence.[36] Prolonged exposure to inhalation anesthetics, without exposure to succinylcholine, may be followed by severe rhabdomyolysis in such patients. To confirm the diagnosis of any form of dystrophinopathy, muscle, even postmortem muscle, can be assayed for dystrophin. Alternately, genetic material can be examined for the characteristic defect on the X chromosome but is less accurate.

The following cases are examples of cases judged to be unlikely or definitely *not* MH by the review committee. Eliminating the diagnosis of MH from the possible explanation of a complication can facilitate the delivery of appropriate treatment.

Case 6

A 6-month-old infant underwent resection of a glioma during an uncomplicated anesthetic that included isoflurane and a nondepolarizing neuromuscular blocker. Three hours after surgery, the heart rate increased to 250 beats per minute and the temperature increased to 42°C. There was questionable rigidity and a seizure occurred. Arterial blood gases included a normal pH and a P_{CO_2} of 36 mmHg. There was no change in vital signs after administration of acetaminophen. Metabolic acidosis was not present and there was no evidence of muscle injury.

One milligram per kilogram of dantrolene was given three times over 30 min. The fever and tachycardia subsided and did not recur. There was no metabolic acidosis, respiratory acidosis, or increase in CK levels. The dantrolene was discontinued.

There was agreement by the review committee regarding the correctness of the diagnosis of neurogenic fever rather than MH. The beneficial effect of dantrolene in this case was a nonspecific decrease in muscle metabolism. Blocking the muscular response to central resetting of thermoregulation decreased the fever. A recommendation was made to check the infant's blood sugar and call the neurosurgeon involved. Anticonvulsants were considered.

Case 7

An 8-year-old adopted female underwent craniotomy for excision of a mass lesion during anesthesia that included thiopental and isoflurane. She had had two previous anesthetics without complications. During surgery, an arterial blood gas analysis showed a pH of 7.45, P_{CO_2} of 25 mmHg, and base deficit of −5.5 meq/L. Two hours later, arterial pH was 7.40, P_{CO_2} of 23 mmHg, and a base deficit of −9 meqv/L. Serum potassium was normal. Ninety minutes later, the pH was 7.29, P_{CO_2} of 26 mmHg, and a base deficit of −12 meqv/L. Postoperatively, she had no respiratory problems, the urine was clear, and the serum glucose, potassium, and sodium concentrations were normal. She was afebrile.

This case is unlikely to be MH because there was no evidence of increased metabolism. Postoperatively, one blood gas had a base deficit of −12 meq/L. Other causes of metabolic acidosis were investigated. Four hours later, after extubation of the trachea, the acidosis had resolved. Blood gases then showed a pH of 7.40, P_{CO_2} of 40 mmHg, and HCO_3 of 25 meqv/L.

In this case, the only sign consistent with MH was metabolic acidosis. Fluid management must be reviewed for hyperchloremic acidosis. Other causes of metabolic acidosis are then investigated. In the absence of fever and other signs of MH, it is not useful to give dantrolene.

Case 8

A 7-year-old female had tonsillectomy, adenoidectomy, and bilateral myringotomy with tympanostomy tube insertion during an anesthetic that included oral midazolam, sevoflurane, and nitrous oxide. During surgery, the child's heart rate increased to 170 beats per minute and then decreased to 160 to 140 beats per minute during stable anesthesia. No anticholinergic was given. The rectal temperature was 36.2°C and the end-tidal CO_2 was normal. The child's heart rate was 120 beats per minute postoperatively in the presence of her mother. Her heart rate remained at 115 to 120 beats per minute.

The child later returned to the emergency room with a temperature of 103°F, which decreased to 101°F with acetaminophen. Blood gases then were a pH of 7.4, P_{CO_2} of 39 mmHg, and HCO_3 of 25 meqv/L. A complete blood count was said to be normal, but the white blood count was 25,500/mL. Myoglobin was not present in the urine. The CK level was 430 IU.

The review committee agreed that the diagnosis of not MH was correct in this case. Persistent tachycardia and a fever near 103°C are of concern, but these seemed more likely to be due to a bacteremia from a cryptic infection than secondary to MH. The clinical course of the patient and the laboratory data helped to document that this was not an episode of MH.

Case 9

An 8-year-old male had pressure-equalizing tube placement during an anesthetic that included oral midazolam preoperatively, 70% N_2O/O_2, and propofol because of a family history of MH. The child did well intraoperatively. Postoperatively, he was observed for 3 h in the recovery room. His temperature was 98°F at the time of discharge from the hospital. Three hours later, his mother reported that the child's temperature increased to 101°F. The child was admitted to the intensive care unit for observation and a cooling blanket was placed over him. His temperature decreased from 101.8°F to 101.1°F. His heart rate was 160 beats per minute. An intravenous catheter was inserted.

There was agreement by the review committee regarding the correct diagnosis of not MH. The patient's increased temperature was more likely due to an intercurrent infection than to MH. Symptomatic treatment was continued. A complete blood count was recommended to look for evidence of an infection. To document that there was no evidence of MH, blood gases and CK levels should be measured and the urine examined. Families who have experienced MH are likely to have a lower threshold for seeking medical care after anesthesia. If we can help document that MH has *not* occurred, then the family and their providers can be spared a lot of extra effort.

Case 10

A 16-year-old female was receiving haloperidol to treat auditory and visual hallucinations. She was also receiving clonopin, motrin, dilantin, and acyclovir (for herpes encephalitis). She presented with rigidity and a temperature that had been increasing over several days to a week. The haloperidol was discontinued 2 days before. Her heart rate was 106 to 130 beats per minute, blood pressure was 100/60 mmHg, temperature was 38.4°C to 38.0°C, and the CK level was approximately 4000 IU. Arterial blood gas included an HCO_3 of 26 meqv/L. Electroencephalography showed increased β-activity. A lumbar puncture showed 10 white blood cells per milliliter. As time passed, the patient's heart rate increased to 160 beats per minute and a blood gas showed acidosis.

It was agreed that this was a case of neurolept malignant syndrome (NMS) rather than MH. However, NMS is a diagnosis of exclusion. Other neurologic problems, such as encephalitis, should be ruled out before concluding that NMS is the cause of the fever, acidosis, and muscle injury. The NMS Hotline (1-888-667-8367) is a group of voluntary psychiatrists with experience in this syndrome and can be helpful in the management of such cases. Neurolept malignant syndrome can last from days to weeks, depending on the half-life of the causative drug. Dantrolene, 1 to 2.5 mg/kg, can be used to reduce the fever and rigidity at any time. Administration of dantrolene should be given in conjunction with a blood gas analysis so that one can judge whether the dantrolene is effective in relieving acidosis.

Case 11

A 5-year-old male underwent hernia repair under sevoflurane anesthesia. During induction, the patient became rigid and his skin became mottled. These signs resolved as the anesthetic was "deepened." There was no difficulty with jaw opening during intubation, which was accomplished during "deep" sevoflurane without a muscle relaxant. The intraoperative course was normal. Postoperatively, he needed albuterol for an asthma flare-up. His temperature increased from 100.1°F to 101.0°F over 0.5 h and remained at 101°F in the postanesthesia care unit. His heart rate increased to 150 beats per minute and then decreased to 110 beats per minute. His breath sounds were "coarse and junky." The arterial blood gas was normal. The CK level was 72 IU. The myoglobin level was 59 ng/mL. Two hours later, the arterial blood gas showed a pH of 7.39, $P{CO_2}$ of 37 mmHg, $P{O_2}$ of 326 mmHg, HCO_3 of 22 meqv/L, and a base excess of −2.7 meqv/L.

There was complete agreement that this was not a case of MH. Although the rigidity and skin mottling are suspicious, the normal blood gas, CK, and myoglobin levels support the conclusion that this was not MH. Tonic and tonic–clonic movements during exposure to sevoflurane have been reported in children. Perhaps the movements observed in this case were due to sevoflurane rather than to an abnormality in the patient. During anesthetic induction with any drug but especially with irritating vapors, rigidity may be observed if secretions or blood touch the interarytenoid space. Sensory nerves in this area will elicit a reflex increase in chest and abdominal muscle tone, laryngeal closure, and apnea. This reflex protects the trachea from irritating fluids. It is a normal reflex in infants and can persist for years. In children with allergies, asthma, recent upper airway infection, or chronic exposure to tobacco smoke, airway reflexes are often more active. During anesthesia, this reflex produces laryngospasm. Deepening the anesthetic or producing a neuromuscular block will relieve the airway obstruction produced by this reflex. In this case, there were several pulmonary complications that might have produced postoperative fever. A chest x-ray, complete blood count, and the examination of sputum might help to differentiate between aspiration, exacerbation of asthma, atelectasis, and pulmonary infection.

In summary, if end-tidal carbon dioxide tension is increasing or minute ventilation is continually being increased to maintain a constant end-tidal carbon dioxide tension, the anesthesiologist must quickly examine the gas delivery system to identify leaks. The patient must be examined to identify anatomic and physiologic factors that would change the compliance of the respiratory system. Exogenous carbon dioxide may be supplied during laparoscopy while the diaphragm is being elevated by increased intraabdominal pressure. These causes of increasing end-tidal carbon dioxide are not MH.

An increasing heart rate suggests that catecholamines and/or oxygen consumption are increasing. If the administration of an anesthetic or narcotic does not reduce the heart rate and exogenous cooling does not reduce temperature, then blood samples should be obtained to evaluate the acid–base status and serum potassium. If these samples are consistent with MH, then more blood should be obtained to measure myoglobin, CK levels, serum creatinine, and clotting function. These laboratory measures will serve as a baseline so that the effects of treatment can be documented.

TREATMENT

An acute episode of MH is treated in the pediatric patient as it is in the adult. Drugs that trigger MH must be eliminated. Potent inhalation anesthetics must be discontinued. When 10 L/min oxygen passes through the anesthesia machine, inhalation anesthetics are practically eliminated within 10 min. Some ventilators and humidifiers may retain potent vapors for a longer period. If the system in use has not been tested in this regard, it should be replaced, without interfering with administration of dantrolene and other aspects of patient treatment.

Dantrolene, 2.5 mg/kg, mixed with sterile water, should be administered as quickly as possible (Table 21-2). The current formulation of dantrolene contains mannitol. It is irritating if it extravasates. Therefore, it may be helpful to administer this drug by gravity drip into as large a vein as possible. Dantrolene should be repeated until the heart rate decreases and acidosis has resolved.

The patient should be cooled actively. Cold intravenous saline can be given. Ice packs can be placed in the axillae, on the groin, around the neck, and on the forehead. Cold saline can be used to lavage the stomach and the bladder. Active cooling should stop when the temperature drops. Active cooling when the core temperature is below 38°C may result in hypothermia. The temperature should be measured continuously.

Placement of a catheter into the internal jugular or subclavian vein and an arterial catheter will facilitate drawing blood for laboratory tests. A Foley catheter should be placed so that the urine can be tested for myoglobin and the volume of urine output recorded.

Laboratory abnormalities should be treated. Hyperkalemia can be treated with intravenous calcium chloride. This may be the most effective treatment when hyperkalemia has produced EKG abnormalities. Glucose with insulin in addition to epinephrine will promote the movement of plasma potassium into the liver and other tissues. Acidosis should be treated vigorously with bicarbonate and increased ventilation. Coagulation abnormalities should be treated as for any other patient with disseminated intravascular coagulation. Replacement of clotting factors, support of the circulation, and early consul-

TABLE 21–2 Drugs Used to Treat Malignant Hyperthermia

Dantrolene 2.5 mg/kg as initial dose
  Dissolved in sterile water
  Repeat up to ≥15 mg/kg
Bicarbonate, 1–2 meqv/kg or
  (0.3 × weight [kg] × base deficit)/2, as initial dose
  Repeat while monitoring serum sodium
Insulin 10 U regular in 50 mL 50% glucose
Calcium chloride, 10 mg/kg, to treat hyperkalemia in the presence of electro cardiographic changes
  Lidocaine or other antiarrhythmics, as indicated

TABLE 21–3 Directory of the North American Malignant Hyperthermia Muscle Biopsy Centers Active in 2000

U.S. centers	
Mayo Clinic Rochester, MN 55905	Denise Wedel, MD 507-255-4236
Northwestern University Chicago, IL 60611	Silas Glisson, PhD 312-908-2541
Thomas Jefferson University Philadelphia, PA 19107	Henry Rosenberg, MD 215-955-5844
Uniformed Services University of the Health Sciences Bethesda, MD 20014	Sheila Muldoon, MD 301-295-3140
University of California Davis, CA 95616	Joseph Antognini, MD 530-752-7809
University of California Los Angeles, CA 90024	Jordan D. Miller, MD 310-825-7850
University of Minnesota Minneapolis, MN 55455	Paul A. Iaizzo, PhD 612-624-9990
Wake Forest University Winston-Salem, NC 27157	Thomas E. Nelson, PhD 336-716-7194
Canadian centers	
Ottawa Civic Hospital Ottawa, Ontario	Gordon Reid, MD, FRCPC 613-761-4169
Toronto General Hospital Toronto, Ontario	Julian Loke, MD, FRCPC 416-340-3128
University of Manitoba Winnipeg, Manitoba	Leena Patel, MD, FRCPC 204-787-2560

Note: These centers comply with the standardization protocol for the caffeine halothane contracture test that resulted from six conferences held 1987, 1989, 1990, 1991, 1994, and 1998.

tation with the hematology department are indicated. Patients with treated MH have died primarily from disseminated intravascular coagulation.

Administration of β-blockers to decrease heart rate or treat arrhythmias may make treatment of hyperkalemia more difficult. Calcium channel blockers may have unpredictable effects on the cardiovascular system in the presence of dantrolene. Verapamil has produced hyperkalemia and severely decreased cardiac function in the presence of dantrolene in humans[37] and pigs.[38] This effect is not always seen in animals.[39,40]

Despite the treatment of an acute episode of MH, the syndrome may recur. This has been termed *recrudescence*. Recrudescence may occur within hours of the initial treatment and in as many as 25% of patients. For this reason, it is recommended that 1 mg/kg dantrolene be given intravenously every 6 h for 24 h after the initial treatment of MH.

PREVENTION

Acquiring a family anesthetic history is the first step in preventing MH. Many families who have lost members to MH will relate that story whenever surgery is planned. A first-degree relative to a known MH-susceptible individual is considered MH susceptible until proven otherwise by contracture testing of the muscle. If individuals undergo contracture testing and agree to have their names and test results linked in the NAMHR, the results of those evaluations can be made available to health care providers and family members when they are adequately identified to the NAMHR (Table 21–3). The NAMHR is open during business hours, eastern standard time (412-692-5464).

The data regarding results of contracture testing are likely to be incomplete for most MH-susceptible families. If a patient weighs less than 40 kg, some centers may defer biopsy. Therefore, young children are seldom candidates for biopsy. If a family wishes to undergo testing for MH susceptibility, the proband, the individual who experienced an episode of MH, should be tested first. This will produce the optimal predictive value of the contracture test.

The very high sensitivity and low specificity of the caffeine halothane contracture test[41,42] results in a positive predictive value of greater than 50% when the prior probability of MH is greater than 20%.[43] Prior probability is estimated by the characteristics of a clinical episode and family relationships. For example, the parents, siblings, and children of an individual with a contracture test diagnostic of MH have a 50% probability of also being MH susceptible.[18] Therefore, the first-degree relatives of individuals known to be MH susceptible should undergo muscle biopsies and contracture tests because the positive and negative predictive values of the test will be good. This means that, if the test result is positive or negative, there is a greater than 90% chance that this is a true result. An individual who experiences an anesthetic complication that includes hypercarbia, metabolic acidosis, and evidence of muscle injury[44] also may have enough data gathered during that anesthetic to suggest that MH has occurred. Such patients may undergo biopsy and contracture tests with the goal of proving that they are not MH susceptible. If there is no strong evidence in the individual's family history that MH susceptibility may be present, then the contracture test results may be falsely positive. Nevertheless, a negative test result can provide significant reassurance to family members that they do *not* have greatly increased risks during general anesthesia. Families that include individuals with positive results and those with negative test results may provide important information for the development of genetic tests for MH susceptibility.

When in doubt about the MH susceptibility of a potential patient, a nontriggering anesthetic should be planned (Table 21–4). Ideally, this will be "stress free" so that changes in heart rate might be due to changes in oxygen consumption and carbon dioxide production rather than to a response to pain or stimulation during surgery. Therefore, drugs that can increase heart rate may be "safe" for MH-susceptible patients, but their administration can create diagnostic dilemmas for the anesthetist. A useful premedicant is midazolam, which may be given intravenously, sprayed into the nostril (0.3 mg/kg, maximum dose 5 mg), or taken by mouth (0.5 mg/kg, maximum dose 15 mg). Midazolam premedication decreases rigidity produced by synthetic narcotics. Nitrous oxide may increase rigidity produced by synthetic narcotics. Propofol is a useful nontriggering general anesthetic that is synergistic with synthetic narcotics. Nondepolarizing neuromuscular blocking agents, anticholinergics, and anticholinesterases can be used as they would be for other patients, with the caveat that it may be helpful to use as little anticholinergic as is feasible. If fever then occurs, there is no drug-induced impairment to dissipation of heat. Antiemetics and local anesthetics are no longer considered potential triggers of MH. Prophylactic dantrolene is not recommended, although dantrolene should be immediately available, if needed. Certainly, continuous capnographic, EKG, and core temperature monitoring would be used during any anesthetic in a MH-susceptible patient.

Ten minutes of 10 L/min oxygen flushed through an Ohio Modulus 1 anesthesia machine reduced the concentration of halothane to less than 100 parts per million (ppm) at the patient end of the anesthesia circuit.[45] Replacing the carbon dioxide absorber or the Air-Shields disposable ventilator bellows did not speed washout of anesthetic. Replacing the circle system increased the rate of halothane washout to produce less than 10 ppm after 10 min of 10 L fresh gas flow. Replacing the hose delivering gas from the anesthesia machine to the ventilating circuit resulted in less than 1 ppm rather than less than 10 ppm halothane at the end of that hose after 10 min of flushing with 10 L oxygen. Similarly, rapid washout has been observed after replacing the Baine circuit and bypassing the humidifier even when the Drager vaporizer was not removed from a Drager anesthesia machine (my personal observation). Similarly rapid washout was observed from Ohmeda Modulus II machines with vaporizers in place.[46] Halothane concentrations in the recovery room air can be 1 ppm.[47] If the anesthetic vaporizer has been tested as described below, then it does not have to be removed from the system or drained. However, cage-mounted vaporizers and Selectatec mounting systems will continue to contaminate the system with halothane.[47]

Anesthesia ventilation systems can be tested with the Riker gas analyzer to determine the washout of inhalation anesthetics. Unfortunately, this equipment, although it is often used to test the calibration of vaporizers, is rarely used to test anesthetic concentrations in other parts of the anesthesia gas delivery system. A reason for this may be that the Riker gas analyzer will respond to water vapor as if it were anesthetic vapor. A reliable signal is obtained only from dry equipment. Therefore, documentation that the vaporizer does not leak when it is turned off and documentation of the interval

TABLE 21–4 Safe Versus Unsafe Drugs for Individuals Susceptible to Malignant Hyperthermia

Safe	Unsafe
Narcotics	Succinylcholine
Benzodiazepines	Decamethonium
Barbiturates	Potent inhalation agents
Propofol	Sevoflurane
Etomidate	Desflurane
All local anesthetics	Isoflurane
Nondepolarizing blockers	Halothane
Anticholinergics	Enflurane
Ketamine	Ether
Nitrous oxide	Verapamil with dantrolene
Anticholinesterases	
Antiemetics	
Vasopressors	

required to eliminate anesthetic vapor after it is turned off must be done as a maintenance procedure and not during administration of anesthesia.

The stocking of dantrolene and other drugs and equipment used to treat MH should be performed as a maintenance procedure. The MHAUS recently produced manuals that detail plans of treatment for MH in different anesthetizing environments: the hospital, the surgery center, and the office surgical clinic. These manuals are customized for each environment, even to providing specific telephone numbers for services needed. An episode of acute MH is such a rare event that it may be difficult to motivate any preparation for it. However, a practice MH drill, like the practice in resuscitation performed for trauma management, can identify areas that should be improved in the system. In a pediatric hospital one might imagine that fewer than 36 vials of dantrolene could be kept immediately available. However, in many anesthetizing environments that care for pediatric patients, adult-size patients are very common. Be prepared!

OUTPATIENT ANESTHESIA FOR MH-SUSCEPTIBLE PATIENTS

Without physical findings suggestive of MH during 1 h in the recovery room, or after an uncomplicated nontriggering anesthetic, it is very unlikely that MH will develop later. Nevertheless, the more conservative, frequently followed guideline has been to watch the child for 4 h postoperatively, before discharge home. This prolonged observation period allows ample time for rehydration and documentation of adequate oral intake and urine color. If the urine is clear, it is unlikely to contain myoglobin. Myoglobinuria would be a sign of muscle injury and an indication for continued intravenous treatment in the hospital. Febrile respiratory complications may occur in the first few hours postoperatively. It is easier to evaluate these problems when the child remains in the hospital or outpatient clinic. Parents should be counseled that fever may occur in any child after discharge from the hospital. If the child is drinking, producing light colored urine, and the fever decreases at least somewhat after acetaminophen administration, the episode is very unlikely to be due to MH. If the child is lethargic, febrile, or tachypneic, the child should be brought to the emergency room for re-evaluation. Documentation of vital signs, venous blood gas, CK levels, and urinalysis might then show evidence of muscle injury, if this has occurred. Postoperative fever is usually due to an infection or the pyrogens released by surgical injury.

OTHER CONDITIONS ASSOCIATED WITH MH SUSCEPTIBILITY

Is there an increased risk of MH in patients known to have a myopathy, other syndromes, or medical conditions found in pediatric patients? Because classic MH, myopathy, and anesthetic syndromes are rare, there is no well-documented answer to the question. Central core disease is thought to be associated with MH susceptibility. Myotonia congenita has been associated with MH susceptibility.[48] But this is not the case for all families with central core disease or myotonia. Historically, King–Denborough syndrome has been associated with MH.[32] Several other syndromes have had this association. In each case, however, there were many patients with that syndrome, such as arthrogryposis, osteogenesis imperfecta, myotonic dystrophy, and Schwartz–Jampel syndrome, who have had anesthetics with potent inhalation agents and no evidence of MH.

In a patient known to have a myopathy that produces elevated CK levels at rest or reduces energy stores in muscle, it may be prudent to provide a "nontriggering anesthetic." It has been suggested that DMD patients are MH susceptible, but there are some patients with DMD who have had negative contracture tests for MH susceptibility,[49,50] and the dystrophin-deficient mouse muscle does not develop contracture when exposed to caffeine or halothane.[51] A myotonic patient may have hypercarbia after succinylcholine has induced marked rigidity. When muscle is severely injured, for any reason, the same complications that are life threatening in MH, especially renal failure and disseminated intravascular coagulation, may occur. Hyperkalemia may be more life threatening and common during anesthesia-induced exacerbations of rhabdomyolysis in myopathy patients than during an episode of classic MH.

REFERENCES

1. MacLennan DH, Duff C, Zortazo F, et al: Ryanodine receptor gene is a candidate for predisposition to malignant hyperthermia. *Nature* 343(6258):559, 1990.
2. McCarthy TV, Healy JM, Heffron JJ, et al: Localization of the malignant hyperthermia susceptibility locus to human chromosome 19q12-13.2. *Nature* 343 (6258): 562, 1990.
3. Manning B, Quanne KA, Ording H, et al: Identification of novel mutations in the ryanodine-receptor gene (RYR1) in malignant hyperthermia: genotype-phenotype correlation. *Am J Hum Genet* 62:599, 1998.
4. Brandt A, Schleithoff L, Jurkat-Rott K, et al: Screening of the ryanodine receptor gene in 105 malignant hyperthermia families: novel mutations and concordance with the in vitro contracture test. *Hum Mol Genet* 8:2055, 1999.
5. McCarthy T, Quane K, Lynch P: Ryanodine receptor mutations in malignant hyperthermia and central core disease. *Hum Mutat* 15:410, 2000.
6. Monnier N, Procaccio V, Stieglitz P, Lunardi J: Malignant hyperthermia susceptibility is associated with a mutation of the alpha-1 subunit of the human dihydropyridine sensitive L-type voltage-dependent calcium-channel receptor in skeletal muscle. *Am J Hum Genet* 60:1316, 1997.
7. Robinson RL, Monnier N, Wolz W, et al: A genome wide search for susceptibility loci in three European malignant hyperthermia pedigrees. *Hum Mol Genet* 6:953, 1997.
8. Sudbrak R, Procaccio V, Klausnitzer M, et al: Mapping of a further malignant hyperthermia susceptibility locus to chromosome 3q13.1. *Am J Hum Genet* 56:684, 1995.
9. Iles DE, Lehmann-Horn F, Scherer SW, et al: Localization of the gene encoding the $\alpha 2/\delta$-subunits of the L-type voltage-dependent calcium channel to chromosome 7q and analysis of the segregation of flanking markers in malignant hyperthermia susceptible families. *Hum Mol Genet* 3:969, 1994.
10. Levitt RC, Olckers A, Meyers S, et al: Evidence for the localization of a malignant hyperthermia susceptibility locus (MHS2) to chromosome 17q. *Genomics* 14:562, 1992.
11. Bendixen D, Skovgaard LT, Ording H: Analysis of anaesthesia in patients suspected to be susceptible to malignant hyperthermia before diagnostic in vitro contracture test. *Acta Anaesthesiol Scand* 41:480, 1997.
12. Hartmann S, Otten W, Kratzmair M, et al: Influences of breed, sex, and susceptibility to malignant hyperthermia on lipid composition of skeletal muscle and adipose tissue in swine. *Am J Vet Res* 58:738, 1997.
13. Iaizzo PA, Kehler CH, Carr RJ, et al: Prior hypothermia attenuates malignant hyperthermia in susceptible swine. *Anesth Analg* 82:803, 1996.
14. Dantrolene sodium approved for malignant hyperthermia. *FDA Drug Bull* 9:27, 1979.
15. Schwartz L, Rockoff MA, Koka V: Masseter spasm with anesthesia: incidence and implications. *Anesthesiology* 61:772, 1984.
16. Pryn SJ, van der Spek AFL: Comparative pharmacology of succinylcholine on jaw, eye and tibialis muscle [abstract]. *Anesthesiology* 73:A59, 1990.

17. Larach MG: Standardization of the caffeine halothane muscle contracture test. *Anesth Analg* 69:511, 1989.
18. Loke J, MacLennan DH: Bayesian modeling of muscle biopsy contracture testing for malignant hyperthermia hyperthermia susceptibility. *Anesthesiology* 88:589, 1998.
19. Oka S, Igarashi Y, Takagi A, et al: Malignant hyperthermia and Duchenne muscular dystrophy: a case report. *Can Anaesth Soc J* 29:627, 1982.
20. Brownell AKW, Paasuke RT, Elash A, et al: Malignant hyperthermia in Duchenne muscular dystrophy. *Anesthesiology* 58:180, 1983.
21. Kelfer HM, Singer WD, Reynolds RN: Malignant hyperthermia in a child with Duchenne muscular dystrophy. *Pediatrics* 71:118, 1983.
22. Wang JM, Stanley TH: Duchenne muscular dystrophy and malignant hyperthermia—two case reports. *Can Anaesth Soc J* 33:492, 1986.
23. Larach M, Rosenberg H, Gronert GA, Allen GC: Hyperkalemic cardiac arrest during anesthesia in infants and children with occult myopathies. *Clin Pediatr* 36:9, 1997.
24. Karan SM, Crowl F, Muldoon SM: Malignant hyperthermia masked by capnographic monitoring. *Anesth Analg* 78:590, 1994.
25. Antognini JF: Creatine kinase alterations after acute malignant hyperthermia episodes and common surgical procedures. *Anesth Analg* 81:1039, 1995.
26. Musley SK, Beebe DS, Komanduri V, et al: Hemodynamic and metabolic manifestations of acute endotoxin infusion in pigs with and without the malignant hyperthermia mutation. *Anesthesiology* 91:833, 1999.
27. Shailesh Kumar MV, Carr RJ, Komanduri V, et al: Differential diagnosis of thyroid crisis and malignant hyperthermia in an anesthetized porcine model. *Endocr Res* 25:87, 1999.
28. Dunford J: Fatal ascending tonic-clonic seizure syndrome. *Ann Emerg Med* 32:624, 1998.
29. Kotani N, Kushikata T, Matsukawa T, et al: A rapid increase in foot tissue temperature predicts cardiovascular collapse during anaphylactic and anaphylactiod reactions. *Anesthesiology* 87:559, 1997.
30. Bhattacharyya KB, Basu N, Ray TN, Maity B: Profile of electrocardiographic changes in Duchenne muscular dystrophy. *J Indian Med Assoc* 95:40, 1997.
31. Heymsfield SB, McNish T, Perkins JV, Felner JM: Sequence of cardiac changes in Duchenne muscular dystrophy. *Am Heart J* 95:283, 1978.
32. King JO, Denborough MA: Anesthetic-induced malignant hyperthermia in children. *J Pediatr* 83:37, 1973.
33. Storella RJ, Keykhah MM, Rosenberg H: Halothane and temperature interact to increase succinylcholine-induced jaw contracture in the rat. *Anesthesiology* 79:1261, 1993.
34. Van der Spek AFL, Fang WB, Ashton-Miller JA, et al: The effects of succinylcholine on mouth opening. *Anesthesiology* 67:459, 1987.
35. Van der Spek AFL, Fang WB, Ashton-Miller JA, et al: Increased masticatory muscle stiffness during limb muscle flaccidity associated with succinylcholine administration. *Anesthesiology* 69:11, 1988.
36. Engel AG, Yamamoto M, Fischbeck KH: Dystrophinopathies. In *Myology, Basic and Clinical*, 2nd ed. Engel AG, Franzini-Armstrong C, eds. New York, McGraw-Hill, 1994, p 1143.
37. Rubin AS, Zablocki AD: Hyperkalemia, verapamil and dantrolene. *Anesthesiology* 66:246, 1987.
38. Saltzman LS, Kates RA, Corke BC, et al: Hyperkalemia and cardiovascular collapse in after verapamil and dantrolene administration in swine. *Anesth Analg* 63:473, 1984.
39. San Juan AC, Wong KC, Port JD: Hyperkalemia after dantrolene and verapamil-dantrolene administration in dogs. *Anesth Analg* 67:759, 1988.
40. Lynch C, Durbin CG, Fisher NA, et al: Effects of dantrolene and verapamil on atrioventricular conduction and cardiovascular performance in dogs. *Anesth Analg* 65:252, 1986.

41. Allen GC, Larach MG, Kunselman AR: The sensitivity and specificity of the caffeine-halothane contracture test: a report from the North American Malignant Hyperthermia Registry. *Anesthesiology* 88:579, 1998.
42. Larach MG, Landis JR, Bunn JS, Diaz M: The North American Malignant Hyperthermia Registry: prediction of malignant hyperthermia susceptibility in low-risk subjects. *Anesthesiology* 76:16, 1992.
43. Brandom BW, Gronert GA: Malignant hyperthermia. *Smith's Anesthesia for Infants and Children,* 6th ed. Motoyama EK, Davis PJ, eds. New York, Mosby-Year Book, 1996, p 816.
44. Larach MG, Localio AR, Allen GC, et al: A clinical grading scale to predict malignant hyperthermia susceptibility. *Anesthesiology* 80:771, 1994.
45. Beebe JJ, Sessler DI: Preparation of anesthesia machines for patients susceptible to malignant hyperthermia. *Anesthesiology* 69:395, 1988.
46. McGraw TT, Keon TP: Malignant hyperthermia and the clean machine. *Can Anaesth J* 36:530, 1989.
47. Ritchie PA, Cheshire MA, Pearce NH: Decontamination of halothane from anaesthesia machines achieved by flushing with oxygen. *Br J Anaesth* 60:859, 1988.
48. Heiman-Patterson TD, Martino C, Rosenberg H, et al: Malignant hyperthermia in myotonia congenita. *Neurology* 38:810, 1988.
49. Heiman-Patterson TD, Natter HM, Rosenberg H, Tahmoush AJ: Malignant hyperthermia susceptibility in X-linked muscle dystrophies. *Pediatr Neurosci* 2:356, 1986.
50. Gronert GA, Fowler W, Cardinet GH III, et al: Absence of malignant hyperthermia contractures in Becker–Duchenne dystrophy at age 2. *Muscle Nerve* 15:52, 1992.
51. Mader N, Gilly H, Bottner RE: Dystrophin deficient muscle is not prone to MH susceptibility: an in vitro study. *Br J Anaesth* 79:125, 1997.

APPENDIX: EMERGENCY MANAGEMENT OF MH AND MH-LIKE SITUATIONS

Diagnosis

Signs of MH	Sudden/unexpected cardiac arrest in young patients	Trismus or masseter spasm with succinylcholine
Increased EtCO$_2$ Trunk or limb rigidity Masseter spasm or trismus Tachycardia/tachypnea Increased temperature (late sign) Acidosis	Presume hyperkalemia and initiate treatment* Usually secondary to occult myopathy (e.g., muscular dystrophy) Measure CK, myoglobin, and ABGs until normalized Consider dantrolene Resuscitation may be difficult and prolonged	Early sign of MH in many patients If limb muscle is rigid, begin treatment with dantrolene For emergent procedures, continue with nontriggering agents; consider dantrolene Follow CK and urine myoglobin ≥36 h

ABG, arterial blood gas; CK, creatine kinase; EtCO$_2$, end-tidal carbon dioxide.
*See point 7 in Acute-Phase Treatment to follow.

Acute-Phase Treatment

1. *Notify surgeon;* **get help; get dantrolene**
   Discontinue volatile agents and succinylcholine
   Hyperventilate with 100% oxygen at flows ≥10 L/min
   Halt the procedure as soon as possible; if emergent, use nontriggers
2. *Dantrolene 2.5 mg/kg with rapid IV*
   Repeat until there is control of the signs of MH
   Sometimes >10 mg/kg is necessary
   Dissolve 20 mg in each vial with at least 60 mL **sterile distilled water** for injection
   The crystals also contain NaOH for a pH of 9, mannitol 3 g
3. *Bicarbonate for metabolic acidosis*
   1–2 meq/kg if blood gas values are not yet available
4. *Cool the patient with core temperature >39°C with cold saline IV, surface, open body cavities, stomach, bladder, or rectum*
   Avoid excess cooling to prevent drift <36°C
5. *Dysrhythmias usually respond to treatment of acidosis and hyperkalemia*
   Use standard drug therapy **except calcium channel blockers that may cause hyperkalemia or cardiac arrest in the presence of dantrolene sodium**
6. *Hyperkalemia: Rx hyperventilation, bicarbonate, glucose/insulin, calcium*
   10 U regular insulin and 50 mL 50% glucose (adult)
   or
   0.15 U/kg insulin and 1 mL/kg 50% glucose (pediatric)
   Calcium chloride 10 mg/kg or calcium gluconate 10–50 mg/kg for life-threatening hyperkalemia
7. *Follow EtCO$_2$, blood gases, electrolytes, CK, core temperature, urine output and color, coagulation factors*
   Venous blood gas (e.g., femoral vein) values may document hypermetabolism better than arterial values
   Central venous or pulmonary arterial monitoring, as needed

CK, creatine kinase; EtCO$_2$, end-tidal carbon dioxide; IV, intravenously.

Post Acute Phase

Observe the patient in an intensive care unit ≥36 h
Dantrolene 1 mg/kg q 4–6 h for 24–48 h, depending on recovery phase
*Follow vital signs and laboratory results**
   Frequent ABG
   CK every 6–8 h
Counsel the patient and family regarding MH and further precautions. Refer them to MHAUS, fill out and send in the AMRA and send a letter to the patient and the patient's physician. Refer patient to the nearest biopsy center for follow-up

---

ABG, arterial blood gas; AMRA, Adverse Metabolic Reaction to Anesthesia Report; CK, creatine kinase; MHAUS, Malignant Hyperthermia Association of the United States.
*See point 6 in Acute-Phase Treatment table.

22 Monitoring and Discharge Criteria From the Recovery Room

Denise Joffe, MD

The recovery room, or postanesthesia care unit (PACU), is a vital component of the pediatric operating room complex. Many of the successes and failures of pediatric anesthesia are directly attributable to the care and course of action taken during the recovery period. It is unfortunate that many anesthesiologists tend to defer a considerable portion of this care and decision-making to others. This chapter addresses those issues important to the everyday care of the immediate postoperative child.

The course of the patient in the PACU of most hospitals depends on whether the patient is an inpatient or outpatient. Most pediatric procedures are performed on outpatients (>70%) and in many institutions patients are monitored in two phases during their postanesthetic course. The first, called phase 1, is the initial recovery period when patients are first brought from the operating room. During this phase of recovery, patients regain consciousness, they regain their protective airway reflexes, and their vital signs should return to within about 20% to 40% of baseline; in short, they "wake up." These patients are in the acute phase of recovery when the nurse-to-patient ratio is highest and the monitoring is most intense. The second phase is where patients recover to the point of street readiness.[1] Patients regain their coordination, and an absence of severe pain, nausea, or vomiting is assured. They or their family receive information about their postoperative surgical and anesthetic course. This stage is usually slightly more prolonged but patients require less observation from the medical staff.

The definition of street readiness depends on the institution. For example, some centers require that all outpatients are able to drink and void before discharge, whereas others do not. The decision seems mostly historical and, although it may be appropriate to ensure that some patients can drink and void before discharge (e.g., patients who have far to travel), recent literature suggests that for most outpatients this stringent policy is unnecessary (see Factors Affecting Discharge). The Joint Commission of Accreditation of Hospitals (JCAH) has established certain policies regarding patient discharge from hospitals, such as: patients require an examination before discharge, they require escorts home, and they must have written postoperative instructions and a contact for questions, but JCAH does not set the criteria for discharge.[1] It has, however, endorsed Aldrete's discharge criteria (see below).[2] Although the criteria for discharge home from the PACU are evolving, in general they are chosen to enable the rapid and safe discharge of patients with the least likelihood of readmission.

Inpatients usually are sent to their rooms after fulfilling criteria for discharge from the phase 1 unit.

Institutions without two separate facilities for the postanesthetic care of their ambulatory patients often treat them in a fashion similar to that described above by organizing the unit into separate sections. An area of the single PACU would admit "sleepy" patients from the operating room and the patients would be moved to a different part of the unit as they recover. Some variation of these recovery room arrangements enables most institutions to handle the multiple ways that inpatient and outpatient surgical services might be organized.

Some PACUs have been set up to keep patients for up to 23 h without "formally" admitting them to the hospital. The phase 2 unit would keep those patients who require minimal nursing care but are not ready for discharge; e.g., patients suffering from postoperative nausea and vomiting or from pain requiring parenteral narcotics.

DIFFERENCES BETWEEN THE PEDIATRIC AND ADULT PACU

Apart from the obvious difference in noise level between adult and pediatric units, there are several other differences which deserve comment. The rapid and pleasant recovery of the pediatric patient depends very much on the presence of the family. As soon as the patient is awake and deemed stable enough for visitors, the parents or a family member should be allowed to join the child. This is especially true for young children who may wake up to strange faces and unfamiliar surroundings. Further, the parents are often the only people who understand the early language of their child!

Assessing pain in young children (especially those younger than 6 years) also can be more challenging. Behavioral features are used to interpret pain levels in the preverbal child. Factors such as facial grimacing, motor movement, sweating, crying, and ease of comforting are important but are indirect and may be affected by conditions other than pain.[3] Aberrations in vital signs may not be as useful in the very young because their normal heart rates are high and their blood pressures and heart rates can be affected by multiple factors unrelated to pain such as fear, anxiety, medications, and fever.

Several different scales are used to assess pain in the verbal child, although these scales have a degree of inaccuracy compared with assessments in older pediatric patients and adults.[4] Younger children also may minimize their pain because they fear having to be administered "medicine."

Children often have graphic imaginations. In the case of combined adult and pediatric PACUs, it often helps to have an area that is child-friendly to distract the child's attention from the surrounding commotion.

MONITORING IN THE RECOVERY ROOM

The American Society of Anesthesiologists guidelines on the standards for PACU care suggest that patients should be transferred to the PACU from the location where they were anesthetized, with equipment and monitoring appropriate for the patient's condition.[5] Studies have shown that up to 28% of healthy pediatric patients desaturate to less than 90% during the short transport from the operating room to the PACU.[6,7] The risk increases with younger age (neonates and infants have less pulmonary reserve and higher oxygen consumption than older children do) and longer transport times. Common sense should prevail when deciding whether oxygen is necessary and what monitoring is required for transport but a conservative policy is suggested. Factors such as the patient's age, coexisting diseases, present illness, intraoperative course, and the distance to the PACU should be considered.

On admission to the PACU, patients should have their vital signs recorded. This includes blood pressure, heart rate, temperature, and oxygen saturation. An aberration in any of these vital signs may prompt further measurements, but in the absence of changes the healthy pediatric patient can be observed with a pulse oximeter. In many institutions, blood pressure measurements are attempted every 15 min if the patient cooperates, and are repeated before discharge. The pulse oximeter is usually left on for the duration of the patient's stay or until the patient no longer tolerates the probe. If, after that, the patient is still thought to require saturation checks, then intermittent monitoring can be used.

Patients who cooperate should have blow-by oxygen. If necessary, a more regulated quantity of oxygen can be administered by face mask. In fact, despite the "diluted" oxygen concentrations delivered with blow-by systems, children generally have higher saturations compared with a face mask because children do not tolerate the mask well.[8] Suprisingly, it has been shown that the degree of wakefulness as measured by a higher postanesthesia recovery score does not always correlate with acceptable saturations.[9] Changes in functional residual capacity,[10] diffusion hypoxia,[11,12] and alterations in baroreceptor function[13] contribute to desaturations that are commonly seen in postoperative patients. In addition, pediatric patients have other physiologic factors related to their cardiorespiratory systems that may contribute to postoperative hypoxia. Pediatric patients have high metabolic rates, increased closing volumes, smaller caliber airways whose resistance increases exponentially with decreasing size, compliant chest walls, and fatigue-prone diaphragms, all of which contribute to a decrease in pulmonary reserve compared with adults. Most studies show that desaturation in the PACU occurs in up to 50% of patients.[14–16] Xue et al. studied more than 1000 healthy patients undergoing superficial plastic surgery procedures and found that up to 30% of pediatric patients develope hypoxia in the PACU.[15] Patients at highest risk of desaturating were younger than 3 years. Consistent saturations over 90% occurred within 1 h of surgery, although saturations were below preoperative values for as long as 3 h.[14,15] These studies made no attempt to use anesthetic agents with short half-lives and this may have some effect on the incidence of desaturation compared with medications with longer-lasting effects.

The use of electrocardiography (EKG) can be safely limited to a subgroup of pediatric patients because dysrhythmias are not a common problem in healthy children. A patient with a history of dysrhythmias should be monitored continuously, and patients with heart disease or previously repaired congenital heart disease also should be monitored, except if they have had repair of uncomplicated heart lesions. Uncomplicated heart lesions include but are not limited to atrial and ventricular septal defect repairs and ligation of patent ductus arteriosus. If a cardiologist or cardiac surgeon is following a patient, then it seems prudent to consider the heart disease "complicated" unless details of the cardiac history dictate otherwise. It is not clear how long these patients should be observed in the PACU, especially if they had uncomplicated intraoperative courses, but it is probably judicious to keep them monitored until they no longer cooperate or until they are ready for discharge to phase 2.

Other patients who occasionally may require EKG monitoring include patients receiving therapy known to cause dysrhythmias such as inhaled medications for the treatment of asthma or post-intubation croup. The routine use of these medications does not warrant EKG monitoring but at times patients become very tachycardic, in which case monitoring may be useful.

DISCHARGE CRITERIA

Recovery Room Scores

Although several different discharge criteria exist, the Aldrete criteria are the "gold standard." Aldrete was the first to publish a functional scoring system to assess a patient's readiness for discharge from the PACU to the floor, and it has been found to be an accurate indicator of discharge eligibility.[17] When pulse oximetry became standard, Aldrete modified the scoring system to include a measure of the patient's saturation instead of using the patient's color as an estimate of oxygenation.[2,18] More recently, Aldrete proposed a further modification of the score for use specifically in the ambulatory population that considers factors thought to be necessary to ensure a safe discharge home.[19]

Fast-tracking (see below) has generated a scoring system that is used intraoperatively to assess readiness for bypassing the phase 1 PACU.[20] All discharge criteria require that the patient's cardiorespiratory status be within approximately 10% to 20% of baseline state and the neurologic condition return to preoperative levels. In addition, ambulatory discharge criteria have to ensure that patients are not in excessive pain or have nausea or vomiting that will lead to dehydration. Further, the surgical procedure should not endanger the patient because of excess bleeding or other complications.

Other ambulatory scoring systems include the postanesthetic discharge scoring system (PADDS)[21] and modified PADDS[22] and multiple clinical recovery scores (CRS) devised by various institutions.[1,21,23] These criteria are similar (Table 22-1) and allow for the safe discharge of patients to the ward (modified Aldrete[2]) or home ("ambulatory" Aldrete, PADDS, and CRS). It has been demonstrated that discharge classifications that assign numerical values to criteria rather than a subjective assessment of criteria have improved interobserver variability and thus are probably more accurate.[21] Despite the development of criteria that are specifically designed for the ambulatory population, the modified Aldrete criteria (not ambulatory criteria) continue to be the most commonly used to discharge day surgery patients.[24]

Fast-Tracking

A recent trend in adult ambulatory anesthesia is fast-tracking patients so that they bypass the phase 1 PACU altogether. Presumably, the decrease in the number of nurses required for a phase 2 PACU translates into cost savings. A recent computer analysis of the potential savings from fast-tracking adults suggests that this assumption may be valid only under certain circumstances. Factors such as how nurses are compensated, the number of operating rooms running concurrently, and the number of patients receiving general anesthesia are the major economic determinants of the cost of running the units.[25]

To succeed in fast-tracking patients, the patient must meet phase 1 discharge criteria in the operating room. Recently, fast-track discharge criteria have been developed that are used intraoperatively to assess these patients.[20] They include not only the usual phase 1 discharge criteria but also an assessment of the patient's pain and nausea or vomiting.[20] Fast-tracking will not be successful if patients require additional intensive nursing care in the PACU.

Although there are few, if any, published studies of fast-tracking pediatric patients, they are likely to be forthcoming. However, there are differences that may make fast-tracking more challenging in the pediatric population. First, almost all procedures require a general anesthetic in children, whereas

TABLE 22–1 Comparison of the Criteria Used to Assess Eligibility for Discharge With Different Scoring Systems

Modified Aldrete[†]	Score	Ambulatory Aldrete[‡]	Score	PADDS[§]	Score	Modified PADDS[¶]	Score	CDC[¶]
Activity		*Activity*		*Vital signs*		*Vital signs*		*Vital signs*
Able to move four extremities voluntarily or on command	2	Able to move four extremities voluntarily or on command	2	Within 20% of preoperative value	2	Within 20% of preoperative value	2	Stable
Able to move two extremities voluntarily or on command	1	Able to move two extremities voluntarily or on command	1	20–40% of preoperative value	1	20–40% of preoperative value	1	
Unable to move extremities voluntarily or on command	0	Unable to move extremities voluntarily or on command	0	40% of preoperative value	0	40% of preoperative value	0	
Respiration		*Respiration*		*Ambulation and mental status*		*Ambulation*		*Ambulation*
Able to breathe deeply and cough freely	2	Able to breathe deeply and cough freely	2	Oriented ×3 has a steady gait	2	Steady gait/no dizziness	2	Steady gait
Dyspnea or limited breathing	1	Dyspnea or limited breathing	1	Oriented ×3 or has a steady gait	1	With assistance	1	
Apneic	0	Apneic	0	Neither	0	None/dizziness	0	
Circulation		*Circulation*		*Pain or nausea/vomiting*		*Nausea/vomiting*		*Nausea/vomiting*
BP ± 20% of preanesthetic level	2	BP ± 20% of preanesthetic level	2	Minimal	2	Minimal	2	No nausea or vomiting
BP ± 20 to 49% of preanesthetic level	1	BP ± 20 to 49% of preanesthetic level	1	Moderate	1	Moderate	1	
BP ± 50% of preanesthetic level	0	BP ± 50% of preanesthetic level	0	Severe	0	Severe	0	

(*continued*)

Consciousness		*Consciousness*		*Surgical bleeding*		*Consciousness*
Fully awake	2	Fully awake	2	Minimal	2	Alert and oriented
Arousable on calling	1	Arousable on calling	1	Moderate	1	
Not responding	0	Not responding	0	Severe	0	*Surgical bleeding*
O₂ saturation		*O₂ saturation*		*Intake and output*		No significant bleeding
>92% on room air	2	>92% on room air	2	Has had PO fluids and voided	2	
Supplemental O₂ required to maintain SpO₂ >90%	1	Supplemental O₂ required to maintain SpO₂ >90%	1	Has had PO fluids or voided	1	
Decreased SpO₂ with supplemental O₂	0	Decreased SpO₂ with supplemental O₂	0	Neither	0	
		Dressing				
		Dry and clean	2			
		Wet but marked and not increasing	1			
		Growing area of wetness	0			
		Pain				
		Pain free	2	*Pain*		
		Mild pain handled by oral medicine	1	Minimal	2	
				Moderate	1	
		Severe pain requiring parenteral medication	0	Severe	0	
				Surgical bleeding		
				Minimal	2	
				Moderate	1	
				Several	0	

(*continued*)

TABLE 22-1 Comparison of the Criteria Used to Assess Eligibility for Discharge With Different Scoring Systems (continued)

Modified Aldrete[†]	Score	Ambulatory Aldrete[‡]	Score	PADDS[§]	Score	Modified PADDS[¶]	Score	CDC[¶]
		Ambulation						
		Able to stand up and walk straight*	2					
		Vertigo when erect	1					
		Dizziness when supine	0					
		Fast feeding						
		Able to drink fluids	2					
		Nauseated	1					
		Nausea/vomiting	0					
		Urine						
		Has voided	2					
		Unable to void but comfortable	1					
		Unable to void and uncomfortable	0					
Total score	10		20				10	N/A
Total score acceptable for discharge	9		18				9	9

BP, blood pressure; CDC, clinical discharge criteria, which differ across institutions and are subjective (no score); N/A, not available; PADDS, postanesthesia discharge scoring system; modified PADDS, eliminates the need to assess oral intake and urine output; PO, per os (by mouth).

*Oxygen saturation.

[†]*Source*: Xue FS, Huang YG, Luo LK, et al: Observation of early postoperative hypoxaemia in children undergoing elective plastic surgery. *Paediatr Anaesth* 6:21, 1996.

[‡]*Source*: Chung F: Are discharge criteria changing? *J Clin Anesth* 5:64S, 1992.

[§]*Source*: Aldrete JA: Modification to the postanesthesia score for use in ambulatory surgery. *J Perianesth Nurs* 13:148, 1998.

[¶]*Source*: White PF, Song D: New criteria for fast-tracking after outpatient anesthesia: A comparison with the modified Aldrete's scoring system. *Anesth Analg* 88:1069, 1999.

many procedures in the adult population can be performed with a lighter plane of anesthesia using "conscious sedation" and regional anesthesia. Although general anesthesia does not preclude fast-tracking in adults, patients who require sedation and not general anesthesia make up a large percentage of those who are eligible for fast-tracking. This latter group of patients is easier to fast-track and requires less skill on the part of the anesthesiologist. Second, a part of the postanesthetic care of very young patients involves a component of observation ("babysitting"). When these children leave the operating room wide awake, they require diligent observation and comforting, at least until they are reunited with their families.

This is particularly pertinent with some of the more popular agents that are used to fast-track patients. For example, studies have associated the use of desflurane and sevoflurane[26–28] with early awakening and recovery of patients, although the incidence of agitation is very high.[29] The incidence of agitation seems to be inversely related to the degree of early awakening. Consequently, these pediatric patients are likely to require a significant amount of nursing care. It should be appreciated that the incidence of emergence delirium has always been high in children, with an incidence of 20%, or greater, commonly acknowledged. Remarkably, this incidence has change very little over the past 20 years despite the introduction of newer inhalational agents. Although some studies have suggested that the incidence of emergence delirium is higher with sevoflurane than with halothane, the time to recovery and discharge are consistently shorter with sevoflurane.[26–29]

Some clinicians are attempting to address the issue of emergence delirium by determining a dose of narcotic or anxiolytic that will decrease the risk without affecting the favorable early awakening characteristics of the inhalational agent. A preliminary report examining the use of fentanyl during tonsillectomy suggested that the cumulative dose is about 2.5 µg/kg.[30] It is not clear whether the addition of narcotics will affect other aspects of the patient's recovery, such as nausea and vomiting. Further, even though patients were found to awaken and recover more quickly with the use of desflurane and sevoflurane than with the use of halothane, these agents have not decreased discharge times. This is likely the result of a combination of factors such as paperwork that has to be completed, rigid discharge criteria that include the requirement to drink and void, or medication given in the postoperative period that cause sedation and delayed discharge.[28,29]

In the adult patient, the bispectral index monitor enables more controlled titration of medications, which facilitates early awakening, and has been credited with some of the success of fast-tracking in adults.[31,32] The use of this monitor may be forthcoming in children but its accuracy has not been validated in this population.

FACTORS AFFECTING DISCHARGE

Vomiting

Severe nausea or vomiting occurs in up to 9% to 50% of pediatric patients and is the most significant factor contributing to prolonged stay in the PACU or unanticipated admission to the hospital.[33–35] The causes are multifactorial and include the age of the patient (highest in those 3 to 5 years old), the type of procedure (highest in patients undergoing strabismus surgery, middle ear surgery, tonsillectomy, and orchidopexy repair), and the anesthetic technique (lower in patients who have not received narcotics[36,37] and possibly lower in those who have not received nitrous oxide[38] or reversal agents[39]). Some anesthetic agents are also thought to lower the risk of nausea and vomiting and include propofol[34] and the antiemetics metoclopramide, droperidol, and odansetron. Although propofol is thought to have an intrinsic antiemetic effect, studies have not supported the use of small doses of propofol as an antiemetic.[40] Most recently, there is growing evidence that the use of steroids, such as decadron, can be useful as a treatment for nausea and vomiting. Although dose–response curves have not been thoroughly studied at this time, the initial results are encouraging, especially given the lack of adverse side effects noted to date.

There are multiple drug and dosage recommendations for antiemetic medication. Although controversial, prophylactic administration of antiemetics is recommended only for procedures associated with a very high risk of postoperative nausea and vomiting because of their variable effectiveness, side-effects, and cost.[41] Other factors that may help decrease the incidence of nausea and vomiting include providing adequate analgesia with the use of nonnarcotic techniques such as regional anesthesia and nonsteroidal anti-inflammatory medication.[37] One key factor in discharging patients, especially patients who are experiencing some nausea, is ensuring adequate hydration. This may require a bolus of fluid before removing intravenous access. It is also felt by many anesthesiologists that mandating oral fluid intake in patients who do not want to drink actually increases the risk of vomiting.[42,43]

Voiding

Fisher et al.[44] studied young patients having hernia or orchidopexy repairs and found that 92% of pediatric patients void by 8 h postoperatively. All patients in that study voided at home without complications regardless of the anesthetic technique administered. In addition, the use of a regional anesthetic technique (caudal, epidural, or ilioinguinal or iliohypogastric nerve block) was irrelevant. A negligible risk of urinary retention has been corroborated by others who also found that regional anesthesia has no effect on the timing to first void.[45,46] Thus, there seems to be no compelling reason to require that most patients void before discharge, except if there are confounding factors such as instrumentation of the urethra. Parents whose children are discharged without having voided should be advised to contact the surgeon or anesthesiologist if their child has not voided by 8 h postoperatively.

Premature Infants

The option of performing ambulatory surgery on neonates and very young infants depends on the patient's history, postconceptual age (PCA), the presence of anemia, and general medical condition. The risk to these infants is the development of postoperative apnea, which presumably is due to abnormalities in their respiratory drives, and is exacerbated by anesthetics except "pure" neuroaxial anesthesia, which is associated with a smaller risk of apnea.[47] Most episodes of apnea occur in the first postoperative hour,[48] although one-third of infants may have apneic episodes 2 to 12 h postoperatively.[49] However, apneic episodes requiring intubation almost always occur within the first 3 h.[48] Patients younger than 44 weeks PCA are thought to be at highest risk for the development of postoperative apnea,[49] although studies have not defined an age limit for monitoring.[50] Most facilities recommend postoperative apnea monitoring for 12 to 24 h in premature infants who are younger than 44 to 60 weeks PCA[49,50] and in some full-term infants (see Chapter 9). In contrast to the PADDS and CRS criteria, Melone et al.[48] studied 124 patients with histories of prematurity, PCAs of 34 to 59 weeks, and various medical problems (some serious and consistent with their histories of prematurity) who underwent outpatient herniorrhaphy repair without mortality and with minimal morbidity. Although some of their patients did develop apnea (one was at home with an apnea monitor), patients responded with minimal stimulation. The investigators believed that their results were in large part attributable to the absence of the use of narcotics and muscle relaxants. However, their results have not been duplicated and probably few anesthesiologists would be willing to provide outpatient anesthesia to this patient population.

Ear, Nose, and Throat Procedures

Tonsillectomy

Although outpatient tonsillectomy and adenoidectomy are now routinely performed at most centers in the United States and Canada, it was not long ago that the subject created a significant amount of controversy.[51] The issue relates to the high incidence of morbidity, especially postoperative nausea and vomiting (up to 62%)[52] and pain (up to 56%).[36] There is also a small risk of postoperative hemorrhage (<1.5%).[53] There have been multiple studies confirming the feasibility of performing the procedure on an ambulatory basis, with a few caveats.[54] Some investigators believe that the procedure should be offered on an ambulatory basis only to healthy children. They claim that patients with pre-existing medical problems tend to develop complications.[55] Patients who have documented sleep apnea should be admitted. Sleep studies often are not performed and decisions about admission often are made based on the patient's history. Symptoms compatible with sleep apnea such as loud snoring, daytime somnolence, and frequent nighttime arousal may dictate a prolonged PACU stay (23 h) or an admission.[56] A young age (<3 years old) is also a relative contraindication to outpatient tonsillectomy because the indication for the procedure is often related to obstructive symptoms.[55,56] However, if patients are carefully selected, some researchers even advocate day surgery for these young patients.[55,57,58]

Many anesthesiologists administer prophylactic antiemetics to this high-risk group. In addition, studies have shown that dexamethasone administered in doses as high as 1 mg/kg up to 25 mg can decrease late symptoms (the first 24 h after discharge) of nausea and vomiting from 62% to 24% and decrease the incidence of return visits to the hospital for treatment of nausea, vomiting, and dehydration from 8% to 0%.[52]

Although pain is not as common a problem as nausea and vomiting, it can be severe and protracted (7 days). Dexamethasone may offer some pain relief in addition to its antiemetic effects.

Postoperative tonsillectomy bleeding is generally classified as primary postoperative hemorrhage (within 24 h) or secondary postoperative hemorrhage (from 24 h to 10 days postoperatively). The shortest possible stay for an outpatient should include the time necessary to identify patients who will develop a posttonsillectomy bleed, and which as a rule occur within 75 min of arrival in the PACU.[53] It is common practice to ensure the absence of postoperative complications such as bleeding, nausea and vomiting, dehydration, and fever and then discharge these patients home 2 to 6 h postoperatively.[55,59]

Myringotomy and Pressure Equalization Tubes

Bilateral myringotomy and pressure equalization tube placement (PET), or BM&T as it is sometimes called, is one of the most common pediatric procedures performed. It is considered to be a simple, fast, and benign procedure, and in most cases it is. However, an inconsolable child often complicates the postoperative course. The causes are probably multifactorial and may include inadequate pain relief, emergence agitation, fear, and separation anxiety. Analgesic requirements are often underestimated. Studies have shown that oral acetaminophen 10 mg/kg and codeine 1 mg/kg provide good analgesia,[60] whereas acetaminophen 10 to 15 mg/kg orally given preoperatively or the same dose given intraoperatively by the rectal route do not provide adequate analgesia.[60–62] Findings from studies using acetaminophen are limited because blood levels were not measured. It has been demonstrated that a one time rectal dose of 40 mg/kg is necessary to obtain adequate acetaminophen serum levels.[63]

Preoperative ibuprofen was not found to be more efficacious than placebo.[62] In patients having PET, ketorolac 1.0 mg/kg intravenously was shown to have variable effects on postoperative analgesic requirements, and even in the best study at least one-third of patients required additional analgesia.[64–66] With ketorolac the tendency is to provide a short perioperative advantage as far as analgesia is concerned, but no difference in analgesic requirements after discharge. Davis et al. found that ketorolac decreases the incidence of emergence agitation after PET insertion in patients receiving sevoflurane and halothane.[66] This may reflect the fact that some component of the agitation is the result of postoperative pain. Disadvantages of ketorolac administration are the requirement for intravenous access, the cost of the medication, and the questionable efficacy.

Choice of Anesthetic

Studies have associated anesthetic agents that have short half-lives or high blood gas solubilities such as remifentanyl, desflurane, sevoflurane, and propofol[67,68] with a faster early awakening and recovery but, for a variety of reasons previously mentioned, found no change in time to discharge home compared with other agents.[27,28]

Regional Anesthesia and Pain Management

For a multitude of reasons regional anesthesia is very commonly used in addition to general anesthesia in the pediatric population. Factors such as multiple surgical procedures amenable to pain control with regional techniques, blocks that are usually easy to perform, and difficulty in interpreting pain scores in children increase the use of local anesthesia in this group. Even the instillation of local anesthesia into the wound has been shown to provide pain relief for up to 24 h.[69]

The timing of placement of caudal blocks (before or after the surgical procedure) has not been shown to affect the duration of analgesia or the time of patient discharge when used for short procedures such as hernia, orchidopexy, or hydrocelectomy repairs.[70] Bupivacaine 0.125% and bupivacaine 0.25% with or without epinephrine in doses from 0.5 to 1 mL/kg are the most commonly used agents and provide approximately 2 to 12[45,70] h of analgesia before oral medications are required. Bupivacaine 0.125% may offer some advantages over the higher concentration because it is associated with less motor effect without compromising the duration or quality of analgesia.[45]

Regional techniques including caudals and epidurals have not been shown to delay voiding but they may affect motor function. This probably should be considered in the older patient who may be offered an equally effective alternative technique compared with caudal or epidural analgesia. Of course, the older patient is less apt to be in the mood to "run around" but may be bothered by paresthesias. However, the use of ropivicaine may change that philosophy because it causes less of a motor block.[71] The caudal space is more difficult to access in older patients and, because epidural anesthesia is usually more demanding (time and technical expertise), other regional techniques may be more appropriate for the older patient having outpatient surgery.

Malignant Hyperthermia

A susceptibility to malignant hyperthermia is not considered a contraindication to outpatient surgery.[72] Authorities are recommending that patients be observed in the PACU for at least 4 h after surgery (see Chap. 21).[73] They should have regular temperature checks and probably should be monitored with an EKG and pulse oximeter, if tolerated. Otherwise, intermittent checks of vital signs suffice.

The Role of the Anesthesiologist

Most busy PACUs that serve a large volume of pediatric patients can run very efficiently with minimal intervention from the anesthesiologist. In 1990, Cohen et al.[35] reported the complication rate on close to 30,000 pediatric anesthetics performed between 1982 and 1987. They found that children are more likely than adults to experience problems in the perioperative period (35% vs. 17%), although fewer than 4% of healthy outpatient children experience serious side effects. In the postoperative period, these major problems were predominantly respiratory and included laryngospasm, bronchospasm, croup, and apnea. Neonatal patients were most at risk for serious complications, usually respiratory, although, in this age group, hypothermia was also a serious problem. Published reports of closed claims analysis support the findings that in pediatric patients morbidity and mortality in the operating rooms and PACUs are frequently the result of a respiratory complication.[74]

The study by Cohen et al. found that nausea, vomiting, and pain were the most common minor complications that required treatment.[35] In many centers, standing orders exist for the treatment of these problems. However, studies continue to find that pediatric patients are undermedicated for their pain and nausea.[36, 41,75] Fortunately, many pediatric patients have the benefit of regional analgesia. A large part of the etiology of inadequate analgesia and nausea may relate to the difficulty of assessing pain and nausea in young children. Therefore, it is unlikely that a more proactive role in the PACU by anesthesiologists would improve the situation. In the operating room, the use of regional anesthesia whenever possible would help decrease or eliminate pain as a factor. The prophylactic use of antiemetics is not always successful in treating postoperative nausea and vomiting. Overall, a 0.9% incidence of unanticipated admissions has been reported for ambulatory pediatric surgical patients and not all admissions are a result of anesthetic morbidity.[33]

CONCLUSION

Most pediatric surgical procedures can be done in the ambulatory surgical setting, and patients are discharged home from the PACU. Regardless of the multiple arrangements of surgical and anesthesia services in most hospitals and surgical centers, most PACUs are organized into two units. Patients are moved from a phase 1 acute unit, where they wake up, are stabilized, and have acute problems treated, to a phase 2 unit, where patients are prepared for discharge home.

Monitoring in the PACU often depends on the child's cooperation. On admission all vital signs should be recorded; subsequent measurements are often made only when abnormalities are being followed. Ideally, a pulse oximeter should be left on the patient until discharge.

Patient factors that may affect eligibility for discharge include pre-existing medical condition, PCA, the surgical procedure, and the distance of the trip home. Common sense should prevail when deciding eligibility for day surgery.

Nausea and vomiting continue to be the most important factors delaying or postponing discharge, and inadequate pain relief persists as a common complaint. However, in general, pediatric patients benefit from ambulatory surgery and most are readily discharged home without complication.

REFERENCES

1. Chung F: Discharge criteria-a new trend. *Can J Anaesth* 42:1056, 1995.
2. Aldrete JA: The post-anesthesia recovery score revisited [letter]. *J Clin Anesth* 7:89, 1995.
3. Johnston CC, Strada ME: Acute pain response in infants: a multidimensional description. *Pain* 24:373, 1986.
4. Ross DM, Ross SA: Childhood pain: the school-aged child's viewpoint. *Pain* 20:179, 1984.
5. *Standards for Postanesthesia Care* [amended]. American Society of Anesthesiologists, 1994.
6. Fossum SR, Knowles R: Perioperative oxygen saturation levels of pediatric patients. *J Postanesth Nurs* 10:313. 1995.
7. Chripko D, Bevan JC, Archer DP, et al: Decrease in arterial oxygen saturation in paediatric outpatients during transfer to the postanaesthetic recovery room. *Can J Anaesth* 36:128, 1989.
8. Amar D, Brodman LE, Winikoff SA, et al: An alternative oxygen delivery system for infants and children in the post-anaesthesia care unit. *Can J Anaesth* 38:49, 1991.
9. Soliman IE, Patel RI, Ehrenpreis MB, et al: Recovery scores do not correlate with postoperative hypoxemia in children. *Anesth Analg* 67:53, 1988.
10. Hedenstierna G, Strandberg A, Brismar B, et al: Functional residual capacity, thoracoabdominal dimensions, and central blood volume during general anesthesia with muscle paralysis and mechanical ventilation. *Anesthesiology* 62:247, 1985.
11. Einarsson S, Stenqvist O, Bengtsson A, et al: Nitrous oxide elimination and diffusion hypoxia during normo- and hypoventilation. *Br J Anaesth* 71:189, 1993.
12. Murphy IL, Splinter WM: The clinical significance of diffusion hypoxia in children. *Can J Anaesth* 37:S40, 1990.
13. Knill RL, Gelb AW: Ventilatory responses to hypoxia and hypercapnia during halothane sedation and anesthesia in man. *Anesthesiology* 49: 244, 1978.
14. Laycock GJ, McNicol LR: Hypoxaemia during recovery from anaesthesia—an audit of children after general anaesthesia for routine elective surgery. *Anaesthesia* 43:985, 1988.

15. Xue FS, Huang YG, Tong SY, et al: A comparative study of early postoperative hypoxemia in infants, children, and adults undergoing elective plastic surgery. *Anesth Analg* 83:709, 1996.
16. Xue FS, Huang YG, Luo LK, et al: Observation of early postoperative hypoxaemia in children undergoing elective plastic surgery. *Paediatr Anaesth* 6:21, 1996.
17. Aldrete JA, Kroulik D: A postanesthetic recovery score. *Anesth Analg* 49:924, 197.
18. Chung F: Are discharge criteria changing? *J Clin Anesth* 5:64S, 1992.
19. Aldrete JA: Modification to the postanesthesia score for use in ambulatory surgery. *J Perianesth Nurs* 13:148, 1998.
20. White PF, Song D: New criteria for fast-tracking after outpatient anesthesia: a comparison with the modified Aldrete's scoring system. *Anesth Analg* 88:1069, 1999.
21. Chung F, Chan VW, Ong D: A post-anesthetic discharge scoring system for home readiness after ambulatory surgery. *J Clin Anesth* 7:500, 1995.
22. Chung F, Chan VW, Ong D: Discharge criteria—a new trend. *Can J Anesth* 42:1056, 1995.
23. Patel RI: Discharge criteria and postanesthetic complications following pediatric ambulatory surgery. *J Postanesth Nurs* 86:1347, 1986.
24. Marshall SI, Chung F: Discharge criteria and complications after ambulatory surgery. *Anesth Analg* 88:508, 1999.
25. Dexter F, Macario A, Manberg PJ, et al: Computer simulation to determine how rapid anesthetic recovery protocols to decrease the time for emergence or increase the phase I postanesthesia care unit bypass rate affect staffing of an ambulatory surgery center. *Anesth Analg* 88:1053, 1999.
26. Lerman J, Davis PJ, Welborn LG, et al: Induction, recovery and safety characteristics of sevoflurane in children undergoing ambulatory surgery. A comparison with halothane. *Anesthesiology* 84:1332, 1996.
27. Song D, Joshi GP, White P: Fast-track eligibility after ambulatory anesthesia: a comparison of desflurane, sevoflurane, and propofol. *Anesth Analg* 86:267, 1998.
28. Welborn LG, Hannallah RS, Norden JM: Comparison of emergence and recovery characteristics of sevoflurane, desflurane, and halothane in pediatric ambulatory patients. *Anesth Analg* 83:917, 1996.
29. Davis PJ, Cohen IT, McGowan FX, et al: Recovery characteristics of desflurane versus halothane for maintenance of anesthesia in pediatric ambulatory patients. *Anesthesiology* 80:298, 1994.
30. Cohen IT, Hannallah R, Hummer K: The minimal effective dose of fentanyl to prevent emergence agitation following desflurane anesthesia in children [abstract]. *Anesth Analg* 88:S292, 1999.
31. Song D, Joshi GP, White PF: Titration of volatile anesthetics using bispectral index facilitates recovery after ambulatory anesthesia. *Anesthesiology* 87:842, 1997.
32. Song D, van Vlymen J, White P: Is the bispectral index useful in predicting fast-track eligibility after ambulatory anesthesia with propofol and desflurane? *Anesth Analg* 87:1245, 1998.
33. Patel RI, Hannallah RS: Anesthetic complications following pediatric ambulatory surgery: a 3-yr study. *Anesthesiology* 69:1009, 1988.
34. Ved SA, Walden TL, Montana J, et al: Vomiting and recovery after outpatient tonsillectomy and adenoidectomy in children. Comparison of four anesthetic techniques using nitrous oxide with halothane or propofol. *Anesthesiology* 85:4, 1996.
35. Cohen MM, Cameron CB, Duncan PG: Pediatric anesthesia morbidity and mortality in the perioperative period. *Anesth Analg* 70:160, 1990.
36. Kotiniemi LH, Ryhanen PT, Valanne J, et al: Postoperative symptoms at home following day-case surgery in children: a multicenter survey of 551 children. *Anaesthesia* 52:963, 1997.
37. Mendel HG, Guarnieri KM, Sundt LM, et al: The effects of ketorolac and fentanyl on postoperative vomiting and analgesic requirements in children undergoing strabismus surgery. *Anesth Analg* 80:1129, 1995.

38. Pandit UA, Malviya S, Lewis IH: Vomiting after outpatient tonsillectomy and adenoidectomy in children: the role of nitrous oxide. *Anesth Analg* 80:230, 1995.
39. Watcha MF, Safari FZ, McCulloch DA, et al: Effect of antagonism of mivacurium induced neuromuscular block on postoperative emesis in children. *Anesth Analg* 80:713, 1995
40. Zestos MM, Carr AS, McAuliffe G, et al: Subhypnotic propofol does not treat postoperative vomiting in children after adenotonsillectomy. *Can J Anaesth* 44:401, 1997.
41. Watcha MF, White PF: Post-operative nausea and vomiting: do they matter? *Eur J Anaesthesiol* 10 (suppl):18, 1995.
42. Schreiner MS, Nicolson S, Martin T, et al: Should children drink before discharge from day surgery? *Anesthesiology* 76:528, 1992.
43. Kearney R, Mack C, Entwistle L: Withholding oral fluids from children undergoing day surgery reduces vomiting. *Paediatr Anaesth* 8:331, 1998.
44. Fisher QA, McComiskey CM, Hill JL, et al: Postoperative voiding interval and duration of analgesia following peripheral or caudal nerve blocks in children. *Anesth Analg* 76:173, 1993.
45. Wolf AR, Valley RD, Fear DW, et al: Bupivacaine for caudal analgesia in infants and children: the optimal effective concentration. *Anesthesiology* 69:102, 1988.
46. Pappas AL, Sukhani R, Hatch D: Caudal anesthesia and urinary retention in ambulatory surgery [letter]. *Anesth Analg* 85:704, 1997.
47. Wellborn LG, Rice LJ, Hannallah RS, et al: Postoperative apnea in former preterm infants: prospective comparison of spinal and general anesthesia. *Anesthesiology* 72: 832, 1990.
48. Melone JH, Schwartz MZ, Tyson KRT, et al: Outpatient inguinal herniorrhaphy in premature infants: is it safe? *J Pediatr Surg* 27:203, 1992.
49. Malviya S, Swartz J, Lerman J: Are all preterm infants younger than 60 weeks postconceptual age at risk for postanesthetic apnea? *Anesthesiology* 78:1076, 1993.
50. Cote CJ, Zaslavsky A, Downes JJ, et al: Postoperative apnea in former preterm infants after inguinal herniorrhaphy. A combined analysis. *Anesthesiology* 82:809, 1995.
51. Yardley MP. Tonsillectomy, adenoidectomy and adenotonsillectomy: are they safe day case procedures. *J Laryngol Otol* 106:299, 1992.
52. Pappas AL, Sukhani R, Hotaling AJ, et al: The effect of preoperative dexamethasone on the immediate and delayed postoperative morbidity in children undergoing adenotonsillectomy. *Anesth Analg* 87:57, 1998.
53. Nicklaus PJ, Herzon FS, Steinle EW IV: Short-stay outpatient tonsillectomy. *Arch Otolaryngol Head Neck Surg* 121:521, 1995.
54. Schloss MD, Tan AKW, Schloss B, et al: Outpatient tonsillectomy and adenoidectomy: complications and recommendations. *Int J Pediatr Otorhinolaryngol* 30:115, 1994.
55. Tom LW, DeDio RM, Cohen DE, et al: Is outpatient tonsillectomy appropriate for young children? *Laryngoscope* 102:277, 1992.
56. Gerber ME, O'Connor DM, Adler E, et al: Selected risk factors in pediatric adenotonsillectomy. *Arch Otolaryngol Head Neck Surg* 122:811, 1996.
57. Mitchell RB, Pereira KD, Friedman NR, et al: Outpatient adenotonsillectomy. Is it safe in children younger than 3 years? *Arch Otolaryngol Head Neck Surg* 123:681, 1997.
58. Rakover Y, Almog R, Rosen G: The risk of postoperative haemorrhage in tonsillectomy as an outpatient procedure in children. *Int J Pediatr Otorhinolaryngology* 41:29, 1997.
59. Guida RA, Mattucci KF: Tonsillectomy and adenoidectomy: an inpatient or outpatient procedure. *Laryngoscope* 100:491, 1990.
60. Tobias JD, Lowe S, Hersey S, et al: Analgesia after bilateral myringotomy and placement of pressure equalization tubes in children: acetaminophen versus acetaminophen with codeine. *Anesth Analg* 81:496, 1995.
61. Verghese S, Davis R, Patel R: Acetaminophen treatment for pain relief in pediatric patients undergoing myringotomy and tube placement: oral vs rectal [abstract]. *Anesthesiology* 81:A1363, 1994.

62. Bennie R, Boehringer LA, McMahon S, et al: Postoperative analgesia with preoperative oral ibuprofen or acetaminophen in children undergoing myringotomy. *Paediatr Anaesth* 7:399, 1997.
63. Birmingham PK, Tobin MJ, Henthorn TK, et al: Twenty-four-hour pharmacokinetics of rectal acetaminophen in children: an old drug with new recommendations. *Anesthesiology* 87:244, 1997.
64. Watcha MF, Ramirez-Ruiz M, White PF, et al: Perioperative effects of oral ketorolac and acetaminophen in children undergoing bilateral myringotomy. *Can J Anaesth* 39:649, 1992.
65. Bean-Lijewski JD, Stinson J: Acetaminophen or ketorolac for post myringotomy pain in children? A prospective, double-blinded comparison. *Paediatr Anaesth* 7:131, 1997.
66. Davis PJ, Greenberg JA, Gendelman M, et al: Recovery characteristics of sevoflurane and halothane in preschool-aged children undergoing bilateral myringotomy and pressure equalization tube insertion. *Anesth Analg* 88:34, 1999.
67. Schroter J, Motsch J, Hufnagel AR, et al: Recovery of psychomotor function following general anaesthesia in children: a comparison of propofol and thiopentone/halothane. *Paediatr Anaesth* 6:317, 1996.
68. Grundmann U, Uth M, Eichner A, et al: Total intravenous anaesthesia with propofol and remifentanil in paediatric patients: a comparison with a desflurane-nitrous oxide inhalation anaesthesia. *Acta Anaesthesiol Scand* 42:845, 1998.
69. Partridge BL, Stabile BE: The effects of incisional bupivacaine on postoperative narcotic requirements, oxygen saturation and length of stay in the post-anesthesia care unit. *Acta Anaesthesiol Scand* 34:486, 1990.
70. Rice LJ, Pudimat MA, Hannallah RS: Timing of caudal block placement in relation to surgery does not affect duration of postoperative analgesia in paediatric ambulatory patients. *Can J Anaesth* 37:429, 1990.
71. Da Conceicao MJ, Coelho L: Caudal anaesthesia with 0.375% ropivacaine or 0.375% bupivacaine in paediatric patients. *Br J Anaesth* 80:507, 1998.
72. Yentis SM, Levine MF, Hartley EJ: Should all children with suspected or confirmed malignant hyperthermia susceptibility be admitted after surgery? A 10-year review. *Anesth Analg* 75:345, 1992.
73. Kaplan RF: Malignant hyperthermia. *Annu Refresher Course Lect* 226, 1992.
74. Morray JP, Geiduschek JM, Caplan RA, et al: A comparison of pediatric and adult anesthesia closed malpractice claims. *Anesthesiology* 78:461, 1993.
75. Kermode J, Walker S, Webb I: Postoperative vomiting in children. *Anaesth Intens Care* 23:196, 1995.

23 | Problems With Pediatric Postoperative Pain Control

Joëlle F. Desparmet, MD
Terrance A. Yemen, MD

The problems with the treatment of postoperative pain in a child are:

- Acknowledging that neonates, infants, and children do feel and experience pain
- Recognizing the presence and intensity of the pain
- Choosing the route of administration of analgesics for optimal pain relief
- Prescribing pain medication to provide the patient with adequate pain relief and minimize side effects
- Monitoring to ensure the patient effectively gets adequate pain relief with minimal side effects

NEUROBIOLOGY OF THE DEVELOPING CHILD

A discussion of developmental pediatric neurobiology is important in this chapter because it contradicts a common misconception that infants, and even children, neither feel nor experience pain, nor are they able to interpret these noxious stimuli into meaningful expression. Although it may be surprising to some, until the 1980s, medical caregivers were commonly reluctant to treat the signs and symptoms of pediatric pain or to even believe that those expressions existed. In fact, several studies in the preceding 30 years reported that children were considerably less likely than adults to receive pain medications having the very same surgical procedures. Some of this behavior resulted from the concerns about in-hospital addiction, respiratory complications, and general misinformation about the neurobiology and neuroanatomy of young children. Fortunately, there has been significant medical insight gained over the past several years; premature and in particular full-term neonates have neurologic systems that are considerably more advanced than previously thought.

The first aspect to consider is that of the developing neuroanatomy. Neuropathways for pain extending from sensory receptors in the skin to areas in the cerebral cortex have been found in newborn infants.[1-3] In fact, the density of nociceptive nerve endings in the skin of newborn infants is similar to, or greater than, that in adult skin. Cutaneous sensory receptors appear in the perioral area of the human fetus by 7 weeks' gestation. The development of synapses between sensory fibers and interneurons in the dorsal horn of the spinal cord occurs during week 6 of gestation.[4,5] Subsequently, sensory receptors spread throughout the face, palm of the hands, and soles of the feet by 11 weeks and includes the proximal aspects of the arms and legs by 15 weeks' gestation. There is complete spread to all cutaneous and mucous tissues by 20 weeks.[6]

Studies also have shown that many cell types appear in the dorsal horn complete with laminary arrangement, synaptic interconnections, and neurotransmitter vesicles before 13 and 14 weeks' gestation. The development of these structures is actually complete by 30 weeks.[7]

A lack of myelination in newborn infants was proposed to promote the concept suggesting infants are incapable of pain perception.[8] This concept is inaccurate. In adults nociceptive impulses are carried through unmyelinated and thinly myelinated fibers. The presence or absence of myelination relates primarily to the speed of conduction velocity. The most recent neuroanatomic data in infants show that nociceptive nerve tracts in the spinal cord and central nervous system have, in fact, undergone complete myelination by the third trimester and continues into adolescence.[9] The significance of myelination resides in the fact that thinly myelinated nerves are easily blocked. This means that low concentrations of local anesthetics can produce significant blockades of neurotransmission in the neonate and young infant, a fact commonly observed in pediatric anesthesia practice.

Pathways responsible for the transmission of pain are complete between the brainstem and the thalamus by 30 weeks' gestation, and thalamocortical pain fibers of the internal capsule and corona radiata are myelinated by 37 weeks.[7,9] The fetal neocortex begins development at 8 weeks' gestation and by 20 weeks each cortex has a complement of 10^9 neurons. Dendritic arborization of corticoneurons are complete and established by 20 to 24 weeks' gestation. Encephalography has been used to demonstrate functional maturity of the cerebral cortex in the neonatal age group. Intermittent bursts have been shown in both cerebral hemispheres by 20 weeks' gestation and are sustained by 22 weeks. Using this criterion, by 30 weeks, the distinction between wakefulness and sleep can be well defined. Quick sleep, active sleep, and wakefulness have been shown to occur in utero, beginning at approximately 8 weeks' gestation. On the basis of this current information, it is reasonable to believe that newborns have the anatomic and functional capacities required for the perception of painful stimuli and, quite possibly, its memory.

In addressing the functional capacity of the premature and newborn to perceive pain, in vivo measurements of metabolic activity of the neonatal brain are available. They show that regions associated with pain perception, such as the cortex, thalmus, and midbrain region, have the maximum metabolic activity and capability necessary for the interpretation of pain.[9]

In general, all children, even premature infants, have the necessary neurodevelopment to be capable of perceiving and experiencing pain as well as expressing an appropriate age-related response to it. Given this understanding, all children deserve pain relief whether it is induced by procedures or during the perioperative period.

ASSESSMENT OF PAIN

Recognizing pain in the postoperative period is not complicated in most children, even though the expressions of these noxious sensations will differ from one age to another. One should assume that there will be some degree of pain after any surgical procedure and that children, including newborns, are no more immune to pain than adults. There are scales adapted to children of all ages to measure pain. Pain should simply be seen as one of several vital signs that are taken during the postoperative period. The problem with pain is not how to measure it but making sure it is measured.

The simplest way to inquire about pain when talking to children is to simply ask them whether they have pain and where they feel it. This may seem an obvious approach, but it is not simple if the child denies pain because of the fear that a positive answer will result in getting an injection or the child does not understand the question because of developmental or language difficulties. Another way to ask a child about the degree of pain is to use a Visual Analog Scale or to ask the child to score the pain, with 0 being *no pain at all* and 10 being the *worst pain*. Both methods are easy to use and have been validated in children older than 5 years. Remember also that parents, who are directly involved with their children, can be invaluable in aiding in the evaluation of their children's pain.

It is more difficult to measure pain in children who are too young or unable to understand these pain scales. In those children, we commonly use a modified Children's Hospital of Eastern Ontario Pain Scale (Table 23-1), which relies on behavioral and physical parameters and not on cognitive development to obtain a pain score. This scale measures pain behavior such as distress, cry, and agitation and physiologic parameters such as blood pressure, heart rate, and oxygen saturation to determine whether the child is in pain. A score above 3/12 indicates a need for analgesics.

Two points are important concerning the assessment of pain in the postoperative period: these measures should be repeated at regular intervals as other vital signs are, and pain should be assessed before and after the administration of the analgesic to assess its efficacy and adapt dosage when necessary. The best way to manage postoperative pain in children is by the use of an acute pain service with 24-h coverage by pediatric physicians and nurses who are immediately available to optimize analgesia and treat side effects. It is also a good idea to establish protocols permitting nurses to give rescue doses of analgesics or adapt the dosage of analgesics according to sliding scales.

ROUTES OF ADMINISTRATION AND DOSAGES OF ANALGESICS

The Intravenous Route

The intravenous route is the one most readily available in the postoperative period and can be used to give analgesics as repeated boluses, a continuous infusion, or a patient-controlled technique (PCA). Research has shown that repeated boluses do not always provide adequate analgesia because of the delays inherent to the technique that result in periods of analgesia followed by increasing pain while the patient waits for the next dose.[10,11] A continuous infusion of analgesics provides more constant analgesia. However, continuous infusions can be insufficient for breakthrough pain and can lead to accumulation particularly in children younger than 1 year. Nonetheless, it may be the best solution for small children (>6 months of age), provided close monitoring is available and bolus doses of analgesics are given for breakthrough pain.

Continuous infusions of narcotics have a very limited safety margin in spontaneously breathing infants (<6 months of age), and a safe infusion rate for these children remains to be found. The line in this age group between comfort and respiratory depression and/or apnea is very thin indeed. Monitoring must be intensive. At the current time, continuous infusions cannot be recommended in the very young pediatric patient.

Patient-Controlled Analgesia

The use of PCA in children has been well studied and is one of the best ways to deliver analgesics. Patient-controlled analgesia requires that the patient assess the pain and administer the medication, but children younger than 6 or 7 years seldom use it correctly.[12]

TABLE 23–1 Behavioral Definitions and Scoring of Children's Hospital of Eastern Ontario Pain Scale

Item	Behavior	Score	Definition
Cry	No cry	1	Child is not crying
	Moaning	2	Child is moaning or quietly vocalizing; silent crying
	Crying	2	Child is crying, but the cry is gentle or whimpering
	Scream	3	Child is in a full-lunged cry; sobbing; may be scored with/without complaint
Facial	Composed	1	Neutral facial expression
	Grimace	2	Score only if definite negative facial expression
	Smiling	0	Score only if definite positive facial expression
Child verbal	None	1	Child not talking
	Other com-	1	Child complains, but not about pain, e.g., "I want to see mommy" or "I am thirsty"
	Pain complaints	2	Child complains about pain
	Both complaints-	2	Child complains about pain and other things, e.g., "it hurts, I want my mommy"
	Positive	0	Child makes any positive statement or talks without making a complaint
Torso	Neutral	1	Body (not limbs) is at rest; torso is inactive
	Shifting	2	Body is in motion in a shifting or serpentine fashion
	Tense	2	Body is arched or rigid
	Shivering	2	Body is shuddering or shaking involuntarily
	Upright	2	Child is in vertical or upright position
	Restrained	2	Body is restrained
Touch	Not touching	1	Child is not touching or grabbing at wound
	Reach	2	Child is reaching for but not grabbing at wound
	Touch	2	Child is gently touching wound or wound area
	Grab	2	Child is grabbing vigorously at wound
	Restrained	2	Child's arms are restrained
Legs	Neutral	1	Legs may be in any position but are relaxed; includes gentle swimming or serpentinelike movements
	Squirming/kicking	2	Definitive uneasy or restless movements in the legs and/or striking out with foot or feet
	Drawn up/tensed	2	Legs tensed and/or pulled up tightly to body and kept there
	Standing	2	Standing, crouching, or kneeling
	Restrained	2	Child's legs are being held down

Combining different analgesics for use in the same patient results in a synergistic effect.[13,14] This approach can reduce the dose of opioids needed, thereby decreasing some of the side effects such as nausea, pruritus, and somnolence. If these side effects occur with a PCA, adding around-the-clock rectal acetaminophen, intravenous or oral ketorolac, or diclofenac can help the patient reduce PCA demands.

This technique has changed the treatment of pediatric and adult pain.[15–17] It is a safe technique to use in children 5 to 6 years of age and older on the ward, if certain principles are followed (it is said that, if a child can play Nintendo, that child can use a PCA pump). The following principles apply to safe PCA usage in children.

First, boluses alone are preferred to a continuous infusion plus boluses. It is better to maximize the dose and/or intervals of the boluses than to add a predetermined continuous infusion. With boluses alone, a somnolent child will stop pushing the button. If a continuous infusion is added, this safety net no longer exists, resulting in an increased risk of respiratory depression, with no real analgesic benefit according to most studies. An exception would be the first 24 h after a major operation, when a child may be too weak to press the button consistently. However, the indication of the PCA in this particular circumstance could be debated, and administration of the analgesic by the nurse may make more sense until that time when the child can effectively use the PCA.

Nurse-administered analgesia is not well studied but has been used safely in a number of children's hospitals to good effect. Such an approach also can be useful during the night. Parents and children commonly complain that after 1 to 2 h they awake and cannot "catch up" with the small boluses of narcotics administered by the PCA pump. The lockout interval that requires the patient to push the button several times over the ensuing 0.5 to 1 h compounds this difficulty. Nurse-administered analgesia during the night or written orders that allow the use of narcotic boluses for breakthrough pain are effective in managing this problem. Parental use of the PCA pump remains questionable and is used with considerable caution, if at all, in most pediatric institutes.

Second, no sedatives or additional opioids should be given to the child on a PCA without approval by the person responsible for the PCA prescription.

Third, an antagonist such as naloxone and proper resuscitation equipment and expertise should be readily available at all times.

A standard prescription for a morphine PCA would start in the postanesthesia care unit with a loading intravenous dose of morphine titrated to pain relief (usually 2 to 3 doses of 0.05 mg/kg 10 min apart) followed by a maximum of 6 to 10 boluses of 20 $\mu g/(kg \cdot h)$, with a lockout time of 6 to 10 min. A lockout time of less than 6 min would not allow the preceding dose to take full effect.

Nausea, vomiting, and pruritus are problems in 30% to 40 % of patients using intravenous narcotics and can be intense. Some children would rather suffer than be pain free, nauseated, and/or somnolent. These patients commonly complain of intense pruritus and are distressed and agitated despite adequate analgesia. Switching to a fentanyl PCA (boluses of 0.5 to 2 µg/kg every 15 min as needed) often can remedy this problem.[18]

When possible, it is a good idea to prescribe acetaminophen or an nonsteriodal anti-inflammatory drug (NSAID) around the clock for 48 to 72 h to enhance analgesia and decrease the need for opioids.

It is said that the hand that prescribes the opioid should prescribe an antiemetic and an antipruritic. A prescription of 10 µg/kg of intravenous naloxone to be repeated two to three times in case of respiratory depression should also be written with the pain management orders (see the PCA Order Form in the Appendix).

The Rectal Route

The rectal route is useful in small children. It can be used at the start of surgery while the patient is asleep. This is also the best time to give drugs rectally in older children who would not accept that route at other times. Rectal acetaminophen has a 45-min onset time, with a peak analgesic effect at 2 h and provides analgesia for 3 to 4 h after minor surgery. Standard doses of rectal acetaminophen (10 to 15 mg/kg every 4 h) have been shown to be no more effective than placebo because of unreliable rectal absorption. Much higher doses, 35 to 40 mg/kg, given at 6-h intervals in infants do not result in toxic plasma levels and provide serum levels compatible with those when using oral administration.[19–21] We prescribe rectal acetaminophen in the following way: a loading dose of 30 to 40 mg/kg is followed 6 h later by 20 to 25 mg/kg every 4 h, with a maximum total dose of 4 g/day. Rectal preparations of indomethacin are also available. Serum levels obtained with the rectal administration of indomethacin are not well described in the literature at this time.

The Epidural or Caudal Route

Epidurals are an efficient way of providing analgesia in children.[22,23] The caudal approach is easy and will cover surgery below the umbilicus (Table 23-2). Young children (<6 years) have few, if any, changes in blood pressure or heart rate with a central sympathetic block. Epidurals are well tolerated even in children with complex congenital heart disease and may be the technique of choice for the anesthetic and postoperative analgesia. Caudal anesthesia or analgesia has a very good safety record. Neurologic injuries are rare and the inadvertent intravascular injection of local anesthetics remains the single greatest risk factor.

A few differences between neonates and older children with regard to the pharmacokinetics of local anesthetics deserve mention. Most local anesthetics, especially the amide anesthetics, are highly protein bound by α_1-acid glycoprotein. This protein is found at significantly lower levels in neonates and infants and rise to nearly adult levels by age 6 months to 1 year. The result is a higher fraction of amide anesthetic, which is unbound and active. This raises the possibility that the neonate is at greater risk of toxic reactions to amide anesthetics. Offsetting this finding, to an undetermined degree, is

TABLE 23–2 Relationship Between the Volume of Local Anesthetic Solution Administered Caudally and the Level of Analgesia

Volume of local anesthetic (mL/kg)	Level of sensory block	Surgical procedure
0.5	Sacral roots	Circumcision, lower limb orthopedics
1.0	L1–T10	Inguinal hernia repair
1.0–1.25	T10–T8	Orchidoplexy
1.25–1.5	T8–T6 (in infants)	Ureteral reimplant

the greater volume of distribution of amide local anesthetic drugs in the neonate versus the older child and adult. The conclusion is that the neonate might be at a slightly increased risk of local anesthetic toxicity. However, the safe serum levels for amide anesthetics such as bupivacaine and ropivacaine have not been established in neonates. Thus, caution is the key to their safe use in infants.

In addition, the metabolisms of amide and ester local anesthetics are lower in the neonate than in the older child and adult. These differences have a questionable affect on duration of action or dosing of these drugs in clinical practice. It is reasonable to assume that, the younger the gestational age of the infant, the greater the caution with dosing. The safest approach is to use the lowest concentration and mass of drug that will be effective.

With the lumbar approach to extradural analgesia, the level of analgesia will rarely exceed the T6 level and is more likely to do so in young infants than in older children. An epidural catheter sometimes can be threaded to the T4 to T5 level in the younger children, but kinking is often a problem, occurring in at least 20% of cases. Fluroscopy can be used to aid the placement of lumbar catheters into the thoracic levels but is time consuming and laborious. The use of a catheter capable of nerve stimulation at the distal tip to verify proper placement at the thoracic level has been described. Further studies are warranted before their use can be recommended.

Thoracic epidurals, especially those inserted at the thoracic level, should be restricted to experienced practitioners and for specific indications where the benefits outweigh the risks. Considerable controversy exists as to the safety of inserting epidural catheters at the thoracic level in anesthetized children. Although pediatric anesthesiologists commonly condone the insertion of lumbar catheters in anesthetized children, the use of the same technique at the thoracic level cannot be advocated at this time. Most practitioners believe the risk of spinal cord injury outweighs any benefit in this population.

A single-shot caudal or epidural with bupivacaine will provide analgesia for 4 to 12 h postoperatively.[12,24] Therefore, this technique is limited to those whose pain is short-lived (although the addition of 1 μg/mL of clonidine may significantly increase the duration of the block without an increase in side effects such as sedation and urinary retention). The use of "single-shot caudals" is particularly suited to outpatient surgery. It is best placed before the start of surgery to take advantage of anesthetic-sparing properties and demonstrate analgesic before the child's emergence from anesthesia.

All local anesthetic blocks have a period of latency and it depends on the location and type of surgery and the age of the patient. The shortest latency occurs in young infants and with superficial surgeries. The latency for an effective block for bone and/or tendon surgery, e.g., clubfoot repair, is particularly long, in the range of 45 to 60 min. One must be careful in giving narcotic analgesia given the latency of caudal and epidural blocks for these surgeries. A common mistake is to ignore the latency of the block and assume that it does not work and give narcotics as an adjunct. Unfortunately, when the block "sets up," the previously given narcotic often produces profound sedation and respiratory depression. This is the advantage of performing the block at the beginning of the surgery and repeating it, if necessary, at the end of surgery. Doing so ensures adequate analgesia before the child emerges from anesthesia.

Local anesthetics without narcotic additives are best for outpatient cases. The addition of opioids, such as fentanyl or sufentanil, may cause nausea, vomiting, and urinary retention without improving or prolonging the analgesic effect. The addition of morphine into the caudal space necessitates continuous respiratory monitoring overnight. The use of morphine, intrathecal or extradural, is not suitable for outpatient care.

Some surgeons and parents have concerns about urinary retention after a caudal analgesia is given. However, studies have shown that, although caudal analgesia with local anesthetics delays voiding, children do void on an average of approximately 6 to 8 h when using bupivacaine or ropivacaine in concentrations of less than 0.25%.

For major surgery a continuous method is often indicated. Catheters are best placed after induction of anesthesia and before the surgery. The absence of reaction to the surgery at light levels of anesthesia may be proof of proper catheter placement. The need for additional analgesics or high concentrations of halogenated agents during the surgery may indicate that the block is inadequate, i.e., the level of analgesia is too low or the catheter is in the wrong space. However, the real test will be the quality of pain relief once the patient is awake. No child should go to the ward with a continuous epidural when proper catheter placement has not been ascertained. An x-ray of the spine after injection of a radiopaque solution such as Omnipaque sometimes is the only way to make sure the catheter is properly placed.

In most cases a loading dose of a local anesthetic combined with an opioid can be administered at the start of surgery and immediately followed by a continuous infusion of the drugs or by boluses every 2 to 3 h. In children there is no need to use concentrated solutions of local anesthetics because the motor block provided by 0.25% bupivacaine is sufficient to allow good surgical conditions in almost all cases.

Postoperatively lower concentrations (0.125 to 0.1%) suffice for adequate analgesia and reduce the risk of toxicity.[16] As a rule of thumb, the total 24-h dose of bupivacaine should not exceed 10 mg/kg. This dose should be reduced by 30% to 40% in babies.[25-30] Even at those doses, a modest motor block can be demonstrated in infants and young children. All epidural or caudal infusions should be stopped if a child has a profound motor block postoperatively. Discontinuing the infusion allows the anesthesiologist to distinguish between locally induced motor blockade and significant neurologic injuries as a result of direct injury or hematoma.

Fentanyl, being lipophilic, will tend to provide analgesia close to the level of the catheter tip when given extradurally. If desired, a greater spread of analgesia can be achieved by using morphine, which spreads in cephalic and caudal directions.[31]

A typical postoperative epidural infusion would be a solution of 0.1% bupivacaine with 2 µg/mL fentanyl delivered at 0.3 mL/(kg · h). A typical morphine epidural would start with a 25- to 50-µg/kg loading dose followed by a 4 to 8 µm/(kg · h) infusion rate (Table 23-3). To improve analgesia, this dose can be increased by 10% twice, with 2 h between increases. If these increases do not improve analgesia or cause side-effects, the technique should be abandoned. Persistence in using an epidural in the face of failure is demoralizing for the patient and the physician. Such persistence also increases the possibility of complications such as local anesthesia overdose and seizures.

When opioids are given epidurally, pruritus, nausea, somnolence, and urinary retention are frequent problems and will need attention in one-third of cases. Moreover, all caregivers need to remember that a well-functioning caudal or epidural does not necessarily remove the discomfort of an intravenous catheter in the hand, a nasogastric tube, or a headache. It certainly is

TABLE 23–3 Dosage of Epidural Drugs

Drug	Initial bolus	Infusion rate
Bupivacaine*	1.25–2.5 mg/kg	0.4 mg/(kg/h)
Lidocaine*	3.0–7.0 mg/kg	1.6 mg/(kg/h)
Ropivacaine*	1.5–3.0 mg/kg	0.5 mg/(kg/h)
Fentanyl[†]	2.0 μg/kg	0.6 μg/(kg/h)
Morphine[†]	25–50 μg/kg	4.0 μg/(kg/h)
Hydromorphone[†]	6.0 μg/kg	1.5 μg/(kg/h)

*In infants dosage should be halved and infusion rates should be decreased by 40% after 48 h.
[†]In infants doses and rates should be reduced by 30 to 50%.

not anxiolytic. Many children will require adjunctive medicines to alleviate these problems.

Epidurals are high maintenance, and monitoring for efficacy and side effects is essential. In-hospital services, protocols for nurses, and visits by trained professionals are the key to success and the prerequisite to ensure safety (see the Appendix for the Epidural Order Form).

Nonsteroidal Analgesia

Nonsteroidal analgesics can provide good postoperative pain relief from minor and major surgeries. They commonly serve as valuable adjuncts to narcotic and local anesthetic-based pain relief techniques. Benefits may include improved analgesia, shorter discharge times, and a reduced incidence of hospital admissions for postoperative pain in the outpatient setting. Nonsteroidal analgesics such as ketorolac have been shown to reduce the incidence of bladder spasm after ureteral reimplant surgery. The use of preoperative indomethacin and intraoperative ketorolac is associated with decreased emergence delirium after myringotomy and pressure-equalization tube insertion in pediatric patients. These drugs are particularly attractive because of their ability to enhance pain relief without significant changes in sedation and respiratory depression in all age groups. These drugs are equally effective when given orally, rectally, or intravenously (when available in this preparation).

Like all drugs, there are some tradeoffs. The use of NSAIDs has been associated with increased bleeding after major and minor surgeries. Studies in pediatric tonsillectomy patients have reported mixed results, with an increase in postoperative bleeding in some studies and no increase in others. Timing of administration may be important. Bleeding problems with NSAIDs theoretically may be reduced by their administration after surgery is complete. Ketorolac is commonly given after tonsillectomy at Montreal Children's Hospital without problems. Nonsteroidal analgesics are avoided after major surgeries where blood loss is considerable such as craniofacial and scoliosis surgeries until 1 to 2 days postoperatively. In addition, laboratory studies have suggested that NSAIDs such as ketorolac interfere with osteoclast proliferation. These studies have not been translated into human clinical studies and the significance of this finding is unclear. The use of NSAIDs in pediatric patients with renal compromise or failure is cautioned, but studies condemning their use in such patients is lacking. Once again, caution is advised.

In general, NSAIDs are an effective and relatively cheap adjunct to pain relief in pediatric and adult patients. Caution should used in dosing and parents should be instructed in their safe usage in the outpatient setting (Table 23-4).

TABLE 23–4 Dosages of Analgesics

Route	IV	PO	Rectal
Acetaminophen	—	20 mg/kg q 4 h Maximum 4 g/24 h	35–40 mg/kg q 6 h
Diclofenac	1–2 mg/kg q 6–8 h	—	—
Ketorolac	0.5 mg/kg q 6–8 h	0.2 mg/kg q 6–8 h	—
Codeine	—	0.5–1.0 mg/kg q 4 h	—
Meperidine	0.8 mg/kg q 2 h	—	—
Morphine	0.05–0.1 mg/kg Continuous: 0.01–0.06 mg/(kg/h)	0.2–0.4 mg/kg q 4 h	Same as oral
Methadone	0.1 mg/kg q 4–6 h	0.1 mg/kg q 4–12 h	—
Hydromorphone	0.005–0.015 mg/kg Continuous: 0.0025–0.008 mg/(kg/h)	0.04–0.1 mg/kg q 4 h	Same as oral

IV, intravenously; PO, per oral.

Peripheral Blocks

It is beyond the scope of this text to describe all the types and methods of peripheral nerve blocks that can be used in pediatric anesthesia, but a few points deserve mention.

Peripheral nerve blocks can be an invaluable method of pain relief for a variety of surgeries. Practicing pediatric anesthesiologists should take the time to become familiar with most, if not all, of these blocks. The safety of placing these blocks has not been well studied in the United States, but these methods have been used extensively in France with very few complications. Such methods can be used in the outpatient setting, such as a dorsal nerve block for circumcision or ilioinguinal nerve block for hernia repair, and the inpatient setting, such as a femoral nerve block in a child with a leg fracture or a brachial plexus block for a syndactyly repair.

The proper conduct of peripheral nerve blocks in children requires training, proper equipment, and a sound knowledge of the anatomy in question. The use and improvement in peripheral nerve stimulators has greatly enhanced the use and efficacy of peripheral nerve blockade. As always, the dosing of local anesthetics is related to age and weight; one size does not fit all.

Although many peripheral nerve blocks are the responsibility of the pediatric anesthesiologist, in a variety of circumstances the surgeon should be encouraged to supplement our analgesic efforts with on-the-field administration of local anesthetic. Such administration is particularly useful during inguinal and umbilical hernia repairs, the excision of superficial lesions, and the open reduction of a variety of small bone fractures. When the surgical administration is being added to a previously performed peripheral nerve block, then the caregivers must be attuned to the maximum allowable safe dose of local anesthetic.

MONITORING CHILDREN RECEIVING ANALGESICS

Various degrees of monitoring are required depending on the age of the patient and the technique used.[32] All children younger than 1 year who receive intravenous opioids or epidural solutions should be monitored closely for respiratory depression. This can be done in an intensive or semi-intensive setting with increased nursing care but not necessarily on a ward. The monitoring should focus on respiration, hemodynamics, and neurologic status because accumulation of the drug can translate into respiratory depression (rapid and shallow as opposed to slow and deep breathing), decreased oxygen saturation, low blood pressure, tachycardia, or, more frequently, bradycardia and seizures.

Particular attention should be paid to correct dosing in the infant. A baby who is jittery and agitated despite repeated doses of a local anesthetic is probably showing signs of toxicity rather than of poor analgesia.[26]

Children older than 1 year metabolize opioid and local anesthetics as efficiently as older children and adults and can be cared for on a ward. Minimum monitoring should include pain and sedation scores, heart rate, blood pressure, and respiratory rate when awake, and heart rate, respiratory rate, and oxygen saturation when asleep. In case of a change in any of these parameters, the child should be fully awakened to determine the level of consciousness.

An increase in sedation and decreases in oxygen saturation and respiratory rate (or rapid, shallow breathing) should lead to the immediate discontinuation of the PCA, intravenous opioid infusion, or epidural infusion followed by the necessary measures to ensure adequate ventilation (see the Appendix for Montreal Children's Hospital PCA Orders and Epidural Orders for prescription and monitoring procedures).

CONCLUSION

Many options are available to treat pain in children. Familiarity with a variety of drugs and techniques and an obsession for detail are the foundation of acute postoperative pain management in children. To improve the pain management of children, the pain must be first measured. Postoperative pain should be considered the fifth vital sign. Trained personnel capable of intervening quickly, optimizing analgesic plans, and treating side effects must be available at all times for success in this endeavor.

REFERENCES

1. Okado N: Onset of synapse formation in the human spinal cord. *J Comp Neurol* 201:211, 1981.
2. Pernow B: Substance P. *Pharmacol Rev* 35:85, 1983.
3. Charney Y, Paulin C, Chayvialle JA, et al: Distribution of substance P-like immunoreactivity in the spinal cord and dorsal root ganglia of the human foetus and infant. *Neuroscience* 10:41, 1983.
4. Humphrey T: Some correlations between the appearance of human fetal reflexes and the development of the nervous system. *Prog Brain Res* 4:93, 1964.
5. Marin-Padilla M: Structural organization of the human cerebral cortex before the appearance of the cortical plate. *Anat Embryol* 165:21, 1983.
6. Rakic P, Goldman-Rakic PS: Development and modifiability of the cerebral cortex: early developmental effects: cell lineages, acquisition of neuronal positions, and areal and laminar development. *Neurosci Res Prog Bull* 20:433, 1982.
7. Gilles FJ, Shankle W, Dooling EC: Myelinated tracts: growth patterns. In *The Developing Human Brain: Growth and Epidemiologic Neuropathology*. Gilles FH, Leviton A, Dooling EC, eds. Boston, John Wright, 1983, p 117.
8. Jansco G, Kiraly E, Jansco-Garbor A: Pharmacologically induced selective denervation of chemosensitive primary sensory neurons. *Nature* 270:741, 1977.
9. Anand KJS, Hickey PR: Pain and its effects in the human neonate and fetus. *N Engl J Med* 317:1321, 1987.
10. Berde CB, Lehn BM, Yee JD, et al: Patient-controlled analgesia in children and adolescents: a randomized prospective comparison with intramuscular administration of morphine for postoperative analgesia. *J Pediatr* 118:460, 1991.
11. Tyler DC, Krane EJ: Postoperative pain management in children. *Anesth Clin North Am* 7:155, 1989.
12. McQuay H, Moore A: *An Evidence-Based Resource for Pain Relief*. Oxford, Oxford University Press, 1998.
13. Burns JW, Aitken HA, Bullingham RES, et al: Double-blind comparison of the morphine sparing effect of continuous and intermittent I.M. administration of ketorolac. *Br J Anaesth* 67: 325, 1991.
14. Gillies GWA, Kenny GNC, Bullingham RES, et al: The morphine sparing effects of ketorolac tromethamine. A study of a new, parenteral non-steroidal antiinflammatory agent after abdominal surgery. *Anaesthesia* 42:727, 1987.
15. Gaukroger PB, Tomkins DP, Van Der Walt JH: Patient-controlled analgesia in children. *Anaesth Intens Care* 17:264, 1989.
16. Lawrie SC, Forbes DW, Akhtar TM, et al: Patient-controlled analgesia in children. *Anaesthesia* 46:1074, 1990.
17. Tyler DC: Patient-controlled analgesia in adolescents. *J Adolesc Health Care* 11:154, 1990.
18. Tobias JD, Baker, DK: Patient-controlled analgesia with fentanyl in children. *Clin Pediatr* 31:177, 1992.

19. Yuan-Chi Lin, Sussman HH, Benitz WE: Plasma concentrations after rectal administration of acetaminophen in preterm neonates. *Anesthesiology* 85:A1106, 1996.
20. Birmingham P, Tobin M, Henthorn T, et al: Loading and subsequent dosing of rectal acetaminophen in children: a 24 hour pharmacokinetic study of new dose recommendations. *Anesthesiology* 85:A1106, 1996.
21. Hopkins CS, Underhill S, Booker PD: Pharmacokinetic of paracetamol after cardiac surgery. *Arch Dis Child* 65:131, 1990.
22. Yaster M, Maxwell LG: Pediatric regional anesthesia. *Anesthesiology* 70:324, 1989.
23. Schecter NL, Berde CB, Yaster M: *Pain in Infants, Children and Adolescents.* Baltimore, Williams and Wilkins, 1993.
24. Wilson PT, Lloyd-Thomas AR: An audit of extradural infusion analgesia in children using bupivacaine and diamorphine. *Anaesthesia* 48:718, 1993.
25. Wolf AR, Valley RD, Fear W, et al: Bupivacaine for caudal anesthesia in children: the optimal effective concentration. *Anesthesiology* 69:102, 1988.
26. Berde CB: Convulsions associated with pediatric regional anesthesia. *Anesth Analg* 75:164, 1992.
27. Agarwal R, Gutlove DP, Lockhart CH: Seizures occurring in pediatric patients receiving continuous infusions of bupivacaine. *Anesth Analg* 75:284, 1992.
28. Berde CB: Bupivacaine toxicity secondary to continuous caudal epidural infusion in children. In response. *Anesth Analg* 77:1305, 1993.
29. McCloskey JJ, Haun SE, Deshpand JK: Bupivacaine toxicity secondary to continuous caudal epidural infusion in children. *Anesth Analg* 75:287, 1992.
30. Peutrell JM, Holder K, Gregory M: Plasma bupivacaine concentrations associated with extradural infusions in babies. *Br J Anaesth* 78:160, 1997.
31. Shapiro LA, Jedeikin RJ, Shalev D, et al: Epidural morphine analgesia in children. *Anesthesiology* 61:210, 1984.
32. Attia J, Ecoffey C, Sandouk P, et al: Epidural morphine in children: pharmacokinetic and CO_2 sensitivity. *Anesthesiology* 65:590, 1986.

APPENDIX: REPRESENTATIVE PATIENT-CONTROLLED ANESTHESIA AND EPIDURAL ORDER FORMS USED AT THE MONTREAL CHILDREN'S HOSPITAL

MONTREAL CHILDREN'S HOSPITAL DEPARTMENT OF ANAESTHESIA PCA ORDERS				
Date:				
1. a) Medication:				
b) Concentration:				
c) Incremental dose:	mg	mg	mg	mg
d) Dosing interval:	min	min	min	min
e) Maximum 1-h limit:	/h	/h	/h	/h
f) Loading dose by anaesthesia: _____ mg Time: _____				

2. No PO, IM, IV, or SC narcotics or sedatives are to be given while PCA infusion is in progress except if agreed to by the anaesthesia department.

3. Drug record q 1 h: # of doses received
   # of patient's attempts
   Total amount of drug infused (mg)

4. Routine monitoring: O_2 saturation monitor regularly unless ambulating
   Hourly observation
   Monitor q 4 h when awake:
       Pain score   Respiratory rate
       Sedation score Heart rate
       O_2 saturation
   Monitor q 2 h when asleep:
       Heart rate   Respiratory rate
       O_2 saturation
   Infusion catheter site q shift for wet dressing, infiltration, infection

5. Notify physician if: Pain score >3 after 2 observations
   Sedation score <3
   O_2 saturation <92% with O_2
   Respiratory rate <10
   Infusion catheter problems

6. EMERGENCY INTERVENTIONS are required if: O_2 saturation <85%
   Respiratory rate <8
   Sedation score <2

   Should the above situation(s) present:
   a) stop infusion
   b) administer O_2
   c) administer Naloxone _____ mg IV PUSH STAT
   Dose may be repeated every 2–3 min until respiratory rate >8;
   d) notify anaesthesia/in-house physician (if anaesthesia personnel not available)
   e) q 15 min V/S

7. Treatment of side effects: _____ for nausea/vomiting
   _____ for itching
   In and out bladder catheter PRN for urinary retention and indwelling catheter if more than 2 in and out are necessary (to be reassessed after 2 days).

8. Other instructions: _____

   DATE: _____   **TIME:** _____   **SIGNATURE:** _____

   MEDICAL CHART

MONTREAL CHILDREN'S HOSPITAL DEPARTMENT OF ANAESTHESIA EPIDURAL ORDERS	

1. **Pain Medication:**
   A. Local Anaesthetic _____, final concentration: _____ %
   B. Opioid _____, final concentration: _____ mg/(µg·mL)
   Dilution: draw up _____ mL of   A: _____
                  _____ mg/µg of   B: _____ (= _____ mL)
       add+ _____ mL of NS
       Rate: _____ mL/h

2. No PO, IM, IV, or SC narcotics or sedatives are to be given while epidural infusion is in progress except if agreed to by the anaesthesia department, with the exception of diazepam (Valium) and anticonvulsants as ordered by the surgery department.

3. Routine monitoring: O_2 saturation and apnea monitors continously unless ambulating
   Hourly observation of the patient
   Monitor q 4 h when awake:
       Pain score   Respiratory rate
       Sedation score   Heart rate
       O_2 saturation
   Monitor q 2 h when asleep:
       Heart rate   Respiratory rate
       O_2 saturation
   Infusion catheter site q shift for wet dressing, infiltration, infection

4. Notify anaesthesia department if:
   Pain score >3 on Visual Analog Scale, >10 on Children's Hospital of Eastern Ontario Pain Scale after two observations at 5-min intervals
   Sedation score >2
   O_2 saturation <90% on room air (RA)
   Respiratory rate <10
   Infusion catheter problems

5. **EMERGENCY INTERVENTIONS** are required if: O_2 saturation <85% on RA *and/or* respiratory rate <8 *and/or* sedation score ≥3
   Should the above situation(s) present:
     a) Stop infusion;
     b) Administer O_2;
     c) Notify anaesthesia/in-house physician (if anaesthesia personnel not available)
     d) **administer Naloxone ____ mg IV PUSH STAT; (10 µg/kg) to be repeated after 5 min**
     e) q 15 min V/S

6. Treatment of side effects: _____ for nausea/vomiting
                           _____ for itching

DATE: _____   **TIME:** _____   **SIGNATURE:** _____

MEDICAL CHART

24 | The Anesthesiologist and Sedation: Who, What, When, Where, and Why?

Myron Yaster, MD
Lynne G. Maxwell, MD
Richard F. Kaplan, MD

In the past, even when their pain was obvious, children frequently received inadequate or no treatment for pain or painful procedures.[1,2] The "common wisdom" that children, even newborn infants, neither respond to nor remember painful experiences to the same degree that adults do is simply untrue.[3-6] Indeed, it is becoming increasingly clear that the failure to provide adequate analgesia to patients in pain increases morbidity, medical costs, and the duration and intensity of illness.[4]

Over the past 10 years, great progress has been made in the treatment of acute and chronic medical and surgical pain in children.[7] The use of opioids and nonopioid analgesics, local anesthetics, and regional anesthetic techniques in the treatment of pain have become commonplace.[8-10] However, procedure-related pain, which is the pain inflicted on children during their medical or surgical treatments (e.g., bone marrow aspiration, lumbar puncture, repair of minor surgical wounds, insertion of an arterial or venous catheter, burn dressing changes, fracture reduction, pulmonary and gastrointestinal endoscopies), has remained a vexing problem. The time-honored technique of immobilization by physical restraint is simply unacceptable and was made possible only because children were easily overpowered, were not routinely asked if they were in pain, and were unable to withdraw their consent.[1,2]

Sedation and immobility are often required for nonpainful procedures. Patients undergoing diagnostic studies (e.g., computed tomography, magnetic resonance imaging, position emission tomography, electroencephalography, or electromyography) or who require high doses of ionizing radiation to destroy tumors and rapidly dividing cell lines (e.g., in preparation for bone marrow transplantation) must be absolutely motionless and immobile for periods that may last 10 to 90 min or even longer.[2,11] Many patients, e.g., the developmentally and mentally handicapped or young children simply cannot remain motionless for even short (10 min) periods. In addition, many normal older children and adults cannot enter the confined spaces and often frightening environment of diagnostic imaging scanners and lie still because they may be intimidated by (claustrophobia) or are uncomfortable in them. Thus, some form of anxiolysis, sedation, or general anesthesia may be required to perform these nonpainful studies or procedures.

Children undergoing diagnostic or therapeutic procedures, whether or not they are painful, are often frightened and uncooperative. This fear may be exacerbated by parental anxiety, separation from parents, and the pain or the anticipation of pain from the procedure itself. Although distraction, guided imagery, and the use of videos and music have clear and documented benefit, increasingly physicians and dentists are using powerful sedative hypnotics, opioids, and general anesthetic agents (alone or in combination) to provide the sedation, immobility, and analgesia needed to successfully complete procedures and studies. These drugs are administered by anesthesiologists, nurse anesthetists, and nonanesthesiologists in physician offices, dental offices, procedure suites, imaging facilities, catheterization laboratories, endoscopy suites, emergency departments, and ambulatory care centers. Interestingly, there is little effort or desire to provide these services, even when possible, by operating room personnel because of the perception that sedation and/or analgesia can be provided outside of the operating room more cheaply, conveniently, and "efficiently."

The need to provide some form of sedation, anxiolysis, analgesia, and amnesia is clear. How to do it is not. Ideally, the characteristics of the drugs used for sedation and analgesia for procedure-related pain and for immobility for imaging and other diagnostic studies would include safety, ease of administration, predictable onset and duration of action, and reversibility. In addition, the drugs used should have no side effects and cause no residual mental or cardiorespiratory depression at the conclusion of the procedure. Such a drug or drug combination does not exist.[12–16] So how should one provide sedation and/or analgesia safely? What is the role of the anesthesiologist in all of this, particularly if the anesthesiologist is not directly involved in these procedures? The purpose of this chapter is to provide definitions, risks, and management guidelines for the use of sedation and analgesia by our nonanesthesia colleagues. We also hope to set limits that we believe are essential for safe practice.

Why should anesthesiologists be involved? As physicians with expertise in airway management, resuscitation, transport, and monitoring of conscious and unconscious patients and in the use of potent analgesics, sedatives, and muscle relaxants, anesthesiologists have a professional responsibility to patients and their colleagues to ensure that sedation and analgesia are provided safely to children. In addition, in the United States, we have a regulatory requirement that mandates this. The Joint Commission on Accreditation of Healthcare Organizations (JCAHO or the Joint Commission) has recognized that there is considerable variation in the level of care provided to sedated children, depending on where the sedation is administered and who is providing it, even within the same institution.[17] It has mandated that the standard of care for all sedated patients be uniform throughout any one institution and that the department of anesthesiology or its director set this standard of care. Thus, institutionally standardized documentation (medical history, physical status, and record keeping during the procedure and the recovery from the procedure), fasting guidelines, and informed consent procedures are mandatory for all patients regardless of the nature, duration, patient history, and location of the procedure.[17,18] Similarly, the personnel who provide sedation or analgesia for and monitor patients during a procedure, the monitoring equipment used during and after the procedure, and recovery facilities must be credentialed or uniform within an institution. These standards are also the responsibility of the department of anesthesiology. Virtually all of the professional societies that govern and set standards and guidelines in medicine and dentistry also delineate acceptable practice. Thus, although the Joint Commission regulates only hospitals and their affiliated institutions, physicians and dentists are held to "the standard of care of the community and the professional societies." Therefore, physicians and dentists must adhere to the same guidelines that are applicable in hospitals even if they practice in freestanding, unaffiliated institutions or private offices.

How then to proceed? A landmark document first published in 1985 and revised in 1992 by the American Academy of Pediatrics (AAP) established guidelines for the monitoring and treatment of pediatric patients during and after sedation for diagnostic and therapeutic procedures.[19,20] These guidelines formalized and defined the concepts of conscious sedation, deep sedation, and general anesthesia (Figure 24–1) as follows:

Conscious sedation: A medically controlled state of depressed consciousness that allows protective airway reflexes to be maintained; retains the patient's ability to maintain a patent airway independently and continuously; and permits appropriate response by the patient to physical stimulation or a verbal command, e.g., "open your eyes."

Deep sedation: A medically controlled state of depressed consciousness or unconsciousness from which the patient is not easily aroused. It may be accompanied by a partial or complete loss of protective airway reflexes and includes the inability to maintain a patent airway independently and respond purposefully to physical stimulation or verbal command.

General anesthesia: A medically controlled state of unconsciousness accompanied by a loss of protective airway reflexes, including the inability to maintain a patient airway independently and respond purposely to physical stimulation or verbal command.

Many other professional societies have established practice guidelines and standards of care for children and adults who are being sedated for diagnostic or therapeutic procedures. These organizations include the American Society of Anesthesiologists, the American Dental Association, the American Academy of Pediatric Dentistry, the American College of Emergency Physicians, and the American College of Radiologists.[11,21-31] Why so many practice guidelines?[23,32]

In these various schema, patients who undergo procedures while consciously sedated require less stringent monitoring and recovery requirements than patients who are deeply sedated or who have received general anesthesia (Figure 24–2). The fact that this level of sedation requires fewer personnel and less stringent monitoring and recovery facilities has enormous implications to health care providers and health care facility administrators. Not surprisingly, in current practice, nearly all sedation is called *conscious sedation,* regardless of the depth of sedation produced.

Deep sedation leads to significantly increased costs compared with performing procedures without sedation or without following recommended

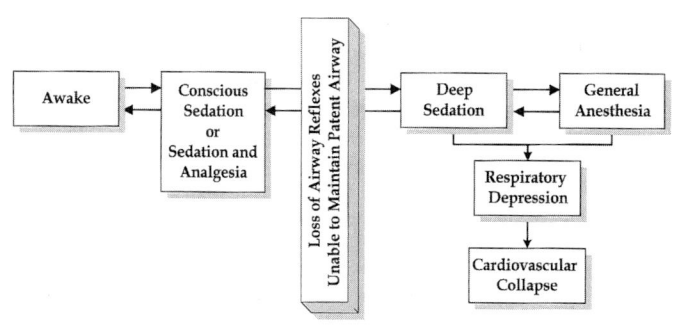

FIG. 24–1 Continuum of drug-induced sedation.

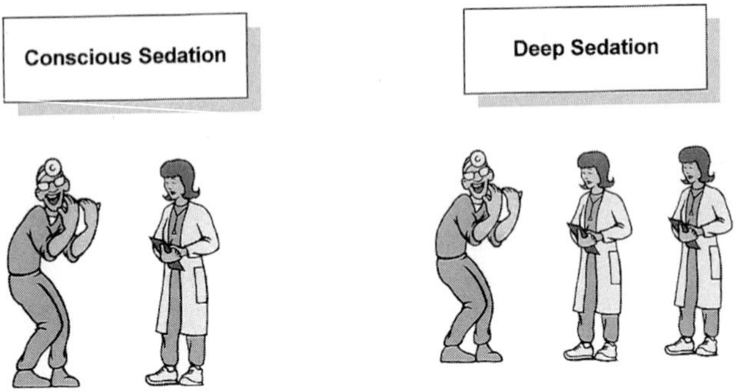

FIG. 24–2 Personnel, monitoring, and record keeping differences based on level of sedation.

guidelines. Patients who are deeply sedated require extra personnel (a second individual who is not performing the procedure but is administering drugs and monitoring the patient), additional training in the use of these drugs, monitoring and resuscitation equipment, recovery facilities, and time. Indeed, many practitioners think that the sedation requirement demanded by the AAP and the Joint Commission are onerous and virtually mandate the use of an anesthesiologist for compliance. The widely publicized and erroneous "excess supply" of anesthesiologists in the United States has led some of our colleagues to suspect that these guidelines, written in large part by anesthesiologists, are a conspiracy to create more jobs for anesthesiologists.[1] This has resulted in attempts to circumvent the guidelines by providing no sedation or referring to deep sedation as conscious sedation. This is a very disturbing mindset because it appears that the needs of the practitioner and the institution may be placed ahead of concerns for the comfort and safety of the child.

Can painful procedures or nonpainful procedures requiring complete immobility (e.g., diagnostic imaging or radiation therapy) be realistically performed in a child who is consciously sedated? We believe the answer is *no*. The myth of the achievability of a state of conscious sedation in which pediatric patients are simultaneously responsive to voice stimulus while immobile in the face of pain is just that—a myth.[1] For example, most practitioners who prescribe chloral hydrate for diagnostic studies believe they are producing conscious sedation. This is a startling concept because chloral hydrate's only effective therapeutic use is to cause unconsciousness. When administered in appropriate doses (50 to 100 mg/kg), it produces unconsciousness and causes respiratory depression.[22,33,34] Further, when administered in doses that are too low to produce unconsciousness (25 mg/kg), paradoxic excitement is common.

We believe that the level of sedation required for most painful procedures in children is deep sedation. In a consciously sedated patient, the appropriate response to a painful stimulus is movement or saying "ouch" (Figure 24–3). This level of sedation is inadequate for most pediatric procedures. Failure to move or respond verbally connotes deep sedation and is the level of sedation required for most pediatric procedures. The AAP guidelines and other professional clinical practice guidelines make an assumption that conscious sedation, deep sedation, and general anesthesia are distinct entities, albeit existing along a continuum, and that monitoring, patient selection, personnel, and equipment can be chosen according to the desired level of sedation (see

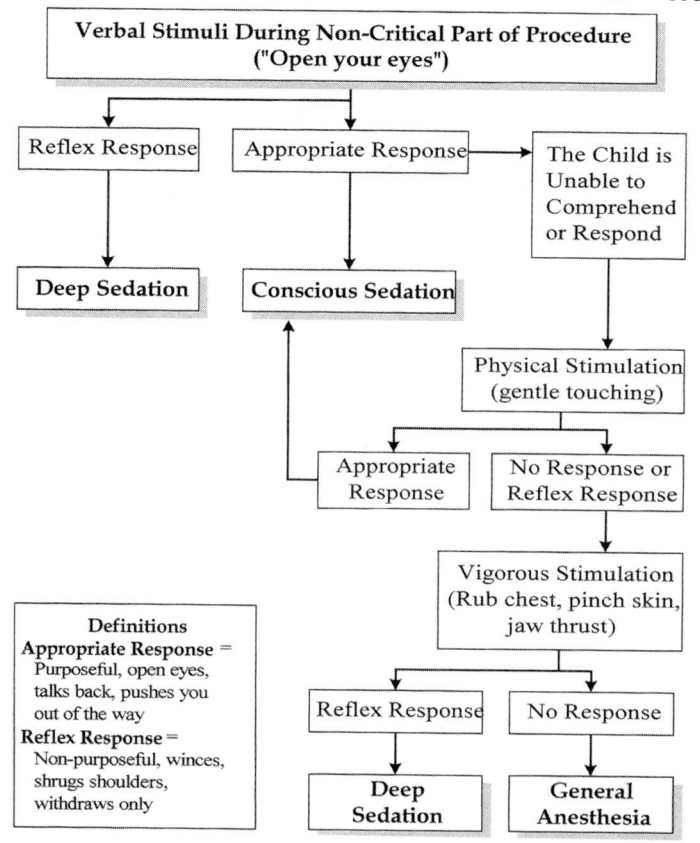

FIG. 24–3 Assessment level of sedation, based on response to stimulation.

Figure 24–1). This assumption is tragically flawed. Conscious sedation can rapidly and unpredictably become deep sedation or general anesthesia.[12,35–37] It is our belief that it is impossible to predict in advance the level of sedation that can be achieved by any single drug or combination of drugs. Therefore, it is our opinion that the practitioner must assume that deep sedation or general anesthesia will occur, that the level of vigilance must be maximal in all cases, and that the area in which a patient is sedated must be fully equipped with monitoring equipment and appropriate personnel.

Physicians, dentists, and nurses who provide sedation for painful procedures must make a series of decisions to do this safely. The choice of drugs must be based on a variety of factors, such as the type, painfulness, and duration of the procedure, as well as the health (including fasting status) and emotional needs of the child. The same individual cannot safely sedate a child and simultaneously perform the procedure. Monitoring by another individual is mandatory. That individual must be capable of recognizing and treating airway obstruction and respiratory and cardiovascular collapse and be knowledgeable about the pharmacodynamics and pharmacokinetics of sedative and/or analgesic drugs alone and in combination. It is important to recognize that the skills of recognizing airway compromise extend beyond merely watching the pulse oximeter, especially in the absence of the use of capnography.[30,31,38–42] It is very difficult, if not impossible, to accurately diagnose desaturation without the use of a pulse oximeter. It must be reemphasized that any drug, even administered in normal doses, may cause complications.[12]

Interestingly, the skill level of the physician, dentist, or nurse providing sedation has never been adequately defined. Current guidelines recommend training in basic life support and perhaps advanced pediatric life support, but fulfillment of this training does not guarantee that an individual possesses the skills necessary to safely administer sedation and detect and treat possible complications. It may be necessary to create a new, separate curriculum for training in sedation practice to ensure patient comfort and safety.

Rather than complaining about the onerousness of the Joint Commission and AAP guidelines, we believe that we have a unique opportunity to significantly improve the safety and comfort of our patients by implementation of institutionwide guidelines. Successful implementation of sedation guidelines will depend to a large part on the environment in which sedation will occur and the governing rules and regulations that apply to the specific environment. A successful sedation policy also must clearly define when the primary practitioner should seek the assistance of and consultation from an anesthesiologist.

The essential elements of a successful institutionwide policy includes organization, education, record keeping, enforcement, and continuing quality improvement.[2,27,43–45] A sedation committee must be carefully constituted and ideally involves many departments, practitioners, and geographic areas. The goal of the committee must be to create a sedation policy that can facilitate patient care without placing undue burdens on the practitioners. An overly burdensome policy may foster the avoidance of sedation and analgesia altogether or circumvention of the policy. Ideally, the committee should be composed of representatives from at least one and preferably two to three sedation practitioner services (e.g., endoscopist, intensive care physician, dentist, surgeon, or emergency medicine physician), anesthesiology, nursing, pharmacy, hospital administration, and risk management. The responsibilities of the sedation committee include the creation of institutionwide sedation policies, determination of institutionwide personnel and equipment needs, creation of educational programs, monitoring of sedation problems, and modification of policies as needed.

The department (or chairman or designate) of the department of anesthesiology plays a pivotal, if not central, role. The department of anesthesiology must help formulate policy, educate nonanesthesia sedation practitioners, act as consultant on difficult patients, and determine when sedation by a nonanesthesiologist is inappropriate. The department of anesthesiology should approve sedation flow sheets and records and be involved, with the committee and the institution's risk management department, in periodic review of the records and compliance with documentation and institutional policies and procedures. A member of the department of anesthesiology also should serve in the process of continuing quality improvement. Continuing quality improvement is needed to review complications, incident reports, and sedation flow sheets to ensure compliance with policy and recommend changes to the sedation committee. Sedation and analgesia also require a treatment plan. The department of anesthesia in each institution must play a decisive role in determining which sedatives, hypnotics, general anesthetics, and analgesics can be used safely alone and in combination. Four drugs in particular can easily produce deep sedation, airway obstruction, an unprotected airway, and cardiorespiratory collapse, namely methohexital, nitrous oxide, ketamine, and propofol. Whether these drugs can, or should be, administered by nonanesthesiologists and, if so, under what conditions, must be determined by individual institutions. There are many studies purporting the safety of these drugs when administered by nonanesthesiologists.[40,41,44,46–53] There are an equal number of case reports documenting catastrophes.[35,54–56]

Interestingly, Cote et al. performed a critical incident analysis of data from the Food and Drug Administration's adverse drug event reporting system.[57] One hundred eighteen reports were reviewed for factors that may have contributed to the adverse sedation event reported. Outcomes ranged in severity from no harm to death. The reports were reviewed by four physicians trained in pediatric anesthesiology, pediatric critical care medicine, or pediatric emergency medicine. Only the reports for which all four reviewers agreed on the contributing factors and outcome were included in the final analysis. They found differences in outcomes for venue: adverse outcomes (permanent neurologic injury or death) occurred more frequently in a nonhospital setting, whereas successful outcomes (prolonged hospitalization or no harm) occurred more frequently in a hospital-based setting. Inadequate resuscitation was more common in nonhospital-based settings. Other factors were inadequate presedation medical evaluation, lack of an independent caregiver providing the sedation, medication errors, and, most importantly, inadequate and inconsistent physiologic monitoring, interpretation, and response.[57] Clearly this report speaks directly to the need for standardized monitoring, equipment, and personnel trained in advanced pediatric resuscitation.

Education is vital. An ongoing institutionwide educational program on sedation emphasizing physician (dentist) responsibilities, nursing responsibilities, guidelines, and pharmacology of drugs should be given frequently enough to train the staff and accommodate staff turnover (usually one to two times a year). Teaching modules, videos, and handouts should supplement this program. Education also must emphasize the limits of sedation by the nonanesthesiologist and criteria for a sedation consult and/or sedation by an anesthesiologist. Medical conditions and management problems that require consultation with an anesthesiologist are listed in Table 24–1. The role of the department of nursing cannot be minimized.[45] The institution's sedation teaching module must be reviewed by newly employed nurses during orientation. Registered nurses must attend the hospital course on sedation once every 2 years or review a nursing module. The nurses must fill out yearly education profiles that include progress on sedation education.

Institutionwide, standardized forms and records for patient prehospital evaluation, fasting guidelines, sedation consent forms, sedation flow sheets, and discharge instructions and precautions are essential to ensure uniform quality of care.[2,41] The sedation flow sheet should be compact and contain a check list for fasting status, consent, review of systems, allergies, and physical examination. It should identify the responsible physician or dentist, assistants, and the person administering the sedation and keeping the record. A time-based record including vital signs (heart rate, blood pressure, respiratory rate, pulse oximetry), level of sedation, drugs administered, complications, and discharge status should be on the same sheet. Abbreviated instructions on how to fill out the form, how to evaluate and score levels of sedation, and an age- and weight-specific pediatric emergency drug quick

TABLE 24–1 Conditions Requiring Consultation With an Anesthesiologist

Medical conditions	Management problems
Airway obstruction, obstructive sleep apnea, severe snoring, large tonsils and adenoids, central (CNS) apnea	Patients who have failed sedation; inability to sedate; paradoxic responses to sedation
Anatomically abnormal airway (tracheomalacia, tracheostenosis, congenital syndromes involving the airway, including Crouzon's disease, trisomy 21, Pierre–Robin syndrome, etc.)	Developmental delay with behavioral problems, severe attention deficit disorders
ASA PS ≥3	
Chronic pulmonary disease (e.g., cystic fibrosis, bronchopulmonary dysplasia)	
Neuromuscular disease	
Poorly controlled seizures	
Poorly controlled GE reflux or patients at risk of pulmonary aspiration of gastric contents (symptoms of reflux between meals, obesity, pregnancy, previous surgical repair of the esophagus)	
Poorly controlled asthma	
Prematurity ≤60 weeks postconceptual age	
Renal or liver disease	
Unrepaired congenital heart disease or clinical congestive heart failure	

ASA PS, American Society of Anesthesiologists' Physical Status score; CNS, central nervous system; GE, gastroesophageal.

reference guide should be printed on the back of the flow sheet for easy review.

Physician, dentist, and nurse compliance with the sedation policy and a system for continuing quality improvement are the final pieces of the puzzle. Compliance can be monitored by the medical and dental staff office, the department of nursing, and a committee charged with the responsibility of continuing quality improvement. Staff privileges should require attendance at an educational program every 2 years and some form of life support credentialing (e.g., basic or advanced life support, pediatric advanced life support, advanced pediatric life support, or advanced cardiac life support). Every 6 months, the medical staff office should report to the department chairman and nursing office a list of individual staff members who need to take an educational course. It is the responsibility of the department chairman and nursing supervisors to secure individual staff compliance. Failure of the individual physician or nurse to meet educational requirements should result in the loss of institutional privileges to administer sedation or analgesia and possible termination of employment. Variance reports should be reported and generated when sedation policy is not followed or when a critical incident occurs. In fact, critical events are regarded as "sentinel events" by the JCAHO. The appropriate institutional review committee reviews the incident and reports to the sedation committee. Educational and corrective action should take place as quickly as possible.

The development of a systems approach to sedation creates a safety net that will protect children and provide anxiolysis, amnesia, analgesia, and possible loss of consciousness. Although individual patient needs, practice requirements, and location limitations produce problems that are individual and specific, the system solution to the problem of pediatric sedation and analgesia as outlined in this chapter is eminently feasible. Perhaps more importantly, it can be accomplished in a way that compromises neither patient safety nor patient comfort.

REFERENCES

1. Maxwell LG, Yaster M: The myth of conscious sedation. *Arch Pediatr Adolesc Med* 150:665, 1996.
2. Yaster M, Krane EJ, Kaplan RF, et al: *Pediatric Pain Management and Sedation Handbook.* St Louis, Mosby Year Book, 1997, p 1.
3. Anand KJ, Sippell WG, Aynsley-Green A: Randomised trial of fentanyl anaesthesia in preterm babies undergoing surgery: effects on the stress response. *Lancet* 1:62, 1987.
4. Anand KJ, Hickey PR: Halothane-morphine compared with high-dose sufentanil for anesthesia and postoperative analgesia in neonatal cardiac surgery. *N Engl J Med* 326:1, 1992.
5. Anand KJ, Hickey PR: Pain and its effects in the human neonate and fetus. *N Engl J Med* 317:1321, 1987.
6. Grunau RV, Whitfield MF, Petrie JH, Fryer EL: Early pain experience, child and family factors, as precursors of somatization: a prospective study of extremely premature and fullterm children. *Pain* 56:353, 1994.
7. Schechter NL, Berde CB, Yaster M: *Pain in Infants, Children, and Adolescents.* Baltimore, Williams and Wilkins, 1993, p 1.
8. Yaster M, Deshpande JK: Mangement of pediatric pain with opioid analgesics. *J Pediatr* 113:421, 1988.
9. Yaster M, Tobin JR, Fisher QA, Maxwell LG: Local anesthetics in the management of acute pain in children. *J Pediatr* 124:165, 1994.
10. Zeltzer LK, Bush JP, Chen E, Riveral A: A psychobiologic approach to pediatric pain: part II. Prevention and treatment. *Curr Probl Pediatr* 27:264, 1997.
11. Nelson MD Jr: Guidelines for the monitoring and care of children during and after sedation for imaging studies. *AJR* 160:581, 1993.
12. Yaster M, Nichols DG, Deshpande JK, Wetzel RC: Midazolam-fentanyl intravenous sedation in children: case report of respiratory arrest. *Pediatrics* 86:463, 1990.
13. Terndrup TE, Dire DJ, Madden CM, et al.: A prospective analysis of intramuscular meperidine, promethazine, and chlorpromazine in pediatric emergency department patients. *Ann Emerg Med* 20:31, 1991.
14. Terndrup TE, Cantor RM, Madden CM: Intramuscular meperidine, promethazine, and chlorpromazine: analysis of use and complications in 487 pediatric emergency department patients. *Ann Emerg Med* 18:528, 1989.
15. Cote CJ: Sedation for the pediatric patient. A review. *Pediatr Clin North Am* 41:31, 1994.
16. Nahata MC, Clotz MA, Krogg EA: Adverse effects of meperidine, promethazine, and chlorpromazine for sedation in pediatric patients. *Clin Pediatr (Phila)* 24:558, 1985.
17. Joint Committee on Accreditation of Healthcare Organizations: *Comprehensive Accreditation Manual for Hospitals.* St Louis, Mosby-YearBook, 1996.
18. Sklar DP: Joint Commission on Accreditation of Healthcare Organizations requirements for sedation. *Ann Emerg Med* 27:412, 1996.
19. Guidelines for the elective use of conscious sedation, deep sedation, and general anesthesia in pediatric patients. Committee on Drugs. Section on anesthesiology. *Pediatrics* 76:317, 1985.

20. American Academy of Pediatrics Committee on Drugs: Guidelines for monitoring and management of pediatric patients during and after sedation for diagnostic and therapeutic procedures. *Pediatrics* 89:1110, 1992.
21. Frush DP, Bisset GS III, Hall SC: Pediatric sedation in radiology: the practice of safe sleep. *AJR* 167:1381, 1996.
22. Egelhoff JC, Ball WS Jr, Koch BL, Parks TD: Safety and efficacy of sedation in children using a structured sedation program. *AJR* 168:1259, 1997.
23. Holzman RS, Cullen DJ, Eichhorn JH, Philip JH: Guidelines for sedation by nonanesthesiologists during diagnostic and therapeutic procedures. The Risk Management Committee of the Department of Anaesthesia of Harvard Medical School. *J Clin Anesth* 6:265, 1994.
24. Ringland R: Creating guidelines for conscious sedation. *Can Nurse* 93:45, 1997.
25. Use of pediatric sedation and analgesia. American College of Emergency Physicians. *Ann Emerg Med* 29:834, 1997.
26. Wilson S, Creedon RL, George M, Troutman K: A history of sedation guidelines: where we are headed in the future. *Pediatr Dent* 18:194, 1996.
27. Rayhorn N: Sedating and monitoring pediatric patients. Defining the nurse's responsibilities from preparation through recovery. *MCN Am J Matern Child Nurs* 23:76, 1998.
28. Use of pediatric sedation and analgesia. American College of Emergency Physicians. *Ann Emerg Med* 29:834, 1997.
29. Society of Gastroenterology Nurses and Associates: Guidelines for nursing care of the patient receiving sedation and analgesia in the gastrointestinal endoscopy setting. *Gastroenterol Nurs* 20 (suppl): 1, 1997.
30. American College of Emergency Physicians: The use of pediatric sedation and analgesia. *Ann Emerg Med* 22:626, 1993.
31. American Academy of Pediatric Dentistry: Guidelines for the elective use of pharmacologic conscious sedation and deep sedation in pediatric dental patients. *Pediatr Dent* 15:297, 1993.
32. Cote CJ: Sedation protocols—why so many variations? *Pediatrics* 94:281, 1994.
33. Weiss S: Sedation of pediatric patients for nuclear medicine procedures. *Semin Nucl Med* 23:190, 1993.
34. Malviya S, Voepel-Lewis T, Tait AR: Adverse events and risk factors associated with the sedation of children by non-anesthesiologists. *Anesth Analg* 85:1207, 1997.
35. Litman RS: Apnea and oxyhemoglobin desaturation after intramuscular ketamine administration in a 2-year-old child. *Am J Emerg Med* 15:547, 1997.
36. Petrack EM, Marx CM, Wright MS: Intramuscular ketamine is superior to meperidine, promethazine, and chlorpromazine for pediatric emergency department sedation. *Arch Pediatr Adolesc Med* 150:676, 1996.
37. Litman RS, Berkowitz RJ, Ward DS: Levels of consciousness and ventilatory parameters in young children during sedation with oral midazolam and nitrous oxide. *Arch Pediatr Adolesc Med* 150:671, 1996.
38. Cote CJ, Rolf N, Liu LM, et al: A single-blind study of combined pulse oximetry and capnography in children. *Anesthesiology* 74:980, 1991.
39. Cote CJ, Goldstein EA, Cote MA, et al: A single-blind study of pulse oximetry in children. *Anesthesiology* 68:184, 1988.
40. Cotsen MR, Donaldson JS, Uejima T, Morello FP: Efficacy of ketamine hydrochloride sedation in children for interventional radiologic procedures. *AJR* 169:1019, 1997.
41. Lowrie L, Weiss AH, Lacombe C: The pediatric sedation unit: a mechanism for pediatric sedation. *Pediatrics* 102:E30, 1998.
42. Council on Scientific Affairs, American Medical Association: The use of pulse oximetry during conscious sedation. *JAMA* 270:1463, 1993.
43. Dlugose D: Risk management considerations in conscious sedation. *Crit Care Nurs Clin North Am* 9:429, 1997.
44. Lund N, Papadakos PJ: Barbiturates, neuroleptics, and propofol for sedation. *Crit Care Clin* 11:875, 1995.

45. Ross PJ, Fochtman D: Conscious sedation: a quality management project. *J Pediatr Oncol Nurs* 12:115, 1995.
46. Parker RI, Mahan RA, Giugliano D, Parker MM: Efficacy and safety of intravenous midazolam and ketamine as sedation for therapeutic and diagnostic procedures in children. *Pediatrics* 99:427, 1997.
47. Shannon M, Albers G, Burkhart K, et al: Safety and efficacy of flumazenil in the reversal of benzodiazepine-induced conscious sedation. The Flumazenil Pediatric Study Group. *J Pediatr* 131:582, 1997.
48. Vade A, Sukhani R: Ketamine hydrochloride for interventional radiology in children: is it sedation or anesthesia by the radiologist? *AJR* 171:265, 1998.
49. Freyer DR, Schwanda AE, Sanfilippo DJ, et al: Intravenous methohexital for brief sedation of pediatric oncology outpatients: physiologic and behavioral responses. *Pediatrics* 99:E8, 1997.
50. Smith I, White PF, Nathanson M, Gouldson R: Propofol. An update on its clinical use. *Anesthesiology* 81:1005, 1994.
51. Bloomfield EL, Masaryk TJ, Caplin A, et al: Intravenous sedation for MR imaging of the brain and spine in children: pentobarbital versus propofol. *Radiology* 186:93, 1993.
52. Swanson ER, Seaberg DC, Mathias S: The use of propofol for sedation in the emergency department. *Acad Emerg Med* 3:234, 1996.
53. Parker RI, Mahan RA, Giugliano D, Parker MM: Efficacy and safety of intravenous midazolam and ketamine as sedation for therapeutic and diagnostic procedures in children. *Pediatrics* 99:427, 1997.
54. Roelofse JA, Roelofse PG: Oxygen desaturation in a child receiving a combination of ketamine and midazolam for dental extractions. *Anesth Prog* 44:68, 1997.
55. Daniels AL, Cote CJ, Polaner DM: Continuous oxygen saturation monitoring following rectal methohexitone induction in paediatric patients. *Can J Anaesth* 39:27, 1992.
56. Mitchell RK, Koury SI, Stone CK: Respiratory arrest after intramuscular ketamine in a 2-year-old child. *Am J Emerg Med* 14:580, 1996.
57. Cote CJ, Notterman DA, Karl HW, et al: Adverse sedation events in pediatrics: a critical incident analysis of contributing factors. *Pediatrics* 105(4 pt 1):805, 2000.

Index

Page numbers followed by letters *f* or *t* denote figures or tables, respectively.

A

AAP. *See* American Academy of Pediatrics
Abdominal trauma, management of, 202–203
Abortion
  adolescent, parental notification or consent for, 20
  refusal of anesthesiologist to provide care in, 24
Abuse, child, ethical and legal issues in, 23
Accessory pathways, in supraventricular tachycardia, 183–187, 192–193
Accidents. *See also* Trauma
  anesthetic, costs in pediatric anesthesia, 9, 9*t*
Acetaminophen
  dosage of, 383*t*
  for enhancement of patient-controlled analgesia, 378
  postoperative
    after myringotomy and pressure equalization tube placement, 368
    after posterior fossa craniotomy, 270
    after supratentorial craniotomy, 268
  rectal, 379
Acetylcholine, in upper respiratory tract infections, 82
Acidosis
  in malignant hyperthermia, 348
  in renal failure, 292
Acoustic neuroma, 268
Actinomycin D
  classification and side effects of, 241*t*
  for Wilms' tumor, 237
Activity level, and eligibility for discharge, 362*t*
Acute hypervolemic hemodilution, 328
Acute lymphoblastic leukemia, 231–232
  bone marrow transplantation for, 232, 250
  chemotherapy for, 232
  clinical presentation of, 231–232
  conditions associated with, 231
  incidence of, 220*t*, 231
  prognosis in
    leukocyte count and, 232
    patient's age and, 232
  tumor lysis syndrome with, 229–230
Acute myelogenous leukemia, 232–233
  bone marrow transplantation for, 233, 250
  chemotherapy for, 233
  clinical presentation of, 232
  coagulopathies with, 230
  conditions associated with, 232
  incidence of, 220*t*, 232
Acute normovolemic hemodilution (ANH), 326–328
  advantages of, 328
  combined with controlled hypotension, 331
  contraindications to, 328
  formula for blood withdrawal in, 327–328
  and hemostasis, 328
Adderall, 62*t*
Adenoidectomy, postoperative pain with, 8–9
Adenoma, hepatic, hepatic failure with, 295*t*
Adenosine, for paroxysmal supraventricular atrial tachycardia, 186–187

Adenotonsillectomy, for obstructive sleep apnea, 101–103
ADHD. *See* Attention-deficit/hyperactivity disorder
Administration. *See also specific drugs and routes of administration*
  by pediatric anesthesiologists, and anesthetic risk, 4
Adolescents
  abortions for, parental notification or consent for, 20
  autologous blood donations from, 322
  behavioral development and responses of, 57, 59*t*
  chronically ill, 67–68
  commonly used stimulants in, 62*t*
  confidentiality of, 19–20
  decision-making and consent by, 15–16, 18–20
  heavy menstruation in, and anemia, 36–37
  pregnancy testing of, 19–20
  preoperative, 38–39
Adrenal insufficiency, hypotension with, 316
β_2-Adrenergic agonists, for upper respiratory tract infections, 85–87
β-Adrenergic receptor(s), in asthma, 93
β_2-Adrenergic receptor(s), in asthma, 92
β-Adrenergic receptor agonists, in head trauma management, 201
β-Adrenergic receptor antagonists
  for long QT syndrome, 189–190
  for malignant hyperthermia, 349
β_2-Adrenergic receptor agonists
  for anaphylactic reactions, 304*t*
  for asthma, 93, 96
Adrenocorticosteroids, classification and side effects of, 242*t*
Adriamycin. *See* Doxorubicin
Adverse Metabolic/Musculoskeletal Reaction to Anesthesia Reports (AMRAs), 339, 341–342
Adverse sedation events, 395–396

Age
  behavioral development and responses by, 59*t*
  blood volume by, 200*t*
  of child with upper respiratory tract infection, and surgical decisions, 84
  of chronically ill child, importance of, 66–67
  and head trauma pathophysiology, 272
  normal pediatric blood pressure by, 313*f*
  patient's, and informed consent, 13, 15–16, 18
  of pediatric outpatients, 27–28
  postconceptional, and complications in former preterm infants, 133–134, 141, 366–367
  and preanesthetic sedation, 42
  and prognosis in acute lymphoblastic leukemia, 232
  vital signs, appropriate, by, 200*t*
Air bubbles, with shunting lesions, 176
Air embolism
  in posterior fossa craniotomy, 269
  risk of, anesthesia and, 3*t*
Air trapping
  in asthma, 92–93
  in bronchopulmonary dysplasia, 99
Airflow, through tube, principles of, and stridor, 108–110
Airway, difficult. *See also* Difficult airway
  management of child with, 143–166
Airway abnormalities, peripheral, with upper respiratory tract infection, 81
Airway distress, in stridor
  assessment of, 113–114, 115*t*, 116*f*
  minimal signs and symptoms of
    with moderately progressive lesion, 116–117
    with nonprogressive lesion, 115–116
    with rapidly progressive lesion, 117–118
  moderate signs and symptoms of

with moderately progressive lesion, 119–121
with nonprogressive lesion, 118–119
with rapidly progressive lesion, 121–123
severe signs and symptoms of
with moderately progressive lesion, 124
with nonprogressive lesion, 123–124
with rapidly progessive lesion, 124–125
Airway edema
in asthma, 92
with thermal, inhalational, or chemical injury, 117–118, 210–211
Airway hyperreactivity
in asthma, 91–92
in bronchopulmonary dysplasia, 99–100
in cystic fibrosis, 88–90
in upper respiratory tract infections, 81, 85
Airway management
anesthesiologist's role in, 107
increased intracranial pressure and, 264–265
in thermal/burn injury, 211, 218
intraoperative, 217
in trauma cases, 196–197
Airway obstruction
in asthma, 91–93
with mediastinal masses, 219
in obstructive sleep apnea, 101
pulmonary edema after, approach to child with, 103–104
risk of, anesthesia and, 3t
stridor with, 101–123. See also Stridor
progression of obstruction in, assessment of, 114–115, 115t, 116f
upper respiratory tract infections and, 82
Airway patency, principles of, and stridor, 110–111
Albumin
decreased levels in thermal/burn injury, 213
in hepatic failure, 296

Albuterol (Proventil, Ventolin)
for asthma, 93, 97
for upper respiratory tract infections, 85–86
Aldosteronism, with hepatic failure, 297
Aldrete's discharge criteria, 358, 361, 362t–364t
Alkyl sulfonates, classification and side effects of, 239t
Allergic reactions/allergies, 300–311
classification of, 301, 302t
clinical manifestations of, 301, 303t
determining cause of, 303–305
epidemiology of, 300
family history and, 300
hypotension with, 314–316
immune system function and, 300
and outpatient surgery, 29
premedication regimes against, 305
requirement for using causative drug in future, 305
specific, often seen by anesthesiologist, 306–309
stridor with, 124–125
treatment of, 301–303, 304t
in vitro immunodiagnostic tests for, 305
in vivo immunodiagnostic tests for, 305
Allergic rhinitis, 300
with asthma, 91
versus pneumonia, 98
versus upper respiratory tract infection, 80–81
Allergic triad, 92
Allogenic bone marrow transplantation, 250–251
Alupent (metaproterenol), for asthma, 93
Amantadine, for upper respiratory tract infections, 85
American Academy of Pediatrics (AAP)
anesthesia resources from, 7
Committee on Bioethics of, elements of consent and assent defined by, 14t
sedation guidelines of, 390–392, 394

American College of Surgeons, endorsement of patient's right to DNR orders, 21
American Heart Association, endocarditis prophylaxis guidelines of, 6, 30, 31*t*, 171, 172*t*–173*t*
American Society of Anesthesiologists (ASA)
  closed claim studies of, 2, 3*t*
  difficult airway algorithm of, 144*f*, 150, 158
  difficult airway task force of, recommendations of, 148, 165
  endorsement of patient's right to DNR orders, 21
  PACU guidelines of, 359
  Physical Status (risk classification) Categories of
    and decisions on proceeding with surgery, in child with upper respiratory tract infection, 84
Amide anesthetics, pharmacokinetics in neonates versus older children, 379–380
Aminophylline
  for anaphylactic reactions, 304*t*
  for postobstructive pulmonary edema, 104
  as respiratory stimulant in former preterm infants, 134
Amiodarone, for bupivacaine-induced dysrhythmia, 181
Ammonia, conversion to urea, hepatic failure and, 296–297
Amphetamine/dextroamphetamine (Adderall), 62*t*
Amputation
  in cancer treatment, pain with, 252*t*
  in thermal/burn injury, 217
AMRAs (Adverse Metabolic/Musculoskeletal Reaction to Anesthesia Reports), 339, 341–342
Analgesic(s)
  combination of, synergistic effect with, 378
  epidural or caudal, 368–369, 379–382
    dosages of, 382*t*
    latency period with, 380
    order forms for, 387–388
    volume of, and level of analgesia, 379*t*
  intravenous, 376
  local, relationship between volume of administered caudally and level of analgesia, 379*t*
  monitoring children receiving, 384–385
  nonsteroidal, 382
  patient-controlled, 215, 255, 376–379
    discontinuation of, 384–385
    nurse-administered analgesia with, 378
    order forms for, 387–388
    parental use of pump for, 378
    side effects of, 378
  peripheral nerve blocks, 384
  rectal, 379
  routes of administration and dosages of, 376–384
Anaphylactic reactions, 300–311
  during anesthesia, 300–301
  clinical manifestations of, 301, 303*t*
  determining cause of, 303–305
  differential diagnosis of, 301, 303*t*
  early recognition of, importance of, 301
  to food, 300
  in hospitalized children, 300–301
  premedication regimes against, 305
  requirement for using causative drug in future, 305
  specific, often seen by anesthesiologist, 306–309
  stridor with, 124–125
  treatment of, 301–303, 304*t*
Anaphylactoid reactions, to radiocontrast media, 308
Anemia
  in adolescent females with heavy menstrual periods, 36–37
  and apnea, 6, 139–141, 366
  with childhood cancer, 223*t*

INDEX

in former preterm infants, and perioperative risk, 139–141, 140t–141t
patients at risk for, 36
physiologic, of prematurity, 139
preoperative testing for, 36–37
with renal failure, 293
with thermal/burn injury, 214
Anesthesiologist(s)
attitude toward parental presence during induction, 72–73
consultation with, conditions requiring, 396t
educational role of, 56, 395
ethical and legal issues of, 13–25
seeking help with, 24–25
excess supply of, erroneous reports of, 392
experience and confidence of, and surgical decisions in upper respiratory tract infections, 84–85
experience of, and anesthetic risk, 4
in management of difficult child or parent, important issues for, 75
pediatric
accessibility to pediatricians, 7
administration of anesthesia by, and anesthetic risk, 4
educational role of, 7
personal integrity issues of, 24
in postanesthesia care unit, role of, 369
production pressure on, 24
refusal of cases by, 24
responsibility in presurgical evaluation of pediatric outpatients, 26
role in airway management, 107
and sedation, 389–399
Aneurysm, incidence of, 180t
Angiotensin II, release in thermal/burn injury, 208–209
ANH. *See* Acute normovolemic hemodilution
Anisocoria, with hematoma and temporal lobe herniation, 271
Anoxia, with thermal/burn injury, 214

Anterior larynx, 157
Anthracycline(s), 243–247
for acute myelogenous leukemia, 233
cardiac toxicity of, 243f, 243–247, 245f
acute, 243f, 243–244
clinically significant late onset cardiomyopathy with, 243f, 244
cumulative dose and, 244–245, 245f
early onset cardiomyopathy with, 243f, 244
late onset asymptomatic cardiomyopathy with, 243f, 244
monitoring for, 245–247, 246f
subacute, 243f, 244
classification and side effects of, 241t
Antibiotic(s)
allergic and anaphylactic reactions to, 301, 306–307
for chemotherapy, classification and side effects of, 241t
parenteral, for thermal/burn injury, 213
Antibiotic prophylaxis
avoidance in thermal/burn injury, 213
for endocarditis, 9, 30, 31t, 171, 172t–173t
Anticholinergic agents
for asthma, 94
for cystic fibrosis, 89–90
in difficult airway cases, 152
dosage, time of onset, and administration of, 152t
in malignant hyperthermia-susceptible patients, 351
side effects of, 94
for upper respiratory tract infections, 81, 85
Anticholinesterases, in malignant hyperthermia-susceptible patients, 351
Anticonvulsants
gingival hypertrophy with, 286
for neurosurgical patients, 263, 268

Antidepressants, tricyclic, for cancer pain, 254
Antidiuretic hormone, inappropriate secretion of, hydrocephalus with, 266
Antidromic reciprocating tachycardia, 183, 184f–185f, 185
Antiemetics, 366, 368, 370
  with patient-controlled analgesia, 379
Antiepileptic drugs, for cancer pain, 254
Antifibrinolytics, decrease in blood loss with, 331–333
Antihistamines
  for anaphylactic reactions, 304t
  for asthma, 97
Antimetabolites, for chemotherapy, classification and side effects of, 240t
Antimitotic drugs, classification and side effects of, 240t–241t
Antisialagogues
  for cerebral palsy patients, 286
  in difficult airway cases, 152
    in fiberoptic intubation, 160
  dosage, time of onset, and administration of, 152t
Anxiety
  parental presence and, 41–42, 72
  sedation for, 41–42, 389–390
Anxiolytic(s)
  for decreasing risk of emergence delirium, 365
  for frightened or anxious children, 41–42, 389–390
Aorta, origin of right pulmonary artery from, 180t
Aorta coarctation, 180t, 312
Aortic valve, bicuspid, 180t
Aortic valve abnormality, 180t
Aortopulmonary window, 180t
Aplastic crisis, in sickle cell disease, 276, 278t
Apnea
  brief, definition of, 131
  with cervical spinal injury, 201–202
  intranasal midazolam and, 48
  in neonates, inhaled anesthesia and, 130
  obstructive sleep, 100–103
    adenotonsillectomy for, 101–103
    diagnosis of, 102
    with hemifacial disorders, 102
    pathophysiologic consequences of, 101
    in syndrome-affected children, 102
  in postanesthesia care unit, 369
  in preterm and former preterm infants, 6, 29, 130
    anemia and, 6, 139–141, 140t–141t, 366
    caffeine for prevention of, 6, 29, 134–136, 135t–137t, 141
    management of, 134–138
    monitoring in postanesthesia care unit, 366–367
    perioperative, 131–134
    postconceptional age and, 133–134, 141, 366–367
    predisposing factors to, 133
    spinal anesthesia versus general anesthesia and, 136–138, 138t
  prolonged, definition of, 131
  rectal methohexital and, 50
  and sudden infant death syndrome, 28
  upper respiratory tract infections and, 82, 86
Aprotinin, decrease in blood loss with, 332
Arnold-Chiari malformations, 268, 270
Arrhythmias, 180t
  with burn injury, 206–207
  in pediatric patients, 179–195
Arterial blood gases
  in asthma, 95
  in bronchopulmonary dysplasia, 100
  in thermal/burn injury, 217
Arteriovenous fistula, systemic, 180t
Artery anomaly, systemic, 180t
ASA. *See* American Society of Anesthesiologists
Ascites, with hepatic failure, 297
Asparaginase
  for acute lymphoblastic leukemia, 232

classification and side effects of, 241*t*
Asperger's syndrome, 64–65
  prevalence of, 64–65
  providing care for children with, 65
Aspergillus fumigatus infection, in cystic fibrosis, 88
Aspiration
  hepatic failure and, 297
  incidence of, 3
  risk of, anesthesia and, 3*t*
  in trauma cases, 198
Aspiration syndrome, versus postobstructive pulmonary edema, 103
Aspirin sensitivity, in allergic triad, 92
Assent
  elements of, 14*t*
  informed, 15–16
  use of, 18
Asthma, 91–97
  categories of, 32
  cold-induced, 92
  with congenital heart disease (cardiac asthma), 169
  exacerbation of, upper respiratory tract infections and, 82, 92
  exercise-induced, 92
  helium and oxygen therapy for, 110
  incidence and prevalence of, 32, 91
  intraoperative management of, 96–97
  mortality from, 91
  outpatient surgery in children with, 32
  pathophysiology of, 92
  physiological differences between children and adults with, 92
  preoperative evaluation in, 94–95
  preoperative management in, 95
  radiographic findings in, 95
  regional versus general anesthesia in, 95
  steroid therapy for, neurologic sequelae of, 68
  treatment of, 94–95
Astrocytoma, 229, 233, 268
Asystole
  with bradycardia, 4
  with long QT syndrome, 189–190
Ataxic cerebral palsy, 284*t*, 285
Atelectasis
  in asthma, 91–92, 95
  in cystic fibrosis, 91
  with inhalational injury, 210
  in upper respiratory tract infections, 82, 85–86
Athetosis, in cerebral palsy, 284
Atlantoaxial subluxation, with cervical spinal injury, 201–202
Atopic disease, with allergies, 300
Atrial contractions, premature, 182
Atrial dysrhythmias, 182–188, 192–193
Atrial fibrillation and atrial flutter, 179, 187–188, 192–193
  accessory pathway and, 186
  acute termination of, 188
  chronic therapy for, 188
  electrocardiogram of, 187, 187*f*
  mechanism of, 184*f*, 187
  with Wolff-Parkinson-White syndrome, 186
Atrial re-entrant tachycardia, 187
Atrial septal defect, 180*t*, 360
Atrioventricular block, 179, 191
  with long QT syndrome, 189
Atrioventricular canal, unrepaired, 175*t*
Atrioventricular conduction abnormalities, 191
Atrioventricular node dysfunction, 179, 183, 184*f*, 186
Atropine
  for acquired long QT syndrome, 190
  for asthma, 95
  co-administration of, with pre-anesthetic sedation, 42
  contraindications in long QT syndrome, 190
  in difficult airway cases, 152
  dosage, time of onset, and administration of, 152*t*
  in head trauma, 272
  in myelodysplasia, 270
  for patients with increased intracranial pressure, 264
  for prevention of dysrhythmia, 181–182
  rectal versus oral, 42

Atropine (*continued*)
  for upper respiratory tract infections, 81, 85
Attention-deficit/hyperactivity disorder, 57–63
  comorbid with learning disabilities, 63
  continuance versus withholding of medication for, before surgery, 61–63
  DSM-IV diagnostic criteria for, 60, 61*t*
  prevalence of, 60
  providing care for children with, 61–63
  stimulant therapy for, 60, 62*t*
  treatment of, 60
Australian Incident Monitoring Study, 2–3
Autism, 63–65
  clinical presentation of, 65
  definition of, 63–64
  DSM-IV diagnostic criteria for, 64*t*
  prevalence of, 64–65
  providing care for children with, 65
  seizures with, 65
Autologous blood donations, 322–325
  advantages of, 323
  collection techniques in selected surgical procedures, 332*t*
  contraindications to, 324
  criteria for, versus criteria for allogenic red cells, 325
  cryopreservation of, 324–325
  from infected patients, ethical issues of, 325
  risks of, 323–324
Autologous bone marrow transplantation, 250
Awake intubation
  in cervical spinal injury, 202
  in trauma management, 198
Azathioprine, classification and side effects of, 240*t*

B

B-cell leukemia, 232
Backward upward right pressure, in laryngoscopy, 158
Baclofen, for cerebral palsy patients, 287
Bacterial endocarditis prophylaxis
  cardiac conditions requiring, 173*t*
  in congenital heart disease, 171, 172*t*–173*t*
  for dental, oral, respiratory tract, and esophageal procedures, 31*t*, 172*t*
  for genitourinary and gastrointestinal procedures, 172*t*
  guidelines for, 9, 30, 31*t*, 172*t*–173*t*
  in outpatient surgery, 30
  procedures not recommended for, 173*t*
  procedures recommended in, 31*t*, 172*t*–173*t*
Barbiturate(s)
  allergic and anaphylactic reactions to, 305, 307
  in former preterm infants, 131
  in head trauma management, 201
  potentiation of effects of, cyclosporine and, 298
BCNU (chemotherapy), classification and side effects of, 239*t*–240*t*
Becker's muscular dystrophy, 344
Beckwith-Wiedemann syndrome, 145, 146*f*
Beclomethasone, for asthma, 94
Behavior, and pain assessment, 376, 377*t*
Behavioral development, 56–57
  by age, 59*t*
  chronic illness and, 66*t*
  models of, 58*t*
Behavioral disorders/problems, 57–65
  in cerebral palsy patients, 285
  postoperative, 8
    preanesthetic sedation and, 41
Benzodiazepine(s)
  allergic and anaphylactic reactions to, 301
  and malignant hyperthermia, 340
  for thermal/burn injury patients, 215
  for trauma patients, 203
Best-interests standard, 14–15
Bicarbonate

for malignant hyperthermia, 348, 348t, 356t
for renal failure, 293
Bilateral myringotomy and pressure equalization tube placement, postanesthesia care in, monitoring in and discharge from, 368
Biliary atresia, hepatic failure with, 295t
Birthweight. *See also* Preterm infants
very low or extremely low, neurologic sequelae of, 67
Bispectral index monitoring, 365
Bleeding, surgical, and eligibility for discharge, 363t
Bleomycin
classification and side effects of, 241t
for Hodgkin's disease, 235
toxicity of, 247–248
Blind intubation
nasotracheal, in trauma cases, 199
oral or nasal, in difficult airway, 159, 161–163
Blood donations, autologous, 322–325
advantages of, 323
collection techniques in selected surgical procedures, 332t
contraindications to, 324
criteria for, versus criteria for allogenic red cells, 325
cryopreservation of, 324–325
from infected patients, ethical issues of, 325
risks of, 323–324
Blood loss, excessive, risk of, anesthesia and, 3t
Blood pressure
depressed. *See* Hypotension
elevated. *See* Hypertension
monitoring in postanesthesia care unit, 360
normal pediatric, by age, 313f
Blood salvage and conservation
antifibrinolytics and other pharmacologic means in, 331–333
combined techniques for, 331
intraoperative, 325–326
combined with hemodilution, 331
postoperative, 326
techniques in children, 322–337, 324t
Blood transfusion
autologous, 322–325
complications of, 200
directed, 325
homologous, alternatives to, 322–337
infectious risks for, 322, 323t
in myelodysplasia surgery, 270
perioperative, for sickle cell disease, 279–280
safety of, concerns over, 322
side effects associated with, 322, 323t
for thermal/burn injury patients, 213–214, 217–218
in trauma management, 199–200, 200t–201t
Blood volume, related to age, 200t
Blow-by oxygen, in postanesthesia care unit, 360
BM&T (bilateral myringotomy and pressure equalization tube placement), postanesthesia care in, monitoring in and discharge from, 368
Bone marrow suppression, with chemotherapy, 238–243
Bone marrow transplantation, 250–251
for acute lymphoblastic leukemia, 232, 250
for acute myelogenous leukemia, 233, 250
allogenic, 250–251
autologous, 250
complications of, 251
for Hodgkin's disease, 235
for neuroblastoma, 236, 250
for non-Hodgkin's lymphoma, 234
preparation for
chemotherapy for, 251
radiation therapy for, 248
Botoxin (botulinum neurotoxin), for cerebral palsy patients, 287

Box diagrams, of physiology in congenital heart disease, 167, 168f
Bradycardia
  with cervical spinal injury, 201–202
  epinephrine-induced, 182
  etiologies of, 4
  halothane-induced, 181
  incidence of, 3–4
  with long QT syndrome, 189
  morbidity with, 4
  in preterm and former preterm infants
    anemia and, 139–141, 140t–141t
    perioperative, 131–134
    spinal versus general anesthesia and, 136–138, 138t
  risk of, administration of anesthesia by pediatric anesthesiologists and, 4
  succinylcholine-induced, 182
  with thermal/burn injury, 212
Bradysdysrhythmias, 191, 193
Brain herniation, with cancer, 222t
Brain metastases, 233
Brain tumors, 233, 266–267
  bone marrow transplantation for, 250
  incidence of, 233
  infratentorial, 233
  neurologic symptoms with, 233
  posterior fossa craniotomy for, 268–270
  supratentorial, 233
  supratentorial craniotomy for, 267–268
  treatment of, 233
Breach of duty, 17t
Breath-holding
  in asthma, 96
  in bronchopulmonary dysplasia, 100
  in upper respiratory tract infections, 82, 86
Brethine (terbutaline), for asthma, 93
Bretylium
  for bupivacaine-induced dysrhythmia, 181
  in long QT syndrome, 190
Bronchiectasis, in cystic fibrosis, 88

Bronchiolitis, 97–98
Bronchoconstriction, vagally mediated reflex, in upper respiratory tract infections, 81
Bronchodilators
  for asthma, 94, 96–97
  for cystic fibrosis, 89–90
  for thermal/burn injury, 211
  for upper respiratory tract infections, 85–87
Bronchopulmonary dysplasia, 98–100
  in asymptomatic patient, 100
  coexisting conditions with, 99
  definitions of, 99
  intraoperative management of, 100
  and outpatient surgery, 29–30
  preoperative evaluation in, 100
  school-age children with history of, 99
  "stupid premie tricks" with, 100
  in symptomatic patient, 100
Bronchoscopy
  fiberoptic, mediastinal masses and, 228–229
  in inhalational injury evaluation, 211
  rigid, availability in surgery for mediastinal masses, 227
Bronchospasm
  in asthma, 96–97
  in bronchopulmonary dysplasia, 100
  hypoxia with, 317
  incidence of, 3
  postoperative, 369
  risk of, anesthesia and, 3t
  in upper respiratory tract infections, 85
Bronkosol (isoetharine), for asthma, 93
Bullard laryngoscope
  in difficult airway, 158
  in thermal/burn injury, 211
Bupivacaine, 368–369
  dysrhythmia induced by, 181
  epidural, 380–381, 382t
  single-shot, 380
Burkitt's lymphoma, 234
  tumor lysis syndrome with, 229

Burn injury
  airway and ventilation in, 211, 218
    intraoperative, 217
  anesthesia induction and maintenance in, 216–217
  anesthetic planning for, 216
  body surface area involved in, 207, 208f–209f
  cardiovascular effects of, 208–209, 212
  chemical, 207
  contraindication to succinylcholine in, 216
  electrical, 206–207
  electrolytes in, 213
  first-degree, 207
  fluid management/resuscitation in, 212–213, 217–218
  hematologic problems with, 214
  infection in, 213–214
  management issues in, 211–215
  management of child with, 206–218
  monitoring, intraoperative, in, 217
  neurologic problems with, 214
  nutrition in, 213
  operating room management of, 215–218
  operating room preparation for, 216
  pain management in, 215
  patient positioning, intraoperative, in, 216
  renal issues with, 214
  second-degree, 207
  skin injury with, 207
  stridor with, 117–118, 211
  surgical procedures for, 215–216
  third-degree, 207
Burn shock, 208–209
Busulfan
  classification and side effects of, 239t
  in preparative regime for bone marrow transplantation, 251

C

Caffeine
  preparations of, 136
  as respiratory stimulant, in former preterm infants, 6, 29, 134–136, 135t–137t, 141
Caffeine citrate, 136
Caffeine halothane contracture test, for malignant hyperthermia susceptibility, 350
Caffeine sodium benzoate, contraindications in infants, 136
Calcium
  decreased levels of
    hypotension with, 316
    in renal failure, 293
    in thermal/burn injury, 213
    with tumor lysis syndrome, 229–230
  elevated levels of, with childhood cancer, 223t
  intracellular, in malignant hyperthermia, 338
Calcium channel blockers
  for controlled hypotension, 329, 330t
  for long QT syndrome, 189
  in malignant hyperthermia, 349
Calcium chloride, for malignant hyperthermia, 348, 348t
cAMP (cyclic adenosine monophosphate), in asthma, 92–93
Cancer, in children, 219–260
  anesthesiologist's approach to, 257
  bone marrow transplantation for, 250–251
  chemotherapy for, 238–248
    classification and side effects of, 239t–242t
  coagulopathy with, 223t, 230–231
  diagnoses of, 231–238
  emotional stress of, 255–257
  hyperleukocytosis with, 222t, 231
  incidence of, 219, 220t
  mortality from, 219
  oncologic emergencies with, 219–230, 222t–223t
    caused by blood and blood vessel abnormalities, 223t
    metabolic, 223t

412 INDEX

Cancer, in children *(continued)*
  pain management in, 254–255
    insufficient, 251–252
    WHO stepwise approach in, 254, 255f
  pain with, 251–255
    elements of, 254, 254f
    treatment-related, 252, 252t
    tumor-related, 252, 253t
  presenting symptoms of, 221t
  radiation therapy for, 248–250
  spinal cord compression with, 222t, 229
  therapies for, 238–257
  tumor lysis syndrome with, 223t, 229–230
    management of, 230t
Capnographic monitoring, of malignant hyperthermia-susceptible patients, 351
Carbon dioxide
  arterial partial pressure in neonates, opioids and, 131
  end-tidal
    correlation of, with arterial partial pressure, in congenital heart disease, 177
    increasing, malignant hyperthermia versus other causes of, 347–348
    retention in bronchopulmonary dysplasia, 99
    ventilatory response in neonates, inhaled anesthesia and, 130
Carbon monoxide poisoning, 210, 214, 318
Carboplatin
  classification and side effects of, 242t
  for neuroblastoma, 236
Cardiac arrest
  do-not-resuscitate orders in, 21–23
  hypotension in, 314
  incidence of, 1–2
  with malignant hyperthermia, 356t
  mortality rate due to, 1–2
  neuromuscular disease and, 7
  risk of, administration of anesthesia by pediatric anesthesiologists and, 4
  with tumor lysis syndrome, 230
Cardiac artery, compression of, with mediastinal masses, 219
Cardiac asthma, 169
Cardiac function, in muscular dystrophy, 289–290
Cardiac grid, for summarizing physiologic manipulations required for cardiac lesion, 173, 175t
Cardiac toxicity, of anthracyclines, 243f, 243–247, 245f
  acute, 243f, 243–244
  cumulative dose and, 244–245, 245f
  monitoring for, 245–247, 246f
  subacute, 243f, 244
Cardiac trauma, 203
Cardiac tumor, 180t
Cardiology consultation, need in child with heart murmur, 30, 30t
Cardiomyopathy
  with anthracycline therapy, 243f, 243–247, 245f
    clinically significant late onset, 243f, 244
    cumulative dose and, 244–245, 245f
    early onset, 243f, 244
    late onset asymptomatic, 243f, 244
    monitoring for, 245–247, 246f
  clinical, with muscular dystrophy, 289
  hypertrophic obstructive, pacemaker and cardioverter-defibrillator for, 191
Cardiopulmonary bypass, in surgery for mediastinal masses, 227
Cardiovascular effects, of thermal/burn injury, 208–209, 212
Cardioverter-defibrillators
  anesthetic considerations for pediatric patients with, 192
  for dysrhythmias, 191–193
Carmustine, classification and side effects of, 239t–240t
Caroli's disease, hepatic failure with, 295t

INDEX

Catecholamine(s)
 exogenous, and hypertension, 312
 release in thermal/burn injury, 208–209
Caudal analgesia, 368–369, 379–382
 continuous method for, 381
 dosages of, 382*t*
 latency period with, 380
 lumbar, 380
 monitoring children receiving, 384–385
 order forms for, 387–388
 postoperative, typical, 381
 thoracic, 380
 volume of, and level of analgesia, 379*t*
Causation, in negligence, 17*t*
Cavernous hemangioma, hepatic failure with, 295*t*
CCNU (chemotherapy), classification and side effects of, 239*t*–240*t*
Central core disease, and malignant hyperthermia, 352
Central nervous system tumors, 233, 266–267
 bone marrow transplantation for, 250
 incidence in children, 220*t*, 233
 radiation therapy for, 248–250
Cephalosporins, allergic and anaphylactic reactions to, 306
Cerebral blood flow
 anesthetic effects on, 201, 202*t*
 increased intracranial pressure and, 261–262
Cerebral palsy, 283–288
 anesthetic management in, 285–288
 ataxic, 284*t*, 285
 baclofen for, 287
 behavior and communication problems in, 285
 botoxin for, 287
 classification of, 284*t*, 284–285
 definition of, 283
 dyskinetic, 284*t*, 285
 epilepsy with, 285
 etiology of, 283–284
 gastrointestinal problems with, 285–286
 gingival hypertrophy with, 286
 incidence of, 283–284
 latex allergy with, 288
 malnourishment with, 288
 malocclusion with, 286
 medications for, 285–287
 pain management in, 285, 287–288
 pathophysiology of, 284–285
 preanesthetic evaluation of seven basic problems, 285–288
 respiratory problems with, 285–286
 spastic, 284, 284*t*
 visual and hearing defects in, 285
Cerebral perfusion pressure
 decreased, with brain tumors, 266–267
 in head trauma cases, 200–201
 increased intracranial pressure and, 261–262
Cerebrospinal fluid
 increased, in hydrocephalus, 266
 and intracranial pressure, 261
Cerebrovascular accident, with childhood cancer, 223*t*
Cervical spinal injury, 201–202
CFTR (cystic fibrosis transmembrane conductance regulator), 87–88
Chemical burns, 207
Chemical injury, stridor with, 117–118
Chemotherapy, 238–248
 for acute lymphoblastic leukemia, 232
 for acute myelogenous leukemia, 233
 classification and side effects of, 239*t*–242*t*
 for Hodgkin's disease, 235
 for Langerhans' cell histiocytosis, 238
 for neuroblastoma, 236
 for non-Hodgkin's lymphoma, 234
 pain with, 252*t*
 as preparative regime for bone marrow transplantation, 251

Chemotherapy (*continued*)
for Wilms' tumor, 237
Chest radiograph
of acute chest syndrome, with sickle cell disease, 276
in asthma, 95
in bronchopulmonary dysplasia, 100
of mediastinal masses, 221, 225*t*, 229, 235
in pneumonia, 98
preoperative, 39
in upper respiratory tract infections, 85
Chest syndrome, acute, in sickle cell disease, 276, 278*t*
Child, difficult
identification of, 56–69
management of, 69–75, 153
important issues for anesthesiologist in, 75
parent's perspective on, 76–78
providing care for, 56–79
as temperament type, 67
Child abuse, ethical and legal issues in, 23
Child development, 56–57
by age, 59*t*
chronic illness and, 66*t*
definition of, 56
models of, 58*t*
Chloral hydrate, 263, 392
Chlorambucil, classification and side effects of, 239*t*
Cholecystokinin, in renal failure, 293
Choledochal cyst, hepatic failure with, 295*t*
Chronic illness, 65–68
child's age and, 66–67
definition of, 66
development and behavior of children with, factors influencing, 66*t*
and family dynamics, 68–69
providing care for child with, parent's perspective on, 76–78
temperament and, 67
Chronic myelogenous leukemia, bone marrow transplantation for, 250

Chymopapain, allergic and anaphylactic reactions to, 305
Circulation, and eligibility for discharge, 362*t*
Cisatracurium, 159*t*
Cisplatin
classification and side effects of, 241*t*–242*t*
for neuroblastoma, 236
Clinical recovery scores (CRS), 361, 362*t*–364*t*
Clonazepam, for pervasive developmental disorders, 65
Clonidine
for cancer pain, 254
with epidural analgesia, 380
for premedication in neurosurgery, 263
Closed claim studies
of anesthetic accident costs, 9, 9*t*
of anesthetic risk, 2–3, 3*t*, 369
Closing volume
in asthma, 92
in upper respiratory tract infections, 81
Co-oximeter, in carbon monoxide poisoning, 210
Coagulation testing, preoperative, 37–38
Coagulopathy
with childhood cancer, 223*t*, 230–231
dilutional, in thermal/burn injury patients, 214, 218
in hepatic failure, 296, 296*t*
with malignant hyperthermia, 341, 348–349
Codeine
allergic and anaphylactic reactions to, 308
dosage of, 383*t*
postoperative, after posterior fossa craniotomy, 270
Cold-induced asthma, 92
Colloids, allergic and anaphylactic reactions to, 301
Committee on Professional Liability (ASA), 2
Communication, with cerebral palsy patients, 285
Compartment syndrome, in thermal/burn injury, 215

Complement activation tests, for allergies, 305
Complete blood count
  preoperative, 37
  in thermal/burn injury, 214
Complication(s), 3–4. *See also specific procedures and disorders*
  closed claim studies of, 2–3, 3t
  of postanesthesia care, 7–9
    incidence of, 7–8
Computed tomography
  of head trauma, 200–201
  of increased intracranial pressure, 262–263
  of multiple trauma, 203
  of tracheal size, in cancer studies, 221–226
Computers, in screening of pediatric outpatients, 27
Confidentiality, of adolescents, 19–20
Congenital heart disease. *See* Heart disease, congenital
Conscious sedation, 391f, 391–392
  definition of, 391
  limitations of, 392
  personnel, monitoring, and record keeping required with, 392f
  transition from, to deep sedation or general anesthesia, 393
Consciousness, and eligibility for discharge, 363t
Consent
  informed
    in difficult airway cases, 149–150
    disclosure of risks and, 9
  pediatric, approaches to, 14t
Contact burns, 206
Continuing quality improvement, and sedation policy, 394, 396
Contracture testing, for malignant hyperthermia susceptibility, 340, 350
Convulsion, risk of, anesthesia and, 3t
Cooling, for malignant hyperthermia, 348, 356t

Cooperative Study of Sickle Cell Disease Group, 279
Cor pulmonale
  with asthma, 92, 95
  with bronchopulmonary dysplasia, 99
  with cystic fibrosis, 89
  with obstructive sleep apnea, 101
Core temperature monitoring, of malignant hyperthermia-susceptible patients, 351
Coronary artery, anomalous, from pulmonary artery, 180t
Corticosteroid(s)
  for asthma, 93–94
  for cystic fibrosis, 89
  for increased intracranial pressure, 265
Coughing
  in asthma, 96
  in bronchopulmonary dysplasia, 100
  in cystic fibrosis, 90
  in upper respiratory tract infections, 82, 85–86
Craniopharyngioma, 233, 263
Craniotomy
  for encephalocele, 270
  posterior fossa, 268–270
    anesthesia maintenance in, 269
    emergence from, 269–270
    induction in, 269
    monitoring in, 269
    patient positioning for, 268–269
    preoperative assessment for, 268
  supratentorial, 267–268
    anesthesia induction and maintenance in, 267
    anesthetic considerations in, 267
    emergence from, 267–268
    neurologic assessment after, overaggressive use of opioids and, 268
    preoperative assessment for, 267
Creatine kinase, in malignant hyperthermia, 340–342

Cricoid pressure, for intubation, in trauma management, 197–198
Cricothyroidotomy, in trauma management, 196, 199
Critical events, 396
Cromolyn sodium, for asthma, 94
Croup
  conservative treatment of, 124
  helium and oxygen therapy for, 110
  pulmonary edema after, 103
  in recovery room (postextubation), 127–128, 369
    incidence of, 127
    management of, 128
  stridor with, 112–113, 124
  treatment of, gas flow principles and, 110
  upper respiratory tract infections and, 82
CRS (clinical recovery scores), 361, 362t–364t
Cryoprecipitate, for thermal/burn injury patients, 214
Cryopreservation, of autologous blood donation, 324–325
Cyanide poisoning, 210–211, 214, 318
Cyanosis, in congenital heart disease, 170
Cyclophosphamide
  for acute lymphoblastic leukemia, 232
  classification and side effects of, 239t
  for neuroblastoma, 236
  in preparative regime for bone marrow transplantation, 251
  for Wilms' tumor, 237
Cyclosporine
  and hypertension, 312
  for immunosuppression, and potentiation of anesthetic drugs, 298
  for Langerhans' cell histiocytosis, 238
Cylert, 62t
Cystic fibrosis, 87–91
  genetics of, 87–88
  incidence of, 87
  induction options in, 90–91
  intraoperative management in, 89–90
  major systemic aberrations in, 88–89
  median survival age in, 87
  postoperative management in, 91
  preoperative evaluation in, 89
  pulmonary therapy for, 89
  surgeries related to, 87
Cystic fibrosis transmembrane conductance regulator (CFTR), 87–88
Cystic hygroma, difficult airway with, 146, 153, 156f
Cytarabine
  for acute lymphoblastic leukemia, 232
  for acute myelogenous leukemia, 233
  classification and side effects of, 240t
  in preparative regime for bone marrow transplantation, 251

D

D-loop transposition, 180t
Dacarbazine, for Hodgkin's disease, 235
Dactinomycin
  classification and side effects of, 241t
  for Wilms' tumor, 237
Damage, proof in negligence, 17t
Dantrolene
  for malignant hyperthermia, 339, 348t, 348–349, 351–352, 356t–357t
  for rhabdomyolysis, 291
Darwin, Charles, 57
Daunorubicin, 243
  for acute lymphoblastic leukemia, 232
  cardiac toxicity of, 243f, 243–247, 245f–246f
  classification and side effects of, 241t
DDAVP
  decrease in blood loss with, 333
  for postoperative diabetes insipidus, 268

Deadspace, increased, hypercarbia with, 320
Debridement, of thermal/burn injury, 213–216
Decadron, for nausea and vomiting, 366
Decision-making, in pediatric care, 13–25
  acceptable, determining parameters of, 15
  best-interests standard for, 14–15
  for forgoing life-sustaining care, 20–23
  by Jehovah's Witnesses, 18–19
  patient's age and maturity and, 13, 15–16, 18
  special situations in, 18–20
Deep sedation, 391f, 391–392
  definition of, 391
  need in painful procedures, 392–393
  personnel, monitoring, and record keeping required in, 392f, 392–393
Defibrillators
  anesthetic considerations for pediatric patients with, 192
  for dysrhythmias, 191–192
Dehydration
  in diabetes mellitus, 283
  in renal failure, 292
  in sickle cell disease, 280
Delirium, emergence, 365, 382
Density, and gas flow through tubes, 110
Department of Anesthesiology, involvement in institution-wide sedation policy, 394–395
1-desamino-8-D-arginine vasopressin. *See* DDAVP
Desaturation events
  in former preterm infants, spinal versus general anesthesia and, 138
  in postanesthesia care unit, 360
  upper respiratory tract infections and, 5, 82–83, 83t, 84f
Desflurane
  dysrhythmia induced by, 181

  and time to recovery and discharge, 365, 368
Development, child, 56–57
  by age, 59t
  chronic illness and, 66t
  definition of, 56
  models of, 58t
Developmental disorders, 57–65
Developmental pediatric neurobiology, 374–375
Developmental psychology, 57
Dexamethasone
  for difficult airway, 165
  for increased intracranial pressure, 265, 269
  for nausea prophylaxis, 368
Dexedrine, 62t
Dextroamphetamine (Dexedrine), 62t
Dextrose infusion, in anesthetic management of diabetes mellitus, 282
Diabetes insipidus
  hydrocephalus with, 266
  postoperative, after supratentorial craniotomy, 268
Diabetes mellitus, 280–283
  anesthetic management in, 282–283
  classification of, 280, 281t
  with cystic fibrosis, 88
  etiology of, 280–281
  fundamentals of care for children with, 282
  goal of pediatric anesthesiologist in, 282
  insulin-dependent (type 1), 280, 281t
  intraoperative monitoring in, 282–283
  non-insulin-dependent (type 2), 280, 281t
  pathophysiology of, 281–282
  scheduling of patients with, early in day, 283
Diagnostic and Statistical Manual of Mental Disorders, 4th edition (DSM-IV), diagnostic criteria
  for attention-deficit/hyperactivity disorder, 60, 61t
  for autism, 64t

Dialysis, for renal failure, 293
  preoperative timing of, 294
Diaphoresis, with congenital heart disease, 169
Diaphragmatic fatigue, in asthma, 92–93
Diaspirin cross-linked hemoglobin solutions, decrease in blood loss with, 333
Diclofenac
  dosage of, 383*t*
  with patient-controlled analgesia, 378
Dietary malabsorption, with cystic fibrosis, 89
Difficult airway
  ASA algorithm for, 144*f*, 150, 158
  clinical management of, 150–165
  with cystic hygroma, 146, 153, 156*f*
  elective tracheotomy for, 149–150, 164
  equipment cart for, 150, 151*f*
  expected, 143
    identification of, 143–149
    and surgery in child with upper respiratory tract infection, 84
  extubation and emergence in cases with, 165
  as foremost challenge in pediatric anesthesia, 143
  with hemifacial microsomia, 145–146, 147*f*, 148*t*, 153–155, 156*f*
  history of difficult intubation and, 143, 148–149
  induction in, 152–153
  informed consent in cases of, 149–150
  intubation in, 153–164
    alternative techniques of, 159–164
    anatomy of, 145, 153–157, 154*f*–155*f*
    blind oral or blind nasal, 159, 161–163
    fiberoptic, 159–160, 160*f*, 161*t*
    retrograde, 159, 163–164, 164*f*
    via laryngeal mask anesthesia, 159, 161, 162*f*
    with Klippel-Feil syndrome, 147, 149*f*
    laryngoscopy in, 153–164, 156*f*
      backward upward right pressure in, 158
      Bullard laryngoscope for, 158
      depth of anesthesia and, 157
      direct, 157–158
      ease of, by mandibular classification, 146, 148*t*
      improving view in, techniques for, 158
      left lateral approach in, 158
      Malimpatti classification of signs predicting, 145, 145*f*
      optimal external laryngeal manipulation in, 158
      space for, potential, assessment of, 155–157
      two-person technique for, 158
  management of child with, 137–160
  mandible assessment and classification in, 145–146, 148*t*
  medical history and, 143–145
  miscellaneous considerations in, 164–165
  mouth assessment in, 145–146
  muscle relaxants for, 153–155, 158–159
  neck assessment in, 145–147
  physical examination in, 143, 145–147
  post case analysis of, 165
  preanesthetic evaluation for, 143–149
  premedication in, 150–152
  preoperative preparation of, 150
  presentation of, 143
  recommendations of ASA task force on, 148, 165
  secretion management in, 150–152, 160
  steroids for, 165
  with thermal/burn injury, 211, 218
  tongue assessment in, 145, 146*f*
  topicalization in, 157, 160
  unexpected, 143, 164–165
Difficult child
  as temperament type, 67

Difficult child, parent, or family
　identification of, 56–69
　management of, 69–75, 153
　　important issues for anesthesiologist in, 75
　parent's perspective on, 76–78
　providing care for, 56–79
Diffusion capacity, in upper respiratory tract infections, 81
Digoxin
　for acute fibrillation and atrial flutter, 188
　for atrioventricular node dysfunction, 186
　for paroxysmal supraventricular atrial tachycardia, 186
　for postobstructive pulmonary edema, 104
Dilantin, prophylactic, in neurosurgery, 268
Dilutional coagulopathy, in thermal/burn injury patients, 214, 218
Diphenhydramine
　for anaphylactic reactions, 304t
　for pretreatment of patients with high risk for radiocontrast media allergy, 308
Directed blood donations, 325
Discharge, from postanesthesia care unit, 358–373
　versus admission, 358–359
　choice of anesthetic and, 368
　criteria for, 358, 361–365
　factors affecting, 365–369
　fast-tracking and, 361–365
　gold standard for, 361
　JCAHO policies on, 358
　malignant hyperthermia and, 369
　nausea/vomiting and, 362t, 365–366, 370
　pain/pain management and, 362t–363t, 368–370
　of preterm infants, 366–367
　recovery room scores and, 361, 362t–364t
　regional anesthesia and, 368–369
　street readiness for, 358
　voiding and, 363t–364t, 366, 369
Disclosure
　of anesthetic risks, 9
　and negligence, 17t
　in pediatric care, 16
Discussion, postoperative, with parents, 75
Disseminated intravascular coagulation, with malignant hyperthermia, 341, 348–349
Diuretics, for increased intracranial pressure, 265
Do-not-resuscitate (DNR) orders
　goal-directed, 21–22
　perioperative, 21–23
　　options for obtaining and documenting, 21–22
　postoperative planning for, 22–23
　procedure-directed, 22
　and response to iatrogenic arrest or emergencies, 23
Dopamine
　for anaphylactic reactions, 304t
　for cardiovascular effects, of thermal/burn injury, 212
Double-outlet right ventricle, 180t
Down's syndrome, cervical spinal injury in children with, 201–202
Doxorubicin, 243
　for acute lymphoblastic leukemia, 232
　cardiac toxicity of, 243f, 243–247, 245f–246f
　　cumulative dose and, 244–245, 245f
　　monitoring for, 245–247, 246f
　classification and side effects of, 241t
　for Hodgkin's disease, 235
　for neuroblastoma, 236
　for Wilms' tumor, 237
Duchenne muscular dystrophy, 288–291
　anesthetic considerations in, 7, 289–291
　diagnosis of, 289
　etiology of, 288
　and malignant hyperthermia, 290–291, 342, 352–353
　pathophysiology of, 288–289
　treatment of, 289
Duodenum injury, 202

Duty
  breach of, 17*t*
  presence of, 17*t*
Dyskinetic cerebral palsy, 284*t*, 285
Dysrhythmias
  anesthetic technique and, 179
  atrial, 182–188, 192–193
  with congenital heart disease, 179–181
  implantable pacemakers and cardioverter-defibrillators for, 191–193
  induced by inhalation anesthesia, 181
  induced by local anesthetics, 181–182
  induced by muscle relaxants, 182
  malignant, 186, 188–189, 192
  with malignant hyperthermia, 340
  monitoring in postanesthesia care unit, 360
  in pediatric patient, acquired, 181
  in pediatric patients, 179–195
    acquired, 181–182
    common, 182–191
    postoperative, 179–181
    types of, 179
  ventricular, 188–190, 193
Dystrophin, in muscular dystrophy, 289, 344

E

e-Aminocaproic acid (EACA), decrease in blood loss with, 333
Ear, nose, and throat procedures, postanesthesia care in, monitoring in and discharge from, 367–368
Easy child, as temperament type, 67
Ebstein-Barr virus, lymphoma with, 233–235
Ebstein's anomaly, 180*t*, 183, 191
Echocardiography, of malignant hyperthermia-susceptible patients, 351
Ectopic atrial tachycardia, 182–183
  mechanism of, 184*f*
Ectopy, as warning sign, 182
Edrophonium, for paroxysmal supraventricular atrial tachycardia, 186
Education
  anesthesiologist's role in, 7, 56, 395
  for patients and families, 56
  on sedation policy, 395–396
Eisenmenger physiology, 167, 176
Electrical burns, 206–207
Electrocardiography
  in anthracycline cardiotoxicity, 243–245
  of atrial fibrillation and atrial flutter, 187, 187*f*
  of junctional ectopic tachycardia, 183*f*
  in malignant hyperthermia, 342, 369
  for monitoring in postanesthesia care unit, 360
  in muscular dystrophy, 289
  of torsade de pointes, 190*f*, 192*f*
  of Wolff-Parkinson-White syndrome, 184–185, 185*f*
Electrolyte(s)
  and anesthetic risk, 3*t*
  in chemotherapy, 243
  in long QT syndrome, 190
  in renal failure, 293
  in thermal/burn injury, 213
Emancipated minors, informed consent of, 18
Embolism
  air
    in posterior fossa craniotomy, 269
    risk of, anesthesia and, 3*t*
  pulmonary, hypotension with, 316
Emergence
  in difficult airway cases, 165
  in head trauma cases, 272
  in hepatic failure, 297
  in hydrocephalic patients, 266
  increased intracranial pressure and, 266
  from posterior fossa craniotomy, 269–270
  after supratentorial craniotomy, 267–268

after surgery for mediastinal masses, 229
Emergence delirium, 365, 382
Emotion, in cancer and cancer treatment, 255–257
Empyema, with cystic fibrosis, 88
Encephalocele, 270
Endobronchial intubation, risk of, anesthesia and, 3*t*
Endocardial cushion defect, 180*t*
Endocarditis prophylaxis
  cardiac conditions requiring, 173*t*
  in congenital heart disease, 171, 172*t*–173*t*
  for dental, oral, respiratory tract, and esophageal procedures, 31*t*, 172*t*
  for genitourinary and gastrointestinal procedures, 172*t*
  guidelines for, 9, 30, 31*t*, 172*t*–173*t*
  in outpatient surgery, 30
  procedures where not recommended, 173*t*
  procedures where recommended, 31*t*, 172*t*–173*t*
Endotracheal tube
  avoidance in asthma, 96
  in cervical spinal injury, 202
  in difficult airway, 153–158
    blind oral and blind nasal insertion of, 161–163
    laryngeal mask airway as conduit for, 161, 162*f*
    retrograde insertion of, 163–164, 164*f*
  kinking or obstruction of
    in posterior fossa craniotomy, 269
    stridor with, 126–127
    upper respiratory tract infections and, 82
  versus laryngeal mask airway, 86, 90, 317
  mediastinal masses and, 228–229
  and postextubation croup, 127–128
  in thermal/burn injury, 217
  in trauma management, 197–199
  in upper respiratory tract infections, 86, 317
Enflurane, dysrhythmia induced by, 181
Enteral nutrition, in thermal/burn injury, 213
Eosinophilic granuloma, 238
Ependymoma, 233, 268
Ephedrine, for pretreatment of patients with high risk for radiocontrast media allergy, 308
Epidural analgesia, 368–369, 379–382
  continuous method for, 381
  dosages of, 382*t*
  latency period with, 380
  lumbar, 380
  monitoring children receiving, 384–385
  order forms for, 387–388
  postoperative, typical, 381
  thoracic, 380
  volume of, and level of analgesia, 379*t*
Epidural hematoma, 271
Epiglottis, visualization in laryngoscopy, in difficult airway, 153–157
Epiglottitis
  protocol for, 120–121
  pulmonary edema after, 103
  stridor with, 112, 119–121
  ventilation in, importance of, 120–121
Epilepsy, in cerebral palsy patients, 285
Epinephrine
  for anaphylactic reactions, 304*t*
  for asthma, 97
  for cardiovascular effects, of thermal/burn injury, 212
  with local anesthetics, dysrhythmias induced by, 181–182
  and masseter muscle rigidity, 339
  racemic, for postextubation croup, 128
  in thermal/burn injury, absorption of, and hypertension, 218

Epipodophyllotoxins, classification and side effects of, 241*t*
Epirubicin, 243
  cardiac toxicity of, 243*f*, 243–247, 245*f*–246*f*
Equipment problems, risk of, anesthesia and, 3*t*
Erythropoietin
  human recombinant, for improving autologous blood donation, 324
  for renal failure, 293
Escharotomies, for thermal/burn injury, 215
Escherichia coli infection, pneumonia with, 97
Esmolol
  for controlled hypotension, 329, 330*t*
  for paroxysmal supraventricular atrial tachycardia, 186–187
Esophageal Intubation, risk of, anesthesia and, 3*t*
Esophageal varices, with hepatic failure, 297
Ether, and malignant hyperthermia, 338
Ethical issues
  in child abuse, 23
  in forgoing life-sustaining care, 20–23
  in informed consent, 13–20
  in pediatric care, 13–25
  in pediatric pain management, 23–24
  in production pressure, 24
  in refusal of cases, 24
  seeking help with, 24–25
Etomidate
  and cerebral blood flow, 201, 202*t*
  for trauma patients, 198, 198*t*, 201, 203–204
Etoposide
  for acute myelogenous leukemia, 233
  classification and side effects of, 241*t*
  for Langerhans' cell histiocytosis, 238
  for neuroblastoma, 236
  in preparative regime for bone marrow transplantation, 251
Ewing's sarcoma, 237
  bone marrow transplantation for, 250
  incidence in children, 220*t*
  radiation therapy for, 248, 250
  spinal cord compression with, 229
Exercise-induced asthma, 92
External beam radiation therapy, 248–250
Extubation
  in difficult airway cases, 165
  in hepatic failure, 297
  in hydrocephalic patients, 266
  inadvertent, risk of, anesthesia and, 3*t*
  increased intracranial pressure and, 266
  and laryngospasm, 127
  after posterior fossa craniotomy, 269–270
  premature, risk of, anesthesia and, 3*t*
  after supratentorial craniotomy, 267–268
  after surgery for mediastinal masses, 229

F

Failure to thrive, with congenital heart disease, 169–170
Family
  of cancer patients, emotional stress of, 255–257
  difficult
    identification of, 56–69
    management of, 69–75
      important issues for anesthesiologist in, 75
    parent's perspective on, 76–78
    providing care for, 56–79
  in postanesthesia care unit, 74–75, 359
Family dynamics, 68–69
Fasciotomies, for thermal/burn injury, 215
Fast-tracking, in postanesthesia care unit, 361–365

Fasting, preoperative, limitation in congenital heart disease, 171
Femoral veins, for intravenous access, in trauma cases, 199
Fentanyl
  epidural, 380–381, 382t
  and intracranial pressure, 264–265
  lollipop formulations of, 45–46, 214
  oral transmucosal
    avoidance in difficult airway cases, 150
    dosage of, 46, 47t
    efficacy of, 47t
    monitoring recommendations for, 47t
    for preanesthetic sedation, 45–46, 47t
    time of onset and peak effect of, 46, 47t
  patient-controlled, 378
  in posterior fossa craniotomy, 269
  potentiation of effects of, cyclosporine and, 298
  in supratentorial craniotomy, 267
  for thermal/burn injury patients, 215
  and time to recovery and discharge, 365
  for trauma patients, 203–204
Fetal hemoglobin, 276
  in preterm infants, 139
  in sickle cell disease, 276
Fever, neurogenic, versus malignant hyperthermia, 345
Fiberoptic bronchoscopy, mediastinal masses and, 228–229
Fiberoptic intubation
  in cervical spinal injury, 202
  in difficult airway, 159–160
  equipment for, 159–160, 160f, 161t
  in thermal/burn injury, 211
  in trauma management, 197
Firearm injuries, 196
Flame burns, 206
Fluid management
  inadequate/inappropriate, risk of, anesthesia and, 3t
  in increased intracranial pressure, 265
  in sickle cell disease, 280
  in thermal/burn injury, intraoperative, 217–218
Fluid resuscitation
  in thermal/burn injury, 212–213, 218
    formulas for, 212
  in trauma management, 199–200
5-Fluorouracil, classification and side effects of, 240t
Fluoxetine, for pervasive developmental disorders, 65
Focal nodular hyperplasia, hepatic failure with, 295t
Folic acid analog, classification and side effects of, 240t
Fontan procedure, 175t, 178, 187–188, 191
Food allergies, 300
Food and Drug Administration, adverse drug event reporting system of, 395
Forced expiratory volume in one second (FEV_1), in upper respiratory tract infections, 81
Forced vital capacity (FVC), in upper respiratory tract infections, 81
Foreign body obstruction, stridor with, 112, 116–117
Four Hs (hypertension, hypotension, hypoxia, hypercarbia), 312–321
Fraction of inspired oxygen (FIO_2), inadequate, risk of, anesthesia and, 3t
Fractionated radiation therapy, 250
Fresh frozen plasma, for thermal/burn injury patients, 214, 217–218
Freud, Sigmund, 58t
Full stomach risk
  in renal failure, 294
  in trauma cases, 198, 272
Fulminant pulmonary edema, 104
Furosemide
  for increased intracranial pressure, 265, 269
  in posterior fossa craniotomy, 269

G

Ganglioma, 236, 268
Ganglioneuroblastoma, 236
Ganglionic blockers, for controlled hypotension, 329, 330*t*
Gas flow, through tubes, principles of, and stridor, 108–110
Gastrin clearance, in renal failure, 293
Gastroesophageal reflux
  with bronchopulmonary dysplasia, 99
  with cerebral palsy, 286
  with cystic fibrosis, 88–90
  incidence of, 3
Gastrointestinal allergies, 300
Gastrointestinal problems, in cerebral palsy patients, 285–286
General anesthesia
  in asthma, versus regional anesthesia, 95
  in continuum of sedation, 391*f*, 391–393
  in preterm and former preterm infants
    versus regional anesthesia, 8–9
    versus spinal anesthesia, 136–138, 138*t*
Germ cell tumors, 237
Gesell, Arnold, 57
Gingival hypertrophy, with cerebral palsy, 286
Glasgow Coma Score, 196, 200, 272
  modified, for infants and younger children, 197*t*
  and trauma outcome, 204, 204*t*
Glenn procedure, 178
Glioma, 233, 268
Globin, 275
Glucocorticoids, for anaphylactic reactions, 304*t*
Glucose infusion, in anesthetic management of diabetes mellitus, 282
Glucose tolerance
  in cystic fibrosis, 88–89, 91
  in diabetes mellitus, 281–282
Glycoprotein(s)
  in hepatic failure, 296
  local anesthetic binding to, 379
Glycopyrrolate
  for asthma, 95, 97
  for cerebral palsy patients, 286
  co-administration of, with preanesthetic sedation, 42
  in difficult airway cases, 152
  dosage, time of onset, and administration of, 152*t*
  for upper respiratory tract infections, 81, 85, 87
Goldenhar's syndrome, 145–146, 147*f*, 164
Gower's maneuver, in muscular dystrophy, 288
Graft versus host disease, 250–251
Granuloma, eosinophilic, 238
Great vessels
  compression of, with mediastinal masses, 219, 229
  transposition of, 175*t*, 180*t*, 191

H

H(s), four (hypertension, hypotension, hypoxia, hypercarbia), 312–321
Haemophilus influenzae infection
  in cystic fibrosis, 88
  immunization against, 119
  pneumonia with, 97
Hagen-Poisseuille equation, of airflow, 108–109
Halothane
  in asthma, 96
  cardiovascular depression with, 1
  in cystic fibrosis, 90
  dysrhythmia induced by, 181
  in hydrocephalic patients, 266
  and intracranial pressure, 265
  in long QT syndrome, 190
  and malignant hyperthermia, 338–339, 342–344
    contracture test for susceptibility to, 350
  in malignant hyperthermia-susceptible patients, 351
  for myringotomy and pressure equalization tube placement, 368
  and rhabdomyolysis, 291
  safety and risks of, 4–5
  and time to recovery and discharge, 365
  in upper respiratory tract infections, 85

Hand-Schuller-Christian syndrome, 238
Head immobilization, for intubation, in cervical spinal injury, 202
Head trauma, 196, 271–272
  age-related pathophysiology in, 272
  anesthesia induction in, 272
  anesthesia maintenance in, 272
  anesthetic considerations in, 271–272
  associated injuries with, 272
  cerebral blood flow in, anesthetic effects on, 201, 202t
  emergence and postoperative management in, 272
  full stomach risk in, 272
  intubation with, 199
  management of, 200–201
  monitoring in, 272
  neurologic status in, 272
  resuscitation and stabilization in, 271
HealthQuiz, in screening of pediatric outpatients, 27
Heart block, congenital complete, 191
Heart disease
  acquired, outpatient surgery in children with, 30–32
  congenital, 167–178
    and anesthetic risk in noncardiac surgery, 5–6
    box diagrams of, 167, 168f
    cardiac grid for summarizing physiologic manipulations in, 173, 175t
    dysrhythmias with, 179–181
    factors in considering patient with, 167–169
    general approaches to physiology in, 174t
    hematologic problems associated with, 170, 170t
    history and physical examination in assessment of, 169–170
    hypoxia with, 318
    important factors in anesthetizing children with, 171, 174t
    incidence of, 167, 180t
    induction and maintenance of anesthesia in, 171–177
    neurologic problems associated with, 67, 171t
    noncardiac manifestations of, 169, 169t–171t
    outpatient surgery in children with, 30–32
    postanesthesia EKG monitoring for patients with, 360
    postoperative care in, 177–178
    preoperative considerations in, 171
    prophylactic antibiotic therapy in, 171, 172t–173t
    pulmonary interactions associated with, 169t
    understanding physiology in, 167, 168f
    vascular access and resistance in, 176t, 176–178
Heart murmur
  evaluation of, 30, 30t
  with mediastinal masses, 221, 226
  and outpatient surgery, 30
Helium and oxygen therapy (Heliox)
  for croup, 110
  for expiratory obstructive diseases, 110
  gas flow principles in, 110
Hemangioendothelioma, hepatic failure with, 295t
Hemangioma, cavernous, hepatic failure with, 295t
Hematocrit
  in asthma, 95
  in congenital heart disease, 170, 170t
  in former preterm infants, and perioperative risk, 139–141, 140t–141t
  minimal acceptable, in acute normovolemic hemodilution, 327
  preoperative testing of, 36–37
  in thermal/burn injury, 214, 217
  in trauma cases, 199
Hematologic problems
  with congenital heart disease, 170, 170t
  with thermal/burn injury, 214

Hematoma(s)
  epidural, 271
  intracerebral, 271
  posttraumatic intracranial, 271–272
  subdural, 271
Hematopoietic malignancies, tumor lysis syndrome with, 229
Hemifacial disorders, obstructive sleep apnea with, 102
Hemifacial microsomia
  classification of, 146
  difficult airway with, 145–146, 147f, 148t, 153–155, 156f
Hemoconcentration, with thermal/burn injury, 214
Hemodilution
  acute hypervolemic, 328
  acute normovolemic, 326–328
    advantages of, 328
    combined with controlled hypotension, 331
    contraindications to, 328
    formula for blood withdrawal in, 327–328
    and hemostasis, 328
    combined with intraoperative blood salvage, 331
Hemodynamic changes, in cardiac defects, 175t
Hemoglobin
  adult, 276
  in congenital heart disease, 170
  fetal, 276
    in preterm infants, 139
  minimum level for autologous blood donation, 322
  preoperative testing of, 36–37
  in sickle cell disease, 275–276
  structure of, 275
  in trauma cases, 199
Hemoglobin-based oxygen carriers, decrease in blood loss with, 333
Hemoglobin electrophoresis, in sickle cell disease, 276–278
Hemoglobinopathies, 275–280
Hemophilia, DDAVP for limiting blood loss in, 333
Hemoptysis, with cystic fibrosis, 88
Hemostatic tests, preoperative, 37–38

Hepatic blastoma, 237
Hepatic failure, 294–298
  acute, 294
  anesthetic considerations in, 296t, 297–298
  cardiopulmonary dysfunction with, 296t
  coagulation problems with, 296, 296t
  etiology of, 294–295, 295t
  and immune status, 296t
  metabolic problems with, 296t, 296–297
  and nutrition status, 296t
  pathophysiology of, 295–297, 296t
  and renal status, 296t
Hepatic fibrosis, congenital, hepatic failure with, 295t
Hepatic transplantation, 298
Hepatitis
  neonatal, hepatic failure with, 295t
  of newborn, hepatic failure with, 295t
  postnatal, hepatic failure with, 295t
Hepatitis A infection, transmission of, via blood transfusion, 322, 323t
Hepatitis B infection
  autologous blood donations from patients with, 325
  transmission of, via blood transfusion, 322, 323t
Hepatitis C infection
  autologous blood donations from patients with, 325
  transmission of, via blood transfusion, 322, 323t
Hepatoblastoma, hepatic failure with, 295t
Hepatocellular carcinoma, 237
  hepatic failure with, 295t
Hepatomegaly, with childhood cancer, 222t, 230
Hepatosplenomegaly
  with acute myelogenous leukemia, 232
  with non-Hodgkin's lymphoma, 234
Histamine, release in thermal/burn injury, 208

Histiocytosis X, 238
History, medical
  in congenital heart disease assessment, 169–170
  and identification of difficult airway, 143–145
  in increased incranial pressure, 261
  in preoperative evaluation, 35
  in stridor, 112–113
HIV infection
  autologous blood donations from patients with, 325
  transmission of, via blood transfusion, 322, 323*t*
Hodgkin's disease, 234–235
  bone marrow transplantation for, 235
  chemotherapy for, 235
  clinical presentation of, 235
  incidence of, 220*t*, 234
  mediastinal masses with, 221
  radiation therapy for, 235, 248
  spinal cord compression with, 229
Human immunodeficiency virus (HIV) infection
  autologous blood donations from patients with, 325
  transmission of, via blood transfusion, 322, 323*t*
Human recombinant erythropoietin, for improving autologous blood donation, 324
Hydralazine, postoperative, after supratentorial craniotomy, 268
Hydrocephalus, 266
  anesthesia induction and maintenance in, 266
  with brain tumors, 267
  emergence in, 266
  myelodysplasia with, 270
  preoperative assessment of, 266
Hydrocortisone
  for anaphylactic reactions, 304*t*
  for asthma, 94
Hydromorphone
  dosage of, 383*t*
  epidural, 382*t*
Hyperaldosteronism, with hepatic failure, 297

Hyperbaric oxygen therapy, in carbon monoxide poisoning, 210
Hypercalcemia, with childhood cancer, 223*t*
Hypercapnia
  in asthma, 92, 95
  response in neonate, 130
Hypercarbia
  with increased intracranial pressure, 262–263
  intraoperative, 319–320
    etiology of, 319*f*, 319–320
    management of, 320, 320*f*
Hypercyanotic "tet" spells, 177, 177*t*
Hyperfractionated radiation therapy, 250
Hyperglycemia, in diabetes mellitus, 281–282
Hyperinflation, in asthma, 92, 95
Hyperkalemia
  controlled, for long QT syndrome, 189
  with increased intracranial pressure, succinylcholine and, 264
  in malignant hyperthermia, 348–349, 356*t*
  in renal failure, 292
  in rhabdomyolysis, 291, 353
  in thermal/burn injury, succinylcholine and, 216
  with tumor lysis syndrome, 229–230
Hyperleukocytosis
  with acute myelogenous leukemia, 232
  with childhood cancer, 222*t*, 231
  definition of, 231
Hypernatremia, in thermal/burn injury, 213
Hyperoxic ventilation, with acute normovolemic hemodilution, 327
Hyperphosphatemia, with tumor lysis syndrome, 229–230
Hypersplenism, with hepatic failure, 297
Hypertension
  definition in pediatric population, 322
  intraoperative, 312–314

Hypertension (*continued*)
    disease states associated with, 312–314, 315t
    etiology of, 312, 313f
    management of, 312, 314f
  in neonates, incidence of, 312
  portal, with hepatic failure, 297
  pulmonary
    in asthma, 92
    in bronchopulmonary dysplasia, 99
    crisis with, in congenital heart disease patients, 178
    incidence of, 180t
    with obstructive sleep apnea, 101
  in renal failure, 293
  systemic, incidence of, 180t
  with thermal/burn injury, 218
Hyperthermia, malignant. *See* Malignant hyperthermia
Hypertrophic obstructive cardiomyopathy, pacemaker and cardioverter-defibrillator for, 191
Hyperuricemia, with tumor lysis syndrome, 229–230
Hypervascularized lesions, 263
Hyperventilation
  for increased intracranial pressure, 265, 269
  in posterior fossa craniotomy, 269
  in supratentorial craniotomy, 267
Hypnotic drugs
  allergic and anaphylactic reactions to, 301
  for pervasive developmental disorders, 65
Hypoalbuminemia, in thermal/burn injury, 213
Hypocalcemia
  hypotension with, 316
  in renal failure, 293
  in thermal/burn injury, 213
  with tumor lysis syndrome, 229–230
Hypomagnesemia, in thermal/burn injury, 213
Hypophosphatemia, in thermal/burn injury, 213
Hypoplastic left ventricle, 180t
Hypotension
  with bradycardia, 4
  controlled, 328–329
    agents used to achieve, 329, 330t
    combined with acute normovolemic hemodilution, 331
    contraindications to, 329
    with increased intracranial pressure, 263
  intraoperative, 314–316
    diagnosis and treatment of, 317f
    etiology of, 314, 316f
  in renal failure, 293
  with thermal/burn injury, 208, 212
  with vancomycin allergy, 306–307
Hypothermia
  in cerebral palsy patients, 288
  in muscular dystrophy, 290
  in sickle cell disease, 280
  with thermal/burn injury, 212, 218
Hypoventilation, hypercarbia with, 320
Hypovolemia
  hypertension with, 312
  postoperative, in congenital heart disease, 178
  in supratentorial craniotomy, 267
  with thermal/burn injury, 208–209, 212
  in trauma patient, drug recommendations for endotracheal intubation for, 198, 198t
Hypoxemia
  in asthma, 92–93, 95
  biphasic response in neonates, 130
  in bronchopulmonary dysplasia, 99–100
  with mediastinal masses, 219, 229
  in pneumonia, 98
  in upper respiratory tract infections, 5, 29, 81–83, 86
Hypoxia
  greater risk in neonate, 316
  with hepatic failure, 297
  increased intracranial pressure and, 262

intraoperative, 316–318
  etiology of, 316–317, 318f
  management of, 319f
  with obstructive sleep apnea, 101
  perinatal, and cerebral palsy, 284
  with postobstructive pulmonary edema, 104
  postoperative, 360
  in sickle cell disease, 280

I

Ibuprofen
  high-dose, for cystic fibrosis, 89
  preoperative, for myringotomy and pressure equalization tube placement, 368
ICP. *See* Intracranial pressure
Idarubicin, 243
  cardiac toxicity of, 243f, 243–247, 245f–246f
  classification and side effects of, 241t
Ifosfamide, classification and side effects of, 239t
Ileum injury, 202
Illness, chronic, 65–68
  child's age and, 66–67
  definition of, 66
  development and behavior of children with, factors influencing, 66t
  and family dynamics, 68–69
  providing care for child with, parent's perspective on, 76–78
  temperament and, 67
Immobilization
  of head and neck, for intubation, in cervical spinal injury, 202
  by physical restraint, unacceptability of, 389
Immune system, immaturity of, and allergies, 300
Immunodiagnostic tests, for allergies, 305
Immunoglobulin E, and allergies, 300, 305, 307
Indomethacin
  and emergence delirium, 382
  rectal, 379

Induction
  allergic and anaphylactic reactions during, 301
  in asthma, 89–96
  for cerebral palsy patients, 287
  in congenital heart disease, 171–177
  in cystic fibrosis, 90–91
  in difficult airway, 152–153
  in difficult child, 74
  in hepatic failure, 297
  in hydrocephalus, 266
  increased intracranial pressure and, 264–265
  in myelodysplasia, 270
  parental presence during, 72–74, 152
    versus preanesthetic sedation, 41–42, 72
  in posterior fossa craniotomy, 269
  in renal failure, 293–294
  sedation before, 41–55, 71
  in supratentorial craniotomy, 267
  in surgery for mediastinal masses, 227–228
  in trauma cases, 198–199, 203, 272
  in upper respiratory tract infections, options in, 85–87
Infants/neonates
  autologous blood donations from, 322
  behavioral development and responses of, 57, 59t
  chronically ill, 66–67
  dosing in, 384
  hypertension in, incidence of, 312
  hypoxia in, greater risk of, 316
  pain perception by, misconceptions about, 374–375, 389
  pharmacokinetics of local anesthetics in, 379–380
  preterm. *See* Preterm infants
  respiratory control and mechanics of, anesthesia and, 130–131
  respiratory function in, 130
  ventricular tachycardia, classification of, 188–189
Infection, in thermal/burn injury, 213
Informed assent, 15–16
  use of, 18

Informed consent
  best-interests standard and, 14–15
  concept of negligence and, 17t
  in difficult airway cases,
      149–150
  disclosure and, 9, 16
  elements of, 14t
  versus informed permission, 13
  of Jehovah's Witnesses, 18–19
  of mature minors and emancipated minors, 18
  patient's age and maturity and,
      13, 15–16, 18
  in pediatric care, 13–20
    approaches to, 14t
    process of, 13–18
    special situations in, 18–20
    use of, 18
Informed permission, 13
  versus informed consent, 13
  use of, 18
Inhalation anesthesia. *See also specific inhalation agents*
  in congenital heart disease,
      174–175
  in difficult airway, 152–153
  dysrhythmias induced by, 181
  effect in neonates, 130
  in long QT syndrome, 190
  malignant hyperthermia with,
      338–340
  in muscular dystrophy patients,
      291
  in trauma cases, 203–204
Inhalational injury, 210–211
  evaluation of, bronchoscopy in,
      211
  neurologic trauma with, 214
Insulin
  allergic and anaphylactic reactions to, 305
  in diabetes mellitus, 280–283
  infusion in anesthetic management of diabetes mellitus,
      282
  for malignant hyperthermia, 348t
Intake and output, and eligibility for discharge, 363t
Integrity, personal, issues of, 24
Interferons, and allergies, 300
Intracerebral hematoma, 271
Intracranial pressure
  increased
    anesthesia maintenance with,
        265
    with brain tumors, 266–269
    with cancer, 222t
    causes of, 261
    child with, 261–266
    clinical presentation of,
        261–262
    emergence with, 266
    fluid management with, 265
    with head trauma, 272
    history and physical examination in, 261
    hypertension with, 314
    imaging in, 262–263
    induction in, 264–265
    laboratory data in, 264
    laryngoscopy and, 264
    monitoring of, 265
    patient positioning in, 264
    physiology of, 261–262
    premedication for, 263
    preoperative assessment of,
        262–263
    supratentorial craniotomy and,
        268
  normal, in adults and children, 261
  succinylcholine and, 264
  in trauma cases, 200–201
    effects of drugs on, 198, 198t,
        203
Intracranial tumors, 266–267
  posterior fossa craniotomy for,
      268–270
  supratentorial craniotomy for,
      267–268
Intramuscular administration, of preanesthetic sedation,
      47t, 52–53
Intramuscular anesthesia, in difficult airway, 152–153
Intraoperative radiation therapy,
      248–250
Intrapulmonary shunting, in asthma,
      92
Intravascular injection, inadvertent, risk of, anesthesia and, 3t
Intravenous access
  pediatric patients lacking, preanesthetic sedation for,
      41–55
  in thermal/burn injury, 212
  in trauma cases, 199

Intravenous analgesia, 376
  monitoring children receiving, 384–385
Intravenous anesthesia
  in difficult airway, 152–153
  effect in neonates, 130
  in muscular dystrophy patients, 291
Intubation
  alignment of axes for, 153, 154*f*
  anatomy of, 145–146, 153–157, 154*f*–155*f*
  difficult
    history of, and identification of difficult airway, 143, 148–149
    risk of, anesthesia and, 3*t*
  in difficult airway, 153–157
    alternative techniques for, 159–164
    blind oral or blind nasal, 159, 161–163
    fiberoptic, 159–160, 160*f*, 161*t*
    retrograde, 159, 163–164, 164*f*
    via laryngeal mask anesthesia, 159, 161, 162*f*
  endobronchial, risk of, anesthesia and, 3*t*
  esophageal, risk of, anesthesia and, 3*t*
  fiberoptic, 197, 211
    in cervical spinal injury, 202
  with mediastinal masses, 228–229
  patient positioning for, 153
  in supratentorial craniotomy, 267
  in thermal/burn injury, 211
    intraoperative, 217
  in trauma management, 197–199, 272
    in cervical spinal injury, 202
    complications of, 199
    uses deemed unnecessary, in case review, 199
Iron therapy
  for anemia, in former preterm infants, 140–141
  for autologous blood donation, 322
  in renal failure, 293
  for thermal/burn injury patients, 214

Isoetharine (Bronkosol), for asthma, 93
Isoflurane
  for controlled hypertension, 330*t*
  dysrhythmia induced by, 181
  and malignant hyperthermia, 341–342
  in posterior fossa craniotomy, 269
  and rhabdomyolysis, 291
  in supratentorial craniotomy, 267
  for trauma patients, 203–204
Isoproterenol, in acquired long QT syndrome, 190

J
Jehovah's Witnesses
  dealing with parents of, 70–71
  decision-making and consent by, 18–19
Jet nebulizer, for asthma, 93
Joint Commission on Accreditation of Healthcare Organizations (JCAHO)
  discharge policies of, 358
  sedation guidelines of, 390, 392, 394
Junctional ectopic tachycardia, 182
  electrocardiogram of, 183*f*
  mechanism of, 184*f*

K
Ketamine
  contraindications to
    in asthma, 96
    in cystic fibrosis, 90
    in long QT syndrome, 190
    in pediatric neuroanesthesia, 263
    in upper respiratory tract infections, 85
  intramuscular
    administration of, 71
    for difficult children, 71, 153
    dosage of, 47*t*, 52
    efficacy of, 47*t*
    monitoring recommendations for, 47*t*
    for preanesthetic sedation, 47*t*, 52, 71
    time of onset and peak effect of, 47*t*, 52
  intranasal

Ketamine (*continued*)
dosage of, 47*t*, 49
efficacy of, 47*t*
monitoring recommendations for, 47*t*
versus other routes of administration, 49, 49*f*
for preanesthetic sedation, 47*t*, 49–50
time to onset and peak effect of, 47*t*
in neonates, effects of, 131
oral
bioavailability of, 44
dosage of, 44–45, 47*t*
efficacy of, 47*t*
monitoring recommendations for, 47*t*
versus oral midazolam, 44–45
with oral midazolam, 46
for preanesthetic sedation, 44–45, 47*t*
redosing with, after expulsion of dose, 45
side effects of, 45
time to onset and peak effect of, 45, 47*t*
rectal
dosage of, 47*t*, 51–52
efficacy of, 47*t*
monitoring recommendations for, 47*t*
for preanesthetic sedation, 47*t*, 51–52
time of onset and peak effect of, 47*t*
sedation with, safety of and policy on, 395
with spinal anesthesia, in preterm and former infants, 6, 136–138
for thermal/burn injury patients, 215
in trauma management, 198, 198*t*, 272
Ketamine-magnesium, postoperative, in difficult airway cases, 165
Ketorolac, 382
dosage of, 383*t*
and emergence delirium, 382
for myringotomy and pressure equalization tube placement, 368
with patient-controlled analgesia, 378
postoperative, after supratentorial craniotomy, 268
Kidney dysfunction
and hypertension, 312
in thermal/burn injury patients, 214
Kidney failure, 292–294
anesthetic considerations in, 293–294
definition in children, 292
effects on medication, 294
etiology of, 291*t*, 292
with malignant hyperthermia, 340
nonsteroidal anti-inflammatory drugs contraindicated in, 382
pathophysiology of, 292–293
in thermal/burn injury patients, 214
treatment of, 293
with tumor lysis syndrome, 230
Kidney transplantation, 293–294
King-Denborough syndrome, malignant hyperthermia with, 343, 352
Klebsiella pneumoniae infection, 97
Klippel-Feil syndrome, difficult airway with, 147, 149*f*

L

L-loop transposition, 180*t*
Labetalol
for controlled hypotension, 329, 330*t*
postoperative, after supratentorial craniotomy, 268
Laboratory testing
appropriate preoperative, in children, 35–40
in increased intracranial pressure, 264
indications for, 35–36
legislative mandate for, 39
for malignant hyperthermia, 341
in trauma cases, 199
β-Lactam antibiotics, allergic and anaphylactic reactions to, 306

Laminar flow, of gas through tubes, 108–110
Langerhans' cell histiocytosis, 238
  chemotherapy for, 238
  clinical presentation of, 238
  disseminated disease in, 238
  solitary lesions with, 238
Language-based learning disabilities, 63
Lap belt syndrome, 202
Laparotomy, in multiple trauma, 202
Larach, Marilyn, 339
Large cell lymphoma, 234
Laryngeal mask airway (LMA)
  in asthma, 96
  in cystic fibrosis, 90
  disadvantages of, 90
  versus endotracheal tube, 86, 90, 317
  introduction of, 161
  intubation via, in difficult airway, 159, 161, 162f
    retrieval of LMA after, 161, 162f
  in newborn resuscitation, limitation of, 161
  popularity of, 161
  stridor with, 126
  in thermal/burn injury, 211
  in tracheomalacia, 119
  in upper respiratory tract infections, 86–87, 317
Laryngeal nerve damage, stridor with, 115–116
Laryngomalacia, stridor with, 112, 114
Laryngoscopy
  in cervical spinal injury, 202
  cystic hygroma and, 153, 156f
  in difficult airway, 153–164, 156f
    alternative techniques for, 159–164
    backward upward right pressure in, 158
    Bullard laryngoscope for, 158
    depth of anesthesia and, 157
    direct, 157–158
    ease of, by mandibular classification, 146, 148t
    improving view in, techniques for, 158
    left lateral approach in, 158
    Malimpatti classification of signs predicting, 145, 145f
    muscle relaxants for, 158–159
    optimal external laryngeal manipulation in, 158
    space for, potential, assessment of, 155–157
    two-person technique for, 158
  displacement of soft tissues of oropharynx in, 153–157, 155f
  increased intracranial pressure with, decrease of, 264
  initial as best, 165
  macroglossia and, 153
  repeated attempts at, damage from, 160, 165
  in thermal/burn injury, 211, 217
Laryngospasm
  in asthma, 96
  in bronchopulmonary dysplasia, 100
  in cystic fibrosis, 90
  extubation management and, 127
  incidence of, 3
  muscle relaxants for, 127
  perioperative stridor and, 125–127
  postoperative, 369
  preanesthetic sedation and, 41
  pulmonary edema after, 103
  in recovery room, 127
  with sevoflurane, 125–126
  in upper respiratory tract infections, 82, 85–86
Larynx, anterior, 157
Lateral pressure, and airway patency, 110–111
Latex allergy, 300–301, 309
  in cerebral palsy patients, 288
  hypotension with, 314–316
  management of, 304t
  populations at high risk for, 309
  testing for, 305
Learning disabilities, 63
  classification of, 63
  comorbid conditions with, 63
  definition of, 63
  providing care for children with, 63
Left-to-right shunts, approach to child with, 173–174, 174t

Left ventricle, hypoplastic, 180*t*
Legal issues
  in child abuse, 23
  in forgoing life-sustaining care, 20–23
  in informed consent, 13–20
  in pediatric care, 13–25
  in pediatric pain management, 23–24
  in production pressure, 24
  seeking help with, 24–25
Letterer-Siwe disease, 238
Leukemia(s)
  acute lymphoblastic, 220*t*, 229, 231–232, 250
  acute myelogenous, 220*t*, 230, 232–233, 250
  central nervous system prophylaxis in, radiation therapy for, 248
  chronic myelogenous, 250
  mediastinal masses with, 221, 229
  recurrent, bone marrow transplantation for, 250
  treatment of, neurologic sequelae of, 68
Leukocytes
  decreased level of, with childhood cancer, 223*t*
  elevated level of
    with acute myelogenous leukemia, 232
    with childhood cancer, 222*t*, 231
    definition of, 231
Lidocaine
  in asthma, 96–97
  and cerebral blood flow, 201, 202*t*
  in cystic fibrosis, 90
  epidural, 382*t*
  for extubation, after posterior fossa craniotomy, 269–270
  in head trauma, 272
  and intracranial pressure, 264
  and laryngospasm, 126
  in long QT syndrome, 190
  postoperative, in difficult airway cases, 165
  in supratentorial craniotomy, 267
  for topicalization, in difficult airway, 157
  in trauma management, 201, 203–204
  in upper respiratory tract infections, 85
Life-sustaining care, decisions to forgo, 20–23
Ligamentous injury, to cervical spine, 202
Listeria infection, pneumonia with, 97
Liver
  in congenital heart disease, 170
  functions of, 296
Liver failure, 294–298
  acute, 294
  anesthetic considerations in, 296*t*, 297–298
  cardiopulmonary dysfunction with, 296*t*
  coagulation problems with, 296, 296*t*
  etiology of, 294–295, 295*t*
  and immune status, 296*t*
  metabolic problems with, 296*t*, 296–297
  and nutrition status, 296*t*
  pathophysiology of, 295–297, 296*t*
  and renal status, 296*t*
Liver injury, 202
Liver transplantation, 298
LMA. *See* Laryngeal mask airway
Local anesthetics
  allergic and anaphylactic reactions to, 307–308
  dysrhythmias induced by, 181–182
  epidural or caudal administration of, 379–382
  latency period with, 380
  metabolism in children older than one year, 384
  with narcotics, 380
  pharmacokinetics in neonates versus older children, 379–380
  relationship between volume of administered caudally and level of analgesia, 379*t*
  without narcotic additives, for outpatient cases, 380

Lollipop formulations, of fentanyl, 45–46, 214
Lomustine, classification and side effects of, 239t–240t
Long QT syndrome, 189–190
  acquired, 190
  congenital, 189–190, 193
    anesthetic management of patients with, 190
    clinical presentation of, 189
    treatment of, 189
    variants of, 189
  congenital versus acquired, 190
  pacemaker and cardioverter defibrillator for, 191–192
  torsade de pointes with, 189, 190f, 193
Loop diuretics, for increased intracranial pressure, 265
Lower respiratory tract, effects of upper respiratory tract infection on, 81
Lower respiratory tract infections
  in cystic fibrosis, 88
  and outpatient surgery, 28
  with upper respiratory tract infection, and surgical decisions, 84
Lown-Ganong-Levine syndrome, 183
Lumbar epidural, 380
Lund and Browder variation, for calculating percentage of body burned, 207, 209f
Lung disease, restrictive
  with cerebral palsy, 285–286
  with muscular dystrophy, 289–290
Lung injury, acute
  with inhalational injury, 210–211
  with thermal/burn injury, intraoperative management of, 217
Lymphoblastic lymphomas, 234
Lymphoma(s), 233–235
  airway obstruction and stridor with, 122–123
  bone marrow transplantation for, 250
  incidence in children, 220t
  large cell, 234
  lymphoblastic, 234
  mediastinal masses with, 122–123, 221, 229, 234
  spinal cord compression with, 229
  tumor lysis syndrome with, 229–230

M

Macroglossia, and difficult airway, 145, 146f
Magnesium, decreased levels in thermal/burn injury, 213
Magnesium sulfate, for acquired long QT syndrome, 190
Magnetic resonance imaging
  in increased intracranial pressure, 262–263
  of spinal cord compression, with childhood cancer, 229
Malabsorption, dietary, with cystic fibrosis, 89
Malignant hyperthermia, 338–353
  acute episode of, diagnosis of, 340–341
  case illustrations of, 341–344
  clinical evidence of, 340t
  directory of biopsy centers, 349t
  disaster in recovery room with, 344
    versus other disorders, 344–348
  and discharge from postanesthesia care unit, 369
  early recognition of, benefits of, 339
  eliminating diagnosis of, case illustrations in, 344–348
  emergency management of, 356t–357t
  genetics of, 338
  historical perspective on, 338–340
  versus intercurrent infection, 346
  masseter muscle spasm/rigidity and, 6, 339, 343–344, 356t
  versus neurogenic fever, 345
  versus neuroleptic malignant syndrome, 346–347
  neuromuscular disorders and, 290–291, 342–344, 352–353
  versus other causes of increasing end-tidal carbon dioxide, 347–348

Malignant hyperthermia (*continued*)
  outpatient surgery in children with, 33, 369
  post-acute phase of, 357*t*
  prevention of, 350–352
  recurrence of (recrudescence), 349
  reports and registry of, 339, 341–342, 350
  versus rhabdomyolysis, 344, 353
  susceptibility to
    conditions associated with, 352–353
    contracture testing for, 340, 350
    families with, identification of, 339–340, 350
    outpatient anesthesia for patients with, 352
    premedication for patients with, 350
    safe versus unsafe drugs for patients with, 351*t*
    use of non-triggering anesthesia in patients with, 350–351
  treatment of, 339, 348–349, 356*t*–357*t*
    drugs used for, 348, 348*t*
  MHAUS manuals on, 352
Malignant Hyperthermia Association of the United States (MHAUS), 339, 352
Malimpatti classification, of signs predicting difficult laryngoscopy, 145, 145*f*
Malocclusion, in cerebral palsy patients, 286
Malpractice
  closed claim studies of
    of anesthetic accident costs, 9, 9*t*
    of anesthetic risk, 2–3, 3*t*, 369
  concept of negligence in, 17*t*
Mandible, assessment and classification in preanesthetic evaluation of difficult airway, 145–146, 148*t*
Mandibular hypoplasia, difficult airway with, 145–146
Mannitol
  in head trauma management, 201
  for increased intracranial pressure, 265, 269
  in posterior fossa craniotomy, 269
  for thermal/burn injury patients, 214
Mask anesthesia. *See also* Laryngeal mask airway
  in asthma, 96
  in upper respiratory tract infections, 85–87
Masseter muscle rigidity (MMR), 6
Masseter muscle spasm (MMS), and malignant hyperthermia, 6, 339, 343–344, 356*t*
Mast cell dysfunction, in asthma, 92
Mature minors, informed consent of, 18
Maxillofacial fractures, nasal intubation contraindicated with, 199
MDI (metered dose inhaler), for asthma, 93
Mean arterial pressure
  acceptable lowest, in controlled hypotension, 328–329
  increased intracranial pressure and, 261–262
Mechanical ventilation, in thermal/burn injury, intraoperative management of, 217
Mechanistic model, of child development, 58*t*
Mechlorethamine, classification and side effects of, 239*t*
Mediastinal masses, 219–229, 234–235
  airway obstruction and stridor with, 121–123, 221
  anesthesia induction in surgery for, 227–228
  anterior, 121–123, 219–224, 234
    anesthetic risk with, assessment of, 221–226, 225*t*, 226*f*–228*f*
    respiratory failure with, pathophysiology of, 226–227
    signs and symptoms of, 221, 225*t*
  extubation and emergence after surgery for, 229

patient positioning in surgery for, 228
types of, 219–224, 225*t*
Medical history
in congenital heart disease assessment, 169–170
and identification of difficult airway, 143–145
in increased incranial pressure, 261
in preoperative evaluation, 35
in stridor, 112–113
Medulloblastoma, 233, 268
Melphalan
classification and side effects of, 239*t*
in preparative regime for bone marrow transplantation, 251
Meningioma, 268
Meningocele, 270
Meningomyelocele, lumbar, stridor with, 123–124
Menstruation, heavy, in adolescents, and anemia, 36–37
Mental impairment
in cerebral palsy, 285
in muscular dystrophy, 289
Meperidine
allergic and anaphylactic reactions to, 308
dosage of, 383*t*
oral
with oral midazolam, for preanesthetic sedation, 46
with phenergan and thorazine, for preanesthetic sedation, 46
Mercaptopurine
classification and side effects of, 240*t*
for Langerhans' cell histiocytosis, 238
Mesenchymoma, hepatic failure with, 295*t*
Metabolic rate, malignant hyperthermia and, 340
Metaproterenol (Alupent), for asthma, 93
Metered dose inhaler (MDI), for asthma, 93
Methadone, dosage of, 383*t*

Methohexital
avoidance in temporal lobe epilepsy, 285
rectal
avoidance in difficult airway cases, 150
dosage of, 47*t*, 50
efficacy of, 47*t*
monitoring recommendations for, 47*t*
for preanesthetic sedation, 47*t*, 50
side effects of, 50
time to onset and peak effect of, 47*t*, 50
sedation with, safety of and policy on, 395
Methotrexate
for acute lymphoblastic leukemia, 232
classification and side effects of, 240*t*
Methylparaben, allergy to, 307
Methylphenidate (Ritalin), 62*t*
Methylprednisolone
for anaphylactic reactions, 304*t*
for asthma, 94
Methylxanthines, as respiratory stimulant in former preterm infants, 134–136
Mexiletine, for cancer pain, 254
MH. *See* Malignant hyperthermia
MH Hotline, 339, 341
MHAUS (Malignant Hyperthermia Association of the United States), 339, 352
Midazolam
co-administration of muscarinic blockers with, 42
intramuscular
dosage of, 47*t*, 52–53
efficacy of, 47*t*
jet injection of, 52
monitoring recommendations for, 47*t*
for preanesthetic sedation, 47*t*, 52–53
time of onset and peak effect of, 47*t*, 52
intranasal
dosage of, 47*t*, 48
efficacy of, 48

Midazolam (*continued*)
  versus intravenous midazolam, 48, 48f
  in patients with hypervascularized lesions, 263
  for preanesthetic sedation, 46–48, 47t, 48f
  time of onset and peak effect of, 47t, 48
  for malignant hyperthermia-susceptible patients, 350
  oral
    for asthmatic child, 95
    in difficult airway cases, 150
    dosage of, 43–44, 45f, 47t
    efficacy of, 43–44, 45f, 47t
    monitoring recommendations for, 47t
    versus oral ketamine, 44–45
    with oral ketamine, 46
    with oral meperidine, 46
    for preanesthetic sedation, 43–44, 45f, 47t, 95, 150
    redosing with, after expulsion of dose, 44
    time to onset and peak effect of, 43–44, 45f, 47t
  versus parental presence during induction, 41–42, 72
  rectal
    dosage of, 47t, 51
    efficacy of, 47t, 51, 51f
    monitoring recommendations for, 47t
    for preanesthetic sedation, 47t, 51, 51f
    time of onset and peak effect of, 47t, 51
  for thermal/burn injury patients, 215
Minors, mature and emancipated, informed consent of, 18
Mitoxanthrone, 243
  cardiac toxicity of, 243f, 243–247, 245f–246f
Mitral valve abnormality, 180t
Mitral valve prolapse, 180t, 188
Mivacurium, 159t
MMS. *See* Masseter muscle spasm
Mobitz type II heart block, 191
Monomorphic ventricular tachycardia, 191, 192f

Morphine
  allergic and anaphylactic reactions to, 308
  dosage of, 383t
  epidural, 381, 382t
  and malignant hyperthermia, 342
  patient-controlled, 378
  postoperative, after posterior fossa craniotomy, 270
  in renal failure, caution with, 294
  for thermal/burn injury patients, 215
Mortality studies, of anesthetic risk, 1–2, 2f
Motor evoked potentials, for intraoperative monitoring of spinal function, 271
Motor vehicle accidents, 196, 201–202
Mouth, assessment in preanesthetic evaluation of difficult airway, 145–146
Mucolytics, for cystic fibrosis, 90
Mucositis, in cancer treatment, pain with, 252t
Mucus plugging, in asthma, 91
Multiple trauma
  anesthetic considerations for child with, 196–205
  strategies for management of, 202–203
Muscarinic blockers, co-administration of, with preanesthetic sedation, 42
Muscle disease
  and anesthetic risk, 7, 291
  and malignant hyperthermia, 290–291, 342–344, 352–353
Muscle relaxant(s). *See also* Succinylcholine
  allergic and anaphylactic reactions to, 301, 305, 307
  for difficult airway, 153–155, 158–159
  dysrhythmias induced by, 182
  and intracranial pressure, 264–265
  for laryngospasm, 127
  in myelodysplasia, 270
  nondepolarizing, 159, 159t
    dose modification in renal failure, 294

and malignant hyperthermia, 340
in malignant hyperthermia-susceptible patients, 351
in posterior fossa craniotomy, 269
in supratentorial craniotomy, 267
in trauma management, 198, 198t, 201, 203, 272
in trauma management, 198, 198t, 201, 203, 272
Muscular dystrophy, 288–291
anesthetic considerations in, 7, 158–159, 289–291
cardiac function in, 289–290
diagnosis of, 289
etiology of, 288
and malignant hyperthermia, 290–291, 342, 344, 352–353
pathophysiology of, 288–289
respiratory function in, 289–290
treatment of, 289
Mustard operation, 187–188, 191
Mycobacterial infection, atypical, in cystic fibrosis, 88
Mycoplasma pneumoniae infection, 97
Myelodysplasia, 270
induction in, 270
monitoring in, 270
patient positioning in, 270
preoperative assessment of, 270
Myelomeningocele, 270
Myelosuppression, with chemotherapy, 238–243
Myoglobin, in malignant hyperthermia, 340–341
Myopathy
and anesthetic risk, 7, 291
and malignant hyperthermia, 290–291, 342–344, 352–353
Myotonia, and anesthetic risk, 7
Myotonia congenita, and malignant hyperthermia, 352
Myringotomy and pressure equalization tube placement
delirium emergence after, 382
postanesthesia care in, monitoring in and discharge from, 368

N

Naloxone, availability in cases using patient-controlled analgesia, 378
Naltrexone, for pervasive developmental disorders, 65
NAMHR (North American Malignant Hyperthermia Registry), 339–342, 350
Narcotic(s)
allergic and anaphylactic reactions to, 308
avoidance of
in difficult airway cases, 150
in patients with increased intracranial pressure, 263
for decreasing risk of emergence delirium, 365
epidural, 380–381, 382t
in former preterm infants, 131
intramuscular, for preanesthetic sedation, 52
and malignant hyperthermia, 340
oral, for preanesthetic sedation, 45–46
for pain management, intravenous, 376
postoperative, in difficult airway cases, 165
for thermal/burn injury patients, 215
for trauma patients, 203–204
Nasal intubation, contraindications to, with maxillofacial fractures and skull-base fractures, 199
Nasal polyps
in allergic triad, 92
with cystic fibrosis, 88, 90
Nasal transmucosal administration, of preanesthetic sedation, 46–50, 47t
Nasogastric tube, in hepatic failure, caution with, 297
Nasopharyngitis, 80. *See also* Upper respiratory tract infections
and outpatient surgery, 29
Natural rubber latex allergy. *See* Latex allergy
Nature versus nurture, 56–57
Nausea
with local anesthetics containing narcotics, 380–381

Nausea (*continued*)
  with oral transmucosal fentanyl citrate, 46
  with patient-controlled analgesia, 378–379
  postanesthesia/postoperative, 8–9
    assessment of, difficulty in children, 369
    causes of, 365–366
    and eligibility for discharge, 362*t*, 365–366, 370
    lowering risk of, 366
    after tonsillectomy, 368
    treatment of, 366, 369
    undermedication for, 369
Neck, assessment in preanesthetic evaluation of difficult airway, 145–147
Neck immobilization, for intubation, in cervical spinal injury, 202
Neck masses
  causes of, 219, 224*t*
  evaluation of, 229
Negligence
  concept of, 17*t*
  and informed consent, 17*t*
Neonate(s)
  hypertension in, incidence of, 312
  hypoxia in, greater risk of, 316
  pain perception by, misconceptions about, 374–375, 389
  pharmacokinetics of local anesthetics in, 379–380
  respiratory control and mechanics of, anesthesia and, 130–131
  respiratory function in, 130
  ventricular tachycardia, classification of, 188–189
Neosynephrine, in head trauma management, 201
Nephroblastoma. *See* Wilms' tumor
Nerve blocks, peripheral, 384
Nerve trauma, in cancer treatment, pain with, 252*t*
Neuraxial agents, for cancer pain, 255
Neurobiology, of developing child, 374–375
Neuroblastoma, 236
  bone marrow transplantation for, 236, 250
  chemotherapy for, 236
  clinical presentation of, 236
  hypertension with, 312
  incidence of, 220*t*, 236
  radiation therapy for, 236, 248, 250
  spinal cord compression with, 229, 236
Neurogenic fever, versus malignant hyperthermia, 345
Neuroleptic agents
  for cancer pain, 255
  for pervasive developmental disorders, 65
Neuroleptic malignant syndrome, 346–347
Neurological problems, 261–274
  associated with congenital heart disease, 171*t*
  with brain tumors, 233
  with thermal/burn injury, 206–207
Neuromuscular disease
  and anesthetic risk, 7, 291
  and malignant hyperthermia, 290–291, 342–344, 352–353
Neurosurgical patient, preoperative assessment of, 262–263
Nicardipine, for controlled hypotension, 329, 330*t*
Nitrogen mustards
  classification and side effects of, 239*t*
  for Hodgkin's disease, 235
Nitroglycerine, for controlled hypotension, 329, 330*t*
Nitrosoureas, classification and side effects of, 239*t*–240*t*
Nitrous oxide
  in congenital heart disease patients, 175–176
  contraindications to
    in cystic fibrosis, 90
    in upper respiratory tract infections, 86
  in hydrocephalic patients, 266
  and intracranial pressure, 264–265
  and malignant hyperthermia, 341–342
  in malignant hyperthermia-susceptible patients, 350

sedation with, safety of and policy on, 395
in supratentorial craniotomy, 267
Non-Hodgkin's lymphoma, 233–234
  bone marrow transplantation for, 234
  chemotherapy for, 234
  complications of, 234, 235t
  histologic subtypes of, 234
  incidence of, 220t, 233
  mediastinal masses with, 221, 234
  radiation therapy for, 234
  spinal cord compression with, 229
Nondepolarizing muscle relaxants, 159, 159t
  dose modification in renal failure, 294
  and malignant hyperthermia, 340
  in malignant hyperthermia-susceptible patients, 351
  in posterior fossa craniotomy, 269
  in supratentorial craniotomy, 267
  in trauma management, 198, 198t, 201, 203, 272
Nonsteroidal anti-inflammatory drugs (NSAIDs), 382
  for cancer pain, 254–255
  for cerebral palsy patients, 287
  contraindications in renal compromise or failure, 382
  dosages of, 383t
  for enhancement of patient-controlled analgesia, 378
  in obstructive sleep apnea, 102
  postoperative, in difficult airway cases, 165
Nonverbal learning disabilities, 63
Norepinephrine
  for anaphylactic reactions, 304t
  for cardiovascular effects, of thermal/burn injury, 212
North American Malignant Hyperthermia Muscle Biopsy Centers, 349t
North American Malignant Hyperthermia Registry (NAMHR), 339–342, 350
Nose, runny, 80. *See also* Upper respiratory tract infections
  outpatient pediatric patients with, 28–29
NSAIDs. *See* Nonsteroidal anti-inflammatory drugs
Nurse(s)
  involvement in sedation policy, 395
  sedation administered by, 394–396
    skill level required for, 394
Nurse-administered analgesia, 378
Nutrition
  in cerebral palsy, 288
  in hepatic failure, 296t
  in renal failure, 293
  in thermal/burn injury, 213

O

Obstructive sleep apnea, 100–103
  adenotonsillectomy for, 101–103
  diagnosis of, 102
  with hemifacial disorders, 102
  pathophysiologic consequences of, 101
  in syndrome-affected children, 102
Oncologic emergencies, in pediatric patients, 219–231, 222t–223t
Oncovin, for Hodgkin's disease, 235
Opiates/opioids
  additional, avoidance of, with patient-controlled analgesia, 378
  allergic and anaphylactic reactions to, 301, 308
  for cancer pain, 254–255
  epidural, 380–382, 382t
  metabolism in children older than one year, 384
  and neonatal respiration, 131
  paraspinal, for trauma patients, 204
  postoperative, and neurologic assessment, 268
  for thermal/burn injury patients, 215
Optimal external laryngeal manipulation, in laryngoscopy, 158
Oral administration, of preanesthetic sedation, 43–46

Oral transmucosal fentanyl citrate (OTFC)
  avoidance in difficult airway cases, 150
  dosage of, 46, 47t
  efficacy of, 47t
  monitoring recommendations for, 47t
  for preanesthetic sedation, 45–46, 47t
  time of onset and peak effect of, 46, 47t
Organismic model, of child development, 58t
Oropharynx, soft tissues of, displacement in laryngoscopy, 153–157, 155f
Orotracheal tube, in posterior fossa craniotomy, 269
Orthodromic reciprocating tachycardia, 183, 184f–185f, 185
Osteosarcoma, 237
  incidence in children, 220t
  spinal cord compression with, 229
OTFC. *See* Oral transmucosal fentanyl citrate
Otitis media, insertion of ventilation tubes in child presenting with runny nose, 29
Outcomes, 1–12
Outpatient management, postanesthesia, risks and complications of, 8–9
Outpatient surgery
  admissions, unanticipated, after, 369
  for ear, nose, and throat procedures, postanesthesia care in, 367–368
  in former premature infants, 29
  pediatric patients for
    age considerations with, 27–28
    with asthma, 32
    with bronchopulmonary dysplasia, 29–30
    classification of, 26
    with congenital or acquired heart disease, 30–32
    criteria for, importance of, 26
    with heart murmur, 30
    with known or suspected malignant hyperthermia, 33, 369
    presurgical evaluation of, 26
    with runny nose, 28–29
    screening methods for, 27–28
    SIDS concerns in, 28
    site considerations for, 27
    special problems in, 28–30
    suitable, selection of, 26–34
  postoperative care in, monitoring and discharge criteria in, 358–373
Oxygen-carrying volume-expanding solutions, decrease in blood loss with, 333
Oxygen saturation
  in bronchopulmonary dysplasia, 100
  and eligibility for discharge, 363t
  monitoring in postanesthesia care unit, 360
  upper respiratory tract infections and, 9, 82–83, 83t, 84f
Oxygen therapy
  and bleomycin toxicity, 247–248
  blow-by, in postanesthesia care unit, 360
  in carbon monoxide poisoning, 210
  for postobstructive pulmonary edema, 104
  during transport to PACU, 359

P

Pacemakers
  anesthetic considerations for pediatric patients with, 192
  for dysrhythmias, 191–193
  for long QT syndrome, 189, 191–192
PACU. *See* Postanesthesia care unit
PADDS (postanesthetic discharge scoring system), 361, 362t–364t
Pain
  assessment in children, 359, 369, 375–376
    Children's Hospital of Eastern Ontario Pain Scale for, 376, 377t
  in cancer patients, 251–255

elements of, 254, 254f
treatment-related, 252, 252t
tumor-related, 252, 253t
perception of, by infants and children, misconceptions about, 374–375, 389
in postanesthesia care unit, and eligibility for discharge, 362t–363t, 368–370
rapidity of recovery/outpatient management and, 8–9
response to, and assessment of sedation, 392, 393f
Pain management
advances in, 389
analgesics for
epidural or caudal, 379–382
intravenous, 376
monitoring children receiving, 384–385
nonsteroidal, 382
order forms for, 387–388
patient-controlled, 215, 255, 376–379
rectal, 379
routes of administration and dosages of, 376–384
neurobiology of developing child and, 374–375
pediatric
in cancer patients, 254–255
insufficient, 251–252
WHO stepwise approach in, 254–255, 255f
in cerebral palsy patients, 285, 287–288
in congenital heart disease patients, 178
deficient, 23, 251–252
in difficult airway cases, 165
ethical and legal issues in, 23–24
postoperative
in cystic fibrosis, 91
and discharge from postanesthesia care unit, 362t–363t, 368–370
after ear, nose, and throat procedures, 367–368
after posterior fossa craniotomy, 270
problems with, 374–386

for trauma patients, 204
in thermal/burn injury, 215
peripheral nerve blocks for, 384
Pancreas, in cystic fibrosis, 87–88
Pancuronium, 159t
contraindications in long QT syndrome, 190
Pansinusitis, with cystic fibrosis, 88
Paraben preservatives, allergy to, 307
Parent(s)
of cancer patients, emotional stress of, 255–257
difficult
identification of, 56–69
management of, 69–75
important issues for anesthesiologist in, 75
providing care for, 56–79
disclosure of anesthetic risks to, 9
informed consent/permission of, 9, 13
versus adolescent confidentiality and autonomy, 19–20
best-interests standard and, 14–15
in difficult airway cases, 149–150
Jehovah's Witness, dealing with, 70–71
perspective of, 76–78
physician bonding with, in preanesthetic evaluation, 70–71
in postanesthetic care unit, 74–75, 359
postoperative discussion with, 75
presence of, during induction, 72–74
attitude of anesthesiologist and other personnel toward, 72–73
in difficult airway cases, 152
effect on child, 72
effect on parent, 72
logistical concerns about, 73
versus preanesthetic sedation, 41–42, 72
use of patient-controlled analgesic pump by, 378
Parkland formula, for fluid resuscitation, 212

Paroxysmal supraventricular atrial
    tachycardia (PSVT),
    183–187
  etiologies of, 183
  management of, 186–187
  mechanism of, 183, 184f
  presentation of
    after 5 years of age, 183–184
    in infancy, 183
Partial thromboplastin time, preoperative assessment of, 37–38
Parvovirus B19 infection, transmission of, via blood transfusion, 323t
Patent ductus arteriosus, 175t, 180t, 360
Patent foramen ovale, 180t
Patient-controlled analgesia, 376–379
  in cancer, 255
  discontinuation of, 384–385
  nurse-administered analgesia with, 378
  order forms for, 387–388
  parental use of pump for, 378
  safety in children, principles of, 378
  side effects of, 378
  in thermal/burn injury, 215
Patient preparation, and anesthetic risk, 7
Pavlov, Ivan, 58t
PCA. See Patient-controlled analgesia
PDDs. See Pervasive developmental disorders
Peak expiratory flow rate (PEFR), in prediction of anesthetic risk, with anterior mediastinal masses, 226, 228f
Pediatric anesthesiologist(s)
  accessibility to pediatricians, 7
  administration of anesthesia by, and anesthetic risk, 4
  educational role of, 7
Pediatric Perioperative Cardiac Arrest Registry (POCA), 1–2
Pediatric Trauma Score, 196, 197t
PEEP (positive end expiratory pressure)
  in posterior fossa craniotomy, 269
  in supratentorial craniotomy, 267

Pemoline (Cylert), 62t
Penicillin(s), allergic and anaphylactic reactions to, 305–306
Pentobarbital
  and metabolism rate of medications, 286
  rectal, in patients with hypervascularized lesions, 263
Pentothal, for patients with increased intracranial pressure, 264
Perfluorocarbon emulsions, decrease in blood loss with, 333
Pericardial abnormality, 180t
Periodic breathing, in preterm and former preterm infants
  anemia and, 139–141, 140t–141t
  management of, 134–138
  perioperative, 131–134, 132t
  postconceptional age and, 134, 141
  spinal versus general anesthesia and, 136–138, 138t
Peripheral airway abnormalities, with upper respiratory tract infections, 81
Peripheral nerve blocks, 384
Permission, informed, 13
  versus informed consent, 13
  use of, 18
Personal integrity issues, 24
Pervasive developmental disorders (PDDs), 63–65
  clinical presentation of, 65
  definition of, 63
  not otherwise specified, 64–65
  prevalence of, 64–65
  providing care for children with, 65
  treatment of, 65
PET (pressure equalization tube placement)
  emergence delirium after, 382
  postanesthesia care in, monitoring in and discharge from, 368
Phenergan, and thorazine, with meperidine, for preanesthetic sedation, 46
Phenylephrine, for paroxysmal supraventricular atrial tachycardia, 186

Phenytoin
    for cerebral palsy, 286
    gingival hypertrophy with, 286
    for long QT syndrome, 189–190
    and metabolism rate of medications, 286
    resistance to nondepolarizing muscle relaxants with, 286
Pheochromocytoma, hypertension with, 312
Phosphates, decreased levels in thermal/burn injury, 213
Physical examination
    in congenital heart disease assessment, 169–170
    and identification of difficult airway, 143, 145–147
    in increased incranial pressure, 261
    in preoperative evaluation, 35
    in stridor, 113
Physical restraint, immobilization by, unacceptability of, 389
Physical Status Categories
    and decisions on proceeding with surgery, in child with upper respiratory tract infection, 84
Piaget, Jean, 58*t*
Pierre-Robin syndrome, 145, 153–155, 156*f*
Pituitary function, in neurosurgical patients, 263
Platelet transfusion
    in childhood cancers, 230–231
    in immunocompromised host, 231
    for thermal/burn injury patients, 214, 218
Pneumocystis carinii infection, 97
Pneumonia, 97–98
    causative organisms of, 97
    complications with, 98
    diagnosis of, 98
    radiographic findings of, 98
    upper respiratory tract infections and, 82
Pneumothorax
    with cystic fibrosis, 88, 90–91
    tension, hypotension with, 316
Point of care testing, in diabetes mellitus, 282

Polysomnography, in obstructive sleep apnea, 102
Portal hypertension, with hepatic failure, 297
Positive end expiratory pressure (PEEP)
    in posterior fossa craniotomy, 269
    in supratentorial craniotomy, 267
Positive pressure ventilation, for postobstructive pulmonary edema, 104
Postanesthesia care, risks and complications of, 7–9
    incidence of, 7–8
Postanesthesia care unit (PACU), 358–373
    admission procedures in, 360
    ASA guidelines for standards in, 359
    child-friendly environment in, 359
    congenital heart disease patients in, 177–178
    course of patient in, 358
    discharge from, 358–359
        versus admission, 358–359
        choice of anesthetic and, 368
        criteria for, 358, 361–365
        factors affecting, 365–369
        gold standard for, 361
        JCAHO policies on, 358
        malignant hyperthermia and, 369
        nausea/vomiting and, 362*t*, 365–366, 370
        pain/pain management and, 362*t*–363*t*, 368–370
        of preterm infants, 366–367
        recovery room scores and, 361, 362*t*–364*t*
        regional anesthesia, 368–369
        street readiness for, 358
        voiding and, 363*t*–364*t*, 366, 369
    ear, nose, and throat patients in, 367–368
    fast-tracking in, 361–365
    monitoring in, 359–360, 370
    pain assessment in, in children, 359, 369
    parents in, 74–75, 359
    pediatric versus adult, 359
    phase 1 unit of, 358, 370

Postanesthesia care unit (PACU) (*continued*)
  phase 2 unit of, 358, 370
  risks and complications in, 7–9
  role of anesthesiologist in, 369
  transport to, care and monitoring in, 359
Postanesthetic discharge scoring system (PADDS), 361, 362*t*–364*t*
Posterior fossa craniotomy, 268–270
  anesthesia maintenance in, 269
  emergence from, 269–270
  induction in, 269
  monitoring in, 269
  patient positioning for, 268–269
  preoperative assessment for, 268
Postobstructive pulmonary edema, 103–104
  versus aspiration syndrome, 103
  classical clinical presentation of, 103
  versus other causes of pulmonary edema, 104
  pathophysiology of, 103–104
  treatment of, 104
Postoperative discussion, with parents, 75
Posttraumatic stress symptoms, cancer and, 255–256
Potassium, elevated levels of (hyperkalemia)
  controlled, for long QT syndrome, 189
  with increased intracranial pressure, succinylcholine and, 264
  in malignant hyperthermia, 340–341, 348–349, 356*t*
  in renal failure, 292
  in rhabdomyolysis, 291, 353
  in thermal/burn injury, succinylcholine and, 216
  with tumor lysis syndrome, 229–230
Pre-excitation syndromes, 179
  tachycardia with, 183–187
Preanesthetic evaluation, 69–71
  assessment of child's behavior and interactions in, 69
  bonding with parents or caregivers in, 70–71
  goals of, 69
  review of illness, previous experiences, and current state of health in, 69
Prednisone
  for acute lymphoblastic leukemia, 232
  for asthma, 94
  for Hodgkin's disease, 235
  for Langerhans' cell histiocytosis, 238
  for pretreatment of patients with high risk for radiocontrast media allergy, 308
Pregnancy testing, of adolescents, 19–20
  preoperative, 38–39
Premature atrial contractions, 182
Premature ventricular contractions (PVCs), 181, 188
Prematurity. *See* Preterm infants
Premedication. *See* Sedation, preanesthetic
Preschool children
  behavioral development and responses of, 57, 59*t*
  chronically ill, 67
Pressure equalization tube placement (PET)
  emergence delirium after, 382
  postanesthesia care in, monitoring in and discharge from, 368
Preterm infants
  apnea in, 6
    monitoring in postanesthesia care unit, 366–367
  cerebral palsy in, 284
  discharge of, from postanesthesia care unit, 366–367
  former
    anemia and perioperative risk in, 139–141, 140*t*–141*t*
    bronchopulmonary dysplasia in, 98–99
    data on, difficulty in interpretation and comparison of, 133
    management of, 134–138
    outpatient surgery in, 29
    perioperative complications in, 131–134, 132*t*
    perioperative management of, 130–142

perioperative use of caffeine in, 6, 29, 134–136, 135t–137t, 141
postconceptional age of, and complications in, 133–134, 141, 366–367
spinal versus general anesthesia in, 136–138, 138t
neurologic sequelae in, 67
regional versus general anesthesia in, 5
respiratory function in, 130
spinal anesthesia in, 6
adjuncts with, caution in using, 6
Primitive neuroectodermal tumors, 233
Procainamide
contraindications in long QT syndrome, 190
for paroxysmal supraventricular atrial tachycardia, 186
Procarbazine
classification and side effects of, 242t
for Hodgkin's disease, 235
Production pressure
definition of, 24
effects of, 24
ethical and legal issues in, 24
management of, techniques for, 24
Proof of damage, in negligence, 17t
Propanolol
for acute fibrillation and atrial flutter, 188
for paroxysmal supraventricular atrial tachycardia, 186
Propofol
antiemetic properties of, 366
intravenous
in cystic fibrosis, 90
in upper respiratory tract infections, 85
and malignant hyperthermia, 340–342
in malignant hyperthermia-susceptible patients, 350–351
sedation with, safety of and policy on, 395
for thermal/burn injury patients, 215
and time to recovery and discharge, 368
for trauma patients, 198, 198t, 203–204, 272
Protamine, allergic and anaphylactic reactions to, 308–309
Prothrombin time, preoperative assessment of, 37–38
Protoheme, 275
Proventil (albuterol)
for asthma, 93, 97
for upper respiratory tract infections, 85–86
Pruritus
with oral transmucosal fentanyl citrate, 46
with patient-controlled analgesia, 378–379
Pseudomonas aeruginosa infection, in cystic fibrosis, 88
Pseudomonas cepacia infection, in cystic fibrosis, 88
PSVT. See Paroxysmal supraventricular atrial tachycardia
Psychoanalytic model, of child development, 58t
Psychological development, 56–57
by age, 59t
chronic illness and, 66t
definition of, 56
models of, 58t
Pulmonary artery
anomalous coronary artery from, 180t
compression of, with mediastinal masses, 219
right, origin of, from aorta, 180t
Pulmonary aspiration, in trauma cases, 198
Pulmonary atresia, 180t
Pulmonary compromise, in cystic fibrosis, 88
Pulmonary edema
fulminant, 104
postobstructive, 103–104
versus aspiration syndrome, 103
classical clinical presentation of, 103
versus other causes of pulmonary edema, 104
pathophysiology of, 103–104
treatment of, 104

448   INDEX

Pulmonary embolism, hypotension with, 316
Pulmonary function tests, in anesthetic risk assessment, with anterior mediastinal masses, 226, 227f
Pulmonary hypertension
  in asthma, 92
  in bronchopulmonary dysplasia, 99
  incidence of, 180t
  with obstructive sleep apnea, 101
Pulmonary hypertensive crisis, in congenital heart disease patients, 178
Pulmonary interactions, associated with congenital heart disease, 169t
Pulmonary toxicity, of bleomycin, 247–248
Pulmonary valve abnormality, 180t
Pulmonary vasoconstriction, in congenital heart disease patients, 178
Pulmonary venous return, total anomalous, 180t
Pulmonic stenosis, 175t
Pulse oximetry
  in cystic fibrosis, 89
  false readings in, in carbon monoxide poisoning, 210
  in malignant hyperthermia, 369
  in postanesthesia care, 7
  in postanesthesia care unit, 360–361
  in upper respiratory tract infections, 86
Purine analogs, classification and side effects of, 240t
Pyelonephritis, chronic, 292
Pyrimidine analogs, classification and side effects of, 240t

Q

QT interval, in long QT syndrome, 189–190

R

Racemic epinephrine, for postextubation croup, 128
Radiation therapy, 248–250
  fractionated, 250
  for Hodgkin's disease, 235, 248
  hyperfractionated, 250
  for neuroblastoma, 236, 248, 250
  for non-Hodgkin's lymphoma, 234
  pain with, 252t
  sequelae of, 248–250, 249t
  for Wilms' tumor, 237, 248, 250
Radioallergosorbent testing (RAST), for allergies, 305, 307
Radiocontrast media, allergic and anaphylactic reactions to, 124–125, 305, 308
Radiologic testing
  in acute chest syndrome, with sickle cell disease, 276
  appropriate preoperative, in children, 35–40
  in asthma, 95
  in bronchopulmonary dysplasia, 100
  indications for, 35–36
  legislative mandate for, 39
  for malignant hyperthermia, 341
  in mediastinal masses, 221, 225t, 229, 235
  in pneumonia, 98
  preoperative, 39
  in upper respiratory tract infections, 85
Ranitidine, for anaphylactic reactions, 304t
Rapacurium, in trauma management, 198, 198t
Rapacuronium, 159, 159t
Rapid sequence induction, increased intracranial pressure and, 264
Rapid sequence intubation, in trauma management, 198, 203
RAST (radioallergosorbent testing), for allergies, 305, 307
Reasonable-person standard, for disclosure, 16
Reciprocating tachycardias, 183, 184f–185f, 185
Recovery, rapidity of, risks and complications in, 8–9
Recovery room, 358–373. *See also* Postanesthesia care unit
  croup in, 127–128

laryngospasm in, 127
  maligant hyperthermia and disaster in, 344
    versus other disorders, 344–348
Recovery room impact events (RRIEs), postanesthesia care and, 7
Recovery room scores, and discharge, 361, 362t–364t
Recrudescence, 349
Rectal analgesia, 379
Rectal transmucosal administration
  advantages and disadvantages of, 50
  of preanesthetic sedation, 47t, 50–52
Red blood cell transfusions
  for anemia, in former premature infants, 139–140
  complications of, 140
  for thermal/burn injury patients, 214, 217–218
Red man's syndrome, with vancomycin allergy, 306–307
Refusal of cases, ethical issues in, 24
Regional anesthesia
  in asthma, versus general, 95
  in cystic fibrosis, 90
  and discharge from postanesthesia care unit, 368–369
  safety and risks of, 5
Remifentanil
  and time to recovery and discharge, 368
  for trauma patients, 204
Renal dysfunction
  and hypertension, 312
  with thermal/burn injury, 214
Renal failure, 292–294
  anesthetic considerations in, 293–294
  definition in children, 292
  effects on medication, 294
  etiology of, 291t, 292
  with malignant hyperthermia, 340
  nonsteroidal anti-inflammatory drugs contraindicated in, 382
  pathophysiology of, 292–293
  in thermal/burn injury patients, 214
  treatment of, 293
  with tumor lysis syndrome, 230
Renal transplantation, 293–294
Resistance, in gas flow through tubes, 108–110
Respiratory acidosis, in asthma, 95
Respiratory complications
  in former preterm infants, 131–134, 132t
  incidence of, 1
  typical, 1
Respiratory distress, in stridor, 113–114, 115t, 116f
  minimal signs and symptoms of
    with moderately progressive lesion, 116–117
    with nonprogressive lesion, 115–116
    with rapidly progressive lesion, 117–118
  moderate signs and symptoms of
    with moderately progressive lesion, 119–121
    with nonprogressive lesion, 118–119
    with rapidly progressive lesion, 121–123
  severe signs and symptoms of
    with moderately progressive lesion, 124
    with nonprogressive lesion, 123–124
    with rapidly progessive lesion, 124–125
Respiratory failure
  in asthma, 92–93
  in cerebral palsy patients, 285–286
  in cystic fibrosis, 89
  with mediastinal masses, pathophysiology of, 226–227
  in muscular dystrophy, 289–290
  in pneumonia, 98
Respiratory function
  and eligibility for discharge, 362t
  in neonate, 130
  in preterm infants, 130
Respiratory problems,, 74–100
Respiratory syncytial virus, 97–98
Respiratory tract infections
  lower
    in cystic fibrosis, 88
    and outpatient surgery, 28

Respiratory tract infections (*continued*)
- with upper respiratory tract infection, and surgical decisions, 84
- upper, 80–87. *See also* Upper respiratory tract infections

Resuscitation
- DNR orders against
  - goal-directed, 21–22
  - perioperative, 21–23
    - options for obtaining and documenting, 21–22
    - postoperative planning for, 22–23
  - procedure-directed, 22
  - and response to iatrogenic arrest or emergencies, 23
- full, 21

Retinoblastoma, 220*t*, 237
- radiation therapy for, 248

Retrograde intubation
- in difficult airway, 159, 163–164, 164*f*
- equipment for, 163, 164*f*

Rhabdomyolysis
- versus malignant hyperthermia, 344, 353
- masseter muscle rigidity and, 344
- muscular dystrophy and, 291
- with thermal/burn injury, 206–207, 214

Rhabdomyosarcoma, 237
- incidence of, 220*t*, 237
- radiation therapy for, 248, 250
- spinal cord compression with, 229

Rheumatic heart disease, 180*t*

Rhinitis, and outpatient surgery, 29

Rhonchi, versus stridor, 108

Right-to-left shunts, 173–176, 174*t*
- postoperative hypovolemia with, 178

Right ventricle, double-outlet, 180*t*

Risk(s), 1–12
- administration of anesthesia by pediatric anesthesiologists and, 4
- anesthesiologist experience and, 4
- anterior mediastinal masses and, 221–226, 225*t*, 226*f*–228*f*
- closed claim and single institutions studies of, 2–3, 3*t*, 369
- coexisting conditions and, 5–7
- congenital heart disease and, 5–6
- disclosure of, 9
- masseter muscle spasm and, 6
- minor, as emerging area of interest, 8
- mortality studies of, 1–2, 2*f*
- neuromuscular disease and, 7, 291
- patient preparation and, 7
- of postanesthesia care, 7–9
  - incidence of, 7–8
- of preanesthetic sedation, 41
- in preterm and former preterm infants, 6, 131–134, 132*t*
- reports of, conceptual and methodologic inconsistencies in, 1
- safety of agents and techniques and, 4–5
- upper respiratory tract infections and, 5, 82–83

Risperidone, for pervasive developmental disorders, 65

Ritalin, 62*t*

Rocuronium, 159*t*
- in head trauma, 272
- and malignant hyperthermia, 342
- in trauma management, 198, 198*t*

Ropivacaine, 5, 369
- decreased cardiac toxicity risk with, 181

RRIEs (recovery room impact events), postanesthesia care and, 7

Rubber latex allergy. *See* Latex allergy

Rule of 9s, for calculating percentage of body burned, 207, 208*f*

Runny nose, 80. *See also* Upper respiratory tract infections
- outpatient pediatric patients with, 28–29

S

Sacrococcygeal teratoma, 237

Safety, of agents and techniques, and anesthetic techniques, 4–5

INDEX 451

Salmeterol (Serevent), for asthma, 93
SBE prophylaxis. *See* Subacute bacterial endocarditis prophylaxis
Scald burns, 206
School-age children
  behavioral development and responses of, 57, 59*t*
  chronically ill, 67
  with history of bronchopulmonary dysplasia, 99
Secretin, in renal failure, 293
Secretion(s)
  in asthma, 91–92
  in cerebral palsy patients, 286
  in cystic fibrosis, 89–90
  in difficult airway cases, management of, 150–152, 160
  in thermal/burn injury, 211, 217–218
  in upper respiratory tract infections, 82
Secundum atrial septal defect, 180*t*
Sedation
  adverse events with, analysis of, 395
  anesthesiologist and, 389–399
  conscious, 391–392, 391*f*–392*f*
  continuum of, 391*f*, 391–392
  contraindications to, with patient-controlled analgesia, 378
  for croup in recovery room (postextubation), 128
  deep, 391*f*–392*f*, 391–393
  for diagnostic or therapeutic procedures, 389–390
  drug selection for, 393–394
  educational programs on, 395–396
  guidelines/policy for
    American Academy of Pediatrics, 390–392, 394
    burden of and complaints about, 392, 394
    compliance with, 396
    continuing quality improvement and, 394, 396
    institutionwide, 394–395
      involvement of department of anesthesiology in, 394–395
      need for, 394
      successful, elements of, 394
    JCAHO, 390, 392, 394
    and supply of anesthesiologists, 392
  level of
    assessment of, based on response to stimulation, 392, 393*f*
    personnel, monitoring, and record keeping based on, 391–393, 392*f*
  nonanesthesiologist administration of, 395
  for nonpainful procedures, 389
  for pervasive developmental disorders, 65
  preanesthetic
    age and, 42
    anxiety level and, 42
    in asthmatic child, 95
    avoidance in pediatric neurosurgical patients, 263
    benefits and risks of, 41
    for cancer patients, 257
    for cerebral palsy patients, caution in, 287
    for children with pervasive developmental disorders, 65
    co-administration of muscarinic blockers with, 42
    deficiency in, in children, 41
    in difficult airway cases, 150
    for difficult children, options in, 71
    ideal, characteristics of, 42–43
    intramuscular administration of, 47*t*, 52–53
    intramuscular ketamine for, 47*t*, 52, 71
    intramuscular midazolam for, 47*t*, 52–53
    intranasal ketamine for, 47*t*, 49–50
    intranasal midazolam for, 46–48, 47*t*, 48*f*
    intranasal sufentanil for, 46–49
    nasal transmucosal administration of, 46–50, 47*t*
    oral and sublingual administration of, 43–46
    oral combinations for, 46
    oral ketamine for, 44–45, 47*t*

Sedation (*continued*)
- oral midazolam for, 43–44, 45*f*, 95, 150
- oral transmucosal fentanyl citrate for, 45–46, 47*t*
- versus parental presence during induction, 41–42, 72
- for pediatric patients lacking intravenous access, 41–55
- rectal ketamine for, 47*t*, 51–52
- rectal methohexital for, 47*t*, 50
- rectal midazolam for, 47*t*, 51, 51*f*
- rectal transmucosal administration of, 47*t*, 50–52
- prehospital evaluation for, forms and records for, 395–396
- for radiation therapy, 250
- skill level of physician, dentist, or nurse providing, 394
- systems approach to, 397

Sedation committee, 394
Sedation flow sheets, 394–396
Seizures
- autism and, 65
- in cerebral palsy patients, 285
- postoperative, after supratentorial craniotomy, 268
- rectal methohexital and, 50

Senning operation, 187–188, 191
Sentinel events, 396
Sepsis
- chemotherapy and, 238
- with thermal/burn injury, 213–214

Serevent (salmeterol), for asthma, 93
Serotonin reuptake inhibitors, for pervasive developmental disorders, 65
Sevoflurane
- advantages of, 152
- in asthma, 96
- in congenital heart disease, 174
- in cystic fibrosis, 90
- in difficult airway, 152–153
- dysrhythmia induced by, 181
- emergence delirium with, 365
- in hydrocephalic patients, 266
- and intracranial pressure, 265
- laryngospasm with, 125–126
- and malignant hyperthermia, 340
- for myringotomy and pressure equalization tube placement, 368
- and rhabdomyolysis, 291
- safety and risks of, 4–5
- in surgery for mediastinal masses, 228
- and time to recovery and discharge, 365, 368
- in upper respiratory tract infections, 85

Shock, with burn injury, 208–209
Sick sinus syndrome, 191
Sickle cell disease, 275–280
- acute crisis in, 276, 278*t*
- anesthetic management in, 276–280
- anesthetic morbidity and mortality in, 278–279
- complete systems review in, 280
- complications of, 276, 278*t*
- etiology of, 275
- hypertension with, 312
- incidence of, 39, 275
- pathophysiology of, 275–276
- perioperative transfusion therapy for, 279–280
- preoperative testing/screening for, 39, 276–278
- various states of, characteristics of, 277*t*

Sickle cell trait, 275
Sickledex (sodium metabisulfite test), in sickle cell disease, 278
SIDS (sudden infant death syndrome), and pediatric outpatient surgery, 28
Single institution studies, of anesthetic risk, 2–3, 3*t*
Single ventricle, 180*t*
Sinoatrial dysfunction, 179
Sinus disease, in cystic fibrosis, 88–89
Sinus node dysfunction, 179, 191
Sinus tachycardia
- in muscular dystrophy, 289
- succinylcholine-induced, 182

Skin graft, for thermal/burn injury, 215–216
Skin injury, with thermal/burn injury, 207
Skin testing, for allergies, 305

Skinner, B. F., 58*t*
Skull-base fractures, nasal intubation contraindicated with, 199
Skull fracture, 271
Skull x-rays, in increased intracranial pressure, 262
Sleep-related breathing disorders, approach to child with, 100–103
Slow-to-warm-up child, as temperament type, 67
Smoke inhalation, 210
Snoring
  with obstructive sleep apnea, 101
  versus stridor, 108
Sodium, elevated levels in thermal/burn injury, 213
Sodium bicarbonate
  for anaphylactic reactions, 304*t*
  for thermal/burn injury patients, 214
Sodium metabisulfite test (Sickledex), in sickle cell disease, 278
Sodium nitrite, for cyanide poisoning, 211
Sodium nitroprusside
  for controlled hypotension, 329, 330*t*
  cyanide poisoning secondary to administration of, 318
  discontinuation of, and hypertension, 312
Sodium thiosulfate, for cyanide poisoning, 211
Somatosensory evoked potentials, for intraoperative monitoring of spinal function, 271
Sore throat, 8
Spastic cerebral palsy, 284, 284*t*
Spina bifida, latex allergy in children with, 309, 314–316
Spinal anesthesia, in preterm and former infants, 6, 136–138, 138*t*
  adjuncts with, caution in using, 6
Spinal cord compression
  with childhood cancer, 222*t*, 229, 236
  surgery for, 271
Spinal cord surgery, 271
  intraoperative monitoring of spinal function in, 271
Spinal injury, cervical, 201–202
Spleen injury, 202
Splenic sequestration, acute, in sickle cell disease, 276, 278*t*
SpO2, upper respiratory tract infections and, 5, 82–83, 83*t*, 84*f*
Staphylococcus aureus infection, in cystic fibrosis, 88
Status asthmaticus, 91, 93
Stellate ganglion blocks, for long QT syndrome, 189
Steroid(s)
  for asthma, 93–94
  for difficult airway, 165
  and hypertension, 312
  for increased intracranial pressure, 265
  for nausea and vomiting, 366
  for postobstructive pulmonary edema, 104
  prophylactic, for prevention of postextubation croup, 128
Stertor, 108
Still, George, 57
Stimulants
  for attention-deficit/hyperactivity disorder, 60, 62*t*
  commonly used, in children, 62*t*
  for pervasive developmental disorders, 65
  side effects of, 60
Stomatitis, with chemotherapy, 243
Street readiness
  definition of, 358
  as discharge criteria, 358
Streptococcus infection, group B, pneumonia with, 97
Streptococcus pneumoniae infection
  in cystic fibrosis, 88
  pneumonia with, 97
Streptokinase, allergic and anaphylactic reactions to, 305
Stress
  on anesthesiologist, from parental presence during induction, 73
  of cancer and cancer treatment, 255–257

454 INDEX

Stress (*continued*)
  on patients and families, 56, 68–69
Stridor, 101–123
  airway distress in, assessment of, 113–114, 115*t*, 116*f*
  airway patency and, 110–111
  with anaphylactic reactions, 124–125
  anatomic location of airway obstruction and, 108
  beyond newborn period, 112
  biphasic, 111
  clinician's challenge in, 107
  congenital, 112
  with croup, 112–113, 124
  definition of, 107
  direct listening in, importance of, 108
  with endotracheal tube kinking, 126–127
  with epiglottitis/supraglottitis, 112, 119–121
  etiologies of, 112
  expiratory, 111
  with fixed anatomic lesion, 123–124
  with foreign body obstruction, 112, 116–117
  gas flow through tubes, principles of, and, 108–110
  during general anesthesia administration, 126
  history of, and difficult airway, 145
  iatrogenic causes of, 112, 115–116
  inspiratory, 111
  in intubated patients under general anesthesia, 126
  with laryngeal mask airway, 126
  management of, 113–115
    key issues in, 113
    proper diagnosis as key element in, 112
  with mediastinal masses, 121–123, 221
  with minimal signs and symptoms of respiratory distress and a nonprogressive lesion (RD-1/NP), 115–116
  with minimal signs and symptoms of respiratory distress and moderately progressive lesion (RD-1/PB), 116–117
  with minimal signs and symptoms of respiratory distress and rapidly progressing lesion (RD-1/PP), 117–118
  with moderate signs and symptoms of respiratory distress and moderately progressive lesion (RD-2/PP), 119–121
  with moderate signs and symptoms of respiratory distress and nonprogressive lesion (RD-2/NP), 118–119
  with moderate signs and symptoms of respiratory distress and rapidly progressive lesion (RD-2/RP), 121–123
  in newborn period, 112
  with obstruction at or above vocal cords, 108
  with obstruction between vocal cords and thoracic inlet, 108
  with obstruction in trachea or bronchus, 108
  with obstruction within thorax, 108
  patient's medical history in, 112–113
  perioperative, and laryngospasm, 125–127
  physical examination in, 113
  physical principles and pathophysiology of, 108–111
  presentations of, 112–113
  progression of airway obstruction in, 114–115, 116*f*
  versus rhonchi, 108
  as sentinel marker of airway obstruction, 107
  with severe signs and symptoms of respiratory distress and moderately progressive lesion (RD-3/PP), 124

with severe signs and symptoms of respiratory distress and nonprogressive lesion (RD-3/NP), 123–124
with severe signs and symptoms of respiratory distress and rapidly progessive lesion (RD-3/PC), 124–125
versus snoring, 108
sound of, 107–108
status of, illustrative case scenarios based on, 115–125
with thermal/burn injury, 117–118, 211
with thermal or chemical injury, 117–118
with tracheomalacia, 118–119
upper respiratory tract infections and, 82
with vocal cord injury or paralysis, 112, 116–117, 123–124
versus wheezes, 107
"Stupid premie tricks," with bronchopulmonary dysplasia, 100
Subacute bacterial endocarditis (SBE) prophylaxis
guidelines for, 6, 30, 31*t*
in outpatient surgery, 30
Subarachnoid hemorrhage, hydrocephalus with, 266
Subdural hematoma, 271
Subglottic stenosis
with bronchopulmonary dysplasia, 100
and difficult airway, 145
stridor with, 112
Subjective-person standard, for disclosure, 16
Sublingual administration, of preanesthetic sedation, 43–46
Succinylcholine
and cerebral blood flow, 201, 202*t*, 203
for cerebral palsy patients, 286–287
contraindications to
with hyperkalemia risks, 216, 264
in neuromuscular disorders, 7, 158–159, 291
in thermal/burn injury, 216

for difficult airway, 158–159
dysrhythmia induced by, 182
in head trauma, 272
interference of, with postoperative chest percussion, 90
and intracranial pressure, 264
for laryngospasm, 127
and malignant hyperthermia, 338–340, 343–344, 353, 356*t*
masseter muscle spasm with, 6, 339
in myelodysplasia, 270
in renal failure, caution with, 294
in trauma management, 198, 198*t*, 203
in head injuries, 201
Sudden cardiac death, 191
Sufentanil
intranasal, for preanesthetic sedation, 46–49
local anesthetics with, 380–381
Superior vena cava syndrome, with childhood cancer, 219, 222*t*, 226–227, 234, 236
Supraglottitis, stridor with, 112, 119–121
Supratentorial craniotomy, 267–268
anesthesia induction and maintenance in, 267
anesthetic considerations in, 267
emergence from, 267–268
neurologic assessment after, overaggressive use of opioids and, 268
preoperative assessment for, 267
Supraventricular tachycardia, 183–187, 192–193
generation of, mechanisms of, 184*f*
Surgical bleeding, and eligibility for discharge, 363*t*
Sweat chloride test, 88
Syndrome of inappropriate secretion of antidiuretic hormone (SIADH), hydrocephalus with, 266
Systemic disorders, commonly seen in pediatric anesthesia, 275–299

T

T-cell function, immaturity of, and allergies, 300
T-cell leukemia, 232
Tachycardia, 179
  antidromic reciprocating, 183, 184f–185f, 185
  atrial re-entrant, 187
  ectopic atrial, 182–183
    mechanism of, 184f
  junctional ectopic, 182
    electrocardiogram of, 183f
    mechanism of, 184f
  with malignant hyperthermia, 340, 342
  in muscular dystrophy, 289
  orthodromic reciprocating, 183, 184f–185f, 185
  paroxysmal supraventricular atrial, 183–187
    etiologies of, 183
    management of, 186–187
    mechanism of, 183, 184f
    presentation of
      after 5 years of age, 183–184
      in infancy, 183
  postanesthesia monitoring for, 360
  sinus, succinylcholine-induced, 182
  supraventricular, 183–187, 192–193
    generation of, mechanisms of, 184f
  with thermal/burn injury, 208, 212
  ventricular, 188–189
    accessory pathway and, 186
    benign, 188
    definition of, 188
    induced by inhalation anesthesia, 181
    monomorphic, 191, 192f
    in neonate, classification of, 188–189
    succinylcholine-induced, 182
Tachykinin, in upper respiratory tract infections, 82
Tachypnea, with congenital heart disease, 169
Tele-Pad, in screening of pediatric outpatients, 27
Temperament
  of chronically ill children, 67
  types of, 67
Temporal lobe, herniation of, with hematoma, 271
Temporal lobe epilepsy, avoidance of methohexital in, 285
Tenoposide, for neuroblastoma, 236
Tension pneumothorax, hypotension with, 316
Terbutaline (Brethine), for asthma, 93, 97
Testicular cancer, radiation therapy in, 248
Tetralogy of Fallot, 175t, 177, 177t, 180t, 189
Theophylline
  for asthma, 93, 96
  cardiovascular toxicity of, 134
  as respiratory stimulant in former preterm infants, 134
Thermal injury, 206
  airway and ventilation in, 211, 218
    intraoperative, 217
  anesthesia induction and maintenance in, 216–217
  anesthetic planning for, 216
  body surface area involved in, 207, 208f–209f
  cardiovascular effects of, 208–209, 212
  contraindication to succinylcholine in, 216
  electrolytes in, 213
  fluid management/resuscitation in, 212–213, 217–218
  hematologic problems with, 214
  infection in, 213–214
  management issues in, 211–215
  management of child with, 206–218
  monitoring, intraoperative, in, 217
  neurologic problems with, 214
  nutrition in, 213
  operating room management of, 215–218
  operating room preparation for, 216
  pain management in, 215
  patient positioning, intraoperative, in, 216

renal issues with, 214
shock with, 207–209
skin injury with, 207
stridor with, 117–118, 211
surgical procedures for, 215–216
Thiobarbiturate(s), allergic and anaphylactic reactions to, 307
6-Thioguanine, for acute myelogenous leukemia, 233
Thiopental
allergic and anaphylactic reactions to, 305, 307
and cerebral blood flow, 201, 202*t*
in myelodysplasia, 270
in supratentorial craniotomy, 267
for trauma patients, 198, 198*t*, 201, 203–204
Thiopentone, in head trauma, 272
Thiotepa, in preparative regime for bone marrow transplantation, 251
Thoracic epidural, 380
Thoracic trauma, management of, 203
Thorazine, phenergan and, with meperidine, for preanesthetic sedation, 46
Thrombocytopenia
with childhood cancer, 230–231
in thermal/burn injury patients, 214
Tiedemann, Dietrich, 57
Toddlers
behavioral development and responses of, 57, 59*t*
chronically ill, 67
Tongue
assessment in preanesthetic evaluation of difficult airway, 145, 146*f*
deflection by, in blind nasal intubation, 163
displacement for laryngoscopy, 153–157, 155*f*
Tonsillectomy
coagulation testing before, 37–38
laryngospasm after, 127
nonsteroidal anti-inflammatory drugs in, 382
for obstructive sleep apnea, 101–103
outpatient, shortest stay possible in, 367
postanesthesia care in, monitoring in and discharge from, 367
postoperative bleeding with, 37, 367
postoperative pain with, 9, 367
Topicalization, in difficult airway, 157, 160
Torsade de pointes, 189, 190*f*,192*f*, 193
Total body irradiation, 248
Total burn surface area, 207
Tracheal size, as predicting factor of anesthetic risk, with anterior mediastinal masses, 221–226, 226*f*, 228*f*
Tracheitis, stridor with, 112
Tracheomalacia
with bronchopulmonary dysplasia, 100
with cerebral palsy, 285–286
stridor with, 118–119
Tracheotomy, elective, in difficult airway, 149–150, 164
Tranexamic acid, decrease in blood loss with, 333
Transposition, of great arteries, 175*t*, 180*t*, 191
Trauma
anesthesia induction in, 198–199, 203, 272
anesthesia maintenance in, 203–204
assessment of, 196–197, 197*t*
blood transfusion in, 199–200, 200*t*–201*t*
cerebral blood flow in, anesthetic effects on, 201, 202*t*
fluid resuscitation in, 199–200
full stomach risks in, 198, 272
head, 196, 199, 201, 202*t*,271–272
incidence of, 196
intravenous access in, 199
intubation in cases of, 198–199, 272
drug recommendations for hypovolemic patient in, 198, 198*t*
uses deemed unnecessary, in case review, 199

Trauma (*continued*)
  management of
    from field to emergency department, 196–200
    from operating room to pediatric intensive care unit, 203–204
    personnel involved in, 196–197
  multiple
    anesthetic considerations for child with, 196–205
    strategies for management of, 202–203
  outcome of, Glasgow Coma Score and, 204, 204*t*
  postoperative care in, 204
  specific injuries in, strategies for management of, 200–203
Treacher-Collins syndrome, 145–146, 147*f,* 161, 164
Tricuspid atresia, 175*t,* 180*t,* 183
Tricuspid valve abnormality, 180*t*
Tricyclic antidepressants, for cancer pain, 254
Trimetaphan, for controlled hypotension, 329, 330*t*
Trismus, 6
Truncus arteriosus, 180*t*
Tryptase, serum levels in allergy testing, 305
Tumor lysis syndrome, 223*t,* 229–230, 236
  management of, 230*t*
Turbulent flow, of gas through tubes, 108–110
Two-person laryngoscopy technique, 158
Tylenol with codeine, for thermal/burn injury patients, 215

U
Ultrasound, in increased intracranial pressure, 262
Umbilical artery catheter, indwelling, and hypertension, 312
Upper respiratory tract infections, 80–87
  versus allergic rhinitis, 80–81
  with allergies, 300
  anesthetic plan in, 86–87
  and anesthetic risk, 5, 29, 82–83
  ASA Physical Status and, 84
  asthma exacerbation with, 82, 92
  with bronchopulmonary dysplasia, 99
  diagnosis of
    clinical criteria for, 80, 81*t*
    gold standard for, 80
  differential diagnosis of, 80–81
  at emergence, management of, 86
  evidence of other infection and, 84
  experience and confidence of anesthesiologist and, 84
  financial considerations in, 85
  hypoxia with, 316–317
  induction options in, 85–87
  intraoperative management of, 85–86
  lower respiratory tract effects of, 81
  nature and severity of infection and, 84
  nature and urgency of surgery and, 83–84
  and outpatient surgery, 29
  patient's age and, 84
  perioperative complications of, 82
    prevention of, 85–86
  perioperative management of, 85
  peripheral airway abnormalities with, 81
  versus pneumonia, 98
  practical considerations in, 84–85
  predicted difficult airway and, 84
  proceeding with surgery in, decisions on
    ASA Physical Status and, 84
    evidence of other infection and, 84
    experience and confidence of anesthesiologist and, 84
    factors influencing, 83–85
    financial considerations in, 85
    nature and severity of infection and, 84
    nature and urgency of surgery and, 83–84
    patient's age and, 84
    practical considerations in, 84–85
    predicted difficult airway and, 84

and SpO2, 9, 82–83, 83*t,* 84*f*
symptoms of, with respiratory syncytial virus infection, 97–98
Urea, conversion of ammonia to, hepatic failure and, 296–297
Ureteral reflux, and renal failure, 292
Urethral valves, posterior, and renal failure, 292
URI. *See* Upper respiratory tract infections
Urination
and eligibility for discharge, 363*t*–364*t,* 366
local anesthetics containing narcotics and, 380–381
Urine analysis
in malignant hyperthermia, 340
preoperative, 37
with thermal/burn injury, 214
Urine output, with thermal/burn injury, 212, 214

V

Vancomycin, allergic and anaphylactic reactions to, 306–307
Vascular resistance
in congenital heart disease, 176*t,* 176–178
in thermal/burn injury, 208
Vasoconstrictors, and hypertension, 312
Vasodilators, for controlled hypotension, 329, 330*t*
Vasopressin
for postoperative diabetes insipidus, 268
release in thermal/burn injury, 208–209
Vasopressors, in renal failure, 293
Vecuronium, 159*t*
Ventilation
in epiglottitis, importance of, 120–121
hyperoxic, with acute normovolemic hemodilution, 327
inadequate, risk of, anesthesia and, 3*t*
in malignant hyperthermia-susceptible patients, 351–352
in neonates, inhaled anesthesia and, 130
in thermal/burn injury, 211, 218
intraoperative, 217
Ventilation:perfusion mismatching
in asthma, 92
in cystic fibrosis, 90
Ventolin (albuterol)
for asthma, 93, 97
for upper respiratory tract infections, 85–86
Ventricle, single, 180*t*
Ventricular arrhythmia, 179
succinylcholine-induced, 182
Ventricular contractions, premature, 181, 188
Ventricular dysfunction, incidence of, 180*t*
Ventricular dysrhythmias, 188–190, 193
Ventricular fibrillation, 179
accessory pathway and, 186
induced by inhalation anesthesia, 181
induced by local anesthetics, 181
with long QT syndrome, 189–190
Ventricular septal defect, 167, 180*t,* 189, 360
Ventricular tachycardia, 188–189
accessory pathway and, 186
benign, 188
definition of, 188
induced by inhalation anesthesia, 181
malignant, 188–189
monomorphic, 191, 192*f*
in neonate, classification of, 188–189
pacemaker and cardioverter-defibrillator for, 191
succinylcholine-induced, 182
Ventriculostomy, 201
Venturi principle, 111
Verapamil
for atrioventricular node dysfunction, 186
for long QT syndrome, 190
in malignant hyperthermia, 349
for paroxysmal supraventricular atrial tachycardia, 186
Vinblastine
classification and side effects of, 240*t*

Vinblastine (*continued*)
  for Hodgkin's disease, 235
  for Langerhans' cell histiocytosis, 238
Vincristine
  for acute lymphoblastic leukemia, 232
  classification and side effects of, 241*t*
  for Hodgkin's disease, 235
  pain with, 252*t*
  for Wilms' tumor, 237
Viscosity, and gas flow through tubes, 110
Visual Analog Scale, for pain assessment, 376
Vital capacity, in upper respiratory tract infections, 81
Vital signs
  age-appropriate, 200*t*
  and eligibility for discharge, 362*t*
  monitoring in postanesthesia care unit, 360
Vitamin D analogs, for renal failure, 293
Vitamin K, and coagulation, in hepatic failure, 296
Vocal cord injury or paralysis, stridor with, 112, 116–117, 123–124
Voiding
  local anesthetics containing narcotics and, 380–381
  in postanesthesia care unit, and eligibility for discharge, 363*t*–364*t*, 366, 369
Vomiting
  with local anesthetics containing narcotics, 380–381
  with oral transmucosal fentanyl citrate, 46
  with patient-controlled analgesia, 378–379
  postanesthesia/postoperative, 8–9
    assessment of, difficulty in children, 369
    causes of, 365–366
    and eligibility for discharge, 362*t*, 365–366, 370
    lowering risk of, 366
    after tonsillectomy, 368
    treatment of, 366, 369
    undermedication for, 369
von Willebrand's disease, DDAVP for limiting blood loss in, 333

W

Wake-up test, for intraoperative monitoring of spinal function, 271
Wheezes
  with congenital heart disease, 169
  versus stridor, 107
When Your Child Needs Anesthesia, 7
White blood cells. *See* Leukocytes
Wilms' tumor, 236–237
  chemotherapy for, 237
  clinical presentation of, 237
  incidence of, 220*t*, 236
  increased risk of, congenital anomalies associated with, 236–237
  platelet dysfunction with, 230
  radiation therapy for, 237, 248, 250
Wolff-Parkinson-White syndrome, 183–187
  electrocardiogram of, 184–185, 185*f*
Work of breathing
  in asthma, 92, 94
  in bronchopulmonary dysplasia, 99
  slower flow rates and, 110
World Health Organization, stepwise approach in pain management, 254–255

X

X-rays. *See* Radiologic testing